Diversity in Deaf Education

Perspectives on Deafness

Series Editors
Marc Marschark
Harry Knoors

The Gestural Origin of Language
David F. Armstrong and Sherman E. Wilcox

Educating Deaf Learners: Creating a Global Evidence Base
Edited by Harry Knoors and Marc Marschark

Teaching Deaf Learners: Psychological and Developmental Foundations
Harry Knoors and Marc Marschark

The People of the Eye: Deaf Ethnicity and Ancestry
Harlan Lane, Richard C. Pillard, and Ulf Hedberg

A Lens on Deaf Identities
Irene W. Leigh

Deaf Cognition: Foundations and Outcomes
Edited by Marc Marschark and Peter C. Hauser

Diversity in Deaf Education
Edited by Marc Marschark, Venetta Lampropoulou, and Emmanouil K. Skordilis

Sign Language Interpreting and Interpreter Education: Directions for Research and Practice
Edited by Marc Marschark, Rico Peterson, and Elizabeth A. Winston

Bilingualism and Bilingual Deaf Education
Edited by Marc Marschark, Gladys Tang, and Harry Knoors

Early Literacy Development in Deaf Children
Connie Mayer and Beverly J. Trezek

The World of Deaf Infants: A Longitudinal Study
Kathryn P. Meadow-Orlans, Patricia Elizabeth Spencer, and Lynn Sanford Koester

Advances in the Sign Language Development of Deaf Children
Edited by Brenda Schick, Marc Marschark, and Patricia Elizabeth Spencer

Advances in the Spoken Language Development of Deaf and Hard-of-Hearing Children
Edited by Patricia Elizabeth Spencer and Marc Marschark

Approaches to Social Research: The Case of Deaf Studies
Alys Young and Bogusia Temple

Diversity in Deaf Education

Edited by

Marc Marschark
Venetta Lampropoulou
Emmanouil K. Skordilis

Oxford University Press is a department of the University of Oxford. It furthers the University's objective of excellence in research, scholarship, and education by publishing worldwide. Oxford is a registered trade mark of Oxford University Press in the UK and certain other countries.

Published in the United States of America by Oxford University Press
198 Madison Avenue, New York, NY 10016, United States of America.

© Oxford University Press 2016

All rights reserved. No part of this publication may be reproduced, stored in a retrieval system, or transmitted, in any form or by any means, without the prior permission in writing of Oxford University Press, or as expressly permitted by law, by license, or under terms agreed with the appropriate reproduction rights organization. Inquiries concerning reproduction outside the scope of the above should be sent to the Rights Department, Oxford University Press, at the address above.

You must not circulate this work in any other form
and you must impose this same condition on any acquirer.

Library of Congress Cataloging-in-Publication Data
Names: Marschark, Marc, editor. | Lampropoulou, Venetta, editor. | Skordilis, Emmanouil K., editor.
Title: Diversity in deaf education / edited by Marc Marschark, Venetta Lampropoulou, Emmanouil K. Skordilis.
Other titles: Perspectives on deafness.
Description: Oxford ; New York : Oxford University Press, [2016] | Series: Perspectives on deafness | Includes bibliographical references.
Identifiers: LCCN 2015037330 | ISBN 9780190493073 (alk. paper)
Subjects: | MESH: Cultural Diversity. | Education of Hearing Disabled—methods. | Cultural Competency. | Early Intervention (Education)--methods. | Mainstreaming (Education)—methods. | Persons With Hearing Impairments—psychology.
Classification: LCC RF291 | NLM HV 2430 | DDC 617.80071—dc23 LC record available at http://lccn.loc.gov/2015037330

9 8 7 6 5 4 3 2 1

Printed by Sheridan Books, Inc., United States of America

Contents

Preface	vii
Contributors	xiii

1. Recognizing Diversity in Deaf Education: From Paris to Athens With a Diversion to Milan — 1
   Greg Leigh and *Marc Marschark*

2. Evidence-Based Practice in Early Intervention: The Proof of the Pudding Is in the Eating — 21
   Marilyn Sass-Lehrer and *Alys Young*

3. The Transition from Early Intervention to School for Deaf and Hard-of-Hearing Children — 49
   Brenda T. Pcon, Janet R. Jamieson, Anat Zaidman-Zait, Deirdre Curle, Nancy Norman, and *Noreen Simmons*

4. School as a Site for Natural Language Learning — 77
   Marlon Kuntze, Debbie Golos, Kimberly Wolbers, Catherine O'Brien, and *David Smith*

5. On the Home Front: Parent Personality, Support, and Deaf Children — 109
   Patrick J. Brice, Rachael M. Plotkin, and *Jennifer Reesman*

6. High Standard Competencies for Teachers of the Deaf and Other Qualified Professionals: Always Necessary, Not Always Guaranteed — 135
   Guido Lichtert, Kevin Miller, Areti Okalidou, Paul Simpson, and *Astrid van Wieringen*

7. Exploring Signed Language Assessment Tools in Europe and North America — 171
   Charlotte Enns, Tobias Haug, Rosalind Herman, Robert Hoffmeister, Wolfgang Mann, and *Lynn McQuarrie*

8. Language Use in the Classroom: Accommodating the Needs of Diverse Deaf and Hard-of-Hearing Learners — 219
   Harry Knoors

9. The Development of Pragmatic Skills in Children
   and Young People Who Are Deaf and Hard of Hearing 247
   Dianne Toe, Pasquale Rinaldi, Maria Cristina Caselli,
   Louise Paatsch, and *Amelia Church*

10. Addressing Diversity in Teaching Deaf Learners to Write 271
    Connie Mayer

11. Many Languages, One Goal: Interventions for Language
    Mastery by School-Age Deaf and Hard-of-Hearing
    Learners 297
    Susan R. Easterbrooks, Joanna E. Cannon, and *Jessica W. Trussell*

12. From Social Periphery to Social Centrality: Building
    Social Capital for Deaf and Hard-of-Hearing Students
    in the 21st Century 325
    Gina A. Oliva, Linda Risser Lytle, Mindy Hopper,
    and *Joan M. Ostrove*

13. The Inclusion of Deaf and Hard-of-Hearing Students
    in Mainstream Classrooms: Classroom Participation
    and Its Relationship to Communication, Academic,
    and Social Performance 355
    Naama Tsach and *Tova Most*

14. Mental Health Problems in Children and Adolescents:
    An Overview 381
    Tiejo van Gent and *Ines Sleeboom-van Raaij*

15. A Comprehensive Reading Intervention: Positive
    Postsecondary Outcomes and a Promising Practice
    for Students Who Are Deaf or Hard of Hearing 417
    Greta Palmberg and *Kendra Rask*

16. Critical Factors Toward the Inclusion of
    Deaf and Hard-of-Hearing Students in Higher Education 441
    Merv Hyde, Magda Nikolaraizi, Denise Powell,
    and *Michael Stinson*

17. 21st-Century Deaf Workers: Going Beyond "Just
    Employed" to Career Growth and Entrepreneurship 473
    Ronald R. Kelly, Andrew B. Quagliata, Richard DeMartino,
    and *Victor Perotti*

18. Recognizing Diversity in Deaf Education: Now What
    Do We Do With It?! 507
    Marc Marschark and *Greg Leigh*

Index 537

Preface

The American educational reformer John Dewey once wrote, "if I were asked to name the most needed of all reforms in the spirit of education, I should say: Cease conceiving of education as mere preparation for later life, and make it the full meaning of the present life" (Dewey, 1893, p. 660). That is, Dewey saw education not only as the acquisition of knowledge and skills obtained from formal schooling, but also the daily application of what every individual has learned—individuals' "fund of knowledge," in current terms—to the benefit both of their daily life and of society.

Some people see education and academic outcomes as pertaining only to the individual learner—a means to the ends of being financially secure, fulfilling one's roles and responsibilities in society, and perhaps just being. Certainly, that is the view of most students while involved in formal education settings who have not yet glimpsed the forest for the trees. For the majority of parents and teachers, however, the education of children and youth, whether formally or informally, is something more. It is not just "preparation for later life" of the individual, but a contribution to society with the ultimate goal of each learner in some way making the world (community, region, culture, nation) a better place.

What is the situation when the learner has some kind of disability? In the case of severe disabilities, it may be appropriate to focus on providing an education that allows the individual simply to enjoy quality of life and perhaps gain employment to a reasonable extent. In the case of mild disabilities, in contrast, it may (indeed, should) be possible to provide accommodations in school, the workplace, and society that allow the individual to lead a life fully commensurate with nondisabled peers. The situation, admittedly, is more complex between these extremes; the extent of an individual's strengths and needs, and the possibilities for accommodating the latter not only vary widely, but also are seen from diverse perspectives—those of the individual and family, school, community, and the larger society (Antia, 2015; Leigh & Crowe, 2015).

Since 1878, through the International Congress on Education of the Deaf (ICED), researchers and educators of deaf or hard-of-hearing (DHH) learners have shared their understanding, their methods, and materials seen as appropriate to the needs of DHH students and, more recently, to their strengths as well. Although intended primarily to be an academic conference focusing on evidence-based practice, ICED has never been immune from the differing philosophies and politics of what is commonly referred to as "deaf education." Indeed, it is frequently noted that deaf education approaches new *méthodes du jour* every few years, even if the evidence to support them is often lacking (Spencer & Marschark, 2010). One reason for this situation, acknowledged by many—if not most—people in the field, is that the DHH population is rather different than other populations identified as "disabled" (Marschark & Knoors, 2012). Among the 13 categories of disability identified by the U.S. government, for example, it is only deaf individuals who sometimes see themselves as a linguistic–cultural minority (instead of or as well as disabled). Historically, this has created significant tension in the field as both deaf and hearing individuals have varied in their acceptance of that view and the extent to which it has been seen as relevant to educational practice.

A second reason for the constant search for new instructional methods in deaf education, simply put, is that despite the myriad approaches, interventions, and educational philosophies that have been offered through the centuries (Lang, 2011), deaf learners continue to lag behind hearing peers in their academic achievement (Marschark, Shaver, Nagle, & Newman, 2015; Qi & Mitchell, 2012). Some individuals within the field seek to attribute the chronic underachievement of DHH learners to a single factor—the "philosophies and politics"—whether related to language, cultural attitudes, school systems, or directly to hearing thresholds. More realistically, and more pertinent in the present context, is recognition that deaf learners comprise an extremely heterogeneous population, and one that is only becoming more diverse over time. Not only does this population vary widely in terms of the extent to which individuals have and/or use residual hearing (in other words, their hearing thresholds) and the presence and severity of secondary disabilities, but, as a function of these factors and associated variability in their early language and educational environments, their use of different language modalities, and social–emotional interactions inside and outside of the family, DHH learners likely are more heterogenous than any other group in the educational system. Adding variability in the quality and appropriateness of instruction, access, and psychosocial functioning and mental health, and the fact that these domains all interact and have cumulative effects, the result is considerable diversity in both deaf learners and the contexts in which they are educated.

As the following chapters illuminate, recognition of the diversity among DHH learners is not new. What perhaps *is* new, or at least is becoming more widely acknowledged, is that the notion of a one-size-fits-all approach to deaf education—a "silver bullet" that is going to result in DHH learners' performing uniformly at the same level as hearing peers—simply is not on the horizon. Throughout the more than 135 years of ICED meetings, advocates of "oral" education, bilingual education, separate education, inclusive education, and any number of variations within and among these have been touted as panaceas for deaf education. Although there is evidence that each and all of these offer benefits to some DHH learners at some ages, the existing evidence base and the 800-lb gorilla that is the missing evidence base indicate there is not a single solution to the many challenges of deaf education. As Marschark and Leigh describe in the final chapter of this volume, interventions that appear to "level the playing field" for some DHH learners are ineffective for others, and some that are effective for young children do not produce lasting gains (at least on average). Like it or not, this is what diversity is all about. The insistence of many in the field that "the one true path" is before us does not change the fact that both history and the existing literature tell us that many paths are needed, even if our goal of optimizing educational opportunities and outcomes for all DHH learners is the same.

There is no doubt that educational, psychological, and linguistic research has provided us with a much better understanding of the foundations and barriers to academic growth by DHH learners. Technology has provided students, parents, and educators with effective teaching–learning tools and communication access (through both signed and spoken language). Meanwhile, societal enlightenment has taught us that diversity with regard to gender, ethnicity, and cultural values can make life more interesting and, in many ways, make us stronger. There is no reason why diversity among DHH learners and the methods used to educate them should be seen as negative or unnecessary. Indeed, the diversity of educational settings and curricula available typically to hearing children serves important societal functions (otherwise we would not have them), and offers the possibility of matching learners to alternative instructional methodologies and settings that allow them to thrive. DHH learners are more diverse than their hearing peers at any age level, and it thus appears evident that, correspondingly, they are likely to need a broader continuum of educational placements if we want them to thrive.

The chapters in this volume—written by deaf and hearing individuals, teachers and parents of deaf learners, and researchers in education, psychology, linguistics, and related fields—barely scratch the surface of the complexity inherent in educating DHH learners. They all bring to the fore, however, that diversity in deaf learners and in deaf education must be acknowledged and perhaps even embraced. If the factors that affect the academic achievement of DHH learners directly are not always obvious or consistent, we need to discover the mediating variables that underlie both variability among learners and variability among instructional approaches that work (or not). As we move beyond obsession with single solutions and single factors accounting for the educational status of DHH learners from primary to postsecondary education, we will no doubt find that some educational approaches work better than others for some learners of some ages in some contexts. What appears simple in theory, however, often becomes more complex (and expensive) in practice. We thus are not suggesting that simply recognizing diversity is sufficient to allow us to accommodate it in the classroom. Nor do we believe that all or even most schools are in a position to provide DHH students with all the resources necessary to optimize the outcomes of each. But, this does not mean we should not try.

As we move toward the goal of educating all DHH learners in a manner that offers each individual the greatest opportunity for academic and personal success, we need research, implementation, and evaluation in practice, and flexibility in the way that we look at deaf learners and deaf education. The chapters in this volume, offered by contributors to ICED 2015 in Athens, Greece, point to several paths forward. They should not be seen as contradictory, but complementary. Diversity in deaf education is largely beyond our control. How we deal with it is not.

Marc Marschark
Venetta Lampropoulou
Emmanouil K. Skordilis

REFERENCES

Antia, S. (2015). Enhancing academic and social outcomes: Balancing individual, family, and school assets and risks for deaf and hard-of-hearing students in general education. In H. Knoors & M. Marschark (Eds.), *Educating deaf learners: Creating a global evidence base* (pp. 527–546). New York, NY: Oxford University Press.

Dewey, J. (1893). Self-realization as the moral ideal. *Philosophical Review, 2*, 652–664.

Lang, H. (2011). Perspectives on the history of deaf education. In M. Marschark & P. Spencer, (Eds.), *The Oxford handbook of deaf studies, language, and education, volume 1, 2nd edition* (pp. 7–17). New York, NY: Oxford University Press.

Leigh, G., & Crowe, K. (2015). Responding to cultural and linguistic diversity among deaf and hard-of-hearing learners. In H. Knoors & M. Marschark (Eds.), *Educating deaf learners: Creating a global evidence base* (pp. 69–92). New York, NY: Oxford University Press.

Marschark, M., & Knoors, H. (2012). Sprache, Kognition und Lernen: Herausforderungen der Inklusion fürgehörlose und schwerhörige. In M. Hintermair (Ed), *Inklusion, Ethik und Hörschädigung* (pp. 129–176). Heidelberg: Median-Verlag.

Marschark, M., Shaver, D. M., Nagle, K., & Newman, L. (2015). Predicting the academic achievement of deaf and hard-of-hearing students from individual, household, communication, and educational factors. *Exceptional Children, 8*, 350–369.

Qi, S., & Mitchell, R. E. (2012). Large-scale academic achievement testing of deaf and hard-of-hearing students: Past, present, and future. *Journal of Deaf Studies and Deaf Education, 17*, 1–18.

Spencer, P. E., & Marschark, M. (2010). *Evidence-based practice in educating deaf and hard-of-hearing students*. New York, NY: Oxford University Press.

Contributors

Patrick J. Brice
Department of Psychology
Gallaudet University
Washington, DC

Joanna E. Cannon
Education of the Deaf and
    Hard-of-Hearing Program
Department of Educational &
    Counselling Psychology &
    Special Education
Faculty of Education
University of British Columbia
Vancouver, British Columbia
Canada

Maria Cristina Caselli
Istituto di Scienze e Tecnologie
    della Cognizione
Consiglio Nazionale delle
    Ricerche
Rome, Italy

Amelia Church
Melbourne Graduate School of
    Education
University of Melbourne
Victoria, Australia

Deirdre Curle
Educational and Counselling
    Psychology, and Special
    Education
University of British Columbia
Vancouver, British Columbia
Canada

Richard DeMartino
E. Phillip Saunders College of
    Business
Rochester Institute of Technology
Rochester, NY

Susan R. Easterbrooks
Program in Education of the Deaf
Educational Psychology,
    Special Education, and
    Communication Disorders
Georgia State University
Atlanta, GA

Charlotte Enns
Faculty of Education
University of Manitoba
Winnipeg, Manitoba, Canada

Debbie Golos
Department of Communicative
    Disorders and Deaf Education
Utah State University
Logan, UT

Tobias Haug
Department of Pedagogical and
    Therapeutic Professions
University of Applied Sciences of
    Special Needs Education
Zurich, Switzerland

Rosalind Herman
Division of Language &
    Communication Science
City University
London, UK

Robert Hoffmeister
Center for the Study of
 Communication & the Deaf
Boston University
Boston, MA

Mindy Hopper
Department of Liberal Studies
National Technical Institute for
 the Deaf
Rochester Institute of Technology
Rochester, NY

Merv Hyde
School of Education
University of the Sunshine
 Coast
Maroochydore, Queensland,
 Australia

Janet R. Jamieson
Educational and Counselling
 Psychology, and Special
 Education
University of British Columbia
Vancouver, British Columbia
Canada

Ronald R. Kelly
REACH Center for Studies on
 Career Success
National Technical Institute for
 the Deaf
Rochester Institute
 of Technology
Rochester, NY

Harry Knoors
Royal Dutch Kentalis
Kentalis Academy
Sint-Michielsgestel,
 The Netherlands
and
Radboud University
Behavioral Science Institute
Nijmegen, The Netherlands

Marlon Kuntze
Department of Government and
 Public Affairs
Burstein Center for Excellence in
 Leadership and Innovation
Gallaudet University
Washington, DC

Venetta Lampropoulou
Deaf Studies Unit
Department of Primary
 Education
University of Patras
Patras, Greece

Greg Leigh
RIDBC Renwick Centre
Royal Institute for Deaf and Blind
 Children
North Rocks, Australia
and
The University of Newcastle
Newcastle, Australia

Guido Lichtert
Research Group
Experimental ORL
Department of Neurosciences
Katholieke Universiteit Leuven
Leuven, Belgium
and
Koninklijk Orthopedagogisch
 Centrum Antwerpen
Antwerp, Belgium

Linda Risser Lytle
Department of Counseling
Gallaudet University
Washington, DC

Wolfgang Mann
Department of Education
University of Roehampton
London, UK
and
City University
London, UK

Marc Marschark
Center for Education Research
 Partnerships
National Technical Institute for
 the Deaf
Rochester Institute of Technology
Rochester, NY

Connie Mayer
Faculty of Education
York University
Toronto, Ontario, Canada

Lynn McQuarrie
Western Canadian Centre for
 Deaf Studies
University of Alberta
Edmonton, Alberta, Canada

Kevin Miller
Department of Special
 Education
Concordia University
Seward, NE

Tova Most
School of Education
Tel-Aviv University
Tel-Aviv, Israel

Magda Nikolaraizi
Department of Special Education
University of Thessaly
Volos, Greece

Nancy Norman
Educational and Counselling
 Psychology, and Special
 Education
University of British Columbia
Vancouver, British Columbia
Canada

Catherine O'Brien
Department of Government and
 Public Affairs
Burstein Center for Excellence in
 Leadership and Innovation
Gallaudet University
Washington, DC

Areti Okalidou
Department of Educational and
 Social Policy
University of Macedonia
Salonika, Greece

Gina A. Oliva
Department of Physical
 Education and Recreation
 (Retired)
Gallaudet University
Washington, DC

Joan M. Ostrove
Department of Psychology
Macalester College
Saint Paul, MN

Louise Paatsch
School of Education
Faculty of Arts and Education
Deakin University
Geelong, Australia

Greta Palmberg
Intermediate District 287
VECTOR Transition Program
Brooklyn Park, MN

Victor Perotti
E. Phillip Saunders College of
 Business
Rochester Institute of Technology
Rochester, NY

Rachael M. Plotkin
Kennedy Krieger Institute
Johns Hopkins University School
 of Medicine
Baltimore, MD

Brenda T. Poon
Human Early Learning
 Partnership, School of
 Population and Public Health
University of British Columbia
Vancouver, British Columbia
Canada

Denise Powell
College of Education, Health and
 Human Development
University of Canterbury
Christchurch, New Zealand

Andrew B. Quagliata
School of Hotel Administration
Cornell University
Ithaca, NY

Kendra Rask
Intermediate District 287
VECTOR Transition Program
Hennepin Technical College
Brooklyn Park, MN

Jennifer Reesman
Kennedy Krieger Institute
Johns Hopkins University School
 of Medicine
Baltimore, MD

Pasquale Rinaldi
Istituto di Scienze e Tecnologie
 della Cognizione
Consiglio Nazionale delle
 Ricerche
Rome, Italy

Penny Roy
Division of Language &
 Communication Science
City University
London, UK

Marilyn Sass-Lehrer
Deaf and Hard-of-Hearing Infants,
 Toddlers, and Their Families
 Interdisciplinary Program
Graduate School and Continuing
 Studies
Gallaudet University
Washington, DC

Noreen Simmons
British Columbia Family Hearing
 Resource Society
Surrey, British Columbia, Canada

Paul Simpson
British Association of Teachers of
 the Deaf
Kent, UK

Emmanouil K. Skordilis
Faculty of Physical Education and
 Sport Science
National and Kapodistrian
 University of Athens
Athens, Greece

Ines Sleeboom-van Raaij
Royal Dutch Kentalis
Sint-Michielsgestel,
 The Netherlands
and
Trajectum Hoeve Boschoord
The Netherlands

David Smith
Department of Theory & Practice
 in Teacher Education
University of Tennessee
Knoxville, TN

Michael Stinson
National Technical Institute for
　the Deaf
Rochester Institute of Technology
Rochester, NY

Dianne Toe
School of Education
Faculty of Arts and Education
Deakin University
Geelong, Australia

Naama Tsach
Department of School
　Counseling and Special
　Education
Tel-Aviv University
Tel-Aviv, Israel

Jessica W. Trussell
National Technical Institute for
　the Deaf
Rochester Institute of Technology
Rochester, NY

Tiejo van Gent
Royal Dutch Kentalis
Sint-Michielsgestel,
　The Netherlands

Astrid van Wieringen
Research Group
Experimental ORL
Department of Neurosciences
Katholieke Universiteit Leuven
Leuven, Belgium

Kimberly Wolbers
Department of Theory & Practice
　in Teacher Education
University of Tennessee
Knoxville, TN

Alys Young
Social Research with Deaf
　People Group
School of Nursing, Midwifery
　and Social Work
University of Manchester
Manchester, UK

Anat Zaidman-Zait
Department of School
　Counseling and Special
　Education
Tel-Aviv University
Tel Aviv, Israel

1

Recognizing Diversity in Deaf Education: From Paris to Athens With a Diversion to Milan

Greg Leigh and Marc Marschark

This chapter is drawn from the opening presentation at the 22nd International Congress on Education of the Deaf (ICED). In that presentation it was our aim to address some of the history of the Congress and, through that, some of the history of the field of education of deaf and hard-of-hearing (DHH) children more broadly as a means to highlight some important issues. In so doing, it was our intention to address the overall theme of the Congress—"Many ways, one goal"—from a historical perspective and to question how effectively the field has accommodated diversity and the need for differentiated approaches for DHH learners. Just as it was in 1878 at the first ICED, in 2015 considerable diversity continues to be the norm within the population of DHH learners on many different levels—from cultural and linguistic diversity, to the diversity associated with the presence of myriad additional disabilities, to the natural variations seen in any population of learners relative to individual cognitive abilities and aptitudes. Some of these are issues are taken up in more detail in Chapter 18. Whatever its basis, diversity has particular consequences for how educators do, or should, approach the task of teaching DHH learners.

Being able to take a historical perspective on educational practice since the first ICED is eminently possible because the field has the benefit of a rich tradition of scholarship, inquiry, and training. Having commenced at that 1878 meeting in Paris, the ICED has been held more or less continuously ever since, albeit with some breaks associated with periods of world wars. It is worthy of note that the conference is almost certainly the world's oldest continuously held conference in any field of education (Leigh & Power, 2004). The history of the Congress, at least for its first 100 years, was recorded rigorously by Brill (1984) in his "Analytical History" of the meetings and has been recorded subsequently through the publication of proceedings and associated edited books of papers (see, for example, Moores, 2011; Power & Leigh, 2004; Weisel, 1998). These records provide a useful lens through which to continue to explore the theme of change and development in deaf education, and how the field responds, or perhaps should be responding, to the diverse nature of DHH learners around the world.

THE VANCOUVER STATEMENT: RESPONDING TO MILAN

The decision to examine the path from 1876 to the 2015 ICED in the opening presentation stemmed from events surrounding the 21st ICED in Vancouver, Canada, and, in particular, a statement that was prepared and delivered to that Congress at the opening ceremony in 2010. The statement was titled "A New Era: Deaf Participation and Collaboration" and was made as a direct, albeit significantly delayed, response to the resolutions made at the 2nd ICED in Milan in 1880. In particular, the statement related to the first two of eight resolutions that were made at the 1880 Congress. Those two resolutions were as follows:

1. The Convention, considering the incontestable superiority of articulation over signs in restoring the deaf-mute to society and giving him a fuller knowledge of language, declares that the oral method should be preferred to that of signs in education and the instruction of deaf-mutes.
2. The Convention, considering that the simultaneous use of articulation and signs has the disadvantage of injuring articulation and lip-reading and the precision of ideas, declares that the pure oral method should be preferred. (Fay, 1881, p. 64).

The statement at the Vancouver Congress was read at the opening ceremony by Dr. Joseph McLaughlin on behalf of the ICED 2010 Vancouver Organizing Committee, the British Columbia Deaf Community, the Canadian Association of the Deaf, and the World Federation of the Deaf. The statement "acknowledged with regret the detrimental effects of the Milan Congress" and issued a call to "accept and respect all languages and all forms of communication" in the education of deaf people. Sinclair (2010) noted that the statement was heralded by "a loud, long-standing and emotional applause" (p. 8). Certainly, anyone present at the ceremony could attest to that being an accurate characterization of the event.

The aims of making the statement were patent and laudable on many different levels—socioculturally, linguistically, and, importantly, educationally. The statement called for the acceptance of cultural and linguistic diversity among DHH people, particularly children. From an educational perspective, the point of the statement was abundantly clear and, at least to these observers, self-evident: that is, it sought to make the point that there cannot be, and never could be, one and only one way to approach the education of all DHH learners. Indeed, the patently self-evident nature of such a statement raises an inevitable and often-overlooked question about the resolutions made in Milan at the 2nd ICED. How was it that such resolutions could have ever been passed in the first place? Given the diversity that must have existed among the population of DHH children at that time, as now, how could it ever have been suggested, much less formally resolved, that there could be just one "true" path to the goal of linguistic and social fulfillment for *all* DHH children? In approaching and seeking to address such a question, it would serve the field well to recall the often-misquoted adage of philosopher and essayist George Santayana who warned that "those who cannot remember the past are condemned to repeat it" (Santayana, 1905, p. 284). So, how did the Milan resolutions come to be?

DECONSTRUCTING THE MILAN RESOLUTIONS

At a political level, the 1880 resolutions in Milan can perhaps best be seen as some skillful lobbying by vested interests to achieve a particular outcome (something not unknown in the field today). It is worthy of note that there were just 164 delegates to that Congress and that those delegates came from just eight countries or regions (Brill, 1984). As was noted by Gallaudet (1881), a clear majority of delegates (87) were from Italy and the majority of those delegates (46) were from just two exclusively oral schools for the deaf in Milan. By any reckoning, the views expressed by such a majority could not have been truly representative of the international zeitgeist in the education of DHH children at the time.

Demonstrably, the first two resolutions passed at the Milan Congress failed to acknowledge the need for educators of deaf children to seek to be responsive to the needs of individual children—that is, the need to match programs to children and not children to programs. Seemingly out of their desire to promote practices and procedures that were being advanced by one part of the educational establishment—however fervently the underpinning beliefs in the correctness of those practices may have been held—the advocates of the resolutions and, in particular, the staff of those two Italian schools actively sought to exclude the potential for alternative approaches to be not only viable, but also perhaps *necessary* for many DHH children to achieve successful linguistic and educational outcomes. Indeed, there appears to have been little consideration of the diversity among the pupils in the broader DHH population that *may not have been*—and almost certainly *were not*—represented in the oral schools in Milan in 1880.

From an empirical perspective, it would also appear the resolutions were based on limited evidence of outcomes for the methods being proposed. There is certainly nothing in the historical record to indicate any formal evidence was advanced in support of the claims of successful application of the methods, other than anecdotes about the speech production abilities of the children in the Milan schools and elsewhere. Based on the records of those who attended the Congress and paid visits to the two schools in question, there is no doubt they were introduced to children who had mastered spoken language successfully and had good spoken communication skills. Buxton (1883, p. 42), for example, noted he had been in Milan and was "officially present when the 'pure oral' method was exemplified by its pupils," but there was no commentary on the nature of the children's hearing loss, their age, or their educational history. The fact that some pupils achieved in this way has never been in doubt. What is absent from the literature and would clearly appear to have been absent from the debate at the time, however, was any evidence to support the notion that the methods were equally applicable to *all* deaf children, as asserted in the ultimate Congress resolutions. Edward Miner Gallaudet (1881) noted this in his reflections on the Congress. He recorded that two of the English delegates to the Congress used "eloquent language" to urge the adoption of exclusively oral teaching methods but that they failed to recognize "the objection which may be raised against the oral method for all deaf-mutes: that, in point of fact, a large proportion of the deaf are incapable of attaining any real success in speech and lip-reading" (p. 5).

The prima facie evidence for the success of the oral methods proclaimed in Milan was the presentation of successfully orally communicating students in the Milan schools. However, there is no evidence that the pupils in the Milan schools were in any way representative of the broader population of DHH children in Italy (or elsewhere in the world) at that time. In all likelihood, that population was rather exclusive with regard to a number of characteristics that would today be recognized as being associated with variance in the linguistic and educational outcomes for children who are deaf or hard of hearing (see Chapter 18).

Quite simply, the full potential for diversity among DHH learners at the time could not have been considered because most of them would not have been enrolled in formal education at all. According to Soysal and Strang (1989), the primary enrollment ratio in Italy in 1870 (i.e., the proportion of all children of school age who were actually enrolled in formal education) was only 29%. Although, as noted by these authors, moves to compulsory education were just beginning around the time of the Milan Congress (i.e., in 1877 in Italy, 1880 in England, and 1882 in France), it is still very likely that a large proportion of deaf children were not engaged in formal education at the time. Furthermore, as would have still been the case for the majority of hearing children at the time, those deaf children who were in schools would almost certainly have been children from higher socioeconomic status backgrounds whose parents were themselves relatively better educated than others in the community. This conclusion is supported by other matters set for debate at the 1880 Congress. Notably, the Congress debated the question of what could be done to provide for the "great number" of deaf children who were not, at that stage, receiving the benefit of instruction "due to the poverty of the families and the want of suitable institutions" (Fay, 1881, p. 64).

In addition to being, disproportionately, from higher socioeconomic status and better educated families, the children in the oral schools of Milan (and elsewhere) would likely also have shared a number of other characteristics. First, it is clear that, relative to modern standards, they would have been identified as being deaf and would have commenced formal education at relatively late ages. This fact is in evidence in another of the debates and subsequent resolutions at the Milan Congress. Resolution 3 centered on the question of the age at which children should commence formal educational intervention with the ultimate resolution being that "the most favourable age at which the deaf can be received in school is 8 to 10 years" (Fay, 1881, p. 64). Clearly, by modern standards, the average age at which most children were afforded educational intervention in 1880 was very late. Another issue that would have defined the population of children in oral schools of the period is the relative absence of children with additional disabilities. Although there is no specific information available about the nature of the population in the schools, it is highly unlikely there was any significant representation of children with disabilities (particularly intellectual or physical disabilities). If such children were in school at all, they would likely have been in entirely separate "institutions" rather than in schools for the deaf, in accordance with the dominant philosophy of the 1880s (Kauffman, 1981; White & Wolfensburger, 1969).

Finally, there is a question around the nature and diversity of hearing loss experienced by children who may have been enrolled in oral schools of the day. Obviously, in the absence of any objective strategies for assessing hearing loss at the time, it is just not possible to know about this issue. However, it is simply logical that (a) there would have been, as there is today, a diverse range of levels of hearing loss among the population of DHH children; and (b) there was no available system of personal amplification that could have enabled children with greater levels and more complex types of hearing loss to access spoken language effectively. Hence, in all likelihood, children with lesser degrees of hearing loss would have been significantly overrepresented among those who had so successfully developed oral language and were the objects of display at the Congress.

So, in summary, it would seem that, in 1880, the pupils for whom a single approach to communication and language acquisition was being deemed to be appropriate by the majority of Congress participants would have been

- From higher socioeconomic and well-educated family backgrounds
- Unlikely to have any disabilities in addition to their deafness
- More likely to have lesser degrees of hearing loss
- Unlikely to have encountered formal education until at least 8 years of age (or potentially older)
- Without any access to amplification that could provide access to spoken language

Notably, these are all factors that we know to be associated with significant variance in the linguistic and educational outcomes achieved by DHH children (Ching et al., 2013a, 2013b). We return to these issues later, but it is important to note here that, although the last factor would clearly have had an equal effect on outcomes for all DHH children during the 19th century, the first four factors would almost certainly have weighed more positively for children in the schools in Milan and more negatively on the developmental outcomes for the large group of DHH children that Gallaudet described as being "incapable of attaining any real success in speech and lip-reading" (Gallaudet, 1881, p. 5).

So, to return to the initial question, how did the Milan resolutions happen? Clearly, whether for political purposes or through lack of awareness and knowledge, there was much about the diverse nature of DHH children at the time that was simply not considered in the framing of the Milan resolutions. Specifically, there was a range of variables among the population of DHH children at the time that should have been considered. Careful consideration of at least some of those issues *would have* made it patently clear there were many students who did not share the characteristics of those who acquired spoken language successfully. These facts alone, we argue, should have suggested the folly in the Milan delegates' dogmatic conclusion about the appropriateness of oral educational methods for all DHH children. Simply put, there was a failure to recognize the diversity that existed within the population of DHH children at the time and, just as significant, there was a rush to embrace an approach on ideological grounds in the absence of hard evidence to support the outcomes of that approach.

RECOGNIZING DIVERSITY IN THE MODERN ERA

From a contemporary perspective, educators and other professionals involved in the identification and education of DHH children should be no less attentive to the diversity that exists among that population of learners today, and should be no less skeptical about suggestions that there should, or could, be any "one true path" to seek language, communication, and educational outcomes for all deaf children. Indeed, just as it should have been in 1880, any claim that there is a single approach that should be applied to the needs of "all deaf children" should be treated with the same degree of skepticism as the pronouncements of the Milan Congress. Having said that, however, we acknowledge there are now greater opportunities for DHH children to develop speech and spoken language that are more commensurate with their hearing counterparts than at any time in history. Without question, those opportunities are the result, in large part, of a number of developments—educational, audiological, technological, and medical. Perhaps the two most notable among these developments have been the advent of universal newborn hearing screening (UNHS) and early access to cochlear implantation. These interventions, perhaps more than any other developments in the history of our field, have had a dramatic impact on children's capacity for spoken language development, and their subsequent educational and vocational opportunities (Leigh, 2008).

In the years since the 2000 ICED was held in Sydney, Australia, the number of DHH children around the world who have been identified early though UNHS has increased dramatically (Leigh et al., 2010). In Australia, for example, in the year following that ICED, just 5% of all children born were screened for birth through such hearing screening programs. Wake (2002) noted that, accordingly, only about 25% of infants born with permanent hearing loss were identified by 12 months of age. In 2015, at the time of the Congress in Athens, that proportion reached 97%, with the vast majority of those children going on to engage with early intervention by 3 months of age.

Increasingly in Australia, as elsewhere in the developed world, children who are identified with severe and profound levels of hearing loss routinely receive one or, more frequently, two (bilateral) cochlear implants. Although far from being universal, this is an internationally observable trend. During the 5 years since the ICED was held in Vancouver, Canada, the number of children younger than 18 years who have received cochlear implants has increased by at least 100,000. According to one maker of implant devices, approximately 30,000 children around the world now receive at least one cochlear implant each year. Significantly, as the number of children receiving cochlear implants increases, the age at which they receive these devices has been decreasing. In Australia, the age at which children, identified through UNHS, receive a cochlear implant continues to decrease. Although exact statistics are not available, it seems reasonable to conclude that the average age of fitting for children whose severe to profound hearing loss is identified through UNHS is now around 9 months.

At this point it is important to note this phenomenon is very much a "first-world" issue. As significant as this trend may be in countries such as Australia, the Netherlands, and the United States, the availability of UNHS and the decreasing age of cochlear implantation are factors that clearly divide the first and developing worlds (Leigh et al., 2010). To account for this dichotomy of opportunity, while ever it exists, there will be the need for a wide variety of responses—both audiological and pedagogical. Such responses will need to be applied differentially according to particular international circumstances. To this end, it behooves us to ensure there is no less emphasis on the development and application of interventions that are applicable and effective in circumstances in which early identification and advanced hearing technologies are not the norm. It should not be that our field simply develops interventions exclusively for the privileged first world, to the detriment of children who are not able to access such advantages (see Chapter 2).

Now, having claimed that two issues—UNHS and early access to cochlear implantation—are dramatically changing outcomes for DHH children, there is an obvious question regarding the extent of available evidence to support this contention. Certainly, we are not suggesting these two developments are a panacea for the linguistic and developmental consequences of deafness, and neither are we of the view that they suggest that "all deaf children" should or even can achieve ideal outcomes via such a route. However, it is, we argue, increasingly apparent that the outcomes of these interventions with DHH children continue to be very positive with regard to speech and spoken language (Dettman & Dowell, 2010; Hammer, 2010; Verbist, 2010), and that there continues to be considerable variability. So, what do we know in this regard?

Accounting for Diversity

The starting premise for these comments is to return to the observations we have already made about the Congress participants in Milan and how they failed to recognize the diversity among the population of DHH learners in 1880. As then, there continues to be a litany of factors that can and do account for diversity of linguistic and educational outcomes in this population, even with the advantages of earlier identification and earlier access to cochlear implantation. Not the least among such factors, and perhaps most commonly cited, is the degree of a child's hearing loss, particularly for those whose hearing loss is insufficient to justify the application of cochlear implants (Sininger et al., 2010). Among others, additional factors that may influence outcomes for deaf children include the following:

- *The presence of additional disabilities*: The degree and consequences of a range of disabilities have been shown to affect the rate and extent of growth in a number of outcomes measures for deaf children (Dammeyer, 2009; Knoors & Vervloed, 2011; Meinzen-Derr et al., 2010).
- *Cognitive ability*: Nonverbal cognitive ability has been shown to be predictive of speech perception (Geers et al., 2003), language

development (Geers, 2006), and reading abilities (Geers, 2003) in deaf children.
- *Socioeconomic status*: There are several issues at play here, some of which impact families' capacities to engage fully in educational and therapeutic processes with their children (Marschark et al., 2015; Powers, 2003);
- *Parental (particularly maternal) level of education*: Higher levels of maternal education have been associated with higher levels of child language ability among both hearing children (Reilly et al., 2010), and DHH children (Pipp-Siegel et al., 2003; Yoshinaga-Itano et al., 1998).
- *Cultural and linguistic background*: Divergent home language backgrounds have been associated with differential levels of achievement in the development of both spoken and signed language (Akamatsu & Cole, 2000; Leigh & Crowe, 2015).
- *Age at time of intervention* (Kennedy et al., 2006; Sininger et al., 2010; Yoshinaga-Itano, 2004).
- *Type and quality of intervention* (Geers & Moog, 1989; Geers et al., 2003). This factor could perhaps be better divided in two: (a) the extent and timeliness of access to a fully available communication mode (regardless of whether that communication is spoken or signed) (Dettman et al., 2007) and (b) the type of assistive hearing device provided for the child and the age at which that device was fitted effectively (Sininger et al., 2010).

Each of these factors, among others, is currently being considered as an independent (predictor) variable in a major investigation of developmental outcomes for DHH children in Australia. The Longitudinal Outcomes of Children with Hearing Impairment (LOCHI) study is a prospective study that aims to identify the effect of numerous variables on outcomes for a large cohort of DHH children from the time of identification of their hearing loss to at least 9 years of age, and potentially beyond.

The LOCHI Study

A succinct overview of the LOCHI study has been provided by Ching et al. (2013b). The study involves more than 450 children, born between 2002 and 2007, in three Australian states (Queensland, New South Wales, and Victoria), who were identified with a hearing loss sufficient to be fitted with a hearing aid. Recruitment was conducted across these three states because of the differential commencement dates and progress of rollout of newborn hearing screening programs during that time. The interstate differences in the rollout of UNHS programs meant that approximately half the children recruited for the study had their hearing loss identified through UNHS before the age of 6 months, thus allowing for an ethical examination of the effects of earlier versus later identification of hearing loss.

As reported by Ching et al. (2013a), at the time of the 3-year assessments, 451 children (54% boys) were enrolled in the study, of whom 56% were identified as having a hearing loss and were fitted with a hearing aid before 6 months of age—on average, by just less than 3 months of age. The remainder of the children were identified, on average, at approximately 8 months of age. At 3 years of age, there were 317 children (70%) who were hearing-aid users and 134 (30%) who had received at least one cochlear implant. There were 107 children (24%) with additional disabilities, 71% who used an aural/oral mode of communication, and 21% who were in environments where a language other than English was spoken language at home. Approximately 33% had parents with university education. All the children in the study received hearing aids and audiological intervention from a common federal government agency—Australian Hearing—which provides free hearing services to Australian children regardless of location and according to a standardized fitting and service regime. Therefore, those aspects of intervention were held constant across the sample (Ching et al., 2013b).

The LOCHI study considers a wide range of predictor variables along with a wide range of outcome variables. The predictor variables include hearing level, additional disability, gender, socioeconomic status, language and mode of communication used at home and in intervention, nonverbal intelligence, and, importantly, the age at which the children received their first hearing aid (i.e., as a proxy for the age at which their hearing loss was identified) and the age at which they received a cochlear implant when applicable. With regard to outcome measures, there is a similar wide range of variables that includes tests of receptive and expressive language, vocabulary, academic achievement, reading ability, and functional communication skills, among others (see Ching et al., 2013a, 2013b). All children enrolled in the study were (or will be) tested 6 months after receiving their hearing aid, 12 months after the first hearing-aid fitting, and then again at 3 years of age, 5 years of age, and, ultimately, at 9 years of age.

Full details of this study have been reported for the assessments at 3 years of age (see Ching & Dillon, 2013; Ching et al., 2013a; Cupples et al., 2013; Leigh et al., 2015). For the purposes of this discussion about diversity among DHH children, we are referencing the reporting of global outcomes for the sample of children at 3 years of age by Ching et al. (2013a). In that analysis, children's outcomes were quantified in terms of *global factor scores*, which, on the basis of factor analysis, were computed for each participant by combining individual test scores across measures of receptive and expressive language, speech production, auditory functional performance, and psychosocial functioning. The global factor score was scaled so that the normative population mean was 100 with a standard deviation (SD) of 15.

For the purposes of this discussion, it is possible to draw some overall conclusions from the findings of the LOCHI study at 3 years of age that clearly point to the impact of particular sources of diversity among outcomes for DHH children. In summary, regression analyses presented by Ching et al. (2013a) revealed that five factors were associated with significantly better global outcomes for DHH children at 3 years. Specifically, the significant predictors of global outcomes were lesser severity of hearing loss, absence of additional disabilities, female gender, higher levels of maternal education, and—for children with cochlear implants—earlier age of implantation. Notably, at least at the 3-year age point, there was no significant effect noted for age of identification of hearing loss as a predictor of global outcomes, although that effect is being noted in the data that are now being reported for the 5-year-old assessment point in the LOCHI study (Ching, 2015). Nevertheless, the significance of the effect of earlier cochlear implantation, which is made possible only by earlier identification of hearing loss through UNHS, provides substantial support for the claims we already made about the "game-changing" significance of the combined effects of earlier identification and earlier cochlear implantation. There are some critical issues to be considered here, however, lest there be any temptation to conclude this path could now be construed as *the* appropriate path for *all* DHH children in this modern era.

First and perhaps foremost, it is important to note that, on average, at 3 years of age, children in the LOCHI study had a global developmental score of 74.6 (SD = 17.1), which is more than 1 SD below the mean for hearing children of the same age (Ching et al., 2013a). This represents a significant gap in development between DHH children and hearing children. There is clearly an issue here with regard to the need for improved interventions to offset the differential in outcomes between DHH children and their hearing peers. It is important to recognize, however, that the findings for these children at 3 years of age should not be generalized to DHH children at other ages. Even within this sample there is the likelihood, if not an expectation, that the average global developmental score will improve at older age levels. To date, this prediction has been supported by early analysis of results for data at the 5-year age level, with Ching (2015) reporting a global language score of 85 for the same sample at that stage. Such a gain is a promising result but, in the context of the current discussion, the issue at point here is not so much about overall mean scores but the dispersion of scores within the sample.

Given the group mean and the size of the SD, it is clear there is a substantial proportion of these 451 children achieving global developmental scores well within the normal range (i.e., with scores between

85 and 115). Similarly, however, there is also a substantial proportion of children with scores considerably less than 1 SD below the normative mean (i.e., less than 70). These results speak to the extent of individual differences within this population. Patently, there are children for whom a combination of factors such as early identification, early access to cochlear implantation, and, among others, an absence of any additional disability, means they are showing developmental outcomes commensurate with or better than their hearing peers. Similarly, there are still children for whom other factors are associated with quite different levels of outcomes. The point here is that there can be no sense in which a single intervention/educational approach could be the appropriate response for all these children. To cater effectively to the developmental needs of a diverse group of learners such as DHH children requires significant differentiation of approaches for individual learners. There can be no basis for a method that advocates a uniform approach for all—whether that uniformity is with regard to language and communication or some other domains of learning.

A DIFFERENTIATED APPROACH

According to Tomlinson and McTighe (2006), a differentiated approach to instruction involves the use of varied processes and procedures to "ensure effective learning for varied individuals" (p. 3). For DHH learners, the logic of using a differentiated approach applies equally to all domains of learning but is particularly applicable for language and communication development (see Chapter 8). In the context of this domain, differentiation involves important decisions and processes to ensure an appropriate match between the personal and ecological communication needs of a learner, and a particular language and mode of communication. As noted by Knoors and Marschark (2012), however, such differentiation of approaches with regard to language and communication remains controversial, with some advocates and practitioners in the fields of early intervention and education for DHH children advocating "that even in this era, all deaf children should be brought up and educated bilingually from an early age" (Knoors & Marschark, 2012, p. 11). From a 2015 perspective, when so many DHH children now gain effective access to spoken language through very early cochlear implantation, any imperative that *all* children should be necessarily taught to communicate via sign language is, we argue, unsustainable. Indeed, it is just as unsustainable as the argument that *all* DHH learners should have been taught using an exclusively oral approach in 1880. In this view, we concur with the perspective of Knoors and Marschark (2012) who argued that "just as education advocates for deaf children argue against a 'one-size-fits-all' approach to school placement, a similar approach to language planning and policy is at best out of date and at worst discriminatory" (p. 8).

In making a case for a differentiated approach to language and communication development for DHH children, it is important to acknowledge this in no way seeks either to *prescribe* or *proscribe* any language or communication choice or possibility for that group. Indeed, to do either would be antithetical to the notion of differentiation and would be contrary to the advice of Santayana (1905) in that we would be forgetting the past and repeating the mistakes of Milan. Rather, in the section that follows, we seek to identify some of the alternative (differentiated) scenarios for the use of sign language that have emerged and/or are likely to become more common in response to the continuing effects of earlier identification of hearing loss and earlier access to improved assistive listening technology for many DHH learners.

Alternative Scenarios for Signed and Spoken Language Use With DHH Learners

As noted previously, DHH learners are now developing listening and spoken language abilities that are more commensurate with their hearing peers than at any time in history (at least in developed countries). Through the benefits of early access to cochlear implantation in particular, spoken language has become accessible as a first language for even the most profoundly deaf children. Perhaps not surprisingly, in the face of such developments, the proportion of children whose parents seek for them to learn sign language as an initial response to the identification of their deafness is decreasing and will almost certainly continue to fall (see Johnston [2006] for a discussion of trends in this regard). This notwithstanding, there continue to be children for whom education involving the use of sign language will still be the most appropriate or viable option because their family has a cultural and linguistic affiliation with the deaf community, their parents (hearing or deaf) simply prefer it, cochlear implants are contraindicated or likely to be of limited application because of physiological or neuropsychological correlates of their hearing loss (Pisoni et al., 2008), or specific language disorders are present that otherwise provide a barrier to spoken language development (Hawker et al., 2008; Quinto-Pozos et al., 2011). Along with the diminution in enrollments, the nature of the programs that involve the use of sign language is changing, with some new conceptions of sign bilingualism emerging (Knoors & Marschark, 2012; Mayer & Leigh, 2010).

For the purposes of this discussion, it is possible to identify several current and emerging possibilities for alternative uses of sign(ed) language and spoken language in early intervention and education for DHH learners. These scenarios certainly differ from the historically dichotomous view of signed and spoken language programs and also from many of the original conceptualizations of sign bilingualism in education (i.e., programs for which the stated aim was typically for learners to acquire a natural sign language and a spoken language sequentially—the latter often being used primarily in its written form). In the sections that follow, we briefly address some alternative conceptions of the use of sign language in the education of DHH learners in the current milieu.

The Use of Sign Language to Support the Development of Spoken Language

Yoshinaga-Itano (2006) argued that, regardless of the application of hearing technologies such as cochlear implants, the use of sign language together with spoken language early in DHH children's development can provide a bridge to the development of spoken language skills. Yoshinaga-Itano (and her colleagues) investigated a population of children who were identified through UNHS in Colorado that included a significant proportion of children who were exposed to both sign language and spoken language from very early infancy—often well before they received a cochlear implant (Yoshinaga-Itano, 2003, 2006; Yoshinaga-Itano & Sedey, 2000). In various reports of this population, it was concluded that contemporaneous exposure to both sign and spoken languages had a positive effect on children's development of their spoken language abilities. Yoshinaga-Itano (2003) noted that children exposed to both languages used their developing sign language skills to supplement their developing expressive speech skills and that "many children who had not yet developed intelligible speech had a significant amount of vocabulary in sign language" (p. 20). She concluded that the sign vocabularies the children acquired early during their infancy were likely to have facilitated the mapping of those lexical items onto their later-developing speech skills (Yoshinaga-Itano, 2006).

Notably, in the population studied by Yoshinaga-Itano and her colleagues, it is apparent that some families combined "services in ASL with services from [other] providers who described their intervention strategies as traditionally auditory-oral or auditory-verbal" (Yoshinaga-Itano, 2003, p. 27). They noted also, however, that some families availed themselves of programs in which speech and signed communication were used simultaneously—in a practice more commonly referred to as *simultaneous communication*. Knoors and Marschark (2012) also noted the potential benefits of DHH children gaining early exposure to both signed and spoken language—either in parallel or in simultaneous communication. They argued that the simultaneous use of both modes of communication (i.e., through the use of sign-supported speech) could "support comprehension and auditory learning ... providing children with greater cloze opportunities and facilitating rather than hindering the acquisition of spoken language" (p. 9). We concur and note there is no empirical evidence that simultaneous communication for these purposes is ineffective, other than evidence that there are *some* teachers who do not use it effectively (Leigh, 1995; Marmor & Pettito, 1979). Given the considerable evidence for the effectiveness of simultaneous communication in the classroom with older deaf learners (see Marschark et al., 2008), there would appear to be no pedagogical or linguistic reason to seek to proscribe or advise against its use for providing children with early exposure to both signed and spoken language (Knoors & Marschark, 2012).

It is worth noting here that there is another situation in which DHH children's contemporaneous development of signed and spoken language is becoming increasingly common—that is, in early intervention for DHH children of Deaf parents (i.e., parents who are themselves users of a natural sign language). In the Australian context, at least, there is considerable anecdotal evidence of Deaf parents opting for cochlear implantation for their deaf children and/or for their enrollment in early intervention programs that focus exclusively on the development of spoken language (Mayer & Leigh, 2010). In these cases, the development of the children's sign language skills as a natural first language is assumed, while the focus of early intervention is on the development of their speech and spoken language skills. In the context of early and effective access to cochlear implants, this is another conception of bilingualism that is both logical and supportable.

Sequential Acquisition of Spoken Language and Sign Language

In another alternative language usage scenario, Knoors and Marschark (2012) noted the potential for increasing numbers of DHH adolescents who have developed spoken language as their first language to seek to acquire sign language as a second language at a later point in their school education. Mayer and Leigh (2010) also noted this potential and observed that this order of language acquisition may "require some redefinition of what it means to be sign bilingual in an educational context" (p. 183). There are many possible reasons for deaf learners approaching the development of the two languages in this order that range from parental motivations for their children with cochlear implants to have access to an alternative language and/or mode of communication for certain purposes to DHH children, adolescents, and young adults themselves desiring to learn sign language later as a basis for access to and cultural identification with the Deaf community. With regard to the latter scenario, Knoors and Marschark (2012) noted the likelihood of an increasing role for continuing education programs to allow orally educated DHH adolescents and adults to acquire and use a sign language as a second language.

We do not contend that the examples of alternative juxtapositions of signed and spoken language in educational contexts presented in this and the previous section are exhaustive of the possible language-use scenarios or the forms of program differentiation that night be pursued actively by schools and services for the deaf to accommodate the changing capacities of children to use spoken language communication. Rather, we seek only to highlight that the current situation with regard to the use of spoken and signed language by DHH learners is becoming increasingly complex—far more complex than the oral language–sign language dichotomy that was at the heart of the disputed resolutions of the Milan Congress in 1880. These scenarios are not described with a view to endorsing them or making any recommendation. Rather, we highlight the potential for differentiated response to the language and communication needs of DHH learners and the issues to which the field must be capable of responding now and in the future.

CONCLUSION

With the passage of time since the first ICED was held in Paris in 1878, two observations about the population of DHH learners can be securely made. First, after more than 135 years, it remains true that considerable diversity exists within the population of DHH learners on many different levels (see Chapter 18). Second, regardless of the resolutions made at the Milan Congress in 1880, there can still be no basis for suggesting that a single approach to the development and use of language by DHH learners is either possible or appropriate. Looking ahead, the issues are whether the field will be able to accept that conclusion by the next ICED (2020) and how it will affect the way we teach DHH learners of all ages.

REFERENCES

Akamatsu, C. T., & Cole, E. (2000). Meeting the psychoeducational needs of deaf immigrant and refugee children. *Canadian Journal of School Psychology, 15*(2), 1–18.

Brill, R. G. (1984). *International Congresses on Education of the Deaf: An analytical history, 1878–1980*. Washington, DC: Gallaudet College Press.

Buxton, D. (1883). Notes of progress in the education of the deaf. *American Annals of the Deaf, 27*, 37–47.

Ching, T. Y. C. (2015). Outcomes of early identified children with hearing impairment at 5 years: The LOCHI study. Paper presented at the 8th Australasian Newborn Hearing Screening Conference (ANHSC 2015). Sydney, Australia.

Ching, T. Y. C., & Dillon, H. (2013). Major findings of the LOCHI study on children at 3 years of age and implications for audiological management. *International Journal of Audiology, 52*(S2), S65–S68.

Ching, T. Y. C., Dillon, H., Marnane, V., Hou, S., Day, J., Seeto, M., . . . Yeh, A. (2013a). Outcomes of early- and late-identified children at 3 years of age: Findings from a prospective population-based study. *Ear and Hearing, 34*(5), 535–552.

Ching, T. Y. C., Leigh, G., & Dillon, H. (2013b). Introduction to the Longitudinal Outcomes of Children with Hearing Impairment (LOCHI) study: Background, design, sample characteristics. *International Journal of Audiology*, 52(S2), S4–S9.

Cupples, L., Ching, T. Y. C., Crowe, K., Seeto, M., Leigh, G., Street, L., Day, J., Marnane, V., & Thomson, J. (2013). Outcomes of children with hearing loss and additional disabilities. *Journal of Deaf Studies and Deaf Education*, 19, 20–39.

Dammeyer, J. (2009). Congenitally deafblind children and cochlear implants: Effects on communication. *Journal of Deaf Studies and Deaf Education*, 14, 278–288.

Dettman, S., & Dowell, R. (2010). Language acquisition and critical periods for children using cochlear implants: The demands of writing and the deaf writer. In M. Marschark & P. Spencer (Eds.), *The Oxford handbook of deaf studies, language, and education* (Vol. 2, pp. 331–342). New York, NY: Oxford University Press.

Dettman, S. J., Pinder, D., Briggs, R. J. S., Dowell, R. C., & Leigh, J. R. (2007). Communication development in children who receive the cochlear implant younger than 12 months: Risks versus benefits. *Ear and Hearing*, 28(2):11S–17S.

Fay, E. A. (1881). Resolutions of the Milan Convention. *American Annals of the Deaf and Dumb*, 26(3), 164–165.

Geers, A. E. (2003). Predictors of reading skill development in children with early cochlear implantation. *Ear and Hearing*, 24, 59S–68S.

Geers, A. (2006). Factors influencing spoken language outcomes in children following early cochlear implantation. In A. R. Moeller (Ed.), *Cochlear and brainstem implants* (pp. 50–65). Basel: Karger.

Geers, A., Brenner, C., & Davidson, L. (2003). Factors associated with development of speech perception skills in children implanted by age five. *Ear and Hearing*, 24, 24S–35S.

Geers, A., & Moog, J. S. (1989). Factors predictive of the development of literacy in hearing-impaired adolescents. *Volta Review*, 91, 69–86.

Hammer, A. (2010). The acquisition of verbal morphology in cochlear-implanted and specific language impaired children. PhD dissertation, Leiden University. LOT Dissertational Series 255. Retrieved from http://www.lotpublications.nl.

Hawker, K., Ramirez-Inscoe, J., Bishop, D. V. M., Twomey, T., O'Donognue, G., & Moore, D. R. (2008). Disproportionate language impairment in children using cochlear implants. *Ear and Hearing*, 2, 467–471.

ICED Vancouver 2010 Organizing Committee (2010). *Vancouver 2010: A new era: Deaf participation and collaboration*. Vancouver, BC: Author.

Johnston, T. (2006). W(h)ither the Deaf community? Population, genetics, and the future of Australian Sign Language. *Sign Language Studies*, 6(2), 137–173.

Kauffman, J. M. (1981). Introduction: Historical issues and contemporary trends in special education in the United States. In J. M. Kauffman & D. P. Hallahan (Eds.), *Handbook of special education* (pp. 3–23). Englewood Cliffs, NJ: Prentice Hall.

Kennedy, C. R., McCann, D. C., Campbell, M. J., Law, C. M., Mullee, M., Petro, S., et al. (2006). Language ability after early detection of permanent childhood hearing impairment. *New England Journal of Medicine*, 354(20), 2131–2141.

Knoors, H., & Marschark, M. (2012). Language planning for the 21st century: Revisiting bilingual language policy for deaf children. *Journal of Deaf Studies and Deaf Education, 17*(3), 291–305.

Knoors, H., & Vervloed, M. P. J. (2011). Educational programming for deaf children with multiple disabilities. In M. Marschark & P. E. Spencer (Eds.), *The Oxford handbook of deaf studies, language and education* (pp. 82–96). New York, NY: Oxford University Press.

Leigh, G. R. (1995). Teachers' use of the Australasian Signed English system for simultaneous communication with their hearing-impaired students. Unpublished Doctoral Thesis. Monash University, Australia.

Leigh, G. (2008). Changing parameters in deafness and deaf education: Greater opportunity but continuing diversity. In M. Marschark & P. Hauser (Eds.), *Deaf cognition: Foundations and outcomes* (pp. 24–51). New York, NY: Oxford University Press.

Leigh, G. (2010). The changing context for education of the deaf in Australia: New imperatives for teacher education. *Japanese Journal of Special Education, 47*(6), 427–441.

Leigh, G., Ching, T. Y. C., Crowe, K., Cupples, L., Marnane, V., & Seeto, M. (2015). Factors affecting psychosocial and motor development in 3-year-old children who are deaf or hard of hearing. *Journal of Deaf Studies and Deaf Education, 20*(4), 331–342.

Leigh, G., & Crowe, K. (2015). Responding to cultural and linguistic diversity among deaf and hard-of-hearing learners. In M. Marschark & H. Knoors (Eds.), *Educating deaf learners: Global perspectives* (pp. 69–92) New York, NY: Oxford University Press.

Leigh, G., Newall, J. P., & Newall, A. T. (2010). Newborn screening and earlier intervention with deaf children: Issues for the developing world. In M. Marschark & P. E. Spencer (Eds.), *The Oxford handbook of deaf studies, language, and education* (Vol. 2, pp. 345–359). New York, NY: Oxford University Press.

Leigh, G., & Power, D. (2004). Education of deaf children at the turn of the 21st century. In D. J. Power & G. R. Leigh (Eds.), *Educating deaf students: Global Perspectives* (pp. xi–xx). Washington, DC: Gallaudet University Press.

Marmor, G., & Pettito, L. (1979). Simultaneous communication in the classroom: How well is English grammar represented? *Sign Language Studies, 23*, 99–136.

Marschark, M., Sapere, P., Convertino, C. M., & Pelz, J. (2008). Learning via direct and mediated instruction by deaf students. *Journal of Deaf Studies and Deaf Education, 13*, 446–461.

Marschark, M., Shaver, D. M., Nagle, K., & Newman, L. (2015). Predicting the academic achievement of deaf and hard-of-hearing students from individual, household, communication, and educational factors. *Exceptional Children, 8*, 350–369.

Mayer, C., & Leigh, G. (2010). The changing context for sign bilingual education programs: Issues in language and the development of literacy. *International Journal of Bilingual Education and Bilingualis, 13*(2), 175–186.

Meinzen-Derr, J., Wiley, S., Grether, S., & Choo, D. I. (2010). Language performance in children with cochlear implants and additional disabilities. *The Laryngoscope, 120*, 405–413.

Moores, D. F. (Ed.) (2011). *Partners in education: Issues and trends from the 21st International Congress on the Education of the Deaf.* Washington, DC: Gallaudet University Press.

Pipp-Siegel, S., Sedey, A. L., VanLeeuwen, A., & Yoshinaga-Itano, C. (2003). Mastery motivation predicts expressive language in children with hearing loss. *Journal of Deaf Studies and Deaf Education, 8*(2), 133–145.

Pisoni, D. B., Conway, C. M., Kronenberger, W., Horn, D. L., Karpicke, J., & Henning, S. (2008). Efficacy and effectiveness of cochlear implants in deaf children. In M. Marschark & P. C. Hauser (Eds.), *Deaf cognition: Foundations and outcomes* (pp. 52–101). New York, NY: Oxford University Press.

Power, D., & Leigh, G. (Eds.) (2004). *Educating deaf students: Global perspectives.* Washington, DC: Gallaudet University Press.

Powers, S. (2003). Influences of student and family factors on academic outcomes of mainstream secondary school deaf students. *Journal of Deaf Studies and Deaf Education, 8,* 57–78.

Quinto-Pozos, D., Forber-Pratt, A. J., & Singleton, J. L. (2011). Do developmental communication disorders exist in the signed modality? Perspectives from professionals. *Language, Speech, and Hearing Services in Schools, 42,* 423–443.

Reilly, S., Wake, M., Ukoumunne, O. C., Bavin, E., Prior, M., Cini, E., ... Bretherton, L. (2010). Predicting language outcomes at four years of age: Findings from early language in Victoria study. *Pediatrics, 126,* e1530–e1537.

Santayana, G. (1905). *The life of reason, volume 1: Reason in common sense.* New York, NY: C. Scribner's & Sons.

Sinclair, W. (2010). We did it! The rejection of Milan resolutions. *Deaf History International Newsletter, 42/43,* 6–9. Retrieved from http://www.deafhistory-international.com/wp-content/uploads/2012/08/2010-42-43.pdf

Sininger, Y. S., Grimes, A., & Christensen, E. (2010). Auditory development in early amplified children: Factors influencing auditory-based communication outcomes in children with hearing loss. *Ear and Hearing, 31*(2), 166–185.

Soysal, Y. N., & Strang, D. (1989) Construction of the first mass education systems in nineteenth-century Europe. *Sociology of Education, 62*(4), 277–288.

Tomlinson, C. A., & McTighe, J. (2006). *Integrating differentiated instruction and understanding by design: Connecting content and kids.* Alexandria, VA: Association for Supervision and Curriculum Development.

Verbist, A. (2010). The acquisition of personal pronouns in cochlear-implanted children. (Dissertation). Leiden University. LOT Dissertational Series 242. Retrieved from http://www.lotpublications.nl.

Wake, M. A. (2002). Newborn hearing screening: Decision time for Australia. *The Medical Journal of Australia, 177*(4), 172–173.

Weisel, A. (Ed.) (1998). *Issues unresolved: New perspectives on language and deaf education.* Washington, DC: Gallaudet University Press.

White, W. D., & Wolfensburger, W. (1969). The evolution of dehumanization in our institutions. *Mental Retardation, 7,* 5–9.

Yoshinaga-Itano, C. (2003). From screening to early identification and intervention: Discovering predictors to successful outcomes for children with significant hearing loss. *Journal of Deaf Studies and Deaf Education, 8*(1), 11–30.

Yoshinaga-Itano, C. (2004). Earlier identification for earlier intervention. In D. Power & G. Leigh (Eds.), *Educating deaf students: Global perspectives* (pp. 69–84). Washington, DC: Gallaudet University Press.

Yoshinaga-Itano, C. (2006). Early identification, communication modality, and the development of speech and spoken language skills: Patterns and considerations. In P. E. Spencer & M. Marschark (Eds.), *Advances in the spoken language development of deaf and hard-of-hearing children* (pp. 298–327). New York, NY: Oxford University Press.

Yoshinaga-Itano, C., & Sedey, A. (2000). Early speech development in children who are deaf or hard of hearing: Interrelationships with language and hearing. *The Volta Review, 100*(5), 181–211.

Yoshinaga-Itano, C., Sedey, A., Coulter, D., & Mehl, A. (1998). Language of early- and later-identified children with hearing loss. *Pediatrics, 102*(5), 1161–1171.

2

Evidence-Based Practice in Early Intervention: The Proof of the Pudding Is in the Eating

Marilyn Sass-Lehrer and Alys Young

The field of early intervention for deaf and hard-of-hearing infants and toddlers has come a long way. In many countries of the developed world, the vast majority of newborns who are deaf or hard of hearing are identified during the first few weeks of life, and their families are referred quickly for early intervention services. Families work with specialists who are knowledgeable about being deaf or hard of hearing and have access to resources that provide them with information as well as social and emotional support.

Deaf children and their families around the world have benefited from advances in neuroscience and linguistics, as well as insights into child and family development. In many resource-rich countries, families have been able to take advantage of improvements in technology that maximize access to language—whether through sound or sight. As a result of the increased number of very young deaf and hard-of-hearing children receiving early intervention services, it is now possible to examine the efficacy of select early intervention practices and propose recommendations for program policies and practices.

Recently published seminal documents addressing best practices in early intervention have shed much needed light on the question: What works in early intervention and why (Joint Committee on Infant Hearing, 2013; Moeller et al., 2013)? The recommendations for best practices in early intervention are based both on review of relevant research and on consensus among experienced practitioners and researchers in this field. The result is two excellent guides to what best practice might look like and why. However, before implementing these recommendations in practice, we must learn how they actually work by examining their implementation in a wide variety of contexts. The best-practice recommendations are not applicable universally to the diversity of children, families, and communities around the globe without proof testing. Program practice recommendations that are perfectly suited for many children and families may prove to be ineffective in some cases, potentially harmful in others, or simply not tuned in to the strengths and diversity of the contexts in which they seek to make a difference. Examples of selected recommended practices that have led to positive outcomes for young children and their families in some contexts are described in this chapter, and questions are raised about what we can learn from the translation of these same practices within diverse cultural contexts and geographic circumstances. We set out to do this, not to demonstrate that the recommendations of the two documents are limited in their relevance, but rather to point to the next phase in strengthening their relevance—the evidence base for their application and translation into practice.

"The proof of the pudding is in the eating," an age-old proverb that dates to at least the 14th century in its English form, is what we use to describe this phenomenon. These best-practice documents may be today's "pudding" in that their effectiveness can only be determined by the consumers who actually use and are impacted by them—that is, early intervention professionals, deaf and hard-of-hearing children, their families, and communities.

The most recent, early-intervention, best-practice documents are described in this chapter along with the processes used to identify their recommended goals, principles, and suggested benchmarks for achievement. Five common principles from these documents were selected for discussion in this chapter because of their comprehensiveness as well as their widespread acceptance as key elements of early-intervention practices (CAHE Review Team, 2007; Individuals with Disabilities Education Improvement Act, 2004 [http://www.idea.gov]; Joint Committee on Infant Hearing, 2007; Nelson et al., 2008; Yoshinaga-Itano, 2003). These five principles are subjected to a bit of "proof-testing" from the perspectives of different geographic, cultural, and political contexts, as well as regions where resources and support systems vary greatly. Unlike in its original usage, proof-testing is not required to determine whether the "pudding" is poisonous! Rather, we use it to determine its quality and how that might be enhanced. Recommendations for research and testing are presented along with a reiteration from one of the documents for a "Call to Action."

BEST PRACTICES IN EARLY-INTERVENTION DOCUMENTS

Two documents published in 2013, one in the United States and one in Europe, detail effective practices in early intervention and spell out the elements for what works, and to some extent why, for young children who are deaf or hard of hearing and their families. Teams of professionals, both deaf and hearing, with expertise in early intervention led by the Joint Committee on Infant Hearing (JCIH) in the United States crafted the *Supplement to the 2007 JCIH Position Statement: Principles and Guidelines for Early Intervention After Confirmation That a Child Is Deaf or Hard of Hearing* (2013). This document is intended to provide guidance to the Early Hearing Detection and Intervention (EHDI) programs in the United States to "optimize the development and well-being of infants/children and their families" (Joint Committee on Infant Hearing, 2013, p. e1326). The JCIH 2013 document focuses on early-intervention practices rather than medical, audiological, or specialized educational interventions for young children. The document identifies 12 goals, guidelines, and benchmarks to assist states in collecting data to monitor "how well" they are doing, and to document their progress toward the attainment of each of the JCIH goals. The overall aim of this document is to improve the quality of care for deaf and hard-of-hearing infants, children, and their families (Yoshinaga-Itano, 2014) while introducing an element of audit and quality assurance to both programs and service providers. Appendix 1 lists the 12 JCIH goals.

Across the Atlantic Ocean from the United States, in Europe, an international panel of experts from 10 countries, including the United States as well as parents of deaf and hard-of-hearing children, identified 10 foundational principles to guide the development of early intervention programs and practices (Moeller et al., 2013). It is referred to as a "principles statement" in its published form, but has been promoted as an "international consensus statement." It suggests that the goal of the Best Practices in Family-Centered Early Intervention is to "promote widespread implementation of validated, evidence-based principles for family-centered early intervention with children who are deaf and hard of hearing and their families" (Moeller et al., 2013, p. 429). Despite differences among nations in the implementation of family-centered practices, the panel agreed on overarching concepts of family-centered programming that guided the development of the 10 principles, and provider and program behaviors. Appendix 2 lists the 10 foundational principles in this document.

EVIDENCE-BASED PRACTICE

There are many similarities in the content of these documents as well as the processes for their development. For example, experts in early intervention for deaf and hard-of-hearing children and family members were involved in the development of these documents, and both involved a process for validating the content, which included professional and consumer perspectives along with the best research evidence available. This research evidence encompassed quasi-experimental designs, qualitative studies and metareviews, and analyses respected within the specialist field. In this regard, the JCIH 2013 and the Best Practices international consensus statement were influenced by an evidence-based practice model that uses three sources of information: (a) clinical expertise, (b) best research evidence, and (c) consumer values and preferences (Buysse, & Wesley, 2006; Sackett, 2002). An evidence-based research model recognizes that the "best" data sources for examining questions of what works and why comes from randomized controlled research studies, observational studies, systematic reviews and metareviews of scientifically based research and qualitative studies, as well as clinical and consumer wisdom. The vast experience of professionals and consumers provide eyewitness accounts of the outcomes of specific early-intervention practices and, together, provide the most authentic evidence of what works for children and their families, and why.

The JCIH 2013 document acknowledged gaps in the research evidence as well as the limited availability of comparative effectiveness studies—for example, comparing one language development approach with another for specific cohorts of children. Nonetheless, the JCIH document noted there is much to be learned from studies of early-intervention programs that have demonstrated positive outcomes for children and their families (Kennedy et al., 2006; Moeller, 2000; Yoshinaga-Itano, 2003), and called on research colleagues to strengthen the evidence base for practice. Moeller et al. (2013) identified 10 family-centered best-practice principles through a consensus process including consumers (families with deaf children) and professionals. The consensus panel agreed "interventions must be based on explicit principles, validated practices and best available research while being respectful of family differences, choices and ways of doing things" (Moeller et al., 2013, p. 430). This is an important statement because it foregrounds the fact that, in addition to "what works and why," we must also ask "for whom and in which circumstances" if we are striving for *the implementation* of effective practice, not just its definition.

Spencer and Marschark (2010) lamented that the field of deaf education has long based educational practices more on beliefs and attitudes than on evidence or educational outcomes. This, they noted, is not uncommon as a result of the differences of opinion in the general field of special education on criteria for evaluating evidence-based practice and the lack of agreement with regard to whether the evidence that exists constitutes a sufficient foundation to guide current practices. Unlike in sister fields of medicine, nursing, or social work, it is rare to subject research studies of early intervention with deaf children and families to standards of systematic review of evidence such as those used in The Cochrane collaboration (2015) or according to principles for the critical appraisal of qualitative research studies and their evidence (Hannes, 2011). The 2008 systematic review to update the 2001 U.S. Preventive Services Task Force recommendation (Nelson et al., 2008) is a rare exception.

In part, the reluctance to do so may arise from concerns that any such systematic approaches to appraising the quality of evidence on which practice is based might be too reductionist in missing a body of knowledge that does not meet the rigorous standards of systematic review but nonetheless constitutes *evidence-informed practice*. Evidence-informed practice, however, is not just based on the available research, but also on clinical and professional expertise and judgment, as well as family and community values and perspectives. One example of this is the conviction that early intervention, when provided by professionals who have expertise in working with young deaf children and their families, results in better outcomes than when providers lack specialized knowledge and skills (Calderon, 2000; Moeller, 2000; Nittrouer & Burton, 2001). Consistently positive outcomes across similar studies lend credence to the idea that early intervention works for the vast majority of young deaf and hard-of-hearing children. Although opinion may differ on what counts as an outcome and whether we might have a limited view of best outcomes for deaf and hard-of-hearing children (which focus more on language/communication and less on social–emotional well-being), nonetheless benefits of early intervention are evident in many areas of development.

The basic "truths" as we know them, sometimes referred to as *practice wisdom*, is not sufficient, however evidence-informed they may be. They must also be subjected continuously to scrutiny for their validity across different populations and in diverse contexts, and fundamentally in light of better evidence. Diversity may indeed arise from the preferences and values of those who are consumers of early intervention services (Young et al., 2006), but it may also arise from considerations that lie outside any notion of personal choice or control. Structural factors such as economic poverty, oppression of minorities, gender bias, political instability, and discrimination may also be factors of the applied contexts worldwide in which early intervention seeks to be effective. Evidence in one context or set of circumstances does not automatically translate to another. We may find the same fundamental evidence-based principles still hold true, but simply have to be applied differently. Or, better evidence arising from new research may cause us to cast off long-held truths about best practice.

Early intervention with deaf and hard-of-hearing children and their families is essentially a practice-based discipline informed by best evidence in the contexts in which it is applied. In this sense, the principles set forth in the two major documents of the past 2 years have high value but require further evidence to be built that arises from their application, if the research base of this discipline is to be strengthened. In other words, *the proof of the pudding may require the tweaking of the "pudding" recipe for different palates, and in light of better ingredients for the varied tables on which it will be served.*

FIVE COMMON PRINCIPLES DESCRIBED

The JCIH 2013 position statement and the Best Practices documents have many similar recommendations. For the purpose of this chapter, five areas have been identified for consideration. Although these are not the only, or arguably the most important, recommendations that came out of these documents, they nonetheless cover a range of topic areas that are mentioned frequently in the literature as critical to the provision of effective early-intervention programming. They include (a) early and timely access to early-intervention services, (b) family social and emotional support, (c) the use of assistive technologies to access language, (d) qualified providers, and (e) provision of services to all children who are deaf or hard of hearing.

Principle 1: Early and Timely Access to Early Intervention

The importance of early identification of hearing and timely access to services for children and their families is a cornerstone of best practices in early intervention. Best practices emphasize the need to establish a system for identifying children who are deaf or hard of hearing as early as possible, and connecting their families to professionals and comprehensive services and resources as quickly as possible. The U.S. JCIH 2007 position statement recommended timelines for hearing screening, identification and confirmation of hearing levels, as well as the initiation of early-intervention services (Joint Committee on Infant Hearing, 2007). The JCIH timelines recommend hearing screening by 1 month of age, confirmation of hearing levels no later than 3 months of age and initiation of early intervention services by 6 months of age. These timelines are based on research that demonstrates positive child outcomes for those children who have had the advantage of comprehensive early intervention. How might this recommendation "play out" in other national contexts in which early hearing screening is not widely available, or in which audiological services and early intervention are not accessible to the majority of the population?

In some nations, an infrastructure for establishing a system for the screening and identification of hearing levels does not exist on a regional—let alone a universal—basis. Identifying hearing ability during the early months of life for every newborn is not a national priority in many low-resource countries because other, more pressing priorities (such as combating life-threatening illnesses) take precedence (Olusanya, 2011). How, then, does one proceed?

In some parts of South Africa, for example, progress toward meeting the goal of universal hearing screening and early identification of hearing abilities is happening, albeit slowly. Although there are some areas in which newborn hearing screenings are being done and audiologists are available to identify hearing levels in very young infants, it is estimated that more than 90% of the 6200 deaf babies born in South Africa annually will not have the prospect of early identification and diagnosis (Swanepoel & Störbeck, 2008; Theunissen & Swanepoel, 2008). Sometimes it is not geography that is the issue; it is the two-tiered health system. Mothers have a far greater chance of their babies' hearing being screened if they have private medical healthcare, but 92% of all babies in South Africa are born in the public healthcare system (Swanepoel et al., 2009). Yet, in responding to the realities of the context in which best practice principles are being applied can yield positive ways forward.

In some parts of sub-Saharan Africa, hearing screening is being coupled with newborn vaccination programs (Olusanya et al., 2009; Swanepoel et al., 2007; Tanon-Anoh et al., 2010). Vaccination programs tend to be government sponsored and have participation because, often, parents are paid to bring their infants for their vaccinations. To combine newborn hearing screening with these events may not tick the box of screening within 1 month of life, but it is the strategy most likely to yield the highest take-up. Many families who might not recognize the serious consequences of later-identified hearing difficulties, recognize the grave importance of vaccinations that prevent serious diseases. Offering hearing screenings in community immunization centers may increase the likelihood of identifying children who are deaf at the earliest time possible, given the resources available and the preferences of the community.

Innovative pudding chefs consider the ingredients available to them and adapt their recipes accordingly. For example, in wartime Britain, fats such as butter were in short supply, but the Ministry of Food encouraged people to continue to enjoy steamed puddings by replacing half the usual fat with grated raw potatoes (Ministry of Food, 1940). *The result might not have been exactly the same, but the intention and impact was. Nonetheless, without the basic ingredients, establishing an early-intervention system is an extremely challenging task but may still bring forth new recipes.*

Principle 2: Family Social and Emotional Support

The JCIH 2013 paper and the Best Practices consensus document concur that social and emotional support helps families adapt to having a deaf child. In this respect, the promotion of a sense of competence and confidence in their child-rearing abilities is vital (Hintermair, 2000). The vast majority of deaf and hard-of-hearing children are born into hearing families who have no experience or understanding of what it means to be deaf (Mitchell & Karchmer, 2004). The discovery in infancy or early childhood that their child's hearing is not within "normal range" often comes as a shock to many hearing families. Families respond to this news in different ways.

Before universal newborn hearing screening, families often described relief when their child's hearing tests confirmed they were deaf because there was an explanation for their child's lack of responsiveness or delays in spoken communication. Parents often had suspicions based on their own watchfulness and instincts that something about their child's development was different long before any confirmation. However, in parts of the world where newborn hearing screening is common, a newborn health check that identifies infants' hearing levels replaces the former, gradual parental awareness that occurs through ongoing parent–child observations and interactions, and typically accelerates the process of discovery. Although this objective measure of hearing ability compresses the time spent worrying about their child's development, family members' adaptation and resolution of their emotional responses are not necessarily less acute or shorter in duration (Young, 2010). In fact, research has confirmed that the shock and, in some cases, disbelief experienced by parents remains the same as in previous times (Fitzpatrick et al., 2007; Young & Tattersall, 2007).

Some families may seek immediate support from professionals, community or spiritual leaders, friends, family members, deaf adults, or other families with deaf children (Jackson, 2011; Meadow-Orlans et al., 2003). Some families may prefer to keep the news private because they are concerned about the implications for their child and family if others learn their child is deaf. Emotional support must be fine-tuned to the diversity of how parents and families react and their own, often highly personal, processes, of coming to terms with a deaf or hard-of-hearing child in the family (Young & Russell, 2016).

In some parts of the world, confirmation that a child is deaf or hard of hearing brings families worries that are very different than those experienced in economically well-resourced nations. For example, families may worry about the safety of their child or their entire family if others discover their child is deaf; they may decide the more prudent response to this news is to keep their child out of sight and do the best they can without the assistance of others who might provide support to them. For these families, participating in early intervention services, even if available, may not appear to be a viable option.

How parents, families, and communities perceive what it means to be deaf is a key variable in understanding parents' reactions and therefore a helpful steer toward culturally sensitive early-intervention practice that is focused on emotional and social support. Although many (but not all) deaf parents may welcome the birth of a child who is "deaf-like-me," the birth of a child with a physical or developmental difference is not necessarily welcome for everyone. From some cultural or religious perspectives, it might be interpreted, for example, as punishment for a frequently unnamed and unfounded offense of the mother, father, or other family members (Lynch & Hanson, 2011). Having a deaf child can be a stress-producing experience for many hearing families (Calderon & Greenberg, 1993; Hintermair, 2006; Pipp-Siegel et al., 2002;

Poon & Zaidman-Zait, 2014). Fear of the unknown or anticipation of the community's rejection may exacerbate feelings of stress and anxiety, or may result in a family's desire to shield the child from public view (Baker et al., 2010).

More generally, families who have negative views about what it means to be deaf or lack understanding of how to communicate with their child may face difficulties in establishing positive family–child relationships, which in turn affect the child's feelings of security, acceptance, and love (Bat-Chava, 2000; Crowe, 2003; Mulcahy, 1998). Although some communities embrace children with exceptionalities and their families, offering extensive support and guidance, other communities and cultures view differences in physical, cognitive, or emotional development as deficits, undesirable, or a drain on national resources. Despite knowing that without provisions for early language learning, people who are deaf are often at risk for a lifetime of poverty or abuse because education and other opportunities are denied or simply unavailable, nations struggling to provide basic health and human services to their populations may choose to spend their limited resources elsewhere (Störbeck & Young, 2016).

The Global Coalition of Parents of Children who are Deaf or Hard of Hearing conducted a worldwide survey of families raising deaf or hard-of-hearing children to understand the support needs of families around the world. Families indicated that professionals and families who understood their unique situation were extremely valuable sources of support and information (Global Coalition of Parents of Children who are Deaf or Hard of Hearing, 2010a). The importance of parent-to-parent support is reinforced by many surveys and focus groups with families who have deaf or hard-of-hearing children. Jackson et al. (2010), Jackson (2011), Meadow-Orlans et al. (2003), and Zaidman-Zait (2007) all identified families with similar experiences as important sources of support. Henderson et al. (2014) conducted a scoping review of the research to identify the thematic concepts of parent-to-parent support. The constructs of parent-to-parent support they identified included (a) well-being: parent, family and child; (b) knowledge: advocacy, system navigation, and education; and (c) empowerment: confidence and competence. They proposed that knowledge and well-being promote a sense of empowerment, which in turn increases well-being. They concluded that parent-to-parent support is a key element to family-centered care that must be provided by experienced parents. Connecting with families who have children who are deaf or hard of hearing, especially those who share similar cultural beliefs and experiences, may be especially helpful to parents (Sass-Lehrer et al., 2016).

In addition to the support that experienced families with deaf or hard-of-hearing children provide, deaf and hard-of-hearing adults are another powerful and often underused resource. Deaf and hard-of-hearing adults help families realize a future for their children and provide an understanding of the experience of *being* deaf or hard of hearing that hearing families and professionals cannot replicate (Mohay et al., 1998; Pittman et al., 2016; Rogers & Young, 2011; Sutherland et al., 2003; Watkins et al., 1998; Young, in press). The JCIH 2013 statement of principles and guidelines as well as the Best Practices international document recommend that adults who are deaf and hard of hearing be involved actively in all aspects of early intervention. Families who have had the opportunity to get to know deaf and hard-of-hearing adults who are living independently and lead fully successful lives often report their fears have been assuaged and they have regained a hopefulness that did not exist before their experience.

Nonetheless, there are places around the world where people who are deaf or hard of hearing face extreme discrimination and are even denied basic human rights. As challenging as these circumstances are, efforts are being made by international organizations such as the World Federation of the Deaf and the European Union of the Deaf to educate governments and political systems to provide improved educational and vocational opportunities to deaf adults so they may take their rightful place as productive citizens of their nations (Pabsch, 2014). Communities of deaf and hard-of-hearing people, whether in sub-Saharan Africa or in other regions of the world, however remote, discover means to connect and extend support and guidance to each other (DeClerck, 2007, 2011; Kusters, 2009). For deaf and hard-of-hearing adults limited in their ability to provide direct in-person language and social support to young deaf children and families, opportunities may be available for these families to connect online with deaf adults through social media.

Establishing family-to-family support networks is challenging in rural or low-resource areas and is especially difficult when families experience a stigma or outright discrimination because they have a deaf or hard-of-hearing child. Community and spiritual leaders are an important resource for these families and are often in a position to establish informal networks of support that include other families with deaf and hard-of-hearing children as well as adults who are deaf or hard of hearing. Community and cultural celebrations might include opportunities for families from different geographic areas to come together to meet, share stories, and offer support to one another. Support from other families with deaf and hard-of-hearing children or from the adult deaf community is far from universal and demands exploration of the community and its cultural resources to provide families with support from others who understand these unique experiences.

One innovative project—The Vietnam Intergenerational Deaf Education Outreach Project, implemented by the World Concern

Development Organization in cooperation with the Ministry of Education and Training in 2011—has provided training and support to the deaf community to work with families with deaf and hard-of-hearing children, schools, and the community to raise awareness and facilitate communication and understanding (World Bank Group, 2015). A major goal of the project is to form family support teams that consist of deaf adults who have been trained as family educators, hearing signing individuals to facilitate communication, and preschool teachers. These teams form collaborative partnerships to support the child, family, and school. The project aims to identify young deaf and hard-of-hearing children, provide home visits, and work with the family, school, and community to prepare these children to be ready to enter primary school.

To return to our pudding metaphor, it is only in recent times that the making of puddings has been an individual activity; throughout history, it was collective. For example, in England, "Stir up Sunday" (the last Sunday before Advent) was always the time when whole families would come together to make their Christmas pudding, sharing ingredients, with each taking a stir and making a wish (Lemm, 2015). *The making of a good pudding requires the emotional and social support of others to ensure the best shared outcome.*

Principle 3: Use of Assistive Technologies

The international consensus document (Moeller et al., 2013) and the JCIH principles and guidelines both identify the importance of assistive technologies not only to enhance access to communication, but also to be used as an educational and social–emotional support avenue for families. Advances in technology are widening the gap between resource-rich and low-resource nations. Assistive listening technologies, such as hearing aids and cochlear implants; visual technologies, such as savvy visual communication devices; and alternative and augmentative communication technologies enhance opportunities for people who are deaf or hard of hearing and those with low vision to access language and expand their communication opportunities.

In addition to these communication-enhancing technologies, Internet access and telecommunication devices such as cell phones provide families who have these amenities with virtually unlimited access to information and, potentially, to sources of support, such as online forums including, for example, the National Deaf Children's Society Parent Place Forum (https://www.ndcs.org.uk/applications/discussion/) or the Aussie Deaf Kids online group for parents (http://www.aussiedeafkids.org.au/parent-forums.html).Videophones and software applications such as FaceTime and Skype enable families to connect with other families with deaf children, specialists who may not be available geographically, and adults who are deaf or hard of hearing. In addition, social media such as Facebook and Wordpress are creating virtual communities of common interest. They are particularly facilitative because of their ability to host messages in signed as well as written languages.

Lack of Internet connectivity, or hearing or visual technologies that are simply unaffordable or unavailable, prevent children and their families from benefiting from these advances. Best practices emphasize the need to make these technologies available to all families, regardless of their economic resources or geographic location, and provide specialists who can support families in making optimal use of technologies appropriate for them and their children. This, unfortunately, is not the reality for many deaf and hard-of-hearing children and their families in the world today.

The lack of availability of assistive technologies for all is not simply an issue of whether a nation state and its citizens are economically rich or poor. Countries of similar levels of economic development may choose widely different social contracts that, in turn, affect the distribution of technological wealth (Benabou, 2005). Compare, for example, the welfare state approach of the United Kingdom in contrast to the laissez-faire, individualistic wealth-driven approach of the United States. In the United Kingdom, hearing aids and cochlear implants are part of the social contract between the state and its citizens, provided free at the point of need and underpinned by a welfare state to which all contribute to collective funds. What one "gets out" may be less or more than what one "puts in." In the United States, those without sufficient personal financial resources or medical insurance that covers these technologies may not have access to the same degree of care—in this case, the best hearing aids, for example, replaced regularly through childhood, or cochlear implantation. Loans and charitable foundations may be called on to make up the deficit (such as World Wide Hearing [http://www.wwhearing.org/]), but the equal rights of access to the best assistive technologies for all are not guaranteed.

Although best-practice recommendations encourage the use of the most advanced hearing and visual technologies available, in situations where these are not available to children and families there may be useful substitutes that can be helpful. Hearing aids that may not include all the available "bells and whistles" may be obtainable from schools, international service organizations, or other agencies. Some governments or nonprofit organizations may provide children with free hearing aids or may provide stipends for families to purchase low-cost hearing aids.

Hearing aids require regular care and can also be costly. For example, batteries and hearing aid parts may be prohibitive for families with household incomes that barely provide for their basic needs, and for those who do not have financial assistance to maintain their child's assistive technologies. In addition, hearing aids are breakable and parts can be lost or damaged easily. By following a solution-focused perspective, the World Health Organization is taking the lead in encouraging the development of low-cost, digital, and, in some cases, solar-powered hearing aids specifically for the developing world (Humphreys, 2013).

Assistive listening technologies require support from specialists who can ensure the device is appropriate and provides benefit for the child. Specialists are also necessary to help families learn how best to care for these devices and use them. Families with young children need to have their child's hearing tested regularly to be sure the hearing aid or cochlear implant is working effectively. Tele-intervention, during which specialists are available to work virtually with families, may be a reasonable and accessible solution to this problem. Although families' and providers' perspectives indicate multiple benefits to the use of tele-intervention via telehealth technology to promote their child's listening skills—for example, more frequency of services, increased skills, increased parental engagement (Blaiser et al., 2013; Houston & Behl, 2011)—effectiveness studies need to be undertaken that examine the broader use of tele-intervention approaches, outcomes for children and their families, and measures of cost–benefits. For listening devices to provide effective access to sound, families need to find qualified specialists either online, at their nearest school for the deaf, or at another location where specialists can show them how to support their child's development of listening skills.

Visual technologies should also be available for all deaf and hard-of-hearing children and their families. Technological innovations such as the Internet enables access to visual languages such as signed languages as never before (Crace & Nathanson, 2015). For hearing families wishing to develop their own sign language learning, and for early-intervention professionals who support children's signed language development, easy access to communication, interactions, and resources online to support their child's signing development make a huge difference (see the Royal Institute for Deaf and Blind Children information on their teleschool at http://www.ridbc.org.au/teleschool). Easy access to video recording, playback, and hosting of visual (signed) media also support children's and families' signed development. Furthermore, all these benefits are available remotely, provided there is access to the Internet. Families may need to travel to find the nearest available services if Internet connectivity, computers, or cell phones with video access are not available locally. Community health or government organizations or schools may have services that families can use. Families may be able to borrow cell phones or computers that can provide at least some limited access from time to time. Although all children and families should have the right to select the technologies best for them, in reality circumstances beyond the control of the individual—such as poverty and geographic location—may reduce the opportunity to use technologies in ways that support language development and overall well-being.

Although pudding makers throughout the world might try to substitute some ingredients when others are in short supply, there is always a point reached when this will not do. Cherry pie cannot be made without cherries. So, too, with assistive technologies designed to support hearing and speech development. There is a bottom line where no substitutes will do, but alternatives might need to be considered. Make apple pie instead?

Principle 4: Qualified Providers

According to the recommendations from the JCIH 2013 and Moeller et al. (2013), young children who are deaf or hard of hearing and their families need providers with specialized knowledge and skills to promote their child's early development, enhance family–child interactions, and provide families with resources to support their positive adaptation to raising a deaf child. Both documents, the JCIH 2013 statement and the Best Practices international consensus document recommend that core competencies be identified for specialists working with families and their children, and that support for ongoing professional development be provided. Direct observations, supervision, and mentoring with specific feedback on providers' performance are recommended to enhance the quality of services.

Sass-Lehrer et al. (2008) identified core competencies of early-intervention specialists based on eight position statements and best-practice documents available at that time. The documents were all developed through a collaborative process reflecting the opinions of researchers, practitioners, and families. These competencies resulted in 116 statements, which are listed in Appendix 1 of the JCIH 2013 document (Joint Committee on Infant Hearing, 2013). Sass-Lehrer et al. (2011) recommended that these competencies be used as (a) a tool to hire "competent providers," (b) a way for providers to assess their own strengths and areas of needs for training, (c) a guide for the development of professional training activities, (d) a method to identify and verify effective practices, and (e) a way to inform policy initiatives related to effective practices.

How can families with deaf and hard-of-hearing children—in places where there are no programs to prepare early-intervention specialists—be sure that early-intervention professionals are providing the guidance they need to support their families and promote their children's development? How can these recommendations be implemented without an infrastructure in place to support professionals and monitor the quality of the services provided?

Some nations are establishing innovative approaches that take advantage of the resources available to meet these challenges. South Africa established a program known as Home Intervention Hearing and Language Opportunities Parent Education Services, or HI HOPES, based on the SKI-HI curriculum model in the United States (Störbeck & Pittman, 2008). Grants and donations, primarily from the business sector, provide funding for free services to families with deaf or hard-of-hearing children younger than 3 years old in the regions where it operates. Specialists, who are known as *parent advisors*, receive training in family-centered early-intervention practices and deliver services in families' homes, in their preferred language. Deaf mentors are also available who use spoken and/or sign language. Working in partnership with families in their own homes helps providers appreciate the supports available to the family and match their recommendations to the family's resources, interests, and priorities. For example, there is little point in recommending costly toys that might be helpful in supporting a child's hearing awareness if there is little money for food. Learning how to use metal cooking pots and other everyday objects to achieve the same effect may be more realistic and consistent with families' resources (Störbeck & Young, 2016).

Internet technology is another encouraging approach to support the training and development of early-intervention specialists. Professionals can access an increasing number of online training programs, webinars, and video conferencing opportunities to promote their knowledge of child development, family-centered practices, sign language and bilingual early intervention, listening and spoken language, assessment, and early educational practices for infants and toddlers who are deaf or hard of hearing. Webinars are offered periodically through centers such as the National Center for Hearing Assessment and Management (http://www.infanthearing.org) and the Laurent Clerc National Deaf Education Center (http://www.gallaudet.edu/clerc_center/webinars.html), both of which are in the United States. In addition, the Victorian Deaf Education Institute in Australia offers professional education in partnership with schools, universities, and professional organizations (http://www.deafeducation.vic.edu.au/Pages/home.aspx). Professionals can improve their sign language skills through computer programs and video technology, and can capture their interactions with families through video on cell phones and then share them with experts in another (distant) location to enhance their own professional skills.

Mentoring relationships between experienced and novice professionals supports the transfer of knowledge and skills, beliefs, and attitudes in working with families and young deaf and hard-of-hearing children. An effective mentoring relationship requires a trusting partnership between the mentor and mentee, as well as a positive attitude and desire for learning (Nevins & Sass-Lehrer, 2016). Conferencing online via Skype or other video technology provides a mechanism for trainers and professionals to reflect on their practices and discuss helpful resources and alternative approaches. Although mentoring relationships hold promise to expand the knowledge and skill levels of professionals providing services, research in examining how well different models work in a diversity of contexts holds the key to their ultimate proof of effectiveness.

The effectiveness of services provided by early-intervention specialists requires a partnership approach in which all parties involved collaborate to document child outcomes and progress made, consider families' perceptions of the helpfulness of the services provided, and assess the providers' knowledge and the application of their skills to work effectively with families and young children. Parents and families are a central partner in this collaborative process; they are not simply the consumer of services provided by a qualified provider, they are the co-creators of the pathways to successful outcomes. However, more evidence is required of the effectiveness of partnership approaches from family perspectives in relation to outcomes for deaf and hard-of-hearing children (Young et al., 2009).

Making a successful pudding not only requires a recipe to follow, but also the skill cooks bring to following it. These skills are built through training and experience, but also include knowing the tastes of those for whom they cook and matching them in the execution of the recipe.

Principle 5: Providing Equitable Services to Children With All Levels of Hearing Abilities

The equitable distribution of resources to all families and children with varying levels of hearing is a concern echoed in the recommendations of both best-practice documents. Young children who are deaf or hard of hearing and their families are an extremely heterogeneous group that reflects the cultural, linguistic, ethnic, socioeconomic, and religious diversity of people internationally. In addition, very young children who are deaf or hard of hearing are also diversely able in terms of their sensory and physical abilities, such as hearing, vision, motor skills, and cognitive potentials. Some deaf infants have family members who are also deaf and who experience fluent, natural communication from the time they are born. Others are born into hearing families with a limited understanding of how to communicate with an infant or toddler who is not able to hear. These differences call for different types and levels of services and resources to maximize each child's potential and the family's overall well-being.

When resources are limited, difficult decisions are often made regarding who receives services and who does not. Although the research available is clear that children with any limitations in their hearing ability who are raised in a predominately hearing environment face challenges acquiring language without specialized services, not all children and families have available to them the resources they need and not all needs are necessarily prioritized in the distribution of resources.

In England, all children identified through newborn hearing screening programs are referred immediately to an early-intervention service and receive contact from a qualified provider (usually a teacher of the deaf). The extent of ongoing direct involvement between provider and child, however, does vary. Rodd and Young (2009) for example, found that, in the face of limited resources, infants with hearing in the severe/profound hearing range would be prioritized by visiting teacher services over those with more hearing. Yet, the complexity and difficulty of some family situations of children with mild/moderate hearing might suggest a more urgent need to facilitate optimal developmental environments, and some families with children who are severely/profoundly deaf might be relatively straightforward by comparison. Although equitable service does not imply equal use of resources, the basis on which scarce resources are used, for whom, and according to which criteria are a legitimate source of inquiry, even within a welfare state that operates as a universal service provider.

Because early-intervention services are often costly, families with children who do not qualify for free or low-cost services may pay for services that are not available, or may have to travel long distances to receive specialized services. Ideally, a range of programs and services is available to meet the individual and unique needs of all children and families. Children who have multiple developmental challenges, for example, may need specialists who have expertise in different areas and/or require costly treatment options and equipment. Young children who are deaf typically require access to native sign language users and professionals who are skilled in offering bilingual early intervention services. Others need assistive listening technologies and specialists to support their abilities to acquire language through listening and spoken language. Programs and services are often not available that provide the full range of communication opportunities to young children and their families that facilitate the acquisition of language through sign language as well as through spoken language.

The provision of comprehensive services to all children who are deaf as well as those who are hard of hearing is a standard that is not easily obtained, but there are some excellent examples where it has been achieved, such as in British Columbia's early hearing service (http://www.phsa.ca/our-services/programs-services/bc-early-hearing-program). Creative programming and distribution of scarce resources may help defray costs and deliver services to more children and their families. Professionals with very specialized skills—for example, specialists whose expertise is in working with deaf children with CHARGE syndrome[1] may be able to train other providers through workshops and webinars, and mentor others with less expertise in a particular area as a consultant. In another example of creative programming, deaf adults who have expertise in working with families may not have the ability to meet each family individually in their home on a regular basis, but may be able to provide monthly weekend retreats or other events where groups of families can participate and interact for extensive periods of time with signing deaf adults.

There is little point in providing an equal slice of only one pudding if not everyone likes that pudding. Innovative chefs are required to provide multiple puddings, sometimes initially on taster menus, later as full-size delights that are available to all who dine. But, if everyone does not have access to the restaurant, not everyone gets to taste and choose.

RECOMMENDATIONS FOR RESEARCH AND FURTHER ACTION

With obesity the new scourge of economically rich countries, we are mindful not to suggest too much eating of puddings to develop proof! Instead, we might rely on the restaurant reports of others, or those chefs and food writers who offer us their "tried and tested recipes." But, what works in one kitchen does not always work in another, and it is not until you try to make that darn pudding that you really know if the recipe works for you! So, too, is the difference between efficacy and effectiveness.

Efficacy refers to the proven beneficial effects of a given intervention or practice; *effectiveness* refers to its demonstration in the circumstances in which it is being implemented. JCIH 2013 and the international consensus statement (Moeller et al., 2013) may both point us to efficacy, but they do not guarantee effectiveness. That needs to be striven for and built in *the application* of the recommendations that have been set forth. This is true in the diversity of arenas of practice in the United States and Europe, where both these documents were engendered, as well as in more challenging circumstances elsewhere. As Störbeck & Young (2016) stated, "Fundamentally early intervention practices must be culturally meaningful to be embraced in cultures and contexts far removed from the western ones in which they were developed" (p. 314). Also, as we discussed earlier, currently there are significant gaps in the evidence base of effective practices, although many highly skilled practitioners are working with effectiveness in mind and are asking: What works in this context and for this particular child and family?

---

[1] The letters in CHARGE stand for coloboma of the eye, heart defects, atresia of the choanae, retardation of growth and/or development, genital and/or urinary abnormalities, and ear abnormalities and deafness (http://www.chargesyndrome.org/about-charge.asp).

Given the focus on the application of best practice and building the evidence base of effectiveness, what can be done? In line with the principles of practitioner research programs in other fields, we suggest a fundamental stance of *constant inquiry*. That is to say, both routine program-level evaluation as well as curiosity-driven practitioner inquiry is built in to how early-intervention programs and individual practitioners perform their daily work. At a program level, collecting and documenting basic information about the effectiveness of programs and services for individual families can be helpful in shaping services.

For example, in England there is a national and ongoing process of audit of the quality and delivery of newborn hearing screen and early-intervention services (NHSP, 2015). The parent-report questionnaire on the effectiveness of multiprofessional early-intervention services—the MVOS (My Views on Services)—was designed specifically for families with deaf and hard-of-hearing children engaging with services (Young et al., 2009). Originating in the United Kingdom, it has been adapted for use in the United States, Canada, and Australia.

The Early Childhood Technical Assistance Center/Early Childhood Outcomes Center (http://www.ectacenter.org/eco/) in the United States requires early-childhood programs to report on the effectiveness of early intervention for both children and their families. To this end, families are asked to indicate how helpful early intervention has been in the following areas:

- Understanding your child's strengths and abilities and special needs
- Knowing your rights and being able to advocate effectively for your child
- Helping your child develop and learn

Programs are also required to report child outcomes in the following areas:

- Social relationships, which includes getting along with other children and relating well with adults
- Use of knowledge and skills, which refers to thinking, reasoning, problem solving, and early literacy and math skills
- Taking action to meet needs, which includes feeding, dressing, self-care, and following rules related to health and safety

Although some large-scale research studies of effectiveness are under way using a variety of research designs from the experimental to the exploratory (such as Ching et al. [2013] in Australia; see also Yoshinaga-Itano & Sedey [2013] in the United States), there is very little use currently being made in our field of practitioner researcher work despite being well established and popular in other disciplines such as social work and education (Fox et al., 2007; Shaw, 2005; Stockton & Morran, 2010; Wolkenhauer et al., 2011). Practitioner research exploits the unique position in which practitioners find themselves. They have situated and contextual knowledge of how an intervention is working in practice in highly specific contexts. They are able to formulate commonsense research questions that address everyday issues of practice as well as contribute to the wider research base. They are able to access easily relevant samples and build trust with participants to engage with a process of constant evaluation and questioning of effectiveness over a long period of time of engagement with a child and family. Ethical safeguards are required, of course, as well as specialized research advice and support, but there is a large workforce of potential applied researchers who are currently underused and able to deliver results of effectiveness of best-practice standards in a wide variety of contexts. Furthermore, a small number of parent researchers are also appearing in pockets of practice around the world who are taking up formal research projects that actively use their unique epistemological positioning in the development of research studies. They are "knowers" on very different grounds than the majority of those working in this field, and their contribution is nonetheless valid.

CONCLUSION: THE PROOF OF THE PUDDING IS IN THE EATING

The JCIH 2013 document identifies 12 goals and recommendations for each of the goals. The JCIH suggests that U.S. states establish a baseline for each of the goals and report annually on the progress made toward achievement of the goals. A team of early hearing detection and intervention specialists in Minnesota has developed an assessment tool based on the JCIH goals (Brown & Davies, 2015). The purpose of the assessment is for stakeholders to identify priorities within their individual states and establish a foundation for measuring their state's progress as they work systematically toward quality improvement of their early-intervention programs.

The international consensus document takes a slightly different approach. This document identifies 10 principles and related provider and program behaviors, and concludes with a "Call to Action" that was adapted from the Global Coalition of Parents of Children Who Are Deaf or Hard of Hearing position statement and recommendation for family support in the development of newborn hearing screening systems and early hearing detection and intervention systems worldwide (GPOD, 2010b). The Call to Action requests that all those with a stake in the improvement of early-intervention programs leading to positive outcomes for children and families (a) endorse the international consensus statement, (b) share the document with colleagues and leaders in the field, (c) recruit parent leaders, (d) support a research agenda examining practices in each respective country, and, last, (e) embed these principles in legislation, guidelines, consensus papers, and positions papers regarding early intervention services and models.

We submit that these documents outline what might be considered the basic ingredients for pudding making. The goals and principles are fundamental to the making of an effective early-intervention system, but require an understanding of the diversity of each national context, geographic setting, awareness of the resources available, and consideration of the unique characteristics of each child and family. Only when the outcomes achieved for all deaf children and their families around the world are aligned with the individual hopes and dreams of these consumers can we know that effectiveness has been achieved—just as the proof-testing of the pudding is in the eating.

APPENDIX 1: GOALS FOR THE IMPLEMENTATION OF BEST PRACTICE IN EARLY INTERVENTION SERVICES

Goal 1: All Children Who Are D/HH and Their Families Have Access to Timely and Coordinated Entry Into EI Programs Supported by a Data Management System Capable of Tracking Families and Children From Confirmation of Hearing Loss to Enrollment Into EI Services

Goal 2: All Children Who Are D/HH and Their Families Experience Timely Access to Service Coordinators Who Have Specialized Knowledge and Skills Related to Working With Individuals Who Are D/HH

Goal 3: All Children Who Are D/HH From Birth to 3 Years of Age and Their Families Have EI Providers Who Have the Professional Qualifications and Core Knowledge and Skills to Optimize the Child's Development and Child/Family Well-being

Goal 3a: Intervention Services to Teach ASL Will Be Provided by Professionals Who Have Native or Fluent Skills and Are Trained to Teach Parents/Families and Young Children

Goal 3b: Intervention Services to Develop Listening and Spoken Language Will Be Provided by Professionals Who Have Specialized Skills and Knowledge

Goal 4: All Children Who Are D/HH With Additional Disabilities and Their Families Have Access to Specialists Who Have the Professional Qualifications and Specialized Knowledge and Skills to Support and Promote Optimal Developmental Outcomes

Goal 5: All Children Who Are D/HH and Their Families From Culturally Diverse Backgrounds and/or From Non–English-Speaking Homes Have Access to Culturally Competent Services With Provision of the Same Quality and Quantity of Information Given to Families From the Majority Culture

Goal 6: All Children Who Are D/HH Should Have Their Progress Monitored Every 6 Months From Birth to 36 Months of Age, Through a Protocol That Includes the Use of Standardized, Norm-Referenced Developmental Evaluations, for Language (Spoken and/or Signed), the Modality of Communication (Auditory, Visual, and/or Augmentative), Social–Emotional, Cognitive, and Fine and Gross Motor Skills

Goal 7: All Children Who Are Identified With Hearing Loss of Any Degree, Including Those With Unilateral or Slight Hearing Loss, Those With Auditory Neural Hearing Loss (Auditory Neuropathy), and Those With Progressive or Fluctuating Hearing Loss, Receive Appropriate Monitoring and Immediate Follow-up Intervention Services Where Appropriate

Goal 8: Families Will Be Active Participants in the Development and Implementation of EHDI Systems at the State/Territory and Local Levels

Goal 9: All Families Will Have Access to Other Families Who Have Children Who Are D/HH and Who Are Appropriately Trained to Provide Culturally and Linguistically Sensitive Support, Mentorship, and Guidance

Goal 10: Individuals Who Are D/HH Will Be Active Participants in the Development and Implementation of EHDI Systems at the National, State/Territory, and Local Levels; Their Participation Will Be an Expected and Integral Component of the EHDI Systems

Goal 11: All Children Who Are D/HH and Their Families Have Access to Support, Mentorship, and Guidance From Individuals Who Are D/HH

Goal 12: As Best Practices Are Increasingly Identified and Implemented, All Children Who Are D/HH and Their Families Will Be Ensured of Fidelity in the Implementation of the Intervention They Receive

Source: Joint Committee on Infant Hearing. 2013. Supplement to the 2007 JCIH position statement: Principles and guidelines for early intervention after confirmation that a child is deaf or hard of hearing. *Pediatrics* 131(4):e1324–e1349. http://pediatrics.aappublications.org/content/131/4/e1324. Accessed January 7, 2016.

APPENDIX 2: BEST PRACTICES IN FAMILY-CENTERED EARLY INTERVENTION: FOUNDATIONAL PRINCIPLES

Principle 1: Early, Timely, and Equitable Access to Services
Principle 2: Family/Provider Partnerships
Principle 3: Informed Choice and Decision Making
Principle 4: Family Social and Emotional Support
Principle 5: Family Infant Interaction
Principle 6: Use of Assistive Technologies and Supporting Means of Communication
Principle 7: Qualified Providers
Principle 8: Collaborative Teamwork
Principle 9: Progress Monitoring
Principle 10: Program Monitoring

Source: Moeller, M. P., Carr, G., Seaver, L., Stredler-Brown, A., & Holzinger, D. (2013). Best practices in family-centered early intervention for children who are deaf or hard of hearing an international consensus statement. *Journal of Deaf Studies and Deaf Education, 18*(4), 429–445. http://jdsde.oxfordjournals.org/content/18/4/429.full.pdf+html. Accessed January 7, 2016.

REFERENCES

Baker, D. L., Miller, E., Dang, M. T., Yang, C.-S., & Hansen, R. L. (2010). Developing culturally responsive approaches with Southeast Asian American families experiencing developmental disabilities. *Pediatrics, 126,* S146–S150. Pediatrics.aappublications.org. Accessed March 19, 2015.

Bat-Chava, Y. (2000). Diversity of deaf identities. *American Annals of the Deaf, 145,* 420–428.

Benabou, R. (2005). Inequality, technology and the social contract. In P. Aghion & S. Durlauf (Eds.), *Handbook of economic growth* (1st ed., Vol. 1, pp. 1595–1638). Oxford North Holland Imprint, Elsevier.

Blaiser, K. M., Behl, D. D., Callow-Heuser, C., & White, K. R. (2013). Measuring costs and outcomes of tele-intervention when serving families of children who are deaf/hard of hearing. *International Journal of Telerehabilitation, 5*(2), 3–10.

Brown, N., & Lindow-Davies, C. (2015). EHDI system self-assessment using JCIH early intervention recommendations: A foundation for continuous improvement. http://www.infanthearing.org/elearning/index.html#webinars [webinar]. Accessed December 24, 2015.

Buysse, V. A., & Wesley, P. W. (2006). *Evidence-based practice in the early childhood field*. Washington, DC: Zero to Three.

CAHE Review Team (2007). A systematic review of the literature for children with permanent hearing loss. http://www.health.qld.gov.au/healthyhearing/pages/publications.asp. Accessed December 24, 2015.

Calderon, R. (2000). Parent involvement in deaf children's educational programs as a predictor of child's language, early reading and social–emotional development. *Journal of Deaf Studies and Deaf Education, 5*(2),140–155.

Calderon, R., & Greenberg, M. T. (1993). Consideration in the adaptation of families with school-aged deaf children. In M. Marschark & M. D. Clark (Eds.), *Psychological perspectives on deafness* (pp. 27–48). Hillsdale, NJ: Erlbaum.

Ching, T. Y., Dillon, H., Marnane, V., Hou, S., Day, J., Seeto, M., Crowe, K., Street, L., Thomson, J., Van Buynder, P., Zhang, V., Wong, A., Burns, L., Flynn, C., Cupples, L., Cowan, R. S., Leigh, G., Sjahalam-King, J., & Yeh, A. (2013). Outcomes of early- and late-identified children at 3 years of age: Findings from a prospective population-based study. *Ear and Hear, 34*(5), 535–552.

Cochrane Collaboration (2015). The Cochrane Library. http://cochranelibrary.com. Accessed January 7, 2016.

Crace, J., & Nathanson, G. (2015). Deaf adults connecting with birth to 3 families. *The NCHAM E-Book*. http://infanthearing.org/ehdi-ebook/2015_ebook/19-Chapter19DeafAdultsConnecting2015.pdf. Accessed December 24, 2015.

Crowe, T. V. (2003). Self-esteem scores among deaf college students: An examination of gender and parents' hearing status and signing ability on self-esteem. *Journal of Deaf Studies and Deaf Education, 8*(2), 199–206.

De Clerck, G. A. (2007). Meeting global deaf peers, visiting ideal deaf places: Deaf ways of education leading to empowerment, an exploratory case study. *American Annals of the Deaf, 152*(1), 5–19.

De Clerck, G. A. (2011). Fostering deaf people's empowerment: The Cameroonian deaf community and epistemological equity. *Third World Quarterly, 32*(8), 1419–1435.

Fitzpatrick, E., Graham, I. D., Durieux-Smith, A., Angus, D., & Coyle, D. (2007). Parents' perspectives on the impact of early diagnosis of childhood hearing loss. *International Journal of Audiology, 46*, 97–106.

Fox, M., Martin, P., & Green, G. (2007). *Doing practitioner research*. London: Sage.

Global Coalition of Parents of Children Who Are Deaf and Hard of Hearing (June 2010a). Support needs of families: Results of a worldwide survey of parents of deaf and hard of hearing children. Poster session presented at the Newborn Hearing Symposium. Como, Italy.

Global Coalition of Parents of Children Who Are Deaf and Hard of Hearing (2010b). *Position statement and recommendations for family support in the development of newborn hearing screening systems (NHS)/early hearing detection and intervention systems (EHDI) worldwide*. https://sites.google.com/site/gpodhh/Home/position_statement. Accessed January 7, 2016.

Hannes, K. (2011). Critical appraisal of qualitative research. In J. Noyes, A. Booth, K. Hannes, A. Harden, J. Harris, S. Lewin, & G. Lockwood. (Eds.), *Supplementary guidance for inclusion of qualitative research in cochrane systematic reviews of interventions*. Version 1. http://cqrmg.cochrane.org/supplemental-handbook-guidance. Accessed January 7, 2016.

Henderson, R. J., Johnson, A., & Moodie, S. (2014). Parent-to-parent support for parents with children who are deaf or hard of hearing: A conceptual framework. *American Journal of Audiology, 23*(4), 437–448.

Hintermair, M. (2000). Hearing impairment, social networks, and coping: The need for families with hearing-impaired children to relate to other parents and to hearing-impaired adults. *American Annals of the Deaf, 145*(1), 41–53.

Hintermair, M. (2006). Parental resources, parental stress, and socioemotional development of deaf and hard of hearing children. *Journal of Deaf Studies and Deaf Education, 11*(4), 493–513.

Houston, K. T., & Behl, D. D. (February 2011). Tele-intervention: A model program of service delivery. Paper presented at the Early Hearing Detection and Intervention Meeting. Atlanta, GA.

Humphreys, G. (2013). Technology transfer aids hearing. *Bulletin of the World Health Organization, 91,* 471–472.

Individuals with Disabilities Education Improvement Act of 2004 (2004). Publication L no. 108-446, 118 Stat 2647.

Jackson, C. W. (2011). Family supports and resources for parents of children who are deaf or hard of hearing. *American Annals of the Deaf, 156*(4), 343–362.

Jackson, C., Wegner, J. R., and Turnbull, A. P. (2010). Family quality of life following early identification of deafness. *Language, Speech and Hearing Services in Schools, 41*(2), 194–205.

Joint Committee on Infant Hearing (2007). Year 2007 position statement: Principles and guidelines for early hearing detection and intervention programs. *Pediatrics, 120,* 898–921.

Joint Committee on Infant Hearing (2013). Supplement to the JCIH 2007 position statement: Principles and guidelines for intervention after confirmation that a child is deaf or hard of hearing. *Pediatrics, 131*(4), e1324–e1349.

Kennedy, C. R., McCann, D. C., Campbell, M. J., Law, C. M., Mullee, M., Petrou, S. et al. (2006). Language ability after early detection of permanent child hearing impairment. *The New England Journal of Medicine, 354,* 2131–2141.

Kusters, A. (2009). Deaf on the Lifeline of Mumbai. *Sign Language Studies, 10*(1), 36–68.

Lemm, E. (2015). Stir up Sunday and Christmas pudding traditions. http://britishfood.about.com/od/Christmas/a/xmaspud.htm. Accessed January 7, 2016.

Lynch, E. W., & Hanson, M. (2011). *Developing cross-cultural competence: A guide for working with children and their families* (3rd ed.). Baltimore, MD: Brookes Publishing.

Meadow-Orlans, K. P., Mertens, D. M., & Sass-Lehrer, M. A. (2003). *Parents and their deaf children: The early years.* Washington, DC: Gallaudet University Press.

Mitchell, R. E., & Karchmer, M. A. (2004). Chasing the mythical ten percent: Parental hearing status of deaf and hard-of-hearing students in the United States. *Sign Language Studies, 4*(2), 138–163.

Ministry of Food (1940). War Cookery Leaflet 13, June 18, 1940. http://recipespastandpresent.org.uk/wartime2.php. Accessed January 7, 2016.

Moeller, M. P. (2000). Early intervention and language development in children who are deaf and hard of hearing. *Pediatrics, 106*(3), e43–e51.

Moeller, M. P., Carr, G., Seaver, L., Stredler-Brown, A., & Holzinger, D. (2013). Best practices in family-centered early intervention for children who are deaf or hard of hearing an international consensus statement. *Journal of Deaf Studies and Deaf Education, 18*(4), 429–445.

Mohay, H., Milton, L., Hindmarsh, G., & Ganley, K. (1998). Deaf models as communication models for hearing families with deaf children. In A. Weisel (Ed.), *Issues Unresolved: New Perspectives on Language and Deaf Education* (pp. 76–87). Washington, DC: Gallaudet University Press.

Mulcahy, R. T. (1998). Cognitive self-appraisal of depression and self-concept: Measurement alternatives for evaluating affective states. PhD dissertation, Gallaudet University.

Nelson, H. D., Bougatsos, C., & Nygren, P. (2008). Universal newborn hearing screening: Systematic review to update the 2001 US Preventive Services Task Force recommendation. *Pediatrics, 122*, e266–e276.

Nevins, M. E., & Sass-Lehrer, M. (2016). Developing and sustaining exemplary practice through professional learning. In M. Sass-Lehrer (Ed.), *Early intervention for deaf and hard-of-hearing infants, toddlers and their families: Interdisciplinary perspectives.* New York, NY: Oxford University Press.

Nittrouer, S., & Burton, L. (2001). The role of early language experience in the development of speech perception and language processing abilities in children with hearing loss. *The Volta Review, 103*, 5–37.

NHSP (2015). Newborn Hearing Screening Programme quality assurance round 4 reports. http://webarchive.nationalarchives.gov.uk/20150408175925/http://hearing.screening.nhs.uk.qualityassurance. Accessed January 7, 2016.

Olusanya, B. O. (2011). Highlights of the new WHO report on newborn and infant hearing screening and implications for developing countries. *International Journal of Pediatric Otorhinolaryngology, 75*(6), 75–78.

Olusanya, B. O., Ebuehi, O. M., & Somefun, A. O. (2009). Universal infant hearing screening programme in a community with predominant non-hospital births: A three-year experience. *Journal of Epidemiology and Community Health, 63*, 481–487.

Pabsch, A. (Ed.) (2014). *UNCRPD implementation in Europe: A deaf perspective.* Brussels, Belgium: European Union of the Deaf.

Pipp-Siegel, S., Sedey, A. L., & Yoshinaga-Itano, C. (2002). Predictors of parental stress in mothers of young children with hearing loss. *Journal of Deaf Studies and Deaf Education, 7*(1), 1–17.

Pittman, P., Benedict, B. S., Olson, S., & Sass-Lehrer, M. (2016). Collaboration with deaf and hard-of-hearing communities. In M. Sass-Lehrer (Ed.), *Early intervention for deaf and hard-of-hearing infants, toddlers and their families: Interdisciplinary perspectives* (pp. 135–166). New York, NY: Oxford University Press.

Poon, P. T., & Zaidman-Zait, A. (2014). Social support for parents of deaf children: Moving toward contextualized understanding. *Journal of Deaf Studies and Deaf Education, 19*(2), 176–188.

Rodd, C., & Young, A. M. (2009). Hearing impaired (HI) support services and caseload prioritization. *Deafness and Education International, 11*(1), 2–20.

Rogers, K. D., & Young, A. (2011). Being a role model: Deaf peoples' experiences of working with families with young deaf people. *Deafness and Education International, 13*(1), 2–16.

Sackett, D. (2002). *Evidence-based medicine: How to practise and teach EBM* (2nd ed.). London: Churchill Livingstone.

Sass-Lehrer, M., Moeller, M. P., Stredler-Brown, A., Clark, K., & Hutchinson, N. (February 2011). Defining core competencies: A three year investigation. Paper presented at the Early Hearing Detection and Intervention Conference. Atlanta, GA.

Sass-Lehrer, M., Porter, A., & Wu, C. (2016). Families: Partnerships in practice. In M. Sass-Lehrer (Ed.), *Early intervention for deaf and hard-of-hearing infants, toddlers and their families: Interdisciplinary perspectives* (pp. 65–103). New York, NY: Oxford University Press.

Sass-Lehrer, M., Stredler-Brown, A., & Moeller, M. P. (February 2008). Focusing on the "I" in EHDI. Paper presented at the Early Hearing Detection and Intervention Conference. New Orleans, LA.

Shaw, I. (2005). Practitioner research: Evidence or critique? *The British Journal of Social Work, 35*(8), 1231–1248.

Spencer, P. E., & Marschark, M. (2010). *Evidence-based practice in educating deaf and hard-of-hearing students.* New York, NY: Oxford University Press.

Stockton, R., & Morran, K. (2010). Reflections on practitioner-researcher collaborative inquiry. *International Journal of Group Psychotherapy, 60*(2), 295–305.

Störbeck, C., & Pittman, P. (2008). Early intervention in South Africa: Moving beyond hearing screening. *International Journal of Audiology, 47*(Suppl. 1), S36–S43.

Störbeck, C., & Young, A. (2016). Early intervention in challenging international contexts. In M. Sass-Lehrer (Ed.), *Early intervention for deaf and hard-of-hearing infants, toddlers and their families: Interdisciplinary perspectives* (pp. 305–327). New York, NY: Oxford University Press.

Sutherland, H., Griggs, M., & Young, A. (2003). Deaf adults and family intervention projects. In C. Gallaway & A. Young (Eds.), *Deafness and education in the UK: Research perspectives* (pp. 5–20). London, England: Whurr Publishers.

Swanepoel, D. W., Louw, B., & Hugo, R. (2007). A novel service delivery model for infant hearing screening in developing countries. *International Journal of Audiology, 46*(6), 321–327.

Swanepoel, D. W., & Störbeck, C. (2008). EHDI Africa: Advocating for infants with hearing loss in Africa. *International Journal of Audiology, 47*(1), S1–S2.

Swanepoel, D. W., Störbeck, C., & Friedland, P. (2009). Early hearing detection and intervention in South Africa. *International Journal of Pediatric Otorhinolaryngology, 73,* 783–786.

Tanon-Anoh, M. J., Sanogo-Gone, D., & Kouassi, K. B. (2010). Newborn hearing screening in a developing country: Results of a pilot study in Abidjan, Cote d'Ivoire. *International Journal of Pediatric Otorhinolaryngology, 74*(2),188–191.

Theunissen, M., & Swanepoel, D. W. (2008). Early hearing detection and intervention services in the public health sector of South Africa. *International Journal of Audiology, 47*(Suppl. 1), S23–S29.

Watkins, S., Pitman, P., & Walden, B. (1998). The deaf mentor experimental project for young children who are deaf and their families. *American Annals of the Deaf, 143*(1), 29–34.

Wolkenhauer, R., Boynton, S., & Dana, N. F. (2011). The power of practitioner research and development of an inquiry stance in teacher education programs. *Teacher Education and Practice, 24*(4), 388–404.

World Bank Group (2015). Vietnam Intergenerational Deaf Education Project; P125581 – Implementation Status Report: Sequence 04. Washington, DC: World Bank Group. http://documents.worldbank.org/curated/en/2015/06/24727418/vietnam-vietnam-intergenerational-deaf-education-outreach-project-p125581-implementation-status-results-report-sequence-04. Accessed January 7, 2016.

Yoshinaga-Itano, C. (2003). From screening to early identification and intervention: Discovering predictors to successful outcomes for children with significant hearing loss. *Journal of Deaf Studies and Deaf Education, 8*(1), 11–30.

Yoshinaga-Itano, C. (2014). Principles and guidelines for early intervention after confirmation that a child is deaf or hard of hearing. *Journal of Deaf Studies and Deaf Education, 19*(2), 143–175.

Yoshinaga-Itano, C., & Sedey, A. (2013). *Outcomes of children who are deaf or hard of hearing*. Paper presented at the Connecticut Early Hearing Detection and Intervention (EHDI) Conference. Hartford, CT.

Young, A. M. (2010). Universal newborn hearing screening: The impact of early identification of deafness on hearing parents. In M. Marschark & P. Spencer (Eds.), *Oxford handbook in deaf studies* (Vol. 2, pp. 241–250). New York, NY: Oxford University Press.

Young, A. (in press). Deaf children and their families: Sustainability, sign language and equality. In G. DeClerck & P. Paul (Eds.), *Proceedings of the International Conference on Sustainability, Sign Language and Equal Opportunities*. Ghent: Academia Press.

Young, A. M., Carr, G., Hunt, R., McCracken, W., Skipp, A., & Tattersall, H. (2006). Informed choice and deaf children—underpinning concepts and enduring concerns. *Journal of Deaf Studies and Deaf Education, 11*, 322–336.

Young, A. M., Gascon-Ramos, M., Campbell, M., & Bamford, J. (2009). The design and validation of a Parent-Report Questionnaire for assessing the characteristics and quality of early intervention over time. *The Journal of Deaf Studies and Deaf Education, 14*(4), 422–435.

Young, A. M., & Russell, J. (2016). Building foundations in family support. In M. Moeller, D. Ertmer, & C. Stoel-Gammon (Eds.), *Contemporary methods of promoting speech and language development in children who are deaf and hard of hearing* (pp. 51–76). Baltimore, MD: Brookes.

Young, A. M., & Tattersall, H. (2007). Universal newborn hearing screening and early identification of deafness: Parents' responses to knowing early and their expectations of child communication development. *Journal of Deaf Studies and Deaf Education, 12*(2), 209–220.

Zaidman-Zait, A. (2007). Parenting a child with a cochlear implant: A critical incident study. *Journal of Deaf Studies and Deaf Education, 12*(2), 221–241.

3

The Transition From Early Intervention to School for Deaf and Hard-of-Hearing Children

Brenda T. Poon, Janet R. Jamieson, Anat Zaidman-Zait, Deirdre Curle, Nancy Norman, and Noreen Simmons

The transition to school is, arguably, the first major transition in the lives of children. Most children first enter school at kindergarten, which is a markedly different environment from home or early-childhood settings such as preschool or daycare. In addition to the move to a new and often more structured physical environment, kindergarten typically has intentional goals for the child's social and academic development that are not usually associated with preschool or home (Haines et al., 1989). Teacher–child interactions in kindergarten are more intentionally focused on academic outcomes than adult–child interactions in home, daycare, or preschool settings (Rimm-Kaufman & Pianta, 2000). Taken together, the change in physical environment, academic focus, and nature of teacher–child interactions render the transition to school to be a qualitative shift for children, families, and teachers (Belsky & MacKinnon, 1994; Bredekamp & Copple, 1997; Love et al., 1992; Pianta & Kraft-Sayre, 1999).

A successful transition to kindergarten is an important investment in a child's later school years. Children's achievement in school remains very stable after the first few years in school (Alexander & Entwisle, 1988) and, from this perspective, the transition to kindergarten is a period when a developing system (defined here by Pianta and Walsh [1996] as a child and his or her social and physical environment) is particularly open to outside influence. The implication is that even small adjustments or impacts on the developing system during the transition may have significant and long-lasting effects on the child's school career.

For children who are deaf or hard of hearing, their families, and the teachers, the transition to school may be experienced as a particularly dramatic departure from home and early-childhood settings. Most deaf and hard-of-hearing children and their families have received some sort of specialized early-intervention services, with the goals of providing the parents with information, support, and skills to accept their child's hearing loss; providing accessible language in the home environment; and facilitating the child's language, social, and cognitive development (Sass-Lehrer & Bodner-Johnson, 2003). In this way, early-intervention services are focused on both the family and child (see Chapter 2). In contrast, school is focused primarily on the child only, with academic performance and socialization strongly emphasized, and so it seems reasonable to assume the qualitative shift to school entry may be more jarring and confusing for all stakeholders—deaf and hard-of-hearing children, their teachers, and their families—than for typically developing children and the adults who surround them. The complexity of the transition may be complicated further by the current widespread placement of deaf and hard-of-hearing children into regular classroom settings (e.g., Gallaudet Research Institute, 2013). Each deaf or hard-of-hearing child presents a unique learning and social–emotional profile shaped in large part by the idiosyncratic combination of cognitive and social–emotional development, all of which has been strongly impacted by the nature and degree of the child's hearing loss. Deaf and hard-of-hearing children in mainstream educational settings may spend most of their time with classroom teachers who are unfamiliar with the learning strengths and needs of students with hearing loss. Nevertheless, in spite of the apparent challenges to the transition process for deaf and hard-of-hearing children, virtually no documented research has examined this important point of transition in the lives of these children and their families. The significance of this major transition justifies consideration of factors that may facilitate—and hinder—a smooth transition for children with hearing loss, their teachers, and families across the varied school contexts that these children may enter.

The purpose of this chapter is twofold: first, to identify facilitators and challenges to building relationships across home, early intervention, and educational contexts, with the aim of facilitating a smooth transition for deaf and hard-of-hearing children and their families; and second, to encourage research across disciplines and contexts within this multifarious process, with a particular emphasis upon strengthening the relationships and interconnectedness of the key stakeholders surrounding the child and family during the transition process.

THE TRANSITION TO SCHOOL: WHAT WE KNOW

The sections that follow provide an overview of what has been documented about the transition to school for three groups of children: those who are typically developing, those who have special needs, and those who are deaf or hard of hearing. As becomes evident, there is a dearth of research on the experience of the transition to kindergarten for children with hearing loss, their families, and educators.

Transition to School for Typically Developing Children

On entry to school, children who transition from home or early-education settings may experience classroom environments that are often more demanding, with greater expectations for children in school to get along with adults and peers, adhere to routines, and remain alert and active for longer periods of time (McIntyre et al., 2006; Rimm-Kaufman & Pianta, 2000). Children typically engage in fewer free-play activities when they start kindergarten, and they participate in more structured, academic learning and group-based activities (Ray & Smith, 2010). Contact between teachers and parents is more formalized than in early-intervention and preschool environments, with less parent–teacher contact (Rimm-Kaufman & Pianta, 1999).

With the changes involved in adjusting to a new environment and expectations of kindergarten, it is not uncommon for children and their parents to experience some anxiety when starting school. McIntyre et al. (2007) found that 80% of the parents they surveyed whose children were moving from early-education environments to kindergarten wished they had more information about academic expectations, their children's kindergarten teacher, and what they could do to help prepare their child. Many of these parents also had concerns about their child's behavior and their ability to follow directions, get along with peers, and meet academic expectations. Findings indicated that parents wanted to be involved in their child's transition to kindergarten, but needed more information about the transition, especially about classroom expectations, classroom placement, and their child's teacher.

In terms of school-based supports for the transition, a number of studies have examined practices that aim to facilitate the school entry process. Pianta et al. (1999) reported that low-intensity, generic contact, such as flyers, brochures, and open houses were used most often by American kindergarten teachers, especially in urban areas with low socioeconomic status. In contrast, high-intensity practices, such as home visits, phone calls, or teacher visits to the child's preschool before school entry were practiced least. Barriers to high-intensity practices included lack of time, funding, and late generation of class lists.

Petrakos and Lehrer (2011) examined parent and teacher perceptions of transition to kindergarten practices in Quebec, Canada. Common transition-to-school practices included kindergarten orientation meetings for parents and children, gradual entry during the first week, and small group meetings with parents and children on the first day of school. Methods of communication were open houses, phone calls, parent–teacher meetings, informal conversations, newsletters, and report cards. Despite the numerous communication methods used, most parents reported not feeling informed of their child's day-to-day activities and progress at school. In addition, both parents and teachers noted that parents of first-born children were more nervous about school entry versus parents who had older children already in the school system.

A study in Finland (Ahtola et al., 2011) revealed that high-intensity practices facilitated the transition. The researchers found that the more preschool and elementary school teachers implemented transition practices (such as child visits to the new classroom, meetings between teachers, sharing of documents such as education plans, and collaborative curriculum development), the faster the children's skills developed during their first year of school. Sharing curricula and other written information about the child, such as educational goals, between the two teachers were the best predictors of the children's skills, although the least commonly used practices. Thus, although low-intensity practices are most often used, it appears that high-intensity practices are most effective in supporting children and families as the children enter the school system.

Transition to School for Children With Special Needs

One of the distinguishing features between the transition to school for children with and without special needs is the potential for involvement of specialized early-intervention programs. The transition from early intervention to school typically represents a shift from one setting that typically has a developmental and family-needs orientation to one that is primarily child focused and oriented to the acquisition of skills to perform well in school. Also, unlike the transition process for typically developing children, in the case of transitioning children with exceptionalities, parents and schools must consider specific ways the special needs will affect learning and, in turn, identify strategies that accommodate and support these needs in the classroom environment.

In many countries, children who are identified with a disability or special need at an early age qualify for services from early-intervention programs. These programs typically apply a family-centered approach, in which the focus is not only on supporting the development of at-risk children, but also on meeting their families' needs through collaborative goal planning, education, and resource provision (Dunst et al., 1994). Parents may perceive the collaborative process of family-centered practices and the deep knowledge acquired of their children's development to be empowering (Pighini et al., 2014).

As children transition to school, however, parents may experience stress and anxiety as their children shift from specialized early-intervention settings, which are tailored primarily to children with special needs, to settings that are child focused and designed for typical children's learning. Mawdsley and Hauser-Cram (2013) investigated perceived benefits of school and worries about school for parents of children with disabilities. They found that mothers who had children with lower functional skills (such as measures of cognitive performance and adaptive skills) perceived that school would benefit their child, but were worried by larger class size and lower proportions of typically developing children in the classroom. Similarly, McIntyre et al. (2010) indicated that caregivers of children entering kindergarten who were receiving special education services had greater concerns about their children's behavior, communication, and academic readiness compared with parents of general-education students. With respect to strategies to offset parents' concerns about the transition, Schischka et al. (2012) found that certain high-intensity practices, such as transition meetings with parents, early-intervention and school team members, as well as preentry visits by the child and parent to the school, helped to smooth the transition.

Parents' perceptions of degree of involvement and decision-making power with the school team also affect the ease of transition. Families often feel they have shifted roles from an "insider" with the early-intervention team to an "outsider" with the school team (Povdey et al., 2013). Many parents of children with disabilities are less satisfied with the transition process compared with parents of children without disabilities, perceiving a less than desired amount of communication from school personnel (Janus et al., 2007; Villeneuve et al., 2013).

Another factor affecting parents' preparedness for the transition is the nature of the child's disability (Briody & Martone, 2010). For example, if the child has a congenital or degenerative condition (such as muscular dystrophy), the parents may be familiar enough with the child's disability to develop a good understanding of the types of supports the child will need in the school environment. In contrast, if the condition is traumatic or recently diagnosed, the parents may require a greater degree of information and support through the transition process. Thus, parents of young children with disabilities often have more worries associated with the transition to school than parents of young children who are typically developing, with the stress increasing when parents lack information about both their child's condition and the school system.

Transition for Children Who Are Deaf or Hard of Hearing

As stated previously, there is little information available regarding the transition from early intervention to school for children with hearing loss; however, Jamieson et al. (2011) found in their investigation of support needs of parents with deaf and hard-of-hearing preadolescents and adolescents that families' needs for information peaked during points of transition. Similarly, Zaidman-Zait (2007) found that parents of children with cochlear implants needed a wide range of information and practical guidance not only for themselves, but also for educating others in the community, including classroom teachers. These informational supports are essential for fostering parents' advocacy roles in the transition process. Thus, it is likely that parents of children who are deaf or hard of hearing are in need of clear communication and information about school services and supports as their children transition from early intervention to school.

Decisions about educational placement are likely to arise during the transition to school. The educational placement choices for deaf or hard-of-hearing children range from specialized programs, to a resource room setting, to integration in general-education classes, reflecting the diversity of deaf learners as well as program availability. Specialized private day schools or public school resource room programs are still the choice for many children who are deaf or hard of hearing, but the majority of these children attend general-education classrooms alongside hearing peers (Luckner & Ayanotoye, 2013; National Center for Education Statistics, 2011). Parents' decision making regarding an educational context that is best suited to meets the needs of the child can be difficult, and may be influenced by factors such as the extent the setting (a) is rigorous academically, (b) provides the child with a sense of belonging among peers, and (c) provides opportunities for interpersonal relations and direct communication with teachers and peers (Angelides & Aravi, 2006).

For children with hearing loss who also have other disabilities, such as autism, intellectual disability, or severe health impairment, the placement decision can be even more difficult. An estimated 35% to 40% of children who are deaf or hard of hearing have an additional disability (Gallaudet Research Institute, 2013). Despite this high percentage of additional special needs among this population, many teachers of the deaf and hard of hearing are not well prepared to work with students with additional disabilities, because their preparation programs tend to focus primarily on the educational needs and issues relevant to hearing loss alone (Luckner & Carter, 2001; Moores et al., 2001). Likewise, teachers who teach in general-education classrooms have reported their teacher education program prepared them insufficiently to work with children who are deaf or hard of hearing (Eriks-Brophy & Whittingham, 2013). Children may begin in one type of classroom and be moved to another, as educators and parents struggle to find the right fit for classroom environment and service provision (Guardino, 2008). For children with hearing loss and additional disabilities, a team approach is often necessary to meet all the child's needs. However, in their examination of the experiences of families with children with a dual diagnosis of hearing loss and autism, Myck-Wayne et al. (2011) found there was often little coordination between services for hearing loss and those for autism. Thus, placement decisions and service coordination in kindergarten can be confusing and frustrating both to parents and professionals when an additional special need is involved.

In summary, the transition to school typically represents the developing child's transition to a new setting, such as from home or preschool to school, and often new or changing interrelationships with surrounding contexts (Rimm-Kaufman & Pianta, 2000). These new and changing relational contexts can introduce anxiety for families as children transition to school. To deepen and expand understanding of the changing relational contexts before and during the transition to school, researchers have drawn on ecological systems theories (e.g., Bronfenbrenner, 1979; Rimm-Kaufman & Pianta, 2000), particularly in consideration of the transition experiences of typically developing children; however, they have not yet been used as a guiding framework for understanding the transition of children who are deaf or hard of hearing, which, as previously noted, holds unique challenges and opportunities involving multiple contexts and people. In the next section, we provide an overview of the transition to school from an ecological systems theoretical perspective.

UNDERSTANDING THE TRANSITION TO SCHOOL FROM AN ECOLOGICAL SYSTEMS PERSPECTIVE

Ecological systems theories, grounded in the foundational work of Urie Bronfenbrenner (Bronfenbrenner, 1979, 1986, 2005; Bronfenbrenner & Morris, 1998, 2006), place the change and stability of contexts and relationships over time as centrally important aspects of children's transition to school. The interconnected and cumulative influences of diverse contexts and relationships within and across these systems are of particular importance to the ecology that surrounds the child during the transition to kindergarten. From an ecological systems perspective, the immediate surroundings, such as the home and school in which children's interactions and activities occur, constitute the microsystem; the mesosystem is reflective of the relations or linkages occurring among multiple microsystems; the exosystem is reflective of contexts not in the child's immediate surroundings, but still influential on the child's development; and the macrosystem is reflective of the influence of broader, overarching structures on a developing child, such as socioeconomic conditions, cultural and societal norms, and values, policies, ideologies, and organization of civil society (Bronfenbrenner, 1979). For children transitioning into school, key contexts include but are not limited to the following:

- *Home*: includes those supports the family provides to prepare a child for entrance to school. Families nurture children's competencies that promote readiness for school, such as cognitive

readiness, language abilities, and social competence. Parents also form a central and primary part of children's social networks and participate differentially in relationships that facilitate children's transition to school, including those with early-intervention or school personnel.
- *Early intervention or preschool*: includes attributes and programming of preschool or early-intervention environments that help to prepare a child for the transition to school. Supports may include those aimed at promoting children's social and academic competencies (child centered), as well as supports directed to families for the transition process, such as provision of informational resources to families and facilitation of family communications with school personnel.
- *School*: includes preparation of the child for entrance to the school setting and, specifically, planning for the formal instruction and classroom supports required on a child's entry to school. Key relationships for the transition include those established between the school and the child (such as child with classroom teachers, child with peers), between school personnel and parents, as well as between school personnel and early-intervention or preschool programs to support the development of diverse children's cognitive, behavioral, and social competencies deemed important for school success.
- *Policy context*: includes influences of policies (such as educational) at the national, state/provincial, regional, or local levels regarding the transition of children—with and without special needs—to school. For example, school district or school policies and guidelines may influence directly children's transition processes to school through their specification of transition planning and practices, groupings and class size, and children's access to additional resources and supports (Rimm-Kaufman & Pianta, 2000).

Contexts play a key role in influencing the developing child's everyday activities and involvement in progressively more complex reciprocal interactions with other people, objects, and symbols (Bronfenbrenner, 1979). These interactions are critical because they engage children in *proximal processes*, also referred to as the "engines of development" (Bronfenbrenner, 1993), where children learn about "what is expected of them, which activities are considered appropriate or inappropriate for them, how they are expected to engage in those activities, the ways other people will deal with them, and the ways in which they are expected to deal with others" (Doucet & Tudge, 2007, p. 310).

An ecological perspective of the transition period focuses on *relationships* with respect to children's direct linkages to people in their surrounding contexts, such as children with their classroom teachers, and also those indirect linkages when a third party acts as an intermediate link between persons in two or more settings, such as when a preschool teacher helps to establish a connection between parents and school personnel to facilitate the transition to school (Bronfenbrenner, 1979). Ecological perspectives of the transition process highlight the importance of the *interconnectedness* and *interplay* between a child's direct interactions and relationships, including those with parents, peers, and teachers, and also the relationships among those surrounding the child, including parents, preschool teachers, early interventionists, and school personnel who interact to form each child's social network (Rimm-Kaufman & Pianta, 2000).

The relationships that develop across settings are not only influenced by the characteristics of the individuals involved (child, parent, teacher), such as each individual's background, prior experiences, values and beliefs, comfort level, and preferences, but also by the proximal and distal contexts in which the interactions occur (Tudge et al., 2009). These relationships shape the surrounding contexts and, in turn, these contexts influence the individuals and the relationships between them. For example, the school context affects directly the developing child's interactions and exposures to developmentally appropriate and engaging environments during the transition process through its influence on the adequacy of the school facilities, class sizes, presence of adequately paid teachers, and availability of safe and child-friendly features in the classroom and surrounding neighborhood (Doucet & Tudge, 2007; Tudge et al., 2009).

THE TRANSITION TO SCHOOL FOR DEAF AND HARD-OF-HEARING CHILDREN: RELATIONAL ASPECTS OF STAKEHOLDER CONTEXTS

In an effort to address the knowledge gap concerning the transition to kindergarten for children who are deaf or hard of hearing, Jamieson et al. (2014) investigated the transition process from the perspective of the various stakeholders in British Columbia, Canada. The researchers adopted an ecological perspective, acknowledging that the transition process from early intervention to kindergarten represents an ecological shift from one system to another. In particular, they sought to identify the multifarious factors that serve as facilitators or barriers to a smooth transition. Data collection involved a series of extensive parent interviews, representing 13 families, conducted throughout the transitional year (from pretransition, or at least approximately 3 months before the transition; to the period during the transition, which included the summer preceding the transition; and the first year of school); parent surveys (n = 37); interviews with early interventionists (n = 20) from programs representing a range of communication approaches; interviews with teachers of the deaf and hard of hearing (n = 37) who worked with entering kindergarten children in integrated settings (in other words, as itinerant teachers), resource rooms, or schools for the deaf; classroom kindergarten teacher surveys (n = 17); and interviews with early-intervention and educational administrators (n = 11). It is important to note that, in the context of the study by Jamieson et al. (2014), the majority of children diagnosed with hearing loss before the age of 5 years typically enrolled in a specialized early-intervention program for deaf or hard-of-hearing children. Therefore, early-intervention programs were the typical early-education settings from which deaf or hard-of-hearing children would transition to school. Although the transition directly from early intervention programs to school is reflective of the transition process for most deaf or hard-of-hearing children in British Columbia and other parts of Canada, it may not reflect practices in other jurisdictions, such as the United States, where children may transition from specialized early-intervention programs to preschool, then preschool to school. The facilitators and barriers we describe, however, may still hold general relevance to contexts involving deaf or hard-of-hearing children's transition to school from early-education settings, broadly conceptualized as inclusive of early-intervention programs and preschool. In the following sections we present an overview of the relational aspects we found to develop across home and early-intervention contexts, early-intervention and school contexts, and home and school contexts, as well as the influence of policy (or governance) on various aspects of the transition process.

Home and Early Intervention

In preparing for children's entry to kindergarten, there are several key relationships that develop and unfold over time before and during the transition. For deaf or hard-of hearing children, particularly critical are the relationships that have developed between parents and early-intervention programs before a child's transition to kindergarten and ways these relationships carry forward to the child's entrance to school.

The Pretransition Period

Well before kindergarten entry, parents in the study by Jamieson et al. (2014) indicated they felt anxious about the child's adjustment to a new educational environment and, in particular, whether the child had all the supports necessary to do well in school socially, emotionally, and academically. Parents' perspectives of how well their children were doing socially, behaviorally, and academically affected the nature and extent of parents' concerns about the transition. Early-intervention programs provided guidance and key emotional support to parents during this point of the transition, particularly if parents felt uncertain about whether their children were ready developmentally for school in terms of their speech and language development and social skills.

Before children's transition to school, parents' activities centered on information seeking, including accessing additional information about options for schools and the types of supports offered for deaf and hard-of hearing children. Pretransition, early-intervention programs focused efforts on development and dissemination of informational resources to help parents better understand what to expect during the transition process. During this critical preparatory phase of the transition, there were several facilitators and barriers for a smooth transition.

Facilitators

Early-intervention programs played an important role in allaying some of the anxiety parents felt about their child's performance in school by sharing with parents the developmental strengths and progress of the child, providing specific information about the supports that the early-intervention program could provide during the transition, and acting as a bridge between early intervention and school. Preliminary findings from Jamieson et al. (2014) indicated that the more parents felt confident about their children's developmental progress and ability to do well in school, the more parents felt the transition process proceeded smoothly.

Early-intervention programs also provided parents with early and ongoing informational supports in obtaining extensive information about hearing loss and the transition process, and opportunities for parent-to-parent networking and information sharing as well. Specifically, early-intervention programs provided informational resources about the transition options available (such as supports available by school or program), various types of options other parents of children with hearing loss had selected, what had worked and not worked for families during the transition, and a checklist or guide with information about who should be involved, what to do, and what to look for (such as the use of carpeting, small class size) during the transition process. These types of supports contributed to parents' sense of empowerment, because they had specific strategies (such as how to advocate) and knowledge (such as transition timelines and checklists) to help them navigate through diverse sources of information available about the transition.

Barriers

Not all families were able to access transition supports that early-intervention programs provided as a result of distance or travel limitations because they lived outside the vicinity of the early-intervention agency. Some consideration and planning to offer diverse, flexible options to families may help to enhance transition support accessibility.

During the Transition

On entry to kindergarten, personnel in early-intervention programs, who provided supports to families from a philosophy of family-centeredness and understanding children's and family's needs, devoted energy and resources to ensuring the progress of the child continued on entry to school and, also, that there was consistency in supports based on the needs of the child between early intervention and school. During this point of the transition, parents turned to their early-intervention program for emotional support and informational resources.

Facilitators
Many parents experienced uncertainty about the timing and procedural aspects of the transition process. Early-intervention programs played an important role in clarifying with parents the time frames and sequence of steps in the transition. Personnel from early-intervention programs also played a key facilitating role between previous educational and support approaches provided during early intervention and those recommended for the child in kindergarten. This bridging role was enacted through parents' participation in one or more preparatory transition meetings involving personnel from both the early intervention program and the school.

Barriers
Primary barriers in the transition process were noted when parents experienced an end to communications and supports from early-intervention program personnel before a child's entry to school. Some early-intervention programs provided excellent preparation for families pretransition, but challenges emerged when there were gaps in supports in the period after the child's exit from the early-intervention program. Some supports that bridge the gaps between early intervention and the school system are needed.

Early Intervention and School

As deaf and hard-of-hearing children transition from early intervention to school, they are faced with not only a new educational setting, but also changes in the nature of the support provided and teaching delivery model used. The exact nature of the support varies depending on the educational placement chosen. There are three common educational settings for deaf and hard-of-hearing children within the school system: (a) schools or specialized day programs for students who are deaf, where placement is with deaf and hard-of-hearing peers; (b) integrated/inclusive school settings, where students with hearing loss are educated alongside their hearing peers and are supported by specialist teachers on an itinerant basis; and (c) self-contained classrooms or resource programs located within integrated school settings, where students with hearing loss may spend at least part of their school day separately with deaf or hard-of-hearing peers and part integrated into general-education classrooms with hearing peers. In the United States, the majority of students with hearing loss transition to the second setting—namely, integrated general-education classrooms (Gallaudet Research Institute, 2013). This reflects current trends in school educational placements for deaf or hard-of-hearing children in Canada as well (Jamieson et al., 2014), where increasing numbers of children attend general-education classrooms and receive support from itinerant teachers of the deaf, as opposed to attending school in separate educational settings (Luckner & Ayantoye, 2013).

The key relationships that develop between early-intervention programs and school are largely dependent on the type of educational setting to which a child transitions.

The Pretransition Period

Early-intervention programs usually had preexisting knowledge of and relationships with the kindergarten programs to which their transitioning children were entering. The nature of this early-intervention–school relationship, and the way in which parents were drawn into it, is important because it is within the context of that relationship that children and families shifted from one system to another. Specifically, children and parents shifted from a family-centered early-intervention program to a more child-centered school system. In this way, the shift can be pronounced for both children and parents. In the year preceding kindergarten entry, the early-intervention programs typically either encouraged parents to make contact with the programs for which the child was eligible or made the contact collaboratively with the parents. The parents were often accompanied by early-intervention personnel on their first interaction with the school system; when this happened, there was overlap between the two systems (early intervention and school). Sometimes, however, there was very limited communication and information exchange between the early-intervention program and the school about the transition. Parents connected with the school system on their own, and when this occurred they appeared to negotiate the relationship with the new system somewhat independently. Parents often made at least one subsequent formal visit to the school, sometimes with the child, to learn more about school policies and educational services available for their child.

Pretransition activities by the parents included attendance at early-intervention-sponsored workshops aimed at informing parents about the upcoming transition, including providing information about placement choices and helping them develop advocacy skills for themselves and their child. Early-intervention pretransition activities often included individual and group meetings with parents, focused attention on children's development of kindergarten-readiness skills, and meetings with school personnel on the parents' behalf.

Facilitators

Professionals across both early-intervention and school systems reported the smoothest transitions when children and families had been affiliated with a specialized early-intervention program, and when the school system was given a several-month advance notice of a child's upcoming transition. This was particularly important for children with additional needs. The advance notice allowed for more comprehensive transition planning, such as observations and visits to the early-intervention or preschool programs by school-based support personnel, transition meetings before kindergarten entry, hiring of appropriate support personnel (such as sign language interpreters, educational assistants), and overall preparation of school staff. In addition, when children transitioned to specialized programs or classes for the deaf and hard of hearing, school personnel had a knowledge base about the unique strengths and needs of students with hearing loss, and sometimes they also had prior understanding of parental experiences. This specialized knowledge facilitated the timely provision of appropriate educational supports for the child. When the placement was a general-education classroom, the shift to the school system was facilitated by a relationship with an itinerant teacher of the deaf and hard of hearing who had knowledge of the child's learning needs and parent concerns.

Barriers

As previously stated, the majority of deaf and hard-of-hearing children transitioned to general-education classrooms, where school administrators and kindergarten teachers usually had a limited understanding of the impact of hearing loss on learning and social development. In these circumstances, parents were often called on to advocate for their child's right to educational supports more strongly than they would need to in a specialized school or program for the deaf. In addition, it was noted that early-intervention programs rarely shared the individual family service plans (IFSP) with the school programs and, given the diversity among the children, this appeared to impact negatively the continuity of goals and services provided with the shift to the new system.

During the Transition

During the approximately 3 months preceding school entry, school programs and some early-intervention programs typically ended their respective school years, and the assumption was made that all necessary document exchange pertaining to a transition between the two systems had been completed. Except for the case of late-transitioning children, for whom transition activities were still underway, the home–early-intervention relationship was deemphasized as the home–school relationship took root. At the actual point of school entry, school personnel usually arranged a school-based team meeting to discuss assessment and learning needs of the transitioning child.

Facilitators

Strong and long-standing relationships between early-intervention programs and allied professionals such as audiologists and speech–language pathologists facilitated smooth transitions because these relationships helped promote open and timely communication about the unique learning needs of the deaf and hard-of-hearing children transitioning to kindergarten. For some children and their families, these allied professionals were the primary support personnel involved in early intervention, and, therefore, helped bridge the transition into school. These professional relationships and ongoing communication were especially important to the support of children and families in rural and remote areas or for children with additional special needs.

Barriers

Challenges to service provision in school were usually related to late notification of the transitioning child, poor communication between systems, and/or an unclear understanding by each system of the policies and guidelines surrounding transition from or to the other. All these issues impeded a smooth shift from one system to another and often placed additional stress on parents as they navigated the move to a new and unfamiliar system. Also, in the event that the school system did not have information about the child's prior assessments and individual goals in early intervention (as detailed in the IFSP), continuity of goals and services were impeded as the team developed the child's individual education program.

Home and School

The Pretransition Period

Particularly critical in the home–school relational context was that a relationship between home and school was established during the months before the child's transition to school and that communications were maintained on the child's entry to kindergarten. The transition to school added new complexities as parents considered the extent that their children's needs would be met in the school environment. Parents indicated that supports readily available to children and their families in early intervention would need to be planned and organized for the child who was entering a new educational environment for kindergarten. Schools, in turn, indicated a need to assess and identify whether special supports were required and also the person or people on the school-based team who would be responsible for ensuring the preparations and supports were in place for the child from the first day of school onward.

Facilitators

The school-based team played a central role in facilitating the transition before and during the school year. A critical point of contact between parents and schools was before the transition. Optimally, schools (or, rather, a school administrator) established connections with families well before the start of kindergarten and, at a minimum, the season before children's entry to school, whether through home visits, telephone, meetings at the school, school orientation, or school tour. A teacher of the deaf or hard of hearing, as a member of the school-based team, was a primary source of support for families with transition planning by initiating contact with the school pretransition. Smooth transitions were also facilitated and the home–school relationship strengthened when school personnel made contact with the parents—sometimes just a phone call—during the "gray zone" between the completion of the early-intervention school year and the start of the school year, the time during the shift between systems when parents often reported feeling especially vulnerable and stressed.

Barriers

A key barrier for a smooth transition process was lack of or limited communication between the school and parents. Parents did not have any contact with the school pretransition for a variety of reasons, such as lack of communications from the school, scheduling conflicts, and language barriers. In some cases, these barriers translated into parents' experiences of being unsupported and unprepared for the transition process. Furthermore, if the diagnosis of hearing loss was delayed (perhaps because a hearing screening did not identify the hearing loss because of a progressive hearing loss or the family immigrated after the child's birth), parents were then affiliated with an early-intervention program for only a short time and, as a consequence, did not have sufficient time or opportunity to learn about the transition process and develop effective self-advocacy skills. In addition, these barriers were compounded when parents had a different primary language from that of school personnel.

During the Transition

With the child's transition to school, parents and schools typically established a new relationship that involved activities such as becoming more acquainted with each other's roles and responsibilities in the transition process, and also establishing strong lines of communication with each other about the child's progress at home and in school.

Parents were concerned with how well their child was adjusting to the schedule, activities, and social environment of kindergarten. They also were gauging to what extent the school was providing tailored support to their deaf or hard-of-hearing child. Members of the school-based team assessed the child's needs in the classroom context and identified strategies to support the child's learning. There were several aspects of this relational context that enhanced or, inadvertently, undermined a smooth transition experience.

Facilitators
The quality of parents' relationships with school personnel was influenced by each of their respective approaches to the transition. Some parents were proactive in seeking information and were active agents in navigating themselves through the process. Others took on a less active role, either because there was an expectation that the school-based team would take the lead in all aspects of the transition process (a blind trust in the school) or because the system of supports was very strong and they felt their needs were being met. In general, the smoothest transitions occurred when both the school-based teams and the parents were involved actively on an ongoing basis in supporting the transition process, and there was an openness in both communication and in attitudes, where parents felt that they could voice their needs and concerns and, in turn, schools were receptive to parent input and responsive to parents' needs and concerns.

Jamieson et al. (2014) found that the supports schools provided for the transition varied greatly. Contributors to the school transition experience were the nature and quality of the parent–school relationship and parents' views that the school had a welcoming, accessible, and open environment, such as when parents felt welcome to visit the classroom. From the parents' perspective, the transitions were best supported when school administrators, teachers, and staff were responsive to the parents' and child's needs, were open and receptive to parent suggestions, and were willing to accommodate the child's needs. An optimal outcome was when parents and teachers were partners in establishing good relationships and communications with each other, such as meetings, phone calls, communication books, and informal conversation.

Barriers
Barriers for a smooth transition also stemmed from difficulties that parents experienced because they did not have prior knowledge or experience with the transition process, and they also lacked knowledge about how the school and special education systems worked, how to advocate, and what types of services and supports should be in place during the transition. Some schools, in turn, did not have specialized supports available or in place (such as contact time with the teacher of the deaf or hard of hearing), particularly in mainstream school settings

where personnel may have limited training or experience working with deaf or hard-of-hearing children. Parents had misunderstandings about how the school services differed from family-centered early-intervention services, leading to frustration and dissatisfaction about the transition to school for both parents and school personnel. In addition, during the months just preceding and following the transition, some parents reported an unexpected resurgence of grief (similar to their experience after the initial diagnosis of hearing loss); the child-centered nature of school systems did not tend to provide emotional support for parents. In these circumstances, parents reported contacting the early-intervention program—with which there was usually a continuing relationship—for emotional support.

Policy Influences on Home, Early Intervention, and School Contexts

From an ecological systems theory perspective (e.g., Bronfenbrenner, 1979), influences outside the child's immediate setting, such as policymaking bodies that develop laws and regulations, affect deaf and hard-of-hearing children, their families, and the early-intervention and school programs in which they are enrolled, both directly and indirectly. Children with hearing loss and their families are served by various branches of government and/or private agencies, each of which has regulatory oversight and corresponding policies for different aspects of service provision. These policies drive the processes that are aimed at continuity and consistency across systems and influence home–early intervention, early intervention–school, and home–school relationships.

The Pretransition Period

Policies that pertain to the pretransition period were aimed at equipping parents with the requisite knowledge to make informed choices about educational placement for their child, preparing the child for academic and social school readiness, and supporting the parents as they made initial contact with school programs. Each of these activities was guided by curricular or programmatic policies for early-intervention programs. During the same period, school programs/districts were involved in contacting early-intervention programs to determine whether any children would be transitioning during the upcoming year. Although not all school districts made this overture to early-intervention programs, the mutual initiative to contact the sending (early intervention) and receiving (school) programs helped ensure the transition process began in a timely manner for all children.

Facilitators

Although early intervention and school programs operated under different branches of the provincial government, it was possible to maintain clear lines of communication between stakeholders in the different systems. This was especially likely to be the case when children were transitioning into specialized programs, such as a school for the deaf, which were highly accustomed to the transition process for deaf or hard-of-hearing children. Some school districts had designated personnel responsible for coordination of the transition of all children with special needs entering the district; this greatly simplified the process and facilitated a smooth transition for all stakeholders, including the parents and the early-intervention program.

Barriers
Although they operated under one government bureaucracy, the various school districts lacked a standardized transition process to guide early-intervention programs and parents. As a consequence, the early intervention–school relationships developed somewhat idiosyncratically during the transition process, depending on the particular school districts involved. Furthermore, the home–school relationships were sometimes delayed in developing until school district policies were clarified to parents. In addition, parents and children had differential access to specialized school programs, depending on geographic location. This variation in availability of educational options was particularly frustrating to parents whose children had additional learning needs.

During the Transition
During the few months preceding the transition, most school districts had a standardized policy whereby the child visited the kindergarten classroom; and the school administrator, teacher of the deaf and hard of hearing, or school-based team connected with the parents. This policy had the effect of setting in motion a document compilation that included the school assembling records from the early-intervention program and often the child's audiologist. Early during the school year, it was standard practice for assessments to be conducted to determine appropriate educational goals for the child.

Facilitators
The process of ensuring continuity of goals and appropriate educational supports was greatly enhanced when there was timely sharing of documents among all stakeholders, most notably audiology and early intervention (particularly with respect to forwarding the child's IFSP). In particular, educational planning and continuity for students with additional needs was strengthened when all professionals involved in service provision collaborated and shared relevant documents during the transition process.

Barriers
"Silo" approaches are common within governance systems, with separate programs and/or services falling under the jurisdiction of different branches of the government. The policies that emanated from

the various branches were sometimes more reflective of philosophical stances of the branch than of straightforward efforts to meet the needs of children with hearing loss. Top-down policies like this affected the shift across sectors negatively and impacted such functions as documentation sharing and educational planning. Also, the family-centered philosophy that guided practices during early-intervention programs stood in marked contrast to the child-centered approach that dominated education for all children. The latter approach tended to leave parents—who had continuing needs beyond early intervention for instruction (such as learning sign language) and emotional support—without needed support. Last, some school district administrators reported that, despite the efforts of governance structures, there were children whose hearing loss remained unidentified until they entered the school system.

WORKING TOGETHER TOWARD A SMOOTH TRANSITION USING AN ECOLOGICAL FRAMEWORK

The transition process involves children's and families' experiences and interactions in multiple settings, including home, early intervention, and school. The smoothness of the transition process depends in part on the nature and extent of the match (or mismatch) of children's experiences across contexts (Doucet & Tudge, 2007) and, specifically, the extent that there are shared values, beliefs, and practices in ways to promote a smooth transition. The findings of Jamieson et al. (2014) indicated there are several dimensions of the transition process in which potential continuity and discontinuity may occur across home, early intervention, school, and policy contexts. A smooth transition was facilitated when there was continuity in contexts, such as when there was information sharing between early intervention and school personnel or when the developing child entered the new setting (kindergarten, for example) in the company of one or more persons who were participants in prior settings, such as a parent. As was evident in that study's findings, the nature, ease, and extent of two-way communication between persons across multiple settings (home–early intervention–school communications) also facilitates the transition and contributes to the potential for each setting to be supportive developmentally (Bronfenbrenner, 1979, p. 216).

The issues in Table 3.1 were drawn from ecological systems theories to outline key transition dimensions, qualities of ecological contexts that were found to promote a smooth transition, and desired outcomes for the transition to school for deaf or hard-of-hearing children.

Table 3.1 Transition Dimensions, Qualities of Ecological Contexts, and Indicators of a Smooth Transition for Deaf or Hard-of-Hearing Children

Key Transition Dimensions	Qualities of Ecological Contexts That Promote a Smooth Transition	Indicators of a Smooth Transition
Opportunities for transition preparation pretransition	Home • Parents who seek and participate in pretransition preparation opportunities (e.g., workshops, review of transition resources) Early-intervention program • Provision of up-to-date information to parents about the child's developmental progress in different domains • Transition support services and informational resource provision to parents (i.e., regarding policies and practices for the transition) • Advance notice to schools about child's specific needs; opportunities for observations by school-based support personnel • Facilitation of pretransition meetings involving parents and school School • Informational resources shared and discussed with parents before school entry • Organization and facilitation of pretransition meetings with parents and early-intervention program	• Parents have a sense of preparedness and empowerment about the transition process. • Parents feel knowledgeable about the child's progress on various developmental domains and readiness for school. • Parents are certain about educational placement options available and the types of supports each school offers for the transition.

(continued)

Table 3.1 Continued

Key Transition Dimensions	Qualities of Ecological Contexts That Promote a Smooth Transition	Indicators of a Smooth Transition
Opportunities for stakeholder involvement before and during the transition process	**Home** • Parents who seek and participate in transition support services available and acquire knowledge about the school and transition process **Early-intervention program** • Bridging the transition between home, early intervention, and school by facilitating information exchange and communications **School** • Hiring of appropriate support personnel • Preparation of school staff (e.g., in-service training) • Proactive approach by school-based team to specifying the timing and procedures of the transition process (e.g., sequence and schedule of events). • Initiation and maintenance of parent–school communications about the transition and ways the school will support the child's needs **Policy context** • Specification of and consistency in transition policies and procedures to enable equitable access to supports across geographic areas	• Parents are certain about the timing and procedures of the transition process (e.g., sequence and schedule of events). • Across home, early intervention, and school contexts, there is shared knowledge and consistency in supports for the developmental progress of the child. • School-based team personnel have a knowledge base of early educational history, child's developmental progress, learning needs, and optimal supports required in the classroom. • There is timely provision of appropriate educational supports for the child. • Parents, regardless of where they live, have access to supports and informational resources before and during the transition.

Opportunities for establishment of strong home–school partnerships to promote the child's developmental progress and well-being

Home
- Parents who are proactive in information-seeking and knowledgeable about the incoming school and special education system
- Parents who voice their needs and concerns
- Parents and schools are partners in the transition.

Early-intervention program
- Establishment and maintenance of the key informational and emotional support role throughout the transition
- Provision of support for parents in their advocacy role for appropriate educational supports for the child

School
- Proactive approach by school-based team to initiate and maintain parent–school communications about child's needs and progress
- Schools provide a welcoming environment and are receptive to parent input, and are responsive to parents' needs and concerns

- Parents and schools are partners in the transition.
- Parents have knowledge of the school and special education system, and ways the child's experiences in school are contributing to the child's developmental progress.
- Schools have an understanding of the impact of hearing loss on learning and social development.
- Schools build on the early learning foundation provided in the home and early-intervention contexts (e.g., continuity in goals) and are proactive in meeting the child's needs.

SUMMARY AND CONCLUSIONS

The transition to school marks a key milestone for deaf or hard-of-hearing children because it launches and shapes the course of their trajectories in school, both academically and socially. In this chapter, we used an ecological systems theoretical lens to explore and highlight key facilitators and barriers within relational contexts—home–early intervention, early intervention–school, home–school, and overarching policy contexts—that contribute to a smooth transition. Central to the transition are the interrelationships established and maintained across stakeholders in home, early intervention, and school contexts both before and during the transition. Based on the findings of Jamieson et al. (2014), key transition dimensions, qualities of ecological contexts that contribute to a smooth transition, and desired outcomes for the transition process were highlighted. The silos inherent in the policy context for the transition to school for deaf or hard-of-hearing children were an overarching influence that contributed to some parents' experiences of fragmentation during the transition process and also resultant inequities in families' access to support and resources for the transition across geographic areas. The findings were suggestive of ways that interventions that aim to improve the quality of the transition experience for deaf or hard-of-hearing children must operate synchronously at multiple levels—from macro to micro—to have pervasive system-level impacts.

ACKNOWLEDGMENT

This research was supported in part by funding from the Vancouver Coastal Health Authority—Child and Youth Mental Health and a grant from The University of British Columbia Humanities and Social Sciences, both to the second author.

REFERENCES

Ahtola, A., Silinskas, G., Poikonen, P. L., Kontoniemi, M., Niemi, P., & Nurmi, J. E. (2011). Transition to formal schooling: Do transition practices matter for academic performance? *Early Childhood Research Quarterly, 26*(3), 295–302.

Alexander, K., & Entwisle, D. (1988). *Achievement in the first two years of school: Patterns and processes.* Chicago, IL: University of Chicago Press.

Angelides, P., & Aravi, C. (2006). A comparative perspective on the experiences of deaf and hard of hearing individuals as students at mainstream and special schools. *American Annals of the Deaf, 151*(5), 476–487.

Belsky, J., & MacKinnon, C. (1994). Transition to school: Developmental trajectories and school experiences. *Early Education and Development, 5*(2), 106–119.

Bredekamp, S., & Copple, C. (Eds.) (1997). *Developmentally appropriate practice in early childhood programs* (rev. ed.). Washington, DC: National Association for the Education of Young Children.

Briody, M. F., & Martone, J. M. (2010). Challenges and considerations when transitioning preschoolers with complex medical histories to kindergarten. *Journal of Early Childhood & Infant Psychology, 6*, 117–132.

Bronfenbrenner, U. (1979). *The ecology of human development: Experiments by nature and design.* Cambridge, MA: Harvard University Press.

Bronfenbrenner, U. (1986). Ecology of the family as a context for human development: Research perspectives. *Developmental Psychology, 22*(6), 723–742.

Bronfenbrenner, U. (1993). The ecology of cognitive development: Research models and fugitive findings. In R. H. Wozniak & K. W. Fischer (Eds.), *Development in context: Acting and thinking in specific environments* (pp. 3–44). New York, NY: Lawrence Erlbaum Associates.

Bronfenbrenner, U. (2005). *Making human beings human: Bioecological perspectives on human development.* Thousand Oaks, CA: Sage.

Bronfenbrenner, U., & Morris, P. A. (1998). The ecology of developmental processes. In W. Damon & R. M. Lemer (Eds.), *Handbook of child psychology* (Vol. 1, pp. 993–1028). New York, NY: Wiley.

Bronfenbrenner, U., & Morris, P. A. (2006). The bioecological model of human development. In *Handbook of child psychology* (6th ed., Vol. 1). Hoboken, NJ: Wiley.

Doucet, F., & Tudge, J. (2007). Co-constructing the transition to school: Reframing the novice versus expert roles of children, parents, and teachers from a cultural perspective. In R. C. Pianta, M. J. Cox, & K. Snow (Eds.), *School readiness and the transition to kindergarten in the era of accountability* (pp. 307–328). Baltimore, MD: Brookes.

Dunst, C. J., Trivette, C. M., & Deal, A. G. (1994). *Supporting and strengthening families: Methods, strategies and practices.* Cambridge, MA: Brookline.

Eriks-Brophy, A., & Whittingham, J. (2013). Teachers' perceptions of the inclusion of children with hearing loss in general education settings. *American Annals of the Deaf, 158*(1), 63–97.

Gallaudet Research Institute (August 2013). *Regional and National Summary Report of Data from the 2011–12 Annual Survey of Deaf and Hard of Hearing Children and Youth.* Washington, DC: GRI, Gallaudet University.

Guardino, C. A. (2008). Identification and placement for deaf students with multiple disabilities: Choosing the path less followed. *American Annals of the Deaf, 153*(1), 55–64.

Hains, A. H., Fowler, S. A., Schwartz, I. S., Kottwitz, E., & Rosenkoetter, S. (1989). A comparison of preschool and kindergarten teacher expectations for school readiness. *Early Childhood Research Quarterly, 4*(1), 75–88.

Jamieson, J. R., Poon, B. T., Zaidman-Zait, A., Curle, D., Norman, N., & Simmons, N. (2014). *Working together for smooth transitions: The move from early intervention to kindergarten for children who are deaf or hard of hearing in B.C., their families, and teachers.* Vancouver, BC: Vancouver Coastal Health Authority.

Jamieson, J. R., Zaidman-Zait, A., & Poon, B. (2011). Family support needs as perceived by parents of preadolescents and adolescents who are deaf or hard of hearing. *Deafness & Education International, 13*(3), 110–130.

Janus, M., Cameron, R., Lefort, J., & Kopechanski, L. (2007). Starting kindergarten: Transition issues for children with special needs. *Canadian Journal of Education, 30*(3), 628–648.

Love, J. M., Logue, M. E., Trudeau, J., & Thayer, K. (1992). *Transitions to kindergarten in American schools: Final report of the National Transition Study: Report* submitted to *U.S. Department of Education*. Portsmouth, NH: RMC Research Corporation.

Luckner, J. L., & Ayantoye, C. (2013). Itinerant teachers of students who are deaf or hard of hearing: Practices and preparation. *Journal of Deaf Studies and Deaf Education, 18*(3), 409–423.

Luckner, J. L., & Carter, K. (2001). Essential competencies for teaching students with hearing loss and additional disabilities. *American Annals of the Deaf, 146*(1), 7–15.

Mawdsley, H. P., & Hauser-Cram, P. (2013). Mothers of young children with disabilities: Perceived benefits and worries about preschool. *Early Child Development and Care, 183*(9), 1258–1275.

McIntyre, L. L., Blacher, J., & Baker, B. L. (2006). The transition to school: Adaptation in young children with and without intellectual disability. *Journal of Intellectual Disability Research, 50*, 349–361.

McIntyre, L. L., Eckert, T. L., Fiese, B. H., DiGennaro, F. D., & Wildenger, L. K. (2007). Transition to kindergarten: Family experiences and involvement. *Early Childhood Education Journal, 35*(1), 83–88.

McIntyre, L. L., Eckert, T. L., Fiese, B. H., Reed, F. D. D., & Wildenger, L. K. (2010). Family concerns surrounding kindergarten transition: A comparison of students in special and general education. *Early Childhood Education Journal, 38*(4), 259–263.

Moores, D. F., Jatho, J., Creech, B. (2001). Issues and trends in instruction and deafness: *American Annals of the Deaf* 1996 to 2000. *American Annals of the Deaf, 146*(2), 71–76.

Myck-Wayne, J., Robinson, S., & Henson, E. (2011). Serving and supporting young children with a dual diagnosis of hearing loss and autism: The stories of four families. *American Annals of the Deaf, 156*(4), 379–390.

National Center for Education Statistics (2011). The condition of education. http://nces.ed.gov.

Petrakos, H. H., & Lehrer, J. S. (2011). Parents' and teachers' perceptions of transition practices in kindergarten. *Exceptionality Education International, 21*(2), 62–73. http://ir.lib.uwo.ca/eei/vol21/iss2/7.

Pianta, R. C., Cox, M. J., Taylor, L., & Early, D. (1999). Kindergarten teachers' practices related to transition into school: Results of a national survey. *Elementary School Journal, 100*(1), 71–86.

Pianta, R. C., & Kraft-Sayre, M. (1999). Parents' observations about their children's transitions to kindergarten. *Young Children, 54*(3), 7–52.

Pianta, R. C., & Walsh, D. J. (1996). *High-risk children in schools: Constructing sustaining relationships*. New York, NY: Routledge.

Pighini, M. J., Goelman, H., Buchanan, M., Schonert-Reichl, K., & Brynelsen, D. (2014). Learning from parents' stories about what works in early intervention. *International Journal of Psychology, 49*(4), 263–270.

Podvey, M., Hinojosa, J., & Koenig, K. (2013). Reconsidering insider status for families during the transition from early intervention to preschool special education. *The Journal of Special Education, 46*, 211–222.

Ray, K. & Smith, M. (2010). The kindergarten child: What teachers and administrators need to know to promote academic success. *Early Childhood Education Journal, 38*, 5–18.

Rimm-Kaufman, S. E., & Pianta, R. C. (1999). Patterns of family-school contact in preschool and kindergarten. *School Psychology Review, 28*(3), 426–438.

Rimm-Kaufman, S. E., & Pianta, R. C. (2000). An ecological perspective on children's transition to kindergarten: A theoretical framework to guide empirical research. *Journal of Applied Developmental Psychology, 21*(5), 491–511.

Sass-Lehrer, M., & Bodner-Johnson, B. (2003). Early intervention: Current approaches to family-centered programming. In M. Marschark & P. E. Spencer (Eds.), *Oxford handbook of deaf studies, language and education* (pp. 65–81). New York, NY: Oxford University Press.

Schischka, J., Rawlinson, C., & Hamilton, R. (2012). Factors affecting the transition to school for young children with disabilities [online]. *Australasian Journal of Early Childhood, 37*(4), 15–23.

Tudge, J. R. H., Freitas, L. B. L., & Doucet, F. (2009). The transition to school: Reflections from a contextualist perspective. In H. Daniels, H. Lauder, and J. Porter (Eds.), *Educational theories, cultures and learning: A critical perspective* (pp. 117–133). New York, NY: Routledge.

Villeneuve, M., Chatenoud, C., Hutchinson, N. L., Minnes, P., Perry, A., Carmen, D., Frankel, E. B., Isaacs, B., Loh, A., Versnel, J., & Weiss J. (2013). The experience of parents as their children with developmental disabilities transition from early intervention to kindergarten. *Canadian Journal of Education, 36*(1), 4–43.

Zaidman-Zait, A. (2007). Parenting a child with a cochlear implant: A critical incident study. *Journal of Deaf Studies and Deaf Education, 12*(2), 221–241.

4

School as a Site for Natural Language Learning

Marlon Kuntze, Debbie Golos, Kimberly Wolbers, Catherine O'Brien, and David Smith

Children in general cannot help but acquire language, and they do it in leaps and bounds. At the same time, they are mostly unaware they are learning language, and it is because it is happening without any effort on their part. The progress they make is amazing, yet it is imperceptible. We can see a lot of progress only by comparing two different points in development. Young children do make grammatical errors, but it is almost useless to try to teach or correct them directly because they are impervious to language instruction (James, 2004; Schlesinger, 1975). It is only through sustained use of language with more skilled language users that they eventually figure it out. Humans are wired to learn language as much as they are wired to learn how to walk. Just as children need to be in contact with the ground to learn to walk, they need to be in social contact with others to learn language.

Although deaf children grow up surrounded by others, the typical social contact most of them experience largely circumvents the use of language. The language of the home most deaf children are born into and the language of the community most of them grow up in is spoken. For many deaf children, including those with cochlear implants, spoken language is not adequately accessible for the purpose of optimal natural language learning. Also, without a language the child can fully share with others, the child does not have an opportunity for the full development of intellectual and emotional relationship with others. Communication that does take place is usually enabled by anchoring it in the concrete world of "here and now," and it is often facilitated through pointing and gesticulation.

Being deaf is not the cause of delays in language development; rather, the delays are the direct manifestations of a social world in which language is not fully accessible and thus largely incomprehensible (Hoff, 2006; Meristo et al., 2007). Some hearing parents put a premium on quality communication with their deaf child and, without much, hesitation embark on making communication as accessible as possible. Some of them, for example, may decide to learn sign language right away. Making a concerted effort to communicate with a deaf child does make a difference. However, as is often the case, communication at home—for one reason or the other—is less than adequate. It is common that communication with deaf children is limited mostly to topics related to what they are doing or what they can see in their immediate surroundings. With communication limited to superficial topics, any opportunity to share thoughts, memories, intentions, and beliefs with their deaf children is forfeited (Meadow, 1975). Communicative interaction is often restricted to routines or behavior management such as telling the deaf child what to do or that certain behaviors are not acceptable. For these families, playful or inquisitive conversational exchange simply does not take place (Courtin & Melot, 1998). When deaf children have limited linguistic access to their parents, be it spoken or signed, it is next to impossible for the parents to engage their deaf children in explanations about emotions, reasons for actions, expected roles, and the consequences of various behaviors (Marschark, 1993).

Language development is prodded simply as a consequence of the need to communicate. Language learning takes place more optimally when the context of communication is less familiar such as when the topic of the conversation is new, when there is a need to understand what is going on, or when there is a new interlocutor with whom to engage in a dialogue. An effort to converse in contexts like those is an opportunity to figure how to use or to experience language in a new way. When communication takes place with comprehension, we are subconsciously exposed to how language works, and it is when language learning takes place. When we figure out how to express our ideas, our emotions, our beliefs, and intentions, we do not realize we are also figuring out how language works and, as a result, our skills with language grow. Many deaf children, are simply not provided access to quality communication without which it is not possible to adequately experience a wide variety of language use and to experiment with how language may be produced. Linguistic access to others is often restricted or is, in some cases, nonexistent.

With opportunities for natural language learning limited in the home, many deaf children arrive at school without adequate foundations in language. Educators commonly agree that without adequate language, learning is limited, and they usually respond to this predicament through remedial measures. Often this involves teaching language directly. Unfortunately that is not how language acquisition normally works. This is a misguided approach because young deaf children, just like any children, do have a natural language-learning capability, and it stands to reason they are similarly impervious to language instruction. The best way to support their language development is to give them accessible means to communicate. Often the language-learning capabilities of deaf children have been left fallow as a result of the mismatch between deaf children's linguistic needs and the modality of the language in their midst both in the home and in the community. It is a situation that is often aggravated by parents being unaware of the need to find ways to include their deaf child in high-quality communication. In essence, when deaf children are in linguistically impoverished setting, the language-learning capacities that they are born with will not be fully tapped and in some cases may atrophy.

A small part of the deaf children population grow up with optimal access to the language in their environment (either signed or spoken language). Those who do are able to enjoy a robust process of language learning that takes place naturally. Some of these children may have parents who are deaf, so they are already immersed in an accessible communicative environment whereas others may have hearing parents who do not hesitate to learn sign language and are able to learn it fairly well and fast enough to keep up with their child's developing signing skills. Some of these children may live in close proximity to schools where sign language is used and where sizable number of deaf student peers attend. Some of them may be able to benefit adequately from residual hearing, amplification, or accommodation in communication to ensure minimally meaningful access to spoken language.

The vast majority of deaf children, however, simply do not have access to the social milieu in which communication is at levels that are necessary for making language development robust. Too rarely are they in a two-way communicative environment where they not only can understand others, but also can be understood. The importance of communicative access cannot be overstated because it is the only way children will know others do talk about thoughts, concerns, or confusion. Equally as important as the opportunity to communicate about these things is the means to get communicative feedback. Feedback helps us figure how to express more completely what we are trying to convey. Successfully conveying what we want to say means figuring how to put ideas, perception, or puzzlement into words. The success of conveying meaning is often aided by the opportunity to respond to questions or comments from others who try to understand what is said (Wells, 1981). That is how language learning works. The importance of shared language between a child and others in the child's social milieu lies in the fact that it is through language that we gain access to the minds of others. When an adult is able to get into the child's mind, the adult is in a privileged position to appreciate more fully the child's current stage of development and how the child views and understands the world. As a result, the adult is able to guide the child in successfully expressing what he or she may not be able to convey successfully on his or her own. Each successful articulation, aided or not, of what the child wants to say helps the child become more competent in language.

Ideally, the lack of access to language should be addressed *before* deaf children start school, but unfortunately usually not much is done until they are *in* school. Educators are cognizant that, without language learning, these children will be severely constrained. They are right for looking at schools as the only and probably the last chance to remediate language delays. However, paradoxical as it may seem, schools may unwittingly conspire against giving deaf children what they really need to catch up with language learning. School as a place of instruction is tasked with the expectations that teachers teach what students need to learn. Natural language learning does happen at schools, but it is rarely designated as an important function of school. Curricula emphasize language teaching rather than spontaneous language use. In the case of a child being delayed in language development, the typical course of responding to the situation is to remediate. To remediate means to instruct; instruction too often results in less opportunity for spontaneous communication. If psycholinguistics tell us that children are impervious to efforts to correct their grammar (e.g., Jackendoff, 1994; McNeill, 1970; Pinker, 1995), it would seem reasonable to extend that observation to the idea that teaching them language directly would not work either. We often perceive the problem to be the children themselves; however, the real problem is the social world in which they grow up. Actually, the best way schools can help support deaf children's language development is most likely by examining the ways they can promote authentic communication and by striving to promote the kind of pedagogy that incorporates authentic communication. School should become the place where deaf children thrive in accessible and engaging communication with others.

This chapter is a compilation of individual research conducted by each of the five authors whose work draws from sociocultural theories of language development and learning. Put together, their research serves to examine collectively the topic of natural language development for deaf children from across various backgrounds within the framework of (1) access to, (2) implementation of, and (3) impact of communication-rich environments. The common thread uniting the research in the chapter ultimately points to communication-rich schooling as a way of mitigating the impoverished contexts typically experienced by deaf children that have a deleterious impact on their language, literacy, and cognitive development.

We propose that, for deaf and hard-of-hearing students, we should examine school as an essential site of natural language learning. First, we review a case from O'Brien's (2011) research that documents what it was like for a teenage deaf student who had attended school for 12 years without communication access suddenly finding himself in an unfamiliar environment where people use sign to communicate. The point is to highlight that, when communication is accessible, language learning can commence. Then the next investigation, conducted by Kuntze (2008, 2010), offers a contrasting study and gives an example of a rich communicative environment that is too rare in deaf education. It shows what language development can look like for preschool-age deaf children who have access to communication both at home and at school with a teacher who can keep them engaged communicatively. The third study, by Smith (manuscript in preparation), is an attempt to illustrate how the use of dialogic pedagogy, which encourages student thinking, in a high school social studies class provides the students with opportunities to use authentic language while learning about history and important concepts in social studies. The last two studies examine school-based programming informed by sociocultural perspectives of language development and learning. Research by Wolbers (e.g., 2008a) illustrates an interactive approach to children's development of writing skills. It is premised on the understanding that an interactive, communication-based pedagogy can facilitate content and language objectives simultaneously, in that the complex thinking and reasoning associated with school-based learning is linked inextricably with complex expression. Research by Golos (e.g., Golos and Moses, 2013b) on the use of educational media to support language and literacy development is motivated by the challenge of bringing deaf children and language and cultural role models together, and how the use of educational media may help adults (who may not be fluent models of American Sign Language [ASL] or another natural sign language) with the task of supporting deaf children's natural process of language learning.

PEER-SUPPORTED LANGUAGE SOCIALIZATION

The extent to which communication is accessible in schools varies as a function of the ability of the school personnel to accommodate the different communicative needs and abilities across the diverse deaf student population. Schools with a large population of deaf students are usually those in which communication is more accessible, and for a large number of deaf children, these schools serve as an important site of language socialization (Erting & Kuntze, 2008). It is primarily at these schools that there are at least some deaf peers with whom to socialize and through whom language skills of many others develop. O'Brien's (2011) research documented an observation that is representative of the experience that many deaf students with limited language skills may have when they enroll in a school with a large deaf student population. John (a pseudonym) was 16 years old when he accompanied his hearing parents to visit a state school for the deaf. Neither he nor his parents knew sign language, and communication was very difficult, limited, and—at times—frustrating. John's attempts to use spoken language were very difficult to understand, and he and his parents were unable to have meaningful conversations. John failed to achieve academically in various school settings where spoken language is used as the language of instruction and where communication takes place only through speaking and speech reading. Neither he nor his parents were ever exposed to a sign language until this initial visit to the school for the deaf. His parents explained they were told never to let John learn sign language and that, to function in a hearing world, John must learn to speech read and speak. However, after 12 years in school, John's parents were told by the school that he was not learning and they should consider enrolling him in the state school for the deaf.

The family made an appointment to visit the state school for the deaf as a "last resort" and to "investigate" whether he should enroll in a school where sign language is used as the language of instruction. Like John, most students with limited language, on arriving at the school for the first time, are often reserved, and their eyes are wide open. For the most part they do not converse, and they often stay with their parents. However, if given the opportunity, veteran students try to communicate with them and use gestures to establish a connection. Gestures are also used to facilitate the introduction of the signed vocabulary as the new student enters the unfamiliar language community. The way language socialization may begin varies as veteran students try to figure what the newcomer may already know or is able to make sense of.

Even for John, who has limited language skills, a brief exposure to communication that is potentially accessible can result in a rapid transformation. As soon as the assistant superintendent started giving the family a tour of the school, it became obvious to him that John would rather be playing with the boys he saw on a basketball court. John had been watching the boys play while looking out a window in a room where his parents were meeting with the assistant superintendent. After the assistant superintendent made several futile attempts to communicate to John that he may go play basketball, he asked the researcher if she would be willing to take John to the basketball court. One of the players, Mark, saw John watching the boys playing basketball and walked over with a basketball in his hands and signed, BASKETBALL, WANT PLAY? John's blank facial expressions showed that he obviously did not understand. So Mark handed the ball to John and showed the sign for basketball. Mark then took the ball back, waiting for John to sign basketball. When John did not, Mark gave the ball back and repeated the sign for basketball. This time he pointed to the basketball after signing BASKETBALL. John smiled and signed back. Mark then gestured to tell John to join him in the basketball game. After the basketball game, John went to the cafeteria with the boys where he continued learning the language. Mark mimed and gave instructions to John about how to enter the cafeteria line, pick up a tray, and tell the cook what he wanted to eat. Mark, along with the other boys, encouraged John during lunch to copy their signs and learn their meaning as he tried to communicate with his new friends.

Many deaf people acquire sign language naturally as a result of coming into contact with peers and elders in the deaf community, and residential schools have historically been an important site of language socialization process that help new nonsigning students move toward an eventual membership in the larger deaf community outside the school (Erting & Kuntze, 2007). The students who have been at the school for a while usually take it upon themselves to assist new students in starting the process of becoming adjusted to a new language environment and learning ASL. There appears to be an understanding among the students, especially those who had experienced schooling in which no signing was used, of what it was like to be a nonsigner in a signing environment.

A sociocultural perspective on language development is premised on the idea that language and cognitive skills are first nurtured in a social interaction between a child and more competent, diverse partners within the child's cultural environment before they become internalized as part of the child's competency (Kumaravadivelu, 2006; Mead, 1934; Vygotsky, 1962). It is a constant process during which each step in language and cognitive development serves to enrich future social interaction through which the child builds communicative and thinking skills. The vignette about John shows that a brief social interaction with peers was enough to impact his language development positively. This is how many nonsigning deaf students receive support in language development simply by coming into contact with peers who sign. The only requirements are that language is fully accessible and that communication is two-way and genuine.

ADULT-MEDIATED COMMUNICATION

Although interaction with peers is important, it by itself is not enough. Research (Kuntze, 2010; Kuntze et al., 2008) on the conversation interactions in a preschool classroom where everyone signs shows the importance of interactions with partners who have much more mature language skills. The interaction with the more competent communicative partner is an opportunity not only to be exposed to a more complex use of language and a more complex cognitive stance, but also—and more important—to be exposed to the potential of understanding more deeply what is being talked about. The dialogue back and forth between the child and the more advanced partner is an opportunity for the child to make sense of what is being talked about and, if necessary, for the partner to figure out how to help the child make sense of the topic. The object of any conversation is always to get meaning across to the other, and the course the dialogue takes is dictated by what it takes to get the meaning across successfully. Learning language and new cognitive stances is never the goal, but nevertheless an important by-product of the process. The incremental progress in language and cognitive development serves to prepare the child for more advanced topics in the future.

The socially mediated process in which the adult or more competent peer helps the child develop these higher order mental functions takes place in naturally occurring informal settings of the home, school, and community (Tharp & Gallimore, 1988). The child is assisted in the process of making sense of complex information through *scaffolding*—a term first coined by Wood et al. (1976) to describe this tutorial relationship between the adult and child that is critical to language learning. Scaffolding provided on the basis of the developmental needs of the child gives the child just enough assistance to complete the tasks the child could not have done independently. The completion of the task helps the child know how to do it more independently the next time.

There are three important conditions to meet before the more competent other can assist the child's performance effectively. According to Trueba (1988), they include (1) effective communication between the child and the adult, (2) shared cultural values and assumptions, and (3) common goals for the activity. It is "through culturally and linguistically appropriate interaction [that] the child develops a suitable cognitive structure that is continually revised with new experiences and feedback" (Trueba, 1988, p. 181). The conversation that is engaging and anchored in a social context and that ensures understanding is key toward supporting language, cognitive, and social development, and it is an opportunity that is historically not adequately provided to many deaf children in different learning contexts worldwide (Ewoldt & Saulnier, 1992; Keating & Mirus, 2003; Martin et al., 2010; Muma & Teller, 2001; Mweri, 2014; Pribanić, 2006; Silverstre et al., 2007; Wilkens & Hehir, 2008).

The following interaction in ASL—but presented here in English translation—between a signing-fluent teacher and Jill (a pseudonym), a girl of age 3 years and 9 months who has hearing parents is an example of a dialogue that engages the child cognitively. The teacher had asked Jill which cracker she liked. They had already discussed two different flavors of goldfish crackers: cheese and pretzel. Jill said, "Brown" which clearly indicated she understood the teacher and gave an answer that referred unambiguously to a specific type of cracker. The teacher could have ended the conversation by giving Jill what she asked for or better by pointing out that the brown cracker is a pretzel. However, she wanted Jill to identify the cracker by type rather than by color. So she chose to continue the conversation by asking what kind of crackers the brown ones are. Jill said something unintelligible (on the recording).

The teacher responded, "No, what kind of crackers are the brown ones? Are they cheese?" This was a technique for steering Jill to look at the difference between crackers by type rather than by color.

Jill responded correctly by shaking her head that they are not cheese, so the teacher repeated the question. Jill was stumped and started to give random answers: "Pink? Orange?"

The teacher responded, "No, no, no," and pulled out a bag of pretzel goldfish crackers. Using the prop was probably a technique to ask the question in a new way without having to mention color. The teacher asked, "What kind of crackers are these?"

Jill said, "Brown," as before.

The teacher was persistent, saying, "Right, but what are they?"

Jill gave the same answer, "Brown."

The teacher went back to the same question she asked earlier: "Are they cheese?"

Jill quickly blurted, "Pretzel."

When the teacher affirmed Jill's answer was correct, Jill beamed, "I knew it. I am awesome. Super good at this. Pretzel, pretzel, pretzel!"

The learning context in which the language of instruction is accessible to all children means more contact time with the language. The opportunity to eavesdrop is important because it helps augment children's exposure not only to language but also to different topics of conversation that may be going on. In a setting such as school, where the one-on-one contact time between the adult and the child is limited compared with the potential contact time between a parent and a child at home, the ability for a child to eavesdrop on a conversation of which the child is not a part is especially important. For example, the engagement just described between the teacher and Jill about the goldfish cracker caught the attention of another child. Joe, the eavesdropping child, was following each turn of the dialogue. Then, at precisely the same moment Jill said, "Pretzel," Joe said the same thing. A frame-by-frame examination on the videotape of the occurrence shows that both children answered the question at exactly the same split second. Based on the eye contact each child had placed on the teacher, it showed that each child gave the answer independently of each other. Although Joe was not part of the conversation and the questions were not directed to him, he was able to participate in it mentally. An important reason it was possible was because he had access to the language of the conversation and had enough language skills to follow it.

The opportunity to learn as a result of observing what is going on in a conversation depends on whether the activity being observed is meaningful and interesting to the observer (Bandura, 1977). One assumption of social cognitive theory is that learning is based on triadic reciprocity (Bandura, 1986) among cognitive, behavioral, and social factors. In the case of language learning, it means the trajectory of language development (behavior) is affected by the child's thoughts and knowledge (cognitive), and how the social context of the utterance mediates the child's effort either to make sense of what is uttered or what he or she wants to say. For some reason, Joe found the conversation about the pretzel interesting and relevant, possibly because the class just had crackers for their snack and the content was already familiar. Joe probably found the topic of the conversation interesting because he appeared to enjoy following each turn of the conversation between the teacher and Jill. The language context of this particular classroom supported language learning not only through students participating in the conversation directly, but also by participating in it indirectly.

A lot of language learning occurs as a part of the mundane process of everyday communication, and we cannot possibly be aware of each instance the child learns a new word or what a phrase means. Language learning is pervasive, and it takes place as long as the language is accessible and the child participates actively in the conversation. In the following example, at a different time, Jill learned the sign for jellyfish as a result of having misunderstood the teacher and thinking she was talking about a different animal. Challenging the teacher that the animal to which she was referring was not an octopus led to an opportunity to learn the new sign for jellyfish and to distinguish it from the sign for octopus. The sign for jellyfish has a phonological shape that, if someone not familiar with the lexical item tried to guess the meaning on the basis of the form, the possibility of thinking it may mean octopus is not far-fetched. That it happened this way is plausible given the context of the story, which was about what a fish saw as it explored its surroundings. The following exchange (also translated into English) took place while the teacher was reading (signing in ASL) a book (written in English) to the class:

> TEACHER: "The fish saw something he had never seen before: a jellyfish."
> JILL: "No, it's not an octopus. No."
> TEACHER: "You're right. It's not an octopus. It's a jellyfish. They're different. You're right."
> JILL (TO HERSELF): "Jellyfish."

In signing jellyfish to herself, Jill was probably trying to practice forming this new sign while making a mental note to herself that, although its form suggests it refers to an octopus, it actually refers to a different animal. During this process, she probably was also subconsciously reinforcing what she already knew about the sign for octopus.

These vignettes about John and Jill underscore the importance of a community in which communication is accessible and understandable. It is in such a context that dialogic pedagogy becomes possible.

DIALOGIC PEDAGOGY

Dialogic modes of instruction have been linked with higher cognitive capacities and critical thinking (Burbules, 1993; Hillocks, 2002; Nystrand, 1997; Ward, 1994), for language plays a critical role in mediating learning (Kraker, 2000) and transforming action (Wertsch, 1991). Language provides an avenue for accessing others' experiences and points of view (Bruner, 1996; Dewey, 1990; Greeno et al., 1997), and it is through collaborative interactions that students are exposed to the strategies and problem-solving techniques of others (Lantolf, 2000). Dialogic pedagogy not only provides students with an exposure to language associated with higher cognitive activities, but also gives them engaged use of language resulting in further language development (Gavelek & Raphael, 1996; Hartman, 1996). Mayer et al. (2002) observed that exemplary teachers of deaf students are the ones more likely to ask meaningful, authentic questions that engage their students in learning.

Discourse with students gives teachers an invaluable strategy for engaging students supportively at higher levels of thinking and talking, which then leads to the expansion of their linguistic and cognitive capabilities. Outside school, deaf and hard-of-hearing students are less likely to have access to the kind of communicative interactions that allow them to learn from others or that engage them in critical thinking, making it more crucial that schools attempt to maximize these opportunities as a part of pedagogy. Dialogue is an important technique for pinpointing areas of content that students may not comprehend fully or for prompting students to think at a higher cognitive level.

A good instructional conversation is comprised of a discourse led by a teacher who treats students as equal partners. The teacher presents provocative ideas or experiences in a strategic manner and then asks questions, probes for reasons, persuades, or remains quiet. Only when necessary do teachers clarify and give direct instruction, and they do so in an efficient manner, without wasting time or words. Teachers know when to push and probe to draw out a student's ideas, but also know when to back off and allow thought and reflection to occur. Teachers also know when to get involved and when to retreat and not inhibit discussions. The most important thing is to ensure all students are engaged and contributing to a meaningful and extended discussion about ideas that are relevant to them (Goldenberg, 1991).

Although the teacher and students having the same language they can share is obviously essential before dialogic pedagogy can even be considered, it does, however, take more than shared language to make the most out of dialogic approach to teaching. Instructional Conversation (IC) (Goldenberg 1992; Tharp & Gallimore, 1991) is a methodology to gauge the extent to which the teacher listens carefully, makes guesses about intended meaning, and adjusts responses to assist students' efforts. The development of IC evolved out of the Kamehameha Early Education Program (KEEP) in Hawaii in the 1970s as part of an effort to improve teaching of native children (Tharp & Gallimore, 1988). IC provides opportunities for the development of the languages of instruction and subject matter by providing feedback to the teacher's efforts to relate formal, school knowledge to the student's individual, family, and community knowledge. In short, IC is a supportive and collaborative event that builds connections among individuals and nurtures a sense of community. Because IC builds on interpersonal connection, it helps the teacher achieve individualization of conversation. The use of IC results in a setting that fosters language development and stimulating cognitive challenges. IC and other instructional standards, such as child-directed activity, complex thinking, modeling, and language and literacy development, were adapted as best practices for children in indigenous educational settings, including Native American schools (Center for Research on Education, Diversity & Excellence, 2014).

Smith (manuscript in preparation) used the elements of IC as a framework to conduct an analysis of a dialogic approach to instruction in a high school social studies class at a residential school that uses ASL/English bilingual communication. The topic of the lesson was on business monopolies during the early 20th century. The teacher was a fluent user of ASL and a member of the U.S. Deaf community. This teacher had more than seven years of teaching experience at kindergarten through grade 12 residential schools for the deaf. The students in this classroom were diverse in terms of ethnicity, early educational placements, and the age at which they learned ASL. Four of the students were Latino, and one of each of the remainder was African American, Asian American, and European American. The school where the study was conducted used ASL as the language of instruction. Some of the participants in the study had gone to the same school since early elementary ages, a few entered during the middle school years, and one transferred from another school during her freshman year. Some of the students were native ASL users whereas the rest had exposure to various types of bimodal (simultaneously speaking and signing) communication environments in the past. At the time of the study, they all appeared to have fluent ASL skills.

The IC framework is composed of 10 elements considered important for helping to evaluate the robustness and success of a classroom discussion. One objective the investigator had for doing the study was to investigate whether the IC framework, which is designed for classroom conversation in spoken language, is adequate as is for evaluating class discussion that takes place in sign. The second objective was to determine whether the IC framework would still be useful for evaluating a teacher already considered exemplary in leading class discussion.

It was observed during the study that many of these elements were descriptive of the lesson as a whole and included connected discourse, a challenging but nonthreatening atmosphere, and self-selected participation. The dialogue was connected and made coherent by cohesive devices such as BUT, OK, NOW, and READY (Roy, 1989); spatial referents; and nonmanual markers (Smith & Ramsey, 2004). A challenging and nonthreatening atmosphere was apparent. Self-selected participation was evident throughout the lesson as students freely contributed to the discourse in a manner consistent with other studies of deaf classrooms at younger ages (Erting & Kuntze, 2008; Golos, 2010; Ramsey & Padden, 1998). All the students participated at least once, and some more frequently than others. To encourage maximum participation classwide, the teacher used eye gaze to indicate who was being addressed (Mather, 1987), pointing to direct attention, and an upright index finger to indicate waiting.

The thematic focus of the lesson was about the antitrust efforts of the U.S. President Theodore Roosevelt's administration (1901–1909). The discussion evolved into one about deaf-owned small businesses trying to succeed in the face of big business competition, and it helped give context and relevancy to the topic of the lesson, which was about monopoly and the government's response to make business practice more fair and competitive. By allowing the dialogue to be student led, the teacher was able to guide it to issues that aroused students' interest in topics important to them, such as deaf people having a fair break in building businesses. The teacher made a connection between deaf-run businesses and the larger issues such as the monopolistic practice of big business and why the government sees the need to restore competition and fair business practices through antitrust efforts. Ultimately, based on subsequent interviews with students, the dialogic approach helped make the topic meaningful and relevant. The discussion about a new topic such as monopolistic practices and antitrust laws gave the students an opportunity not only to expand their knowledge about the topic, but also to absorb the vocabulary and language for discussing the topic.

The dialogic approach to instruction also helps the teacher monitor student comprehension. By making use of what the students say, how they respond to questions, and what they ask, the teacher is in a privileged position to determine how to use student background knowledge and schemata to help them better understand the topic under discussion. The investigator noted the social studies teacher was able to go back to points covered in the lesson and to tie them to students' current knowledge. Students appeared to have enough background knowledge on which they were able to draw during the discussion, and this suggested that constant access to class discussions to date had helped them build knowledge and participatory skills, which in turn helped make future class discussions more productive and take place at an even deeper level.

In addition to the 10 original IC elements, Smith (manuscript in preparation) added two other elements for classroom interaction conducted in signed languages. Smith and Ramsey (2004) noted that a deaf teacher in their study consistently elicited student responses to clarify content and used specific eye gaze for checking comprehension, which the investigators considered reflective of sociocultural language practices used by Deaf teachers. It was not enough just to rely on how students responded to each other or to the teacher. The teacher tried to elicit student response as a strategy to check comprehension. The teacher did this simply by making pauses and raising her eyebrows, which in effect indicated she was posing the "Are you following me?" question. She did it frequently, and it was followed by a downward head nod, as if asking for affirmation, and maintaining eye-gaze checks. The immediate collection of various forms of student feedback such as head nods, facial expressions, and interjected comments helped the teacher determine the best course to take for continuing the discussion. If all was going well and the students were following with the needed level of comprehension, the teacher continued the discussion. If not, the teacher backtracked to repair the sites of comprehension breakdown.

The IC framework proved useful for identifying areas for improvement even for the teacher considered exemplary in leading class discussion, because it helped the teacher and investigator focus on areas that probably would have escaped scrutiny. The two areas that were noted as needing improvement were related to the missed opportunities to dig deeper via extended discourse: elicitation of bases for statements and elicitation of student response/clarification. Inquiries for bases of statements involved the use of evidence and reasoning to support an argument or position—such as "How do you know?" and "What makes you say that?" Setting up a problem and asking for clarification prompted students to clarify, solve, or provide missing information. Both of these types of elicitations from students involve critical thinking skills. Elicitations also are a means of seeing how much background knowledge students can apply to a situation. These two missing elements from the teacher being observed are related to task persistence. One of the positive attributes of a good teacher of deaf students (or any teacher, in general) is a high level of task persistence in their discourse (Harris, 2010; Kluwin, 1983; Smith & Ramsey, 2004).

The use of IC can help teachers who already use dialogic pedagogy expand their repertoire of extended discourse strategies and give students more opportunities for natural language learning. It can help other teachers, including those who teach younger students, to consider adopting dialogic pedagogy as a part of their teaching practice.

IMPACT OF COMMUNICATION-RICH SCHOOLING

Smith's (manuscript in preparation) analysis in the previous section of dialogic pedagogy in a high school social studies classroom is an example of how content-area instruction may be conducted in a way that students are provided simultaneously with opportunities for language development. The course of students' language development is mediated by the nature of the topics of conversation of which they are a part, and by the extent to which their participation is supported and maintained by the relevance or meaningfulness the conversation has to them. Implementation of dialogic pedagogy then becomes the means through which teaching and learning of social studies is achieved, and can subsequently promote the development of both conceptual knowledge and language. Communication-rich schooling allows for the integration of dialogic pedagogical approaches to every aspect of the deaf child's school day, embedded in the teaching and learning of content areas such as science and math.

One particular challenge for teachers of the deaf is how to teach students to read and write in English when many are still developing expressive and receptive language competency. Traditionally, language has been taught to deaf students using structured curricula, in which grammar aspects are taught explicitly and systematically (Rose et al., 2004). Communication-rich schooling, on the other hand, means the creation of school-based environments where natural language learning can occur, and that embedding dialogic pedagogical approaches into the teaching and learning of any content, including reading and writing, can allow for students to make progress in both language and content. Although such an approach may be deemed time-consuming, we argue that the development of language and critical thinking skills is linked inextricably to the opportunities the child is provided to communicate concepts, perspectives, and ideas. In the next section we illustrate how communication-rich schooling can affect both language as well as literacy-related content objectives, and therefore can be a means to accomplishing content objectives while simultaneously promoting language development.

Wolbers (2007) has developed a communication-based approach to writing instruction—strategic and interactive writing instruction (SIWI)—that encompasses the dual objectives of promoting expressive/receptive language development and writing skill development. For the purpose of this chapter, two elements of SIWI are described in detail. They are (1) the dialogic, interactive format of guided writing; and (2) the use of communication strategies for the purpose of meaning making and meaning sharing in a space called the *language zone*. A full description of the SIWI model can be accessed elsewhere (Wolbers et al., 2012, 2014).

One element of SIWI is a dialogic, interactive approach to guided writing whereby deaf and hard-of-hearing students engage in writing with other students and the teacher. It is through this dialogic, interactive format that students are apprenticed as writers and provided a conversation through which natural language learning can occur. They share their ideas, build on each other's contributions, and determine necessary writing actions cooperatively. The approach is based on dialogic pedagogy principles that purport understanding is constructed through collective problem solving in shared activity (Wells, 2000).

Successful use of dialogic pedagogy is predicated on the teacher having a disposition toward learning that is inquisitive and exploratory (Burbules, 1993) while valuing and encouraging student contributions (Tharp & Gallimore, 1988). It also means the teacher has the ability to orchestrate skillfully students' talk on a moment-to-moment basis by questioning, eliciting, or listening and then contingently reconceptualizing, expanding, clarifying, challenging, offering, or weaving comments into a larger tapestry of meaning (Gavelek & Raphael, 1996; Goldenberg, 1992). In short, the goal is to sustain conversational involvement as a means of advancing understanding (Mariage, 2001). Being engaged in conversation with students helps the teacher monitor the level of independence the students have for an activity, and provide the needed level of support they may need to complete the activity successfully. In other words, by using open-ended questions or providing more subtle prompts, the teacher knows when to "step back" to release control over the learner's activity and when to "step in" by offering guiding comments or modeling when the activity is out of reach (Englert & Dunsmore, 2002). One example of "stepping in" is the teacher communicating what she is thinking if she was in student's shoes at a given moment of the student's writing activity. By thinking aloud, the teacher makes the normally invisible cognitive activity of an expert writer visible through language, and—when done in language students understand—deaf students are able to appreciate the real deliberations, negotiations, and struggles a writer experiences. Therefore, the dialogic exchanges of guided writing allow students to develop their thinking, talking, and actions as mature writers. Mayer et al. (2002) alluded to the dialogic pedagogical practices of exemplary teachers of the deaf as those with the potential to spur the conceptual and linguistic development of deaf children.

A second important element of SIWI is the provision for meaning making and meaning sharing in a space called the *language zone*. Sustained communication between the student and the teacher helps support students in expressing their thoughts, clarifying intended meanings, or repairing communication breakdowns. When meaning is understood and shared between members, concepts can be paired with sign language and/or spoken language. The teacher looks for opportunities to model language around understood concepts, and then encourages students to take up modeled language in their own expressions through natural turn taking about the concepts.

The following dialogue that transpired in a third grade classroom serves to illustrate such a communicative interaction. The students and teacher had baked a pumpkin pie for a Thanksgiving celebration and were in the process of recounting that experience in a newsletter to their parents. While engaged in planning for writing, the students exhibited difficulty explaining in signs what they had done to bake the pie. They revisited digital pictures taken during the baking activity, and the teacher asked open questions such as "What did we do here? What is that?"

Student responses were largely limited or confusing. For example, when pointing at a picture of two students measuring the brown sugar, the teacher asked what they were doing, and a student responded, "Freeze."

The teacher tried to clarify by asking, "Freeze? Like ice?"

The student pointed at the picture and added, "Cold."

The teacher tried to probe deeper into the student's understanding by pointing at the sugar and asking, "Cold?"

At that point, she directed the class to a different student who was signing, "Sugar." She asked, "Do you remember what kind of sugar that was? Which color was it, white or brown?"

The students responded with, "Brown sugar."

The first student again joined the conversation by pointing at the sugar and saying, "Sugar freeze," and he proceeded to communicate something that resembled the claw-shaped hands coming together like a ball and pressing inward.

The teacher then understood what he intended to express and recast his expression by saying, "Yes, the sugar was hard. It was hard." The student copied the teacher's use of the sign "hard" while nodding his head.

While recapping the activity in each of the digital pictures, the teacher asked students to name the items in the pictures and explain what they were doing with those items. Based on students' responses, she was able to support students in their expressions when there were gaps in vocabulary or grammar. Because the teacher's model language was purposefully more complex and complete than the expressive abilities of the students, she carefully grounded newly exposed language to the concrete objects and actions in the pictures by pointing frequently to help connect language with meaning.

After recapping the activity using the digital pictures, the students made decisions about what information they wanted to include in their writing. The events or ideas they wanted to include were drawn on medium-size sticky notes and then ordered on the board the way they would be presented in writing. This activity provided the students with two more opportunities to express the various events of making a pumpkin pie—once while deciding what events to include on the sticky notes and once again when discussing how to order the events.

The teacher used every opportunity to guide the students to describe and express fully the events in ASL. A rule of thumb used by SIWI teachers is to provide sufficient language modeling and supported engagement around understood concepts so that students are able to leave the room with enough linguistic resources acquired to explain the event to someone new with greater clarity and detail than they currently have.

Next, the teacher and students worked on moving the expressed concepts in ASL to writing their ideas in English for the newsletter. They tackled one drawing at a time, labeling the drawing with English words and phrases and then using the notes to construct English sentences. At times, the ASL expression needed to be expanded or clarified further. For example, the teacher asked the students to come to the front of the class to role-play an event that helped them notice actions that were not included in their language expressions. One student became the oven and another student was the teacher who turned on the oven. The teacher pointed at the person role-playing the turning on of the oven, and asked, "Who?"

The students then realized neither their drawing nor their expression included the teacher, so they added a picture of the teacher and also wrote the word *teacher* next to the drawing.

The teacher then asked, "What is the teacher doing?"

She guided the students to express the event by supplementing or supplanting the gesture and role-play actions with ASL: "The teacher turned on the oven."

When expression of the concept in ASL was clear and complete, the teacher began asking for the English words associated with each item or action in the drawing or role-play. She guided them to finding equivalence in English for what they had just fully expressed in ASL.

"When we sign this [turning of knob], what are the words we use in English for that?" asked the teacher.

One student responded with "on" and the teacher reacted positively and provided more scaffolding by relating the concept to turning on the lights.

When they had found the English equivalent and they had labeled the picture with *teacher, oven,* and *turn on,* the teacher requested them to start putting together the ideas into a full English sentence that could be drafted on their English board and revised for their newsletter.

In this example, we see how the teacher and students were engaged in a writing activity; yet, much time and care is taken in the language zone with digital pictures, drawings, role-play, and gestures to clarify, develop, and expand students' expressive language in ASL associated with the shared concepts. Thus, the teacher is intentional in building understanding and skills for writing by first expressing concepts through the air. In that regard, SIWI is premised on the notion that good writing is based on having a clear idea on what to say.

With the embedding of dialogic pedagogical practices during guided writing and the use of meaning making and sharing strategies, SIWI serves as an example of a communication-rich school program that can simultaneously address both content and language objectives. In fact, deaf and hard-of-hearing students receiving SIWI, when ASL is the expressive language of focus, grow in their abilities to express increasingly clear and complex language as measured by gains in mean length of ASL utterances and declines in unintelligible utterances. Furthermore, students—regardless of lower or higher language proficiency at the start of instruction—show similar language growth over time (Dostal & Wolbers, 2014).

At the same time, quasi-experimental research demonstrates that elementary and middle grade students receiving SIWI who are diverse by virtue of hearing loss, school setting, and language mode also make statistically significant literacy gains. Students have evidenced greater improvements with writing skill associated with a taught genre, such as information reports, as measured by primary trait rubrics. They also show greater gains than students in a comparison group with untaught genres of writing (Wolbers, 2008a). Second, there are statistically significant gains in writing fluency as measured with length variables such as total words or number of T-units (Dostal & Wolbers, 2014; Wolbers, 2010). Students have additionally demonstrated significantly greater progress with written language (such as subject/verb agreement, correct use of determiners, number of complex sentences) and conventions (punctuation, for example) than comparison group students (Wolbers, 2008a). Third, there are significantly greater gains in word identification ability among students who receive SIWI compared with those who do not (Wolbers, 2007). Last, SIWI studies, which are exploratory in nature, show similar positive outcomes for primary traits of writing, written language, writing fluency, and word identification (Wolbers, 2008b; Wolbers et al., 2012) while suggesting possible improvements in students' abilities to edit and revise their writing (Wolbers, 2008b), writing with greater sentence complexity and awareness (Wolbers et al., 2012), and reducing the ASL grammatical features present in their writing (Wolbers et al., 2013). All together, we can deduce that the time and care taken to provide a school-based environment conducive to natural language learning does not need to happen at the expense of academic content learning; rather, both can happen jointly. The outcomes of SIWI allude to the importance of accessible, meaningful, and rich communication as the central driving force of effective school-based programming for deaf students. Ultimately, instructional and programmatic approaches should support natural processes of language development. We have illustrated how this occurs in preschool, in a social studies class, and in a writing program. The next section shows how the principle of accessible, meaningful, and rich communication may be applied in the design of video-based educational programming for supporting students' development of ASL and English literacy.

USE OF INTERACTIVE, EDUCATIONAL MEDIA TO BROADEN LANGUAGE INPUT

The greatest challenge in the education of deaf students probably lies in the question of how we can provide deaf children with access to communication that is understandable as well as an environment that allows them to communicate easily with others. Many deaf children start preschool without much language. The children's education is thus held hostage by the limited communicative skills they have. Ideally, they should go to a quality early-childhood education program with highly qualified teachers who not only can communicate well with them and provide rich language and literacy experiences, but also who are knowledgeable of child development especially in the areas of language, literacy, and cognitive development. These teachers would know how best to meet the individual needs of each child by identifying where the children are with regard to their language development, then scaffolding these skills by using strategies such as asking open-ended questions, providing new vocabulary, and connecting classroom activities to the students' everyday lives (e.g., International Reading Association & the National Association for the Education of Young Children, 1998). However, there may not be enough of these types of high-quality settings for deaf children in any type of school, including those that provide fluent sign language models (see Chapter 18).

One way to gauge the quality of language environment in early-childhood education programs for deaf children is by determining the extent to which literacy activities are incorporated throughout the day in various classroom activities. For example, interactive read-alouds provide opportunities for fostering key language and literacy skills, and researchers (such as Trelease [2013]) recommend reading aloud multiple times throughout the day in an early-childhood classroom. Yet, in a recent survey of 70 early-childhood educators of the deaf in the United States, 60% of teachers reported reading aloud to children only 15 minutes or less per day (Golos et al., manuscript in preparation).

Another way to gauge the quality of early-language environments is by determining the number of times teachers include ASL stories such as ABC stories (which are stories that include only the signs whose hand formations match the handshapes of the letters of the alphabet and put them in the alphabetic order), handshape stories (telling a story in a poetic way by using signs formed by a limited range of handshapes and putting them together in a patterned fashion), or number stories (telling a story using signs with the same handshapes that numerical signs use and putting them together in a numerical sequence). These activities provide deaf children an opportunity to become more attuned to the phonological structure of ASL (such as handshape, movement, palm orientation, location), to the letters of the alphabet, and to the numerical symbols. McQuarrie and Abbott (2013) suggested that an increased understanding on language through language play may be an important component to learning to read successfully. However, in the aforementioned survey, responses from 44 schools that used either ASL or Total Communication revealed only six teachers who provided ASL stories daily.

Children greatly benefit from having both linguistic and cultural role models at a young age (e.g., Holcomb, 1997). Although, ideally, all deaf children should be exposed to Deaf role models and fluent users of sign on a daily basis, few teachers reported providing such exposure (Golos et al., manuscript in preparation). Bringing a Deaf person to the classroom as a guest, volunteer, or aide is a good way to supplement deaf children's exposure to adults who can serve as a language model (Erting & Pfau, 1997) and can engage them in extended conversation. Yet, it appears this is not happening as frequently as it should (Golos et al., manuscript in preparation). For some, this may simply be the result of living in areas that do not have easy access to Deaf adult role models.

Although not intended to replace "live" models, research suggests that incorporation of educational media is a promising *supplemental* tool for providing language and cultural role models for those who do not have adequate access to them (e.g., Fisch, 2004). Research on educational media programs such as *Sesame Street* and *Blue's Clues* has long suggested that media can provide rich interactive experiences with language and literacy, particularly for struggling readers (Fisch, 2004), and even more so when teachers encourage interaction with media (e.g., Linebarger, 2009). More recent research reveals the same to be true for interactive educational media in ASL (e.g., Golos & Moses, 2013b). In a series of five studies (Golos & Moses, 2010, 2011, 2013a, 2013b, 2015), when deaf and hard-of-hearing children (n = 75) were exposed to a research-based educational video series (the *Peter's Picture* video series), they made significant gains in language and literacy skills targeted within each episode (such as vocabulary, knowledge of story elements, sequencing skills). This video series (see Golos and Moses [2013b] for a detailed description of the series and research studies) models Deaf characters interacting in ASL and was originally developed for parents and teachers to use in home or classroom settings to supplement "live" fluent language and cultural role models.

Similar to research-based strategies used during shared reading and other literacy activities, these videos incorporate strategies such as chaining and asking questions to elicit interactive behavior between the characters onscreen and the viewing audience. For example, in one episode, the main character, Peter, explains one of the target vocabulary items: *backyard*. After he describes what different types of backyard may look like, he asks both the child characters in the video and, virtually, the audience viewing the video, "What does your backyard look like?" He then pauses to give the viewing audience time to respond. This provides an opportunity for children viewing the video either to think of an answer in their head or respond in sign or spoken language. If not, an adult watching the video alongside the child can stop the video and repeat Peter's question to elicit a response. After the pause, Peter proceeds to answer his own question, providing multiple possible answers: "Maybe your backyard looks like this [followed by a description of a type of backyard such as one that is flat with grass and surrounded by a fence] or that [followed by a description of a different type of backyard such as one with rolling hills, no fence, and lots of trees]." By providing children different possible answers to the question, they are given a chance to affirm or change their answer. More important, the interaction gives children exposure to how language works and how to think, and it helps them realize that, for some questions, there are different possible answers. Not everyone has a backyard, nor do all backyards look the same.

After discussing the meaning of a given target vocabulary item, Peter helps viewers make a connection between the discussion about backyard and the printed English word by asking the viewing audience (along with child characters onscreen) to copy him as he signs the target vocabulary (BACKYARD), then fingerspells (B-A-C-K-Y-A-R-D), and finally repeats the same target sign (BACKYARD) while the printed word appears simultaneously across the screen. This process is repeated multiple times throughout each episode for the target vocabulary.

In each episode, Peter introduces new theme-based vocabulary before taking the onscreen children, along with the viewing audience, on a virtual adventure where he introduces them to one of his deaf friends, each of whom has a different type of job (librarian, chef, and so on). Different events occur, and Peter takes pictures. They then return to Peter's Place, where they sequence the pictures, play a word game, make a book, and retell the story of their adventure. This provides children, their parents, and teachers access to linguistic and cultural models through Deaf children and Deaf adults interacting with one another, as well as techniques on making connections between ASL and written English in different contexts.

This type of interactive medium has been effective in eliciting language and literacy-related behaviors from children who view the program. When viewing in small groups of peers, children engage by answering questions (in sign and/or spoken language), copying target vocabulary by signing or fingerspelling the words, asking questions, making comments related to the story, or pointing to print on screen (see Golos and Moses [2013b], for a review of studies). However, similar to live experiences, children learn and engage even more when adults make use of the media series to encourage communicative interaction with and support and build on the interaction the way educational programs such as *Peter's Picture* are designed to elicit (e.g., Golos & Moses, 2011).

Golos and Moses (2013b) recommended that to use the videos more fully, teachers can facilitate learning by conducting activities before, during, and after video viewing. For example, when teachers promote interaction during video viewing such as encouraging the children to copy Peter's signing or by pausing the video to ask open-ended questions, learning increases (Golos & Moses, 2013b). Furthermore, when teachers were provided with materials and implemented activities after video viewing, teachers reported that not only did children's learning increase, but also they carried over strategies demonstrated in the video into other daily activities (Golos & Moses, 2015).

One particularly interesting finding across studies is that engagement and learning occurred regardless of participants' diverse backgrounds, use of amplification, or amount of prior exposure to ASL such as whether they attended programs using ASL/English, spoken language, or a combination of speaking and signing. In fact, results from a recent study show that educational media in ASL may also benefit hearing children (Moses & Golos, 2015). Results across studies indicate that this type of medium may be of even greater benefit for children who arrive at preschool already delayed in language and literacy skills. It also supports previous research that suggests that exposure to sign language may foster language and literacy development even for children whose primary mode of communication is spoken language (e.g., Mayberry, 2007). These types of materials can be particularly useful for early-childhood educators who do not have access to Deaf adult role models and are thus unable to bring fluent language models into the classroom. Teachers in rural or mainstream settings or teachers who have many language delayed students may benefit particularly from these media as a means of not only providing cultural and linguistic role models, but also building background knowledge. In fact, anecdotal evidence suggests that some teachers are already incorporating these types of videos in the classroom. According to one teacher of deaf students:

> We use the videos as a "virtual" field trip. These videos provide in-depth access to language. Our students are able to "visit" places that are not accessible for them due to low economic status. Also, many of their families are not able to communicate to their children the places where they go (C. Davis, personal communication, October 16, 2014).

PEDAGOGY DRIVEN BY COMMUNICATION THAT IS AUTHENTIC

For the most part, the education of deaf students has been driven by the persistent fact that many deaf children are not making progress in language development, at least at a pace that is commensurate with what is expected of any normally developing child. Children in general are expected to acquire language without any assistance. This is an appropriate perception; however, it also inadvertently fosters a response—which is misinformed—that when a deaf child does not make progress in language development as "expected," something is wrong with the child. Such a perception may be rooted in the fact that people take many things about language development for granted. If we look at the world of deaf children through a sociocultural lens, we begin to understand their anemic progress in language development more broadly. This will help free us from the perception of the child's language-learning capabilities as the site of a problem, and will allow us to move to the language-learning context as the site to address the child's language-learning needs.

Educators are correct when they consider language learning an important area to address. It is likely the most important consideration to make because many things about the child's development and academic achievement are dependent on the level of language skills a child has. Educators, by default, try to address the language delay within the framework of school and instruction. Ideally, deaf children's limited access to language should be remediated in the home and in the community, but it is in school that educators have more leverage to address the problem. The language development difference between deaf children and other children often leads too quickly and uncritically to the notion that deaf children need remediation in language learning.

Throughout the years, professionals working with deaf students have tried to address deaf students' language-learning needs by focusing on approaches that are largely designed to teach language. What we are trying to argue is that instead of the *direct* teaching of language to deaf students, educators should be looking more at the creation of opportunities for *natural* language learning within the classroom and less at the remedial approaches in language instruction. It is necessary to make use of deaf children's inherent language-learning capabilities. If the social context of deaf children's lives in the home and the community does not give deaf children ample opportunities to tap their language-learning capabilities, then school should step in and create the kind of language-learning opportunities deaf children are not provided at home and in the community. Furthermore, the social context of learning is rarely discussed in deaf education (but see Chapter 8) and a possible reason for this is the prevalent perception that the ability to benefit from a social approach to learning presupposes the child has enough language to begin with. Another reason is that the teachers, especially those with limited signing skills, may find it difficult to sustain extended conversation with their deaf students.

The studies discussed in this chapter reveal collectively the importance of access to communication-rich environments, argue for their implementation, and give examples of the impact of providing deaf students with these kind of environments. We have seen from the vignettes about John and Jill about how the parents may vary in how they respond to their children being deaf and how the kind of response that they make has an impact on their children's language development. John's parents decided on a spoken language approach for John as the sole communication mode. They most likely may have wanted what they believed to be in John's best interest and may also have wanted John to learn language the way most children do. Unfortunately, his progress in the development of spoken language was slow and arduous, indicating it was not a feasible way for him to acquire language. John subsequently fell further and further behind. Jill's parents, on the other hand, were under a completely different set of circumstances. The school district where the family lived did not have a program for deaf students because there was a state school for the deaf in the neighborhood. Jill's mother unwittingly set her daughter on the course of learning sign language almost immediately. She was told she needed to learn signs; she just obliged and managed to learn them. The preschool class (in that state school) her daughter attended, which was full of signing deaf peers and a teacher who was a skilled signer, was crucial in keeping Jill engaged constantly in daily communicative interactions and to do so in a way that pushed the limits on Jill's development of language and cognitive abilities.

Some signing teachers unwittingly but fortuitously teach in a way that provides opportunities for students to acquire language skills— that is, through the act of communicating and discussing the content being taught about. Some teachers use dialogic pedagogy without realizing it and, by not being aware of it, they do not know its potential value nor do they try to maximize its use as a teaching methodology. The merits of dialogic pedagogy should be expounded on, its use encouraged, and its practice promulgated more widely. The formal evaluation of dialogic pedagogy using a tool such as IC has the potential not only to help make dialogic pedagogy seen as a viable teaching methodology and but also to help individual teachers develop the fine points of the methodology. Dialogic pedagogy is an effective way to nurture natural language development without making language learning the main focus. Learning about the content is the goal of schooling, and dialogic pedagogy is an effective approach to help students think, understand, and learn about that content. After all, as Tharp and Gallimore (1988, p. 111) put it, "To most truly teach, one must converse; to truly converse is to teach," and we add that teaching that is steeped in authentic communication is the kind of teaching that results in the acquisition of language as a by-product of talking and learning about the content.

Instructional programming for deaf students that is informed by sociocultural theories of language development and learning is in its nascent stage of development. SIWI and educational media-based curricula such as *Peter's Picture* are examples of how instructional innovations for helping students learn written English are designed on the principles of meaningful and understandable communication, and that communication needs to take place in the language that allows students to communicate effectively. Any design of instructional programming for deaf students needs to involve a thoughtful consideration of how the provision of the opportunities to communicate may be a part of the mix. Educators need to consider the value of providing deaf students with an opportunity, not only to express what they want to say or what they are not clear about in ways that others can understand, but also to get information from others that they need in ways they can understand. The effort to support students' development of a sign language such as ASL does not necessarily compete in the use of instructional time with the goals of helping them learn literacy skills. As a matter of fact, the success of both SIWI (which is for helping students develop written English skills) and *Peter's Picture* (which is for helping students acquire key language and early literacy skills in both ASL and English) suggests that using the most accessible language with which students are most comfortable is effective in helping them learn written English efficiently and in helping to bolster their primary language. It is arguably conceivable that instructional programming based on authentic communication using whatever modes required to maximize communication has the potential to support language and literacy learning also for children for whom spoken language is the primary mode of communication.

In summary, we believe firmly that deaf children do not differ from other children in terms of language-learning capabilities. When deaf children are exposed to language that is fully accessible, they exhibit robust language development (Meier, 1991). The challenge is in making sure there is a goodness of fit between a deaf child and the language in the child's environment. Language needs to be accessible, and there needs to be enough people with whom deaf children are able to communicate.

For too long the prospect of language development of deaf children has been left to chance and dictated largely by the sociocultural world into which they are born. Some are born into a world where language in a visually accessible modality is already present. As a result, these children are in an environment where their language-learning abilities flourish naturally. However, for many deaf children, the prospect of natural language learning is determined by different variables that are varingly in place by chance. Some parents may innovate by going ahead and learning sign language or by improvising on the language of the home. Some deaf children have enough residual hearing or are able to benefit from the use of cochlear implants that enable varying levels of development of spoken communication. In short, the scope of language development that each deaf child undergoes is subject not only to the extent of access they have to different formats of communication but also to the frequency of high-quality communicative interactions they can be a part of. The extent of access to understandable communication is the ultimate factor that determines the quality and quantity of language to which they are exposed, and this is what shapes the course of their language development. The most ideal course of action is, of course, to help families figure how to make communication as accessible as possible for their deaf child and how to ensure the deaf child is able to participate in various formats of communicative interaction at home. Despite the best efforts of early-intervention programs, schools will continue to receive deaf students of all ages whose language development reflects the consequences of limited access to communication. Schools need to seek ways to level the playing field for deaf students' language development by providing enriched opportunities for natural language learning. A powerful way of doing this is by shifting to instruction that is driven by authentic communication.

It may be a little unusual for school as the place of instruction to consider being a place for natural language learning. Usually opportunities for natural language learning belong to the domain of home and the community. However, for deaf children school needs to become an extension of home and the community. Schools have the potential to create the needed personnel and resources to become the place where diverse deaf children are provided opportunities not only for natural language learning, but also for catching up with language development. We need to acknowledge that the best course of language development is to acquire it naturally, and schools will go a long way by instituting pedagogical practices that recognize that deaf children need to be provided opportunities for natural language development and by grounding content-area instruction in authentic and meaningful communication.

ACKNOWLEDGMENTS

The research reported by Kuntze was supported by a subaward to Boston University by a National Science Foundation (NSF) grant (no. SBE-0541953) through Gallaudet's Science of Learning Center on Visual Language and Visual Learning (VL2). The research reported by Wolbers was supported by the Institute of Education Sciences, U.S. Department of Education, through grant R324A120085 to the University of Tennessee. The opinions expressed are those of the authors and do not represent views of the National Science Foundation or the U.S. Department of Education.

REFERENCES

Bandura, A. (1977). *Social cognitive theory.* Englewood Cliffs, NJ: Prentice-Hall.

Bandura, A. (1986). *Social foundations of thought and action: A social cognitive theory.* Englewood Cliffs, NJ: Prentice-Hall.

Bruner, J. (1996). *The culture of education.* Cambridge, MA: Harvard University Press.

Burbules, N. (1993). *Dialogue in teaching.* New York: Teachers College Press.

Center for Research on Education, Diversity & Excellence (2014). *Instructional Conversation.* http://manoa.hawaii.edu/coe/crede/sample-page/.

Courtin, C., & Melot, A. M. (1998). Development of theories in deaf children. In M. Marschark (Ed.), *Psychological perspectives of deafness* (pp. 79–102). Malwah, NJ: Erlbaum.

Dewey, J. (1990). *The school and society: The child and the curriculum.* Chicago, IL: University of Chicago Press.

Dostal, H., & Wolbers, K. (2014). Developing language and writing skills of deaf and hard of hearing students: A simultaneous approach. *Literacy Research and Instruction, 53*(3), 245–268.

Englert, C. S., & Dunsmore, K. (2002). A diversity of teaching and learning paths: Teaching writing in situated activity. In J. Brophy (Ed.), *Social constructivist teaching: Affordances and constraints* (pp. 81–130). Boston: JAI.

Erting, C. J., & Kuntze, M. (2008). Language socialization in deaf communities. In P. Duff and N. H. Hornberger (Eds.), *Encyclopedia of language and education* (2nd ed., Vol. 8, pp. 287–300). New York: Springer Science+Business Media.

Erting, L., & Pfau, J. (1997). *Becoming bilingual: Facilitating English literacy development using ASL in preschool.* Sharing Ideas series. Washington, DC: Gallaudet University Pre-College National Mission Programs.

Ewoldt, C., & Saulnier, K. (1992). *Engaging in literacy: A longitudinal study of three- to seven-year-old deaf participants.* Final report for the Gallaudet Research Institute, Center for Studies in Education and Human Development. Washington, DC: Gallaudet University.

Fisch, S. M. (2004). *Children's learning from educational television*. Mahwah, NJ: Routledge.
Gavelek, J. R., & Raphael, T. E. (1996). Changing talk about text: New roles for teachers and students. *Language Arts, 73*(3), 182–192.
Goldenberg, C. (1991). Instructional conversations and their classroom application. Educational practice report: 2. http://files.eric.ed.gov/fulltext/ED341 253.pdf.
Goldenberg, C. (1992). Instructional conversations: Promoting comprehension through discussion. *The Reading Teacher, 46*, 316–326.
Golos, D. (2010). Literacy behaviors of deaf preschoolers during video viewing. *Sign Language Studies, 11*(1), 76–99.
Golos, D., & Moses, A. (2011). How teacher mediation during video viewing facilitates literacy behaviors. *Sign Language Studies, 12*(1), 98–118.
Golos, D., & Moses, A. (2013a). Developing preschool deaf children's language and literacy learning from an educational media series. *American Annals of the Deaf, 158*(4), 411–425.
Golos, D., & Moses, A. (2013b). The benefits of using educational videos in American Sign Language in early childhood settings. *Learning Landscapes, 6*(2), 125–147.
Golos, D., & Moses, A. (2015). Supplementing an educational video series with video-related classroom activities and materials. *Sign Language Studies, 15*(2), 103–125.
Greeno, J. G., Collins, A., & Resnick, L. B. (1997). Cognition and learning. In D. Berliner & R. Calfee (Eds.), *Handbook of educational psychology* (pp. 15–45). New York: Simon & Schuster Macmillan.
Harris, R. L. (2010). *A case study of extended discourse in an ASL/English bilingual preschool classroom*. http://www.gallaudet.edu/documents/rgs/sol/harris-dissertation.pdf
Hartman, M. (1996). Thinking and learning in classroom discourse. *Volta Review, 98*(3), 93–106.
Hillocks, G. (2002). *The testing trap: How state assessments control learning*. New York, NY: Teachers College Press.
Hoff, E. (2006). How social contexts support and shape language development. *Developmental Review, 26*(1), 55–88.
Holcomb, T. (1997). Development of deaf bicultural identity. *American Annals of the Deaf, 142*(2), 89–93.
International Reading Association & National Association for the Education of Young Children (1998). Learning to read and write: Developmentally appropriate practices for young children. A joint position statement of the International Reading Association and the National Association for the Education of Young Children. *Young Children, 53*(4), 30–46.
Jackendoff, R. (1994). *Patterns in the mind*. New York, NY: BasicBooks.
James, S. (2004). Language development in the young child. In T. Maynard & N. Thomas (Eds.) *An introduction to early childhood studies* (pp. 28–38). London: Sage.
Keating, E., & Mirus, G. (2003). Examining interactions across language modalities: Deaf children and hearing peers at school. *Anthropology and Education, 34*(2), 115–135.

Kluwin, T. (1983). Discourse in deaf classrooms: The structure of teaching episodes. *Discourse Processes, 6*, 275–293.
Kraker, M. J. (2000). Classroom discourse: Teaching, learning and learning disabilities. *Teaching and Teacher Education, 16*, 295–313.
Kumaravadivelu, B. (2006). *Understanding language teaching*. Mahwah, NJ: Lawrence Erlbaum Associates.
Kuntze, M., Fish, S., Berlove, N., Goodman, C., & Kim, K. (2008). The longitudinal study on the higher order thinking skills and acquisition of reading skills in children from ages 3–9. Presented at a poster session, NSF Center on Science of Learning annual meeting. Washington, DC.
Kuntze, M. (2010). Tracking the development of language and discourse skills of ASL-competent children. Visual Language and Visual Learning 2009-2010 Presentation Series. Gallaudet University, Washington DC.
Lantolf, J. (2000). *Sociocultural theory and second language learning*. New York: Oxford University Press.
Linebarger, D. (2009). Evaluation of the *Between the Lions* Mississippi literacy initiative. http://pbskids.org/read/files/BTL_Mississippi_April2009.pdf.
Mariage, T. V. (2001). Features of an interactive writing discourse: Conversational involvement, conventional knowledge, and internalization in "Morning Message." *Journal of Learning Disabilities, 34*(2), 172–196.
Marschark, M. (1993). *Psychological development of deaf children*. New York: Oxford University Press.
Martin, D., Bat-Chava, Y., Lalwani, A., & Waltzman, S. B. (2010). Peer relationships of deaf children with cochlear implants: Predictors of peer entry and peer interaction success. *Journal of Deaf Studies and Deaf Education, 16*(1), 108–120.
Mather, S. A. (1987). Eye gaze & communication in a deaf classroom. *Sign Language Studies, 54*(1), 11–30.
Mayberry, R. (2007). When timing is everything: Age of first-language acquisition effects on second-language learning. *Applied Psycholinguistics, 28*, 537–549.
Mayer, C., Akamatsu, C. T., & Stewart, D. (2002). A model for effective practice: Dialogic inquiry with students who are deaf. *Exceptional Children, 68*(4), 485–502.
McNeill, D. (1970). *The acquisition of language: The study of developmental linguistics*. New York: Harper & Row.
McQuarrie, L. M., & Abbott, M. (2013). Bilingual deaf students' phonological awareness in ASL and reading skills in English. *Sign Language Studies 14*(1), 61–81. (special issue on assessment).
Mead, G. H. (1934). *Mind, self and society*. Chicago, IL: Chicago University Press.
Meadow, K. P. (1975). The development of deaf children. In E. M. Hetherington (Ed.), *Review of child development research* (Vol. 5, pp. 441–508). Chicago, IL: University of Chicago Press.
Meier, R. P. (1991). Language acquisition by deaf children. *American Scientist, 79*(1), 60–70.
Meristo, M., Falkman, K. W., Hjelmquist, E., Tedoldi, M., Surian, L., & Siegal, M. (2007). Language access and theory of mind reasoning: Evidence from deaf children in bilingual and oralist environments. *Developmental Psychology, 43*(5), 1156–1169.

Moses, A., & Golos, D. (2015). An alternative approach to early literacy: The effects of ASL on educational media in literacy skills acquisition for hearing children. *Early Childhood Education Journal*.

Muma, J. R., & Teller, H. (2001). Developments in cognitive socialization: Implications for deaf education. *American Annals of the Deaf*, 146(1), 31–38.

Mweri, J. G. (2014). Diversity in education: Kenyan sign language as a medium of instruction in schools for the deaf in Kenya. *Multilingual Education*, 4(1), 1–14.

Nystrand, M. (1997). *Opening dialogue: Understanding the dynamics of language and learning in the English classroom*. New York: Teachers College Press.

O'Brien, C. (2011). The influence of deaf culture on school culture and leadership: A case study of a school for the deaf. PhD dissertation, University of Missouri.

Pinker, S. (1995). *The language instinct: How the mind creates language*. New York, NY: Harper Collins.

Pribanić, L. (2006). Sign language and deaf education: A new tradition. *Sign Language & Linguistics*, 9(1–2), 233–254.

Ramsey, C., & Padden, C. (1998). Natives and newcomers: Gaining access to literacy in a classroom for deaf children. *Anthropology & Education Quarterly*, 29(1), 5–24.

Rose, S., McAnally, P. L., & Quigley, S. P. (2004). *Language learning practices with deaf children* (3rd ed.). Austin, TX: PRO-ED.

Roy, C. (1989). A sociolinguistic analysis of the interpreter's role in the turn exchanges of an interpreted event. PhD Dissertation, Georgetown University.

Schlesinger, I. M. (1975). Grammatical development: The first steps. In E. Lenneberg & E. Lenneberg (Eds.) *Foundations of language development: A multidisciplinary approach* (Vol. 1, pp. 203–223). London: Academic Press.

Silvestre, N., Ramspott, A., & Pareto, I. D. (2007). Conversational skills in a semistructured interview and self-concept in deaf students. *Journal of Deaf Studies and Deaf Education*, 12(1), 38–54.

Smith, D. H., & Ramsey, C. L. (2004). Classroom discourse practices of a deaf teacher using American Sign Language. *Sign Language Studies*, 5(1), 39–62.

Tharp, R. G., & Gallimore, R. (1988). *Rousing minds to life: Teaching, learning, and schooling in social context*. New York: Cambridge University Press.

Tharp, R. G., & Gallimore, R. (1991). The *instructional conversation: Teaching and learning in social activity*. Research report 2. Santa Cruz, CA: National Center for Research on Cultural Diversity and Second Language Learning.

Trelease, J. (2013). *The read aloud handbook*. London: Penguin Books.

Trueba, H. T. (1988). Culturally based explanations of minority students' academic achievement. *Anthropology & Education Quarterly*, 19, 270–287.

Vygotsky, L. S. (1962). *Thought and language*. Cambridge, MA: MIT Press.

Ward, I. (1994). *Literacy ideology, and dialogue: Towards a dialogic pedagogy*. Albany, NY: State University of New York Press.

Wells, G. (1981). *Learning through interaction. Volume 1: The study of language development*. New York: Cambridge University Press.

Wells, G. (2000). Dialogic inquiry in education: Building on the legacy of Vygotsky. In C. D. Lee & P. Smagorinsky (Eds.), *Vygotskian perspectives on literacy research* (pp. 51–85). New York, NY: Cambridge University Press.

Wertsch, J. V. (1991). *Voices of the mind: A sociocultural approach to mediated action*. Cambridge, MA: Harvard University Press.

Wilkens, C. P., & Hehir, T. P. (2008). Deaf education and bridging social capital: A theoretical approach. *American Annals of the Deaf, 153*(3), 275–284.

Wolbers, K. (2007). Strategic and interactive writing instruction (SIWI): Apprenticing deaf students in the construction of informative text. PhD dissertation, Michigan State University.

Wolbers, K. (2008a). Strategic and interactive writing instruction (SIWI): Apprenticing deaf students in the construction of English text. *ITL International Journal of Applied Linguistics, 156*, 299–326.

Wolbers, K. (2008b). Using balanced and interactive writing instruction to improve the higher order and lower order writing skills of deaf students. *Journal of Deaf Studies and Deaf Education, 13*(2), 255–277.

Wolbers, K. (2010). Using ASL and print-based sign to build fluency and greater independence with written English among deaf students. *L1-Educational Studies in Language and Literature, 10*(1), 99–125.

Wolbers, K., Bowers, L., Dostal, H., & Graham, S. C. (2013). Deaf writers' application of ASL knowledge to English. *International Journal of Bilingual Education and Bilingualism, 17*(4), 410–428.

Wolbers, K., Dostal, H., & Bowers, L. (2012). "I was born full deaf." Written language outcomes after one year of strategic and interactive writing instruction (SIWI). *Journal of Deaf Studies and Deaf Education, 17*(1), 19–38.

Wolbers, K., Graham, S. C., Dostal, H., & Bowers, L. (2014). A description of ASL features in writing. *Ampersand, 1*, 19–27.

Wood, D., Bruner, J. S., & Ross, G. (1976). The role of tutoring in problem solving. *Journal of Child Psychology and Psychiatry, 17*(2), 89–100.

5

On the Home Front: Parent Personality, Support, and Deaf Children

Patrick J. Brice, Rachael M. Plotkin, and Jennifer Reesman

Some years ago, Howard Cutler, a psychiatrist, had the opportunity to interview the Dalai Lama (Dalai Lama & Cutler, 2009). He described to his holiness the case of a young woman who seemed to have everything anyone could want—she was bright, attractive, and successful academically, and she had a supportive family—but she was extremely depressed, bordering on suicidal. Cutler asked how the Dalai Lama understood such a situation. After a pause, his holiness replied, "I don't know. People are complicated!" People are complicated indeed. Many people, families and professionals alike, are interested in fostering the well-being and successful outcomes for deaf and hard-of-hearing children, and in studying the factors that affect success. Yet, for almost every finding published that helps in illuminating the factors that contribute to positive outcomes, we can find other results that are inconsistent at best, or completely contradictory at worst.

Our goal in this chapter is to look at our current knowledge on the topic of parents and families with deaf children, and the family factors that have been studied and are thought or found to be related to the success of deaf children. This includes parenting stress, family support, communication, and child characteristics, and all factors that can contribute to diversity in developmental and academic outcomes. Our aim is to point out some important characteristics that are only recently being incorporated into the literature and show how we need a more complex and nuanced understanding of parent–child relationships. It is not simply that parental behavior influences a child's growth and development. Nor is it simply the case that a child's behavior or characteristics influences a parent's stress or adjustment. Parents come to parenting with a lifetime of experiences, understandings, and attitudes. These past learnings, coming out of a family living in a society and culture, influence how parents understand their children and how they perceive of their children's needs. These *perceptions* and dispositions, based on a lifetime of experience, often prove to be more important in determining and shaping the experience of a child than any objective attributes of the child or the family. By taking these understandings into account, those working in the field of deaf education and in the trenches at home raising deaf children, may do a better job of providing the kind of support, service, and advice that foster success. In this chapter, we examine more closely the variables most salient on the home front, and offer a framework and lens for understanding and supporting families of deaf children to develop resilience.

WHAT IS THE EFFECT OF HEARING LOSS?

When it comes to studying deaf children and their families, researchers started with simple questions influenced by simple models of development. In its most basic form, the question was: How does hearing loss affect child development? The dependent variables in question included cognition or intelligence, language, and social behavior. The early studies based on Piaget's theory of cognitive development are examples of this question. Hans Furth's (1966) studies looking at whether deaf children achieved conservation skills illustrate the basic form of this question. Despite his false assumption that deaf children were growing in the absence of language, the efforts to measure conservation in deaf children examined the effects of hearing loss on cognition and cognitive development.

Since those early studies on Piagetian tasks, researchers from countries around the world have proceeded in a systematic and comprehensive manner to examine what may be viewed as qualitative differences in how deaf children process information. Marschark and his colleagues have presented data suggesting that deaf children do not use a top-down strategy in problem solving (Marschark, 2003) or in approaches to reading (Marschark et al., 1993). They suggested that a focus on individual items as opposed to relations between items or items and a larger picture is a difference (Marschark & Wauters, 2008). Similarly, research on short-term or working memory in deaf children (and adults) has found consistent performance differences that appear to reflect dissimilar underlying information-processing strategies (Hall & Bavelier, 2010). Ongoing research programs examining information processing and neurocognitive functioning in deaf children and adults hope to provide a more sophisticated understanding of cognition and language in the future.

Another body of research, on language development in deaf children, exists that comes from the same fundamental question: How does hearing loss affect development of a language? One area of study has been the development of sign language, particularly a native sign language such as American Sign Language, in deaf children with deaf parents. Linguists have studied various aspects of language development, such as babbling (Petitto & Marentette, 1991), phonological development (Marentette & Mayberry, 2000), first words/signs, and development of sentences (Folven & Bonvillian, 1991). The general conclusion in this area of research is that deaf children learn a sign language in the same way that hearing children learn a spoken language, with parallel timing. Schick and Hoffmeister (2001), for example, found that deaf children with hearing parents learn American Sign Language in a way that seems easy and effortless when they are exposed or immersed in it from a young age.

Research on deaf children learning spoken language concludes that, as one would predict, the rate of (spoken) language development is slower in deaf children (Blamey & Sarant, 2011). Blamey and Sarant (2011) noted "there are no simple relationships among spoken language, age, and hearing levels" (p. 250). Perhaps ironically, research does suggest that *nonverbal* intelligence is one of the strongest predictors of language outcomes for deaf children (Mayne et al., 2000). Blamey and Sarant (2011) suggest that it may be a "combination of nonverbal intelligence and cognitive processing strategies such as working memory span and verbal rehearsal" (p. 251) that underlies language learning.

Children, however, develop and learn through relationships (see Chapter 4). It is not just the specific type of communication or the language choice that may or may not make a difference; it is the quality of the relationship in which the communication occurs. Pressman et al. (1999) demonstrated this in a study of families participating in the Colorado Home Intervention Research Project. They monitored 24 deaf and hard-of-hearing toddlers and their families receiving early-intervention services and found that, even after controlling for initial levels of language development, maternal sensitivity, measured by the Sensitivity subscale of the Emotional Availability Scales (Biringen & Robinson, 1991), predicted later language growth significantly. Pressman et al. (1999) proposed that maternal sensitivity could provide a supportive context even when symbolic communication is unclear. Sarant et al. (2009) also found, in an Australian sample, that family member involvement in their child's life and education was a significant predictor of spoken language outcomes in 57 children younger than six years. They concluded that family involvement was one of the most important aspects of early intervention to foster and to which to attend in supporting language development.

COCHLEAR IMPLANTS

Cochlear implantation has changed the experience of hearing loss for many families. Cochlear implants (CIs) are becoming more sophisticated, and children are having them implanted at younger ages to reap the benefits they may provide in language and overall development. As with many areas of research involving deaf and hard-of-hearing children, the results are often inconsistent (see Chapter 18). One of the most obvious questions to ask is whether children who received a CI have better speech and language than children who do not. CIs were developed with exactly this point in mind; by improving auditory skills, the child would develop better speech and language.

The data on CIs thus far are variable. Some studies (Dettman & Dowell, 2010; Svirsky et al., 2010) showed children using CIs do better in spoken language. Other researchers report more variability in outcomes (Dowell et al., 2004). Speech production of children with CIs has been rated to be more intelligible than that of deaf children without CIs (Chin et al., 2003). Children with CIs also seem to be faster learning spoken language than children who use hearing aids (Geers, 2006), although interpretation of these results is complicated by inherent differences between the groups that are unable to be controlled. Not surprisingly, earlier implantation appears to foster improved and faster spoken language development (Svirsky et al., 2004).

CI use also appears to aid academic achievement, although Spencer et al. (2011) point out that the evidence does have inconsistencies and that achievement is still not completely equivalent to that expected for hearing children. Some researchers (e.g., Geers et al., 2008) have reported that reading achievement lagged further and further behind as children with CIs became older. Age of implantation may be playing a role, although data from various studies have suggested better reading outcomes for earlier (Archbold et al., 2008) and later (Geers, 2004) implantation. Spencer et al. (2011) argued convincingly for conceptualizing children with CIs as hard-of-hearing children. They are not functioning like children with typical hearing, but neither are they functioning like deaf children without CIs, requiring a thoughtful and individualized approach to education and intervention.

The impact of CI use on social interaction and social development also shows empirical research with conflicting findings. Interviews with parents of children with CIs done by Bat-Chava and Deignan (2001) and Christiansen and Leigh (2002) found parents generally reported improvement in their children's social life. This included becoming more outgoing, having more hearing friends, and interacting more frequently with hearing children. Some children, though, were reported to still have difficulties in social situations. In contrast, Boyd et al. (2000) conducted a laboratory procedure called the *peer group entry task*. In this measure, a target child is invited to engage or play with two confederate children already involved in an activity. The target child's strategies and successful engagement are assessed. These researchers found that 27% of their "hearing impaired" participants failed the entry task, whereas only 5% of hearing peers failed. The authors found the results "disappointing."

A small number of studies have investigated the experiences within the family of having a deaf child with a CI and, in particular, the process the parents went through as they decided and then experienced the implantation with their child. Archbold et al. (2006) interviewed more than 100 parents of children with CIs using a parental perspectives measure they developed. Parents agreed they needed as much information as they could get and needed to be active in the decision-making process. Parents in this group were not uniform in their perception of the severity of stress in the whole process, but agreed that ongoing support was important.

Overall, research on the level of stress experienced during the cochlear implantation process is inconsistent, and the data are difficult to reconcile. Some studies have reported increased parental stress for families with children who have CIs (Quittner et al., 1991; Spahn et al., 2001). Other studies were not able to find appreciable differences in stress between parents whose children had CIs and those with typically hearing children (Asberg at al., 2008; Horsch et al., 1997; Sarant & Garrad, 2014).

PARENTAL STRESS

The literature suggests that parenting stress may be linked to several negative outcomes. In hearing families, parenting stress is associated with less optimal parenting, lower levels of developmental competence in children, and disrupted family systems (Crnic et al., 2005). In parent–child interactions, parents who are more stressed display more negative interactive patterns with their children (Crnic & Low, 2002). The literature also suggests that parenting stress may be linked to parental dissatisfaction and poor child functioning (Crnic & Low, 2002). Pipp-Siegel et al. (2002) found parenting stress was associated with child behavior problems. Hintermair (2006) reported that hearing parents with deaf children who experience high levels of stress have children with more socioemotional difficulties. In their review of the literature, Calderon and Greenberg (1993) concluded that successful maternal coping skills had a significant influence on the development of their deaf child. The more successful the mothers were in acquiring strategies for coping with their deaf child, the better developed the children's emotional sensitivity, inhibition, and social competence. Similarly, Watson et al. (1990) found that a lack of social competence in deaf children occurred in association with parental stress experience.

In general, parents of children with disabilities report greater parenting stress than parents of children without disabilities (Beckman, 1991). The identification of their child's disability is a critical life event for parents, and it is known that high stress can arise from it. Parents of newly identified deaf children have a persistent feeling of being overwhelmed and inadequate for the task of raising a deaf child. Yoshinga-Itano and Abdala de Uzcategui (2001) surveyed parents after an initial screening indicated a concern with their babies' hearing. Parents in that study reported feelings of shock, anger, confusion, fear, sadness, frustration, depression, loneliness, and blame. At the time of identification, or closely thereafter, parents are presented with technical information and the need to make decisions about a broad range of options. The subsequent decision-making process can be emotional, challenging, and stressful (Calderon & Greenberg, 1993).

Meinzen-Derr et al. (2008) investigated more than 150 families of children with a hearing loss. They divided their sample into three groups based on how long it had been since the child had been identified with a hearing loss, and compared amount and sources of stress. For families with a more recent identification of a hearing loss, healthcare and emotional well-being was the greatest source of stress. In contrast, families with a longer time span from the identification of the hearing loss were most troubled by concerns with education and general support systems. Meinzen-Derr et al. (2008) concluded that parental stressors change over time as the developmental needs of the child changes.

Factors Linked to Parenting Stress

Previous research has identified several factors that contribute to parenting stress in parents of deaf children. These factors can be broadly classified as either demographic characteristics of the child or parent, or factors related to the child's hearing loss. Studies have examined child demographic characteristics that may influence maternal stress as a function of parenting a child with hearing loss, including child age, gender, and the presence of additional disabilities.

Asberg et al. (2008) and Holt et al. (2012) did not find an effect of age on parental stress. Other researchers (Hagborg, 1989; Konstantrareas & Lampropoulou, 1995) did report evidence that stress increases as children age; maternal stress was reported to increase as the child's age increased from 2 to 14 years in a sample of mothers of deaf children. Similarly, Pipp-Siegel et al. (2002) found that mothers of older deaf children reported more stress than mothers of younger children. However, when other variables (such as the presence of another disability, ethnicity, expressive language) were accounted for, there was no relation between parental stress level and the child's age. Conceptually, one would predict parental stress to increase with age as language comes to dominate interpersonal interaction and as more challenging decisions (such as educational placement), become necessary, and children reach adolescence. Until we have longitudinal data that examine the changes or lack of changes systematically in the experiences of families over time, the effect of age will be uncertain.

There also are equivocal results regarding parenting stress as a function of parenting children with disabilities in addition to hearing loss. Pipp-Siegel et al. (2002) found that having additional disabilities was a predictor of elevated stress. Meadow-Orlans et al. (1995) reported no difference between stress scores of mothers whose children were deaf with additional disabilities and those without. These researchers did note, however, that in their extremely small sample of deaf children with other disabilities (n = 5), the stress scores were at both extremes of the range such that the overall means masked great variability.

For children who are deaf, additional factors related specifically to hearing loss have been reported to affect maternal stress, including degree of hearing loss, age of identification of hearing loss, language ability, and mode of communication used. Results regarding the effect of degree of hearing loss on reports of parenting stress are variable. In their study of mothers of children with moderate to profound deafness, Konstantareas and Lampropoulou (1995) found no relationship between degree of hearing loss and maternal stress. However, others have suggested more mild hearing loss may be related to greater stress by way of more dysfunctional parent–child interactions (Pipp-Siegel et al., 2002). Pipp-Siegel et al. (2002) proposed that this counterintuitive finding might be the result of parents of children with milder hearing losses not expecting much of an impact from the hearing loss. This can lead to unexpected problems and perhaps communication that is more confusing, such as when parents speak to their children without accommodating the loss and believing they must have been heard, only to be confronted with behavior that is unexpected. It may also be related to the cultural backgrounds of the samples—that of Pipp-Siegel et al. (2002) from the United States. and that of Konstantareas and Lampropoulou's (1995) from Greece.

Konstantareas and Lampropoulou (1995), in their sample of Greek families, reported that age of hearing loss onset was related to parenting stress, with onset of hearing loss before the age of 18 months being associated with increased maternal stress. In contrast, earlier age of identification could be related to decreased stress, because earlier age of identification is typically related to access to early intervention and increased language ability during infancy and preschool years (Pipp-Siegel et al. 2002; Yoshinaga-Itano et al., 1998).

For hearing parents of deaf children, parent–child communication becomes a central issue because parents must learn actively how to communicate with their child, rather than rely on intuitive communication strategies (Koester et al., 2000). Regarding mode of communication, Greenberg (1983), in an older investigation, reported that mothers who were part of an intervention group that supported total communication were less stressed compared with parents who used either spoken or signed communication. It is perhaps more likely, though, that effectiveness of communication, regardless of the mode or type, is what matters in predicting parenting stress (Ello & Donovan, 2005). Deaf children with language delays may face additional challenges as they grow because their language abilities may not keep pace with the increasing developmental demands on early childhood. Yoshinaga-Itano (2003) reported that language development is one of the variables related most strongly to stress in parents of deaf children. The stress that parents experience is likely tied to the discrepancy between increasing demands, such as playing and interacting with other children in preschool or daycare, managing more activities of daily living, and their child's ability to meet them (Lederberg & Golbach, 2002). Quittner et al. (2010) also noted that language delays influence parenting stress by way of child behavior problems. Children who have significant language delays have difficulty regulating their emotions, attention, and behavior (Barker et al., 2009). They may have difficulty expressing their needs, which has been suggested to lead to frustration and acting out.

Several studies have shown that, compared with hearing children, deaf children of hearing parents exhibit higher rates of behavior problems (Barker et al., 2009). Deaf children have been described as more impulsive and less compliant, less socially mature, and less skilled in social problem solving (Vostanis et al., 1997). Early research by Meadow (1980) and Quittner et al. (1990) reported that the most commonly reported behavior problems in deaf children included attention difficulties, such as impulsivity, distractibility, and short attention span. van Eldik et al. (2004) obtained similar data in a Dutch sample and reported that deaf children exhibited higher rates of behavior problems than hearing children. Quittner et al. (2010) argued that language difficulties and poor parent–child communication can lead to elevated levels of behavior problems, which ultimately leads to greater parenting stress.

Separate from the characteristics of children and their hearing status, some characteristics of mothers that are associated with stress have been investigated. For example, previous research with hearing children has found an inverse relationship between stress and socioeconomic status (Deater-Deckard & Scarr, 1996). An additional factor that has been seen to affect maternal stress is a mother's perception of the amount of support she receives. Increased social support has been found to have a beneficial effect on stress in families of children with disabilities in general (Beckman, 1991) and with hearing loss specifically (Lederberg & Golbach, 2002; Pipp-Siegel et al. 2002).

Parenting Stress Levels with Deaf Versus Hearing Children

To date, several studies have examined the levels of parenting stress among parents of young deaf children and whether these parents experience more stress than parents of young hearing children. Contradictory findings have emerged. The aim of the earliest study in this area (Quittner et al., 1990) was to assess the extent of parenting stress, social support, and psychological adjustment among mothers of deaf and hearing children. To assess parenting stress, both general (Parenting Stress Index [PSI]) (Abidin, 1983) and a context-specific (Family Stress Scale [FSS]) (Quittner et al., 1990) measures of parenting stress were used. The PSI is a 126-item questionnaire designed to identify sources of stress in parent–child subsystems. The FSS consists of 16 items with both general and context-specific stressors. Eleven FSS items address general family stressors (such as finances and discipline) and five items address stressors specific to early-childhood deafness (such as communication and managing hearing aids/cochlear implants). The results of the study provided considerable evidence that mothers of deaf children experienced greater levels of stress in their parenting role and poorer emotional adjustment than mothers of hearing children. Greater levels of stress for both the general and context-specific measures were found.

Meadow-Orlans (1994) assessed the stress levels of parents of nine-month-old infants using the PSI. Contrary to hypotheses based on much of the previous literature, this study found no statistically significant differences in parenting stress scores between mothers with deaf or hearing children. Meadow-Orlans (1994) suggested that parenting stress might increase as the importance of parent–child communication effectiveness increases, and communication difficulties between parents and their children become more pertinent or pronounced.

In a longitudinal study, Lederberg and Golbach (2002) assessed the developmental changes in parenting stress among mothers of deaf and hearing children when the children were 22 months, 3 years, and 4 years of age. When the children were 22 months of age, parenting stress was measured using the short form of the Questionnaire on Resources and Stress (QRS-F [Friedrich et al., 1983]). The QRS-F is a 52-item self-report questionnaire designed specifically to measure stress in families of children with disabilities (including hearing loss). When the children were three and four years old, Lederberg and Golbach (2002) replaced the QRS-F with the PSI because it had become the most commonly used instrument to measure parenting stress within this field of study. The results of their study showed that at the child's age of 22 months, mothers of deaf children indicated more stress than mothers of hearing children. At the child's age of three and four years, however, the amount of stress noted by mothers of deaf children was comparable with the control group of mothers of hearing children and with the normative sample for the PSI. Because different instruments were used to measure stress, it is possible to surmise that the "age effects" could have been the result of either the change in instruments or a decrease in parental stress as deaf children entered preschool.

Pipp-Siegel et al. (2002) examined which factors contributed to stress in mothers of deaf children. To measure contributing factors, they considered three broad categories of potential predictors: demographic characteristics of the child, variables related to hearing loss, and maternal characteristics and perceptions. The Parental Stress Index/Short Form, a measure derived from the full-length PSI, was used. Their results suggested that stress levels among mothers of children who are deaf or hard of hearing were not *clinically* higher than those of mothers of hearing children. On one subscale of the Parental Stress Index/Short Form, Parental Distress, a scale designed to assess the amount of stress an individual is feeling as a parent, a statistically significant but small difference was found, with mothers of deaf children reporting *less* stress than the normative sample of mothers of hearing children. These results were inconsistent with previous research; the majority of studies had reported no differences in general parenting stress in parents of hearing children compared with parents of deaf children, with the exception of Quittner et al. (1990). Pipp-Siegel et al. pointed out, however, that the difference was small (no effect size was provided), even if statistically significant, and only was obtained on one measure. Two other measures of parental stress did not find differences between mothers of deaf as opposed to hearing children.

More recently, Quittner et al. (2010) examined parenting stress using both general and context-specific measures of parenting stress in order to identify key mechanisms underlying parenting stress in a large, national cohort of hearing parents of deaf and hearing children. Context-specific measurement was included because of its sensitivity to the challenges of early childhood deafness compared with general measures of stress (Quittner et al., 1990). The results of the study suggested that parents of deaf children do not report elevated levels of general parenting stress when compared with parents of hearing children, a finding consistent with those of Asberg et al. (2008) and Pipp-Siegel et al. (2002). In contrast, support was found for higher levels of stressors specific to raising a deaf child in parents of deaf versus hearing children. Parents of deaf children reported elevated stress related to communication difficulties, educational concerns, maintenance of assistive listening devices, and the need to be a language teacher for their child. These results converge and support the findings of previous studies conducted by Quittner et al. (1990, 1991). Similarly, the study by Lederberg and Golbach (2002) included a disability-specific measure of parenting stress and found higher levels of parental stress.

COPING IN PARENTS OF DEAF CHILDREN

As described by Lazarus and Folkman (1984), "people and groups differ in their sensitivity and vulnerability to certain types of events, as well as in their interpretations and reactions" (p. 23) to environmental demands and stressors. They described the variations among individuals as related to the cognitive processes or *appraisals* that intervene between the encounter and the reaction. Therefore, it is important to understand the factors that influence parental stress as well as those that contribute to the process of reducing stress by ways of coping. The most widely used definition of coping is that of Lazarus and Folkman (1984), who defined coping as "constantly changing cognitive and behavioral efforts to manage specific external and/or internal demands that are appraised as taxing or exceeding the resources of the person" (p. 141).

A distinction that launched the examination of coping was that between problem-focused and emotion-focused coping (Lazarus & Folkman, 1984). Problem-focused coping is intended to influence the source of stress and is directed at the stressor itself, taking steps to remove or to evade it, or to diminish its impact if it cannot be evaded (Folkman et al., 1991). Emotion-focused coping is intended to alter one's internal reactions to stressors and prevent, minimize, or reduce this distress through applying coping strategies. Because there are many ways to reduce distress, emotion-focused coping comprises a wide range of responses, including self-soothing (such as relaxation and seeking emotional support), expression of negative (yelling or crying, for example) or positive emotions (such as broadening one's outlook in times of stress), positive reinterpretation, a focus on negative thoughts (such as rumination), and attempts to escape stressful situations (including avoidance, denial, and wishful thinking). Which specific strategies are used depend on learned experiences from one's family as well as cultural expectations regarding behavior.

The presence of a child with hearing loss in the family can be a continuous source of potential stress on the hearing family (Calderon & Greenberg, 1999). When an event is evaluated as stressful, individuals respond with coping processes. Coping processes serve two functions or purposes: the regulation of emotion and the adjustment of the person–environment relationship. Parents' emotional responses and how they cope with this stressor affect both family adjustment and child outcomes. Calderon and Greenberg (1993) reviewed the literature available at the time and concluded that successful coping on the mother's part had a significant influence on child development. The more successful the mothers were in acquiring helpful strategies for coping with their deaf child, the better developed their children's emotional sensitivity and problem-solving behavior appeared to be. The children also exhibited less impulsive behavior and better social competence.

As indicated earlier, and in the literature, coping behaviors are described primarily as "emotion focused" or "problem focused" (Folkman & Lazarus, 1985). For example, parents of a newly identified deaf infant often seek out other parents with children who are deaf to validate and manage their feelings toward their child's deafness (see Johnson, DesGeorges, Foster, Kozhevnikova, & Mallabiu, this volume). This is an example of emotion-focused coping. Parents also request and research literature on hearing loss as well as ask numerous questions about communication and educational options. This is an example of problem-focused coping. Ultimately, coping consists of, first, appraising the stressor (for example, hearing loss) and the available resources (support groups, educational programs, early-intervention services, Internet resources) and, second, choosing behaviors to regulate emotions or solve problems.

Despite the common assumption that rearing a child with a disability may put a strain on parents, studies have shown that not all families are at risk. Szarkowski (2002) conducted a qualitative study with parents in the United States and in Italy that identified positive characteristics of hearing parents' relationship with their deaf child. The results identified and described many of the resources and environmental pieces that, when in place, can lead to a more positive experience in parenting a deaf child. Parents from both countries were able to identify positive experiences, and noted support of a significant other and extended family was viewed as critical for raising deaf children. Parents acknowledged that having access to deaf-related services, deaf individuals, trained professionals, and education opportunities for deaf children were all important factors in coping with the stressors they experienced (Meadow-Orlans et al., 2003).

Apparently, the only study to determine which factors (resources) mediate the impact of the stressor (hearing loss) on the outcome (family functioning) was done by Calderon (1988). In that study, she had parents complete numerous questionnaires designed to assess coping resources as well as parents' current level of adjustment to having a deaf child, the current level of personal and family life adjustment, and the negative impact of current life experiences. Home interviews and structured observations of the family were also conducted. Results indicated that mothers who experienced fewer negative life stressors in the past and/or those who reported greater satisfaction with their social support had better personal adjustment. A mother's adjustment to her deaf child was most related to her level of satisfaction with social support. In a related study, Calderon et al. (1991) examined the influence of family coping on the social skills of deaf children. Results indicated that maternal problem-solving skills related positively to the child's emotional understanding and problem-solving skills, as reported by the child's teachers; positive maternal adjustment to the child was also related to lower child impulsivity and greater social understanding, according to teachers' reports.

The work of Calderon et al. (1991) points out the importance of looking beyond demographic characteristics when studying parents and families. Given the complexity of humans and of systems such as families, it is not surprising that so often we obtain conflicting findings from various studies. Simple models of development tend to treat one side or another of an equation as a constant. For example, when looking at the effect of age of the child on stress, the implicit assumption is that this impact will be the same on all parents. The work by Calderon et al. (Calderon, 1988; Calderon et al., 1991) shows that other characteristics of the parent, such as their ability to be creative and systematic in solving problems, are important and must be taken into consideration in designing research and in interpreting results.

A TRANSACTIONAL MODEL OF DEVELOPMENT

Forty years ago, Sameroff and Chandler (1975) pointed out that simple models of development typically fail to explain what we actually observe. For example, there are highly successful children with numerous risk factors that, if added together, would have predicted with certainty that the child would struggle and fail. Yet, resilience literature shows this does not always happen (Sameroff, 2009). We must go beyond even interactions between people to what Sameroff and Chandler (1975) called "transactions"—the changes that happen to *both* people who are interacting as a result of that interaction.

Although these ideas were easy to accept and may have seemed like common sense, they had very little influence on research design. For the past 40 years, most studies of child development continued to focus on either the child or on the parent. Some did add a bit of complexity by adding interaction terms. This added level of complexity was welcome, but very few studies have looked at these changes over time. Thus, there was no way to track how (or whether) the changes in parents and the changes in children were synchronized.

The research designs needed—to incorporate transactions and track the synchrony of changes in functioning—are extremely difficult to carry out. There are, however, a small but growing number of research programs studying hearing children and their development from this perspective that are informative for studies of deaf children and their families. One such program comes from the Michigan Family Study (McDonough, 2000), which monitored approximately 200 families when their children were 7 months to 33 months, assessing a number of child and family characteristics. The longitudinal nature of their data was a crucial component to being able to examine transactions in the family.

MacKenzie and McDonough (2009) investigated the connection between caregiver reports of a child's crying being upsetting for parents and the actual amount of crying. They found practically no relation between the two. What was even more informative, however, was their examination of perceptions of crying according to the caregiver's beliefs about the child. Parental beliefs were categorized as "balanced" versus not. Parents with balanced perceptions saw both positive and negative aspects to their relationship with their child, but also expressed acceptance, respect, and a valuing of the relationship. Parents with a nonbalanced view were emotionally distant, indifferent, or overwhelmed by their child. When the children were seven months of age, caregivers with a balanced view did not find their child's crying upsetting, regardless of the actual amount of crying. When examining the longitudinal data, caregivers with more distorted beliefs who had high-crying infants were substantially less warm and supportive, and these caregivers also rated their children as having more behavior problems at 33 months. This design and data analysis illustrate there is a complex interplay between actual behaviors in the family and perceptions held about children that influence each other mutually and lead to changes in both children and parents at later times.

Very little research on parental stress, including parents of deaf children, has looked at these sorts of *intra*personal factors and interactional characteristics that might affect how situations are perceived or how they may influence the experience of stress. Most of the literature on stress in parents of deaf children has looked at what situational factors might affect stress, and have almost always been external to the parents, such as severity of hearing loss, age of diagnosis, additional child disabilities, or a child's use of a CI.

PARENTAL PERSONALITY

Based on the parenting literature with regard to hearing families, it can be argued that intrapersonal resources play an important role in parenting and determining levels of parenting stress. According to Belsky and colleagues (Belsky & Barends, 2002; Vondra et al., 2005), parent personality is the most important determinant of parenting behavior. Several studies have provided empirical support for their assertion, showing that personality traits play an important role in determining levels of parenting stress (Belsky & Barends, 2002). Personality is known to influence the type of stressors experienced and the appraisals of their severity (Vollrath, 2001).

Broadly, personality is defined as characteristic patterns of thoughts, feelings, and behaviors over time and across situations. To paraphrase Allport (1961), personality is the dynamic organization within the person of the psychological and physical systems that underlie that person's patterns of actions, thoughts, and feelings. Many personality theories assert that people are basically biological, social, self-protective, self-actualizing, and learning creatures. Personality also involves individual differences, which can be found on any dimension; however, the most widely adopted framework is the Big Five-Factor Model.

The Big Five-Factor Model of personality (McCrae & Costa, 2003) is an organization of personality traits in terms of five basic dimensions: neuroticism, extraversion, openness to experience, agreeableness, and conscientiousness. This five-factor structure has since been replicated in diverse samples across numerous raters, including self, peers, and clinicians (John & Srivastava, 1999). Each broad trait is composed of multiple facets that provide a more nuanced picture of what the person is like.

> *Neuroticism (N)*: Neuroticism concerns the ease and frequency with which a person becomes upset and distressed. Anxiety and sensitivity to threat is indeed its emotional core (Caspi et al., 2005). Individuals who are given high ratings on scale N are prone to experience negative emotions such as depression, anxiety, or anger (McCrae, 1992; McCrae & Costa, 1987). N is associated with high rates of stress exposure and intense emotional and physiological reactivity to stress.
>
> *Extraversion (E)*: Extraversion is based on factors of assertiveness, spontaneity, energy, confidence, agency, and happiness (Depue & Collins, 1999). It also tends to be associated with being sociable, warm, cheerful, energetic, and assertive (McCrae, 1992; McCrae & Costa, 1987).
>
> *Openness (O)*: Openness to experience (McCrae & Costa, 1985) involves curiosity, flexibility, imaginativeness, and willingness to immerse oneself in atypical experiences. It also tends to be associated with being creative, imaginative, curious, psychologically minded, and flexible in thinking (Costa & McCrae, 1992).
>
> *Agreeableness (A)*: Agreeable people are friendly and helpful, empathic (Graziano et al., 2007), and able to inhibit their negative feelings (Graziano & Eisenberg, 1999). Agreeableness tends to be associated with being altruistic, acquiescent, trusting, and helpful (McCrae, 1992; McCrae & Costa, 1987).
>
> *Conscientiousness (C)*: Conscientiousness reflects the qualities of planning, persistence, and purposeful striving toward goals. It is often associated with being organized, reliable, hardworking, determined, and self-disciplined (McCrae, 1992; McCrae & Costa, 1987).

Personality and Coping

Personality plays an important role in almost every aspect of the stress and coping process (O'Brien & DeLongis, 1996). Personality has been linked to the likelihood of experiencing stressful situations (Bolger &

Zuckerman, 1995), the appraisal of an event as stressful (Gunthert et al., 1999), the likelihood of engaging in certain coping strategies (David & Suls, 1999; O'Brien & DeLongis, 1996; Watson & Hubbard, 1996), and the effectiveness or outcomes of these coping strategies (Bolger & Zuckerman, 1995; Gunthert et al., 1999). Coping has been described as "personality in action under stress" (Bolger, 1990, p. 525), and theorists have suggested that, "coping ought to be redefined as a personality process" (Vollrath, 2001, p. 341). Neuroticism, for example, has been associated with high rates of stress exposure and intense emotional and physiological reactivity to stress. It predicts exposure to interpersonal stress, and tendencies to appraise events as highly threatening and coping resources as low (Bolger & Zuckerman, 1995; Suls & Martin, 2005). Conscientiousness predicts low-stress exposure (Vollrath, 2001), likely because conscientious persons plan for predictable stressors and avoid impulsive actions that could lead to potential problems (Carver & Connor-Smith, 2010). Agreeableness is linked to low interpersonal conflict and thus less social stress (Asendorpf, 1998). Extraversion is associated with low stress reactivity and positive appraisals of available coping resources (Vollrath, 2001).

PARENTAL PERSONALITY, STRESS, AND CHILD ADJUSTMENT

Plotkin et al. (2013) investigated the interrelationships between parental personality, experience of parental stress, and adjustment in deaf children. One hundred fourteen parents participated. Most of the parent sample was European American with some college education, and most were using spoken language approaches with their deaf children. The researchers administered the FSS (Quittner et al., 1990, 1991), a context-specific measure of perceived parenting stress for parents of deaf children. To assess personality, the NEO was also administered. The NEO Five-Factor Inventory-3 (Costa & McCrae, 1992) is a 60-item self-report measure that captures neuroticism, extraversion, conscientiousness, agreeableness, and openness. Last, child adjustment was measured using the Child Behavior Checklist for two age groups: 1.5 to 5 years and 6 to 18 years (Achenbach & Rescorla, 2001).

The findings of Plotkin et al. (2013) attest to the complicated relationships between parent and child variables. In their study, neuroticism was found to be related significantly to greater levels of parenting stress in everyday activities, including finances, marriage, and daily routines, and, unexpectedly, was associated only with one deaf-specific factor: stress over being their child's teacher of language. This finding suggests that their child's hearing loss is a relatively insignificant factor in terms of their appraisal of stress. The lack of a strong connection between children's hearing loss and parents' appraisal of stress may explain why there have been conflicting reports in the study of parenting stress in parents' raising deaf children, because it appears that stress is not simply manifesting as a result of the *specific* challenges of raising a child with hearing loss. For some parents, the greatest extent of parenting stress appears not to be related to the presence of hearing loss itself, but rather is attributable to the parents' long-standing personality features, which may or may not predispose them to feeling and reporting greater stress. It is likely that deaf-specific challenges are present within each family; however, more anxious parents will report overall higher levels of stress regardless of those deaf-specific issues. In contrast, those with more outgoing personalities may cope more easily, reporting less stress. Still others with different dispositions may be influenced more strongly by dealing with the lives of their deaf children.

In their study (Plotkin et al., 2013), parents who rated themselves as more extraverted reported lower levels of stress in activities that were deaf specific (such as understanding assistive listening devices and performing audiological care) as well as daily stressors related to going on outings and their child's education. This finding is not surprising; it was anticipated that parents who were more extraverted would perceive outings as pleasurable. These findings support that intrapersonal resources regarding being socially inclined have strong potential as a protective factor for parents.

Results of the study by Plotkin et al. (2013) are consistent with Hintermair's (2006) work in Germany examining the relationship between parenting stress and child adjustment, with higher levels of parenting stress associated with higher levels of child externalizing behavior problems (aggression, oppositional behavior, and attention problems). As a result of methodological limitations, it was not possible for Plotkin et al. (2013) to draw implications about the direction of causation between parental stress and child behavior problems. But, parents who reported higher levels of neuroticism were more likely to rate their children as displaying greater behavioral difficulties, consistent with the notion that high levels of parental neuroticism are related to more negative, intrusive, and overcontrolling parenting behavior patterns (Luster & Okagaki, 2005), which, in turn, is believed to lead to poorer child adjustment. In contrast, parents of young children who perceived themselves as high in extroversion rated their children as demonstrating low levels of externalizing, internalizing, and overall behavioral difficulties.

Last, results of a multiple regression analysis in the study by Plotkin et al. (2013) demonstrated that the age of the child plays an important role mediating between stress and personality. Parental neuroticism predicted internalizing problems significantly in children ages three to five years, indicating a strong relationship between parental expressions of emotional distress and early child development of symptoms of anxiety, depression, and somatic complaints. The finding of low ratings of conscientiousness predicting externalizing problems also corroborates prior research linking externalizing problems to parenting stress and offers new insight into how parenting personality can play a significant role in the development of emerging behavioral regulation skills. Lower conscientiousness has been related to parenting behaviors with hearing children that are permissive and inconsistent in discipline; this has been associated consistently with externalizing behaviors (Patterson et al., 1997).

Although not an initial research question in the study by Plotkin et al. (2013), Plotkin et al. (2015) analyzed data separately for families depending on whether the child had received a CI. Regression models to predict child adjustment as measured on the Child Behavior Checklist differed for deaf children with and without CIs. In children without CIs, parent personality was most predictive of adjustment, whereas in children with CI, stress and personality *both* predicted adjustment. One possible interpretation of these data is that when families choose not to have a child undergo cochlear implantation, the general disposition toward the world (personality) is the major influence on a child's behavior. However, in families that chose a CI for their child, the opportunity to experience stressors surrounding the implantation surgery and subsequent interventions are substantial, leading to stress that goes beyond that experienced by other families whose deaf child does not have a CI. This implies that in helping families with young deaf children, for those families in which the child has a CI, both a parent's personality as well as specific support around the CI is necessary to consider. These data appear to suggest that providing developmentally sensitive supports to parents that can empower their support to their young child on the very specific matters associated with a CI (listening checks, basic troubleshooting, device settings, and so on) may be of particular use in promoting child adjustment. In families in which the deaf child does not use a CI, support that focuses on the parent's general approach to the world may prove more beneficial.

IN THE TRENCHES: SUPPORTING FAMILIES AND DEAF STUDENT SUCCESS

The most general implication of the data reviewed in this chapter is that a one-size-fits-all model of support or intervention is not totally effective. Similar to research emerging in the field of temperament and the transactional model (Sameroff, 2009), the question more is goodness-of-fit, rather than that one principle is always correct. MacKenzie and McDonough (2009) further argued that goodness-of-fit is not a coming together of "independent, static characteristics of a caregiver and child" (p. 49). Not all environments are equal and not all families can (or should) respond to children in the same ways. Furthermore, the cultures in which families are living provide an additional influence on expectations regarding behavior and parenting, which have yet to be examined in a systematic fashion.

A program of support that focuses on group support may be most effective for families that tend to be more extraverted—those that gain energy and inspiration from interacting with other people. For other parents who are less bolstered by this, a different, more individually tailored program may be needed. In addition, parents who are inclined to struggle with anxiety and to feel more worry in general need a greater range of support. Their child's hearing loss may be just one more item in a list of things the parent may be finding stressful. Support that focuses on how to help manage a child with hearing loss will be useful, but ultimately limited, because other aspects of life may be equally troubling and continue as a source of stress.

In addition to personality, understanding the parent's perception of the child in general is important, and likely more important than any objective characteristics of the child (MacKenzie & McDonough, 2009; Sameroff, 2009). Degree of hearing loss, innate temperament or difficultness, or other demographic types of characteristics will probably be far less influential than how the parent *interprets* those behaviors. Whether the parent believes or finds them to be troubling, inappropriate, or problematic is more important than what they "actually" may be as witnessed by someone outside the family.

The unifying theme that arises from the multitude of studies reviewed thus far reinforces the notion that people are indeed complicated, as are the families within which people live and grow. Supporting the success of deaf children unites individuals around a common goal. The path that leads to that goal may not be the same for every child or family. Supporting families on their path may require different modalities of interventions. For some, promotion of the positive factors they already have may be sufficient, whereas for others, ameliorating the impact of stress and negative life events may be a primary focus in supporting a family.

Knowledge of the individual factors that contribute to success is a first step in designing programs or meeting the needs of a family with a deaf child. Although many professionals who work with deaf children and their families are well trained to be extremely knowledgeable about specific factors related to deafness, basic knowledge about psychological factors such as personality, coping, and stress may be less familiar. Systems that provide knowledge in these domains and design programs with these factors in mind may find they are able to serve a more diverse community and recognize success more broadly.

Most important, knowledge and appreciation of specific factors will be best used when an understanding of the interaction of both parent and child factors is then applied, and will enhance the development of supports. This is not to shy programs away from the creation of traditional support groups or social opportunities for families, but rather to recognize that this approach should not be expected to demonstrate success with all families. Professionals who take the knowledge base presented within these pages and apply it to their families will be better able to support the "complicated" people within the trenches.

REFERENCES

Abidin, R. R. (1983). *Parenting Stress Index (PSI): Manual and administration booklet*. Charlottesville, VA: Pediatric Psychology Press.

Achenbach, T. M., & Rescorla, L. A. (2001). *Manual for the ASEBA school-age forms & profiles*. Burlington, VT: University of Vermont, Research Center for Children, Youth, & Families.

Allport, G. W. (1961). *Patterns and growth in personality*. New York, NY: Holt, Rinehart & Winston.

Archbold, S., Harris, M., Nikolopoulos, T. P., O'Donoghue, G., White, A., & Lloyd Richmond, H. (2008). Reading abilities after cochlear implantation: The effect of age at implantation on reading age, five and seven years after implantation. *International Journal of Pediatric Otorhinolaryngology, 72,* 1471–1478.

Archbold, S., Sach, T., O'Neill, C., Lutman, M., & Gregory, S. (2006). Deciding to have a cochlear implant and subsequent after-care: Parental perspectives. *Deafness and Education International, 8,* 190–206.

Asberg, K. K., Vogel, J. J., & Bowers, C. A. (2008). Exploring correlates and predictors of stress in parents of children who are deaf: Implications of perceived social support and mode of communication. *Journal of Child and Family Studies, 1,* 486–499.

Asendorpf, J. B. (1998). Personality effects on social relationships. *Journal of Personality and Social Psychology, 74,* 1531–1544.

Ashton, M. C., Lee, K., & Paunonen, S. V. (2002). What is the central feature of extraversion? Social attention versus reward sensitivity. *Journal of Personality and Social Psychology, 83,* 245–252.

Barker, D. H., Quittner, A. L., Fink, N. E., Eisenberg, L. S., Tobey, E. A., & Niparko, J. K. (2009). Predicting behavior problems in deaf and hearing children: the influence of language, attention, and parent–child communication. *Developmental Psychopathology, 21,* 373–392.

Bat-Chava, Y., & Deignan, E. (2001). Peer relationships of children with cochlear implants. *Journal of Deaf Studies and Deaf Education, 6,* 186–199.

Beckman, P. J. (1991). Comparison of mothers' and fathers' perceptions of the effect of young children with and without disabilities. *American Journal on Mental Retardation, 95,* 585–595

Belsky, J., & Barends, N. (2002). Personality and parenting. In M. H. Bornstein (Ed.), *Handbook of parenting: being and becoming a parent* (2nd ed., Vol. III, pp. 415–438). London: Lawrence Erlbaum Associates.

Biringen, Z., & Robinson, J. (1991). Emotional availability in mother–child interactions: A reconceptualization for research. *American Journal of Orthopsychiatry, 61,* 258–271.

Blamey, P., & Sarant, J. Z. (2011). Development of spoken language by deaf children. In M. Marschark & P. E. Spencer, (Eds.), *The Oxford handbook of deaf studies, language and education* (Vol 1., pp. 241–257). New York, NY: Oxford University Press.

Bolger, N. (1990). Coping as a personality process: A prospective study. *Journal of Personality and Social Psychology, 59*, 525–537.

Bolger, N., & Zuckerman, A. (1995). A framework for studying personality in the stress process. *Journal of Personality and Social Psychology, 69*, 890–902.

Boyd, R., Knutson, J., & Dalstrom, A. (2000). Social interaction of pediatric cochlear implant recipients with age-matched peers. *Annals of Otology, Rhinology, and Laryngology, 109*(12, Suppl. 185), 105–109.

Calderon, R. (1988). Stress and coping in hearing families with deaf children. Unpublished PhD dissertation, University of Washington.

Calderon, R., & Greenberg, M. (1993). Considerations in the adaptation of families with school-aged deaf children. In M. Marschark & D. Clark (Eds.), *Psychological perspectives on deafness.* Hillsdale, NJ: Lawrence Erlbaum Associates, pp. 27–48.

Calderon, R., & Greenberg, M. (1999). Social and emotional development of deaf children. In M. Marschark and P. E. Spencer (Eds.), *The Oxford handbook of deaf studies, language, and education* (pp. 177–189). New York, NY: Oxford University Press.

Calderon, R., Greenberg, M. T., & Kusche, C. (1991). The influence of family coping on the cognitive and social skills of deaf children. In D. Martin (Ed.), *Advances in cognitive, education, and deafness* (pp. 195–200). Washington, DC: Gallaudet University Press.

Carver, C. S., & Connor-Smith, J. (2010). Personality and coping. *Annual Review of Psychology, 61*, 679–704.

Caspi, A., Roberts, B. W., & Shiner, R. L. (2005). Personality development: Stability and change. *Annual Review of Psychology, 56*, 453–484.

Cattell, R. (1943). The description of personality: Basic traits resolved into clusters. *Journal of Abnormal and Social Psychology, 38*, 476–506.

Chin, S., Tsai, P., & Gao, S. (2003). Connected speech intelligibility of children with cochlear implants and children with normal hearing. *American Journal of Speech Language Pathology, 12*, 440–451.

Christiansen, J., & Leigh, I. W. (2002). *Cochlear implants in children: Ethics and choices.* Washington, DC: Gallaudet University Press.

Costa, P. T., Jr., McCrae, R. R. (1992). Revised *NEO Personality Inventory (NEO-PI-R) and NEO Five-Factor Inventory (NEO-FFI) professional manual.* Edessa, FL: Psychological Assessment Resources.

Crnic, K. A., Gaze, C., & Hoffman, C, (2005). Cumulative parenting stress across the preschool period: Relations to maternal parenting and child behavior at age 5. *Infant and Child Development, 14*, 117–132.

Crnic, K., & Low, C. (2002). Everyday stresses and parenting. In M. H. Bornstein (Ed.), *Handbook of parenting: Practical issues in parenting* (2nd ed., pp. 243–268). Mahwah, NJ: Lawrence Erlbaum Associates.

Dalai Lama, & Cutler, H. (2009). *The art of happiness in a troubled world.* New York, NY: Harmony Books.

David, J. P., & Suls, J. (1999). Coping efforts in daily life: Role of Big Five traits and problem appraisals. *Journal of Personality, 67*, 265–294.

Deater-Deckard, K., & Scarr, S. (1996). Parenting stress among dual-earner mothers and fathers: Are there gender differences? *Journal of Family Psychology, 10,* 45–59.

Depue, R. A., & Collins, P. F. (1999). Neurobiology of the structure of personality: Dopamine, facilitation of incentive motivation, and extraversion. *Behavioral and Brain Sciences, 22,* 491–517.

Dettman, S., & Dowell, R. (2010). Language acquisition and critical periods for children using cochlear implants. In M. Marschark & P. E. Spencer (Eds.), *The Oxford handbook of deaf studies, language and education* (Vol 2, pp. 331–343). New York, NY: Oxford University Press.

Dowell, R., Blamey, P., & Clark, G. (March 1997). Factors affecting outcomes in children with cochlear implants. Paper presented at the XVI World Congress of Otorhinolaryngology, Head, and Neck Surgery. Sydney, Australia.

Ello, L. M., & Donovan, S. J. (2005). Assessment of the relationship between parenting stress and a child's ability to functionally communicate. *Research on Social Work Practice, 15,* 531–544.

Folkman, S., Chesney, M., McKusick, L., Ironson, G., Johnson, D. S., & Coates, T. J. (1991). Translating coping theory into an intervention. In J. Eckenrode (Ed.), *The Social Context of Coping* (pp. 239–260). New York: Plenum Publishing.

Folkman, S., & Lazarus, R. S. (1985). If it changes it must be a process: Study of emotion and coping during three stages of a college examination. *Journal of Personality and Social Psychology, 48,* 150–170.

Folven, R. J., & Bonvillian, J. D. (1991). The transition from nonreferential to referential language in children acquiring American Sign Language. *Developmental Psychology, 27,* 806–816.

Friedrich, W. N., Greenberg, M. T., & Crnic, K. (1983). A short form of the questionnaire on resources and stress. *American Journal of Mental Deficiency, 88,* 41–48.

Furth, H. G. (1966). *Thinking without language.* New York, NY: Collier-Macmillan.

Geers, A. (2004). Speech, language, and reading skills after early cochlear implantation. *Archives of Otolaryngology Head and Neck Surgery, 130,* 634–638.

Geers, A. (2006). Spoken language in children with cochlear implants. In P. Spencer & M. Marschark (Eds.), *Advances in the spoken language development of deaf and hard-of-hearing children* (pp. 244–270). New York, NY: Oxford University Press.

Geers, A., Tobey, E., Moog, J., & Brenner, C. (2008). Long-term outcomes of cochlear implantation in the preschool years: From elementary grades to high school. *International Journal of Audiology, 47*(Suppl. 2), S21–S30.

Graziano, W. G., & Eisenberg, N. H. (1999). Agreeableness as a dimension of personality. In R. Hogan, J. Johnson, & S. Briggs (Eds.), *Handbook of personality* (pp. 795–825). San Diego, CA: Academic Press.

Graziano, W. G., Habashi, M. M., Sheese, B. E., & Tobin, R. M. (2007). Agreeableness, empathy, and helping: A person X situation perspective. *Journal of Personality and Social Psychology, 93,* 583–599.

Greenberg, M. T. (1983). Family stress and child competence: The effects of early intervention for families with deaf infants. *American Annals of the Deaf, 128,* 407–417.

Gunthert, K. C., Chen, L. H., & Armeli, S. (1999). The role of neuroticism in daily stress and coping. *Journal of Personality and Social Psychology, 77,* 1087–1100.

Hagbor, W. J. (1989). A comparative study of parental stress among mothers and fathers of deaf school-age children. *Journal of Community Psychology, 17,* 220–224.

Hall, M.L., & Bavelier, D. (2010). Working memory, deafness, and sign language. In M. Marschark & P.E. Spencer (Eds.), *The Oxford handbook of deaf studies, language and education* (Vol 2, pp. 458–472). New York, NY: Oxford University Press.

Hintermair, M. (2006). Parental resources, parental stress, and socioemotional development of deaf and hard of hearing children. *Journal of Deaf Studies and Deaf Education, 11,* 493–513.

Holt, R., Beer, J., Kronenberger, W. G., Pisoni, D. B., & Lalonde, K. (2012). Contribution of family environment to pediatric cochlear implant users' speech and language outcomes: Some preliminary findings. *Journal of Speech, Language, & Hearing Research, 55,* 848–864.

Hooker, K., Frazier, I. D., & Monahan, D. J. (1994). Personality and coping among caregivers of spouses with dementia. *The Gerontologist, 34,* 386–392.

Horsch, U., Weber, C., & Detrois, P. (1997). Stress experienced by parents of children with cochlear implants compared with parents of deaf children and hearing children. *American Journal of Otolaryngology, 18*(Suppl.), s161–s163.

Jamieson, J. R. (1994). Instructional discourse strategies: Differences between hearing and deaf mothers of deaf children. *First Language, 14,* 153–171.

John, O. P., & Srivastava, S. (1999). The Big-Five trait taxonomy: History, measurement, and theoretical perspectives. In L. A. Pervin & O. P. John (Eds.), *Handbook of personality: Theory and research* (Vol. 2, pp. 102–138). New York, NY: Guilford Press.

Koester, L. S., Papousek, H., & Smith-Gray, S. (2000). Intuitive parenting communication, and interaction with deaf infants. In P. E. Spencer, C. J. Erting, & M. Marschark (Eds.), *The essays in honor of Kathryn P. Meadow-Orlans: The deaf child in the family and at school* (pp. 55–71). Mahwah, NJ: Lawrence Erlbaum Associates.

Konstantareas, M. M., & Lampropoulou, V. (1995). Stress in Greek mothers and deaf children. *American Annals of the Deaf, 140,* 264–270.

Lazarus, R. S., & Folkman, S. (1984). *Stress, appraisal, and coping.* New York, NY: Springer.

Lederberg, A. R., & Golbach, T. (2002). Parenting stress and social support in hearing mothers of deaf and hearing children: A longitudinal study. *Journal of Deaf Studies and Deaf Education, 7,* 330–345.

Luster, T., & Okagaki, L. (Eds.) (2005). *Parenting: An ecological perspective* (2nd ed.). Mahwah, NJ: Lawrence Erlbaum Associates.

MacKenzie, M. J., & McDonough, S. C. (2009). Transactions between perception and reality: Maternal beliefs and infant regulatory behavior. In A. Sameroff (Ed.), *The transactional model of development: How children and contexts shape each other.* Washington, DC: American Psychological Association.

Maitlin, J. A., Wethington, E. M., & Kesser, R. C. (1990). Situational determinants of coping and coping effectiveness. *Journal of Health and Social Behavior, 31,* 103–122.

Marschark, M. (2003). Cognitive functioning in deaf adults and children. In M. Marschark & P. E. Spencer (Eds.), *The Oxford handbook of deaf studies, language, and education* (pp. 464–477). New York, NY: Oxford University Press.

Marschark, M., DeBeni, R., Polazzo, M. G., & Cornoldi, C. (1993). Deaf and hearing–impaired adolescents' memory for concrete and abstract prose: Effects of relational and distinctive information. *American Annals of the Deaf, 138,* 31–39.

Marschark, M., & Wauters, L. (2008). Language comprehension and learning by deaf students. In M. Marschark & P. C. Hauser (Eds.), *Deaf cognition: Foundations and outcomes* (pp. 309–350). New York, NY: Oxford University Press.

Marentette, P., & Mayberry, R. I. (2000). Principals for an emerging phonological system: A case study of early ASL acquisition. In C. Chamberlain, J. Morford, & R. I. Mayberry (Eds.), *Language acquisition by eye* (pp. 71–90). Mahwah, NJ: Lawrence Erlbaum Associates.

Mayne, A., Yoshinaga-Itano, C., & Sedey, A. (2000). Receptive vocabulary development of infants and toddlers who are deaf or hard of hearing. *The Volta Review, 100*(5), 29–52.

McCrae, R. R. (Ed.) (1992). The five-factor model: Issues and applications [Special issue]. *Journal of Personality, 60*(2), 175–215.

McCrae, R. R., & Costa, P. T., Jr. (1985). Updating Norman's "adequate taxonomy": Intelligence and personality dimensions in natural language and in questionnaires. *Journal of Personality and Social Psychology, 49,* 710–721.

McCrae, R. R. & Costa, P. T., Jr. (1986). Personality, coping, and coping effectiveness in an adult sample. *Journal of Personality, 54,* 385–405.

McCrae, R. R., & Costa, P. T., Jr. (1987). Validation of a five-factor model of personality across instruments and observers. *Journal of Personality and Social Psychology, 52,* 81–90.

McCrae, R. R., & Costa, P. T. (2003). *Personality in adulthood, a five-factor theory perspective* (2nd ed.). New York, NY: Guilford Press.

McDonough, S. C. (2000). Interaction guidance: An approach for difficult-to-engage families. In C. H. Zeanah (Ed.), *Handbook of infant mental health* (2nd ed., pp. 485–493). New York, NY: Guilford Press.

Meadow, K. P. (1980). *Deafness and child development.* Berkeley, CA: University of California Press.

Meadow-Orlans, K. P. (1994). Stress, support, and deafness: Perceptions of infants' mothers and fathers. *Journal of Early Intervention, 18,* 91–102.

Meadow-Orlans, K. P., Mertens, D. M., & Sass-Lehrer, M. A. (2003). *Parents and their deaf children: The early years.* Washington, DC: Gallaudet University Press.

Meadow-Orlans, K. P., Smith-Gray, S., & Dyssegaard, B. (1995). Infants who are deaf or hard of hearing, with and without physical/cognitive disabilities. *American Annals of the Deaf, 140,* 279–286.

Meinzen-Derr, J., Lim, L., Choo, D., Buyniski, S., & Wiley, S. (2008). Pediatric hearing impairment caregiver experience: Impact of duration of hearing loss on parental stress. *International Journal of Pediatric Otorhinolaryngology, 72,* 1693–1703.

O'Brien, T. B., & DeLongis, A. (1997). Coping with chronic stress: An interpersonal perspective. In B. H. Gottlieb (Ed.), *Coping with chronic stress. The Plenum series on stress and coping* (pp. 161–190). New York, NY: Plenum Press.

Patterson, G. R., Reid, J. B., & Dishion, T. J. (1997). *Antisocial boys (A social interactional approach).* Eugene, OR: Castalia Publishing.

Pettito, L. A., & Marentette, P. E. (1991). Babbling in the manual mode: Evidence for the ontogeny of language. *Science, 251,* 1493–1496.

Pipp-Siegal, S., Sedey, A. L., & Yoshinaga-Itano, C. (2002). Predictors of parental stress in mothers of young children with hearing loss. *Journal of Deaf Studies and Deaf Education, 7,* 1–17.

Plotkin, R., Brice, P. J., & Reesman, J. (2013). It is not just stress: Parent personality in raising a deaf child. *Journal of Deaf Studies and Deaf Education, 19*(3), 347–357.

Plotkin, R. M., Reesman, J., & Brice, P. J. (2015). Parent personality and stress as predictors of adjustment in deaf children with or without a cochlear implant. Paper presented at the International Congress on Education of the Deaf. Athens, Greece.

Pressman, L. J., Pipp-Siegel, S., Yoshinaga-Itano, C., & Deas, A. (1999). Maternal sensitivity predicts language gain in preschool children who are deaf and hard of hearing. *Journal of Deaf Studies and Deaf Education, 4*(4), 294–304.

Quittner, A. L., Barker, D. H., Cruz, I., Snell, C., Grimley, M. E., & Botteri, M. (2010). Parenting stress among parents of deaf and hearing children: Association with language delays and behavior problems. *Parenting, 10,* 136–155.

Quittner, A. L., Glueckauf, R. L., & Jackson, D. N. (1990). Chronic parenting stress: Moderating versus mediating effects of social support. *Journal of Personality and Social Psychology, 59,* 1266–1278.

Quittner, A. L., Steck, J. T., & Rouiller, R. I. (1991). Cochlear implants in children: A study of parental stress and adjustment. *American Journal of Otology, 12,* 95–104.

Sameroff, A. (2009). The transactional model. In A. Sameroff (Ed.), *The transactional model of development: How children and contexts shape each other.* Washington, DC: American Psychological Association.

Sameroff, A., & Chandler, M. J. (1975). Reproductive risk and he continuum of caretaking casualty. In F. D. Horowitz, M. Hetherington, S. Scarr-Salapatek, & G. Siegel (Eds.), *Review of child development research* (Vol. 4, pp. 187–244). Chicago, IL: University of Chicago Press.

Sarant, J. Z., & Garrard, P. (2014). Parenting stress in parents of children with cochlear implants: Relationships among parent stress, child language, and unilateral versus bilateral implants. *Journal of Deaf Studies and Deaf Education, 19,* 85–106.

Sarant, J. Z., Holt, C., Dowell, R., Rickards, F., & Blamey, P. J. (2009). Spoken language development in oral preschool children with permanent childhood hearing impairment. *Journal of Deaf Students and Deaf Education, 14*(2), 205–217.

Schick, B., & Hoffmeister, R. (2001). ASL skills in deaf children of deaf parents and of hearing parents. Paper presented at the Society for Research in Child Development International Conference. Minneapolis, MN.

Spahn, C., Richter, B., Zschocke, I., Lohle, E., & Wirsching, M. (2001). The need for psychosocial support in parents with cochlear implant children. *International Journal of Pediatric Otorhinolaryngology, 57,* 45–53.

Spencer, P. (2004). Individual differences in language performance after cochlear implantation at one to three years of age: Child, family, and linguistic factors. *Journal of Deaf Studies and Deaf Education, 9,* 395–412.

Spencer, P. E., Marscharck, M., & Spencer, L. J. (2011). Cochlear implants: Advances, issues, and implications. In M. Marschark & P. E. Spencer, (Eds.), *Oxford handbook of deaf studies, language and education* (pp. 452–472). New York, NY: Oxford University Press.

Suls, J., & Martin, R. (2005). The daily life of the garden-variety neurotic: reactivity, stressor exposure, mood spillover, and maladaptive coping. *Journal of Personality, 73*, 1485–1509.

Svirsky, M., Teoh, S. W., Caldwell, M., & Miyamoto, R. (2010). Speech intelligibility of prelingually deaf children with multichannel cochlear implants. *Annals of Otology, Rhinology, and Laryngology, 109*(12, Suppl. 185), 123–125.

Szarkowski, A. A. (2002). Positive aspects of parenting a deaf child: Development of a positive perspective. Unpublished doctoral dissertation, Gallaudet University.

Tupes, E. C., & Christal, R. E. (1961). *Recurrent personality factors based on trait ratings.* USAF ASD technical report no. 61–97. Lackland Air Force Base, TX: U.S. Air Force.

van Eldik, T., Treffers, P. D. A., Veerman, J. W., & Verhulst, F. C. (2004). Mental health problems of deaf Dutch children as indicated by parents' responses to the child behavior checklist. *American Annals of the Deaf, 148*, 390–395.

Vollrath, M. (2001). Personality and stress. *Scandinavian Journal of Psychology, 42*, 335–347.

Vondra, J., Sysko, H. B., & Belsky, J. (2005). Developmental origins of parenting: personality and relationship factors. In T. Luster, & L. Okagaki (Eds), *Parenting: An ecological perspective* (2nd ed., pp. 35–71). London: Lawrence Erlbaum.

Vostanis, P., Hayes, M., Du Feu, M., & Warren, J. (1997). Detection of behavioral and emotional problems in deaf children and adolescents: Comparison of two rating scales. *Child: Care, Health, and Development, 23*, 233–246.

Watson, S. M., Henggeler, S. W., & Whelan, J. P. (1990). Family functioning and the social adaptation of hearing-impaired youths. *Journal of Abnormal Child Psychology, 18*(2), 143–163.

Watson, D., & Hubbard, B. (1996). Adaptational style and dispositional structure: Coping in the context of the Five-Factor Model. *Journal of Personality, 64*, 737–774.

Yoshinaga-Itano, C. (2003). From screening to early identification and interventions: Discovering predictors to successful outcomes for children with significant hearing loss. *Journal of Deaf Studies and Deaf Education, 8*, 11–30.

Yoshinaga-Itano, C., & Abdala de Uzcategui, C. (2001). Early identification and social-emotional factors of children with hearing loss and children screened for hearing loss. In E. Kurtzer-White & D. Luterman (Eds.), *Early childhood deafness* (pp.13–28). Baltimore, MD: York Press.

Yoshinaga-Itano, C., Sedey, A. L., Coulter, D. K., & Mehl, A. L. (1998). Language of early- and later identified children with hearing loss. *Pediatrics, 102*, 1161–1171.

6

High Standard Competencies for Teachers of the Deaf and Other Qualified Professionals: Always Necessary, Not Always Guaranteed

Guido Lichtert, Kevin Miller, Areti Okalidou,
Paul Simpson, and Astrid van Wieringen

For the child or student who is deaf, there are a variety of factors that influence developmental progress or educational success, whether these services are provided in the home, in preschool, or in elementary or secondary school. Of all these factors, the most powerful is a child's or student's teacher or therapist (Mason-Williams, 2014). An effective teacher or therapist can have a dramatic impact on a child's or student's educational progress and achievements. For example, students of an effective teacher can gain a whole grade level on standardized tests compared with students of the same age with a less effective teacher (Green, 2014). In addition, parents exert an important influence on the development of their children. Moeller (2000), Holzinger et al. (2011), and Sass-Lehrer and Young (see Chapter 2) have evidenced the importance of families and early family-centered intervention with respect to the language development of deaf children.

In a similar fashion, a variety of factors influence the professional's effectiveness. For example, effective teaching, rehabilitating, or coaching families depends on having the essential knowledge and skills needed to work competently with the children, students, or families to whom they are assigned (National Council Accreditation of Teacher Education, 2006). In other words, they have met certain standards or have mastered specific competencies for their area of expertise. It must be kept in mind, however, that expertise is not static. Teaching practices can change as new ideas or methods are adopted or as advances in technology transform the way children and students learn. As a result of developments in hearing screening and hearing technology; the growing body of research in medical, linguistic, and educational topics related to deaf education as well as the changing educational policies; the role and competencies of teachers of the deaf (ToDs) and other qualified professionals (such as speech language therapists [SLTs], audiologists, educational psychologists) change continuously. Thus, it is necessary to update competencies or standards on a regular basis to ensure the effectiveness of these professionals.

Changes in teaching methods and teaching environments, changes in the policy of family-based early intervention, and advances in technology, such as cochlear implants, give rise to the need for teachers, therapists, and other qualified professionals to reassess the current competencies or standards that apply to educating and rehabilitating children and students who are deaf, and to guiding their families. In this chapter, we explore the issue of competencies or standards expected of ToDs and other professionals who work with children or students who are deaf and their families. The necessity of mandatory competencies, as well as the ranking of their importance, was investigated by means of a survey in the framework of a European Leonardo Research project (Leonardo da Vinci Lifelong Learning Project, 2011a, 2011b). In many countries, not only professionals with teaching degrees, but also those with a degree in speech language therapy and educational psychologists have direct and indirect responsibilities with respect to the bringing up and educational progress of deaf children and adolescents. In Flanders, for example, SLTs also work as itinerant professionals in mainstream schools, having the same tasks as an itinerant ToD. Two issues investigated are whether these professionals believe, compared with itinerant ToDs or ToDs in special education, these competencies are necessary and whether these skills should be acquired through specific training.

As a result of neonatal hearing screening and early intervention, the competencies of SLTs are also changing. The need for new competencies and training was explored further in a Greek study. Not only professionals, but especially parents of deaf children play a vital role in the language and academic development of these children (Calderon, 2000, Holzinger et al. 2011; Meadow-Orlans et al., 2003; Moeller, 2000; Yoshinaga-Itano, 2000; also, see Chapter 2). Therefore, it is investigated whether ToDs and other professionals working as home-based providers and, who are considered to empower parents during their upbringing, have the necessary competencies to exchange their knowledge and expertise with parents in partnership. This chapter presents the status of competencies and standards as they affect ToDs and other professionals who educate and support students who are deaf, and their families in Europe. We argue in support of competencies or standards that are mandatory and comparable across countries. We believe every effort should be made to provide the highest standards in deaf education, based on contemporary developments, optimally to empower the children, students, and their families.

THE NEED FOR PAN-EUROPEAN COMPETENCIES FOR TEACHERS OF THE DEAF

In this section we describe the results of a survey carried out within the framework of a European Leonardo da Vinci project concerning the necessary competencies for ToDs. This program was initiated by the United Kingdom. It has long been recognized that the complexity of needs demonstrated by deaf children requires ToDs to have a specific additional qualification to that of being a generally qualified teacher. In the United Kingdom, a qualification for ToDs has been mandatory since the 19th century (McLoughlin, 1987).

It is still a requirement to have a specialist qualification in the United Kingdom, and the regulations are clear that any ToD working with deaf learners must acquire the qualification within 3 years of beginning to work with them. The qualification specification sets out clearly the competencies ToDs need to acquire to achieve the qualification and be accepted as a ToD (Department of Education, Statutory Instrument 2003, No. 1662, The Education [School Teachers' Qualifications] [England] Regulations 2003, 9). Failure to do so terminates this employment.

In 2008, Andrew Broughton—head of specialist services for deaf children in Shropshire, Telford, Wrekin in England—convened a meeting to discuss a European project to consider the need to develop such competencies across Europe. This had been highlighted by a special edition of the British Association of Teachers of the Deaf magazine, which reviewed the educational provision for deaf children in a range of European countries (British Association of Teachers of the Deaf, 2005). This was also stimulated by discussions in the European Union to standardize the competencies needed by mainstream teachers (European Commission, Directorate-General for Education and Culture, 2011).

Five partners came together to make a joint bid for European funding to consider the need for and develop a list of competencies that would be seen as a minimum requirement for all specialist teachers working with deaf children and young people in the European Union. The overarching aim of the project was to reduce the exclusion of deaf children and young people by developing competencies for ToDs applicable in a pan-European context. It would uphold the right of every child to have access to the support and education that would enable them to succeed. In addition to the Sensory Inclusion Service team in Telford and Wrekin (which currently provides specialist support services to deaf children), the University of Malta, the University of Leuven (Belgium), and the Mary Hare School for deaf children in the United Kingdom (which works in collaboration with Oxford Brookes University), were involved. The final partner was la Fédération Européenne des Associations de Professeurs de Déficients Auditifs (FEAPDA), a federation of associations of ToDs in 10 European countries that, at that time, comprised

Belgium, Germany, Italy, Luxembourg, Macedonia, the Netherlands, Poland, Slovenia, Sweden, Switzerland, and the United Kingdom.

The partners agreed they needed more knowledge about the training of ToDs in partner countries and across Europe. Having determined this, the group's intention was to develop a set of core competencies for training ToDs that would be applicable in a pan-European context. Last, it was important to disseminate the findings relating to need and the agreed core competencies to encourage their adoption across Europe in the light of increased interest in standardizing competences for teachers across the community.

Where Are the Teachers of the Deaf in Europe?

A questionnaire was sent out to FEAPDA members and a range of other European countries asking about the numbers of ToDs, and the nature of their ToD training and whether it was mandatory. There is huge variation in terms of numbers and qualification levels across the respondents' countries, but many countries, including Austria, Bulgaria, the Czech Republic, Cyprus, Denmark, Estonia, Greece, Hungary, Ireland, Latvia, Lithuania, Portugal, Romania, the Slovak Republic, and Spain, did not provide information about the status or existence of ToDs. This prevents us from having a clear picture of the overall provision in Europe. Seven countries (France, Finland, Germany, the United Kingdom, Luxembourg, Poland, and Slovenia) indicated that a mandatory specific qualification was needed to teach deaf children, and at different levels—some in the form of a diploma (such as in the United Kingdom, but this can also be done at the master's level); others are available only at the master's level (in Germany and Slovenia, for example). In some cases (such as in Finland), the qualification, for example, did not include any pedagogy, only linguistic elements—sign language. Malta had a specialist qualification, but it was not mandatory, and some countries either had a generic specialist qualification (such as in Flanders, Belgium) or no qualification (such as in Sweden and Italy). In France, the mandatory qualification differs according to whether the teacher is working in mainstream schools or special schools for the deaf.

There was a wide variety of responses to the question about how many ToDs hold a specialist qualification in each country. In Belgium (Flanders), only 10% have a specific qualification for teaching deaf children, whereas in Slovenia, 100% of the ToDs have it. In the United Kingdom, approximately 90% of the ToDs have the mandatory qualification, and most of the others are studying for it.

The nonspecialized ToDs in the various countries had trained in different ways (Leonardo da Vinci Lifelong Learning Project, 2011a). They were trained within the field, took relevant short courses, had general training for the education of children and young people with disabilities, or trained as sign language interpreters. From the responding European countries, only Germany and the United Kingdom had sets of competencies or defined areas of study that were in use in the training of ToDs. The other countries were not able to produce a list of competencies. Despite a low response rate from the different European countries, we concluded there is no regular pattern for the training and employment of ToDs.

Development of a Survey of Competencies

The aim of the survey was to investigate the need for a specialist qualification and to develop a set of competencies that would be common across Europe and agreed to by ToDs as essential for their profession. To examine the issue globally, a study was made of documents used in teacher trainer institutions in Europe—in particular, in Germany (Heidelberg University), the United Kingdom (Teaching Development Agency, 2009), the United States (Easterbrooks, 2008a, 2008b, 2008c), Canada, and Australia, where ToD competencies were already listed in some form. Last, a list of competencies for consultation was drawn up by the different partners during and between meetings. The list was redrafted a number of times—nine in all—over a number of meetings. The principal source of the list was the one in use in the United Kingdom at that time, the latest version having been produced in 2009 after 2 years of consultation and with the approval of the government (Teaching Development Agency, 2009). It was agreed by all to be a good starting point.

Eighty-seven competencies were categorized into three groups: *knowledge and understanding* (for example, understand how children and young people process auditory and visual information, and how this might affect the teaching and learning approach), *professional skills* (for example, provide a wide range of opportunities for the development of receptive and expressive language), and *personal attributes* (for example, has good communication skills, and a knowledge and skills base that inspires confidence from families, children, and other stakeholders).

To evaluate the likely efficacy of the process, a short pilot consultation took place involving ToDs and parents of deaf children and young people, as well as health professionals, psychologists, researchers, and teacher trainers in the partner countries and in the other FEAPDA member countries, demonstrating the survey to them and receiving their feedback about the process. These consultations raised the difficult question concerning the interpretation of the concept "ToD." Some respondents found it difficult to decide whether a given competency was applicable only for a ToD or for the whole range of professionals working with deaf children and young people. Others indicated that the various roles of a ToD are often carried out by different professionals.

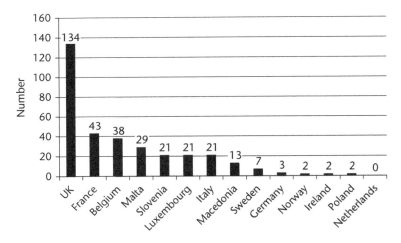

Figure 6.1 Distribution of the complete questionnaires in different European countries.

Taking into account the comments received after the initial pilot, the questionnaire was rewritten and uploaded to an online survey system. The list of questions (see Appendix 1) was then distributed to the ToDs in the 13 European countries listed in Figure 6.1. This was undertaken by the partners of the Leonardo project. In total, 336 surveys were completed.

NEED FOR COMPETENCIES

There were 336 respondents from 13 European countries (Belgium, France, Germany, Ireland, Italy, Luxembourg, Macedonia, Malta, Norway, Poland, Slovenia, Sweden, and the United Kingdom), and the majority in each agreed that such competencies were necessary. In general, they stated that not having specialist training for teachers working with deaf children potentially compromises teachers' ability to educate their students effectively. They also agreed that the development of such competencies, should they be adopted by educational departments in the different countries, would improve European cooperation and parity across the continent in the education of deaf learners, which would be beneficial for both the learners and their teachers, and could increase the effectiveness of deaf education across Europe.

Some respondents stated the need for competencies had increased in the light of early diagnosis of hearing loss, which has become much more common across Europe as a result of the development of newborn hearing screening. It was felt essential that to capitalize on early diagnoses, clear and robust competencies were needed by ToDs to provide the necessary support in those early years and beyond—to preschool settings and school. From the responses of the 336 respondents, 79% of the list of competencies was considered essential, 19% helpful, and 2% not necessary.

Partners sent the final report of the study to their national education departments, and a meeting was held with the Minister of Education in Luxembourg (which is the headquarters of FEAPDA) to secure support. The report was launched at a press conference (February 4, 2014), also in Luxembourg. There are ongoing discussions about taking the work further and developing online training for current course providers to support the delivery of these competencies in countries where they are not currently in use. This would involve conducting a larger scale survey, developing materials online to enable educators working with deaf children to have access to training linked to the competencies, and developing a skills ladder of qualifications that would be linked to the competencies and recognized in all member states. The long-term aim is to encourage Europe-wide acceptance of the necessity of making the specialist qualification mandatory based on these competencies in the interest of the education of deaf children.

THE NEED TO UNDERSTAND WHY THE COMPETENCIES WERE RANKED AS THEY WERE

In Flanders, the Dutch-speaking part of Belgium, ToDs work as teachers in special schools as well as itinerant teachers in mainstream schools. SLTs in Flanders also work in mainstream schools as itinerant professionals, expecting to do the same work as itinerant teachers. Following the previous Leonardo research, an investigation took place into whether people who work as ToDs or SLTs in Flanders also believe that competencies listed in the survey are necessary. As mentioned, a distinction between ToD and SLT has to be made because ToDs in Flanders (as in the United States) can refer either to ToDs in special schools or to itinerant teachers in mainstream schools. SLTs here refers to professionals working as itinerant professionals in mainstream schools but without a qualification as a teacher. In addition to questioning key competencies of a ToD, a survey was carried out regarding whether the skills should be acquired through specific training.

Survey and Respondents

The survey was translated into Dutch and administered (through an online service) to teachers, principals, and teachers in the service centers and schools for the deaf. Two groups of respondents were selected: teachers working in the school for the deaf in Flanders (n = 215) and itinerant teachers (n = 158). The teachers worked full time or part time with children or adolescents with a hearing loss in special elementary education or special secondary education, and all had a generic teaching degree and a teaching degree for special education. Through in-service training or training as a sign language interpreter, additional competencies are acquired to work with children with hearing loss. This training varies from school to school. Itinerant professionals work full time or part time with children or young people with a hearing loss in regular primary, secondary, and higher education. Only itinerant professionals with a teaching degree for special education or a degree as an SLT and/or audiologist were included in the study (n = 108). In Flanders, SLTs are trained for at least 3 years in speech, language, and audiology—domains not taught in the generic teacher's curriculum. The SLTs, however, lack knowledge and skills in didactics (teaching). The survey was distributed to 373 persons (215 teachers and 108 itinerant professionals).

The results are based on the data from 66 respondents, indicating a response rate of approximately 20% (completed questionnaires). A number of respondents were not included because they did not answer at least one category (A, knowledge and understanding; B, professional skills; C, personal attributes; see Appendix 1). Half of the respondents (n = 33) practiced as teachers within a special school (primary and secondary), and the other half worked as itinerant professionals in primary or secondary schools. Seventeen itinerant professionals (52%) had a teaching degree, 13 (39%) had an SLT degree, and three persons (9%) had both degrees. One person working at a school of the deaf also had two degrees. Twenty teachers (61%) were employed in special secondary education, 12 (36%) in special elementary education, and one person (3%) in both. With regard to the itinerant professionals, 17 (52%) were employed on several educational levels.

Because of the relatively small sample size, only results from teachers in special education (n = 33) and itinerant professionals (teachers and SLTs, n = 33) are considered here. Persons with two degrees (n = 3) were added to the group of SLTs/itinerant professionals, so the group of itinerant professionals consisted of 18 teachers (54%) and 15 SLTs (46%)

Specific Skills and Training

One hundred percent of respondents (n = 66) replied that the ToDs or SLTs should have special competencies. With the exception of one respondent, all considered specialized training for working with children with hearing loss necessary. The only respondent who replied "no" considered internal (school) training to be sufficient. The need for specific skills is situated mainly in the area of communication, deaf awareness, and didactics.

Core Competencies

Of the total group of teachers in special and itinerant education, 62% of competencies were ranked as essential (E), 34% were ranked as a plus (P), which means "a benefit but not essential," and 4% were ranked as neither essential nor plus (N). Figure 6.2 shows the distribution of the rankings of E, P, and N for the three categories (A, B, and C) of questions of the survey (see Appendix 1) for teachers in special education (Figure 6.2a) and for the itinerant professionals (Figure 6.2b). The competencies of the items in groups A, B, and C were ranked significantly differently by both teachers in special education and the itinerant professionals. Both groups of respondents gave more E rankings to category B than to the other two categories. In this sense, the distribution pattern for both

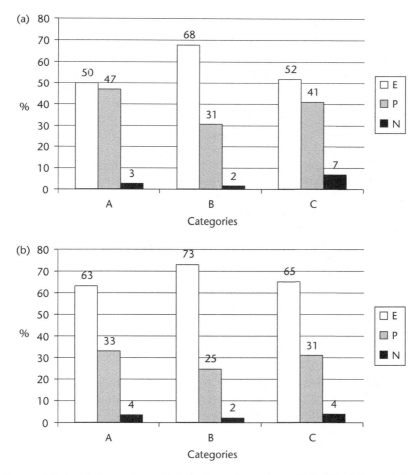

Figure 6.2 (a, b) Percentage distribution of rankings (E, P, N) of the competencies of the three categories (A, knowledge and understanding; B, professional skills; C, personal attributes, see previous part) for teachers of the deaf (n = 33) (a) and for itinerant professionals (n = 33) (b). E, essential; N, neither; P, plus.

categories was similar. Yet, the difference in distribution of the rankings was most diverse within the group of teachers in special education.

In general, itinerant teachers ranked significantly more competencies as essential compared with the teachers in special education in categories A, B, and C. For the P and N scores, no significant differences between the three categories were observed, with the exception of the P scores in category A, reflecting that the itinerant teachers scored significantly lower than the teachers in special education. This finding is not surprising, because a higher percentage of E rankings results in a lower percentage of P and N rankings.

Qualifications and Experience

To know whether the aforementioned difference in opinion is the result of training, the data of itinerant professionals with a degree as a teacher ($n = 18$) were compared with those with a degree in speech–language therapy ($n = 15$). Again, the itinerant professionals with a degree in speech–language therapy ranked significantly more competencies as essential than itinerant professionals with a degree as teacher in special education. This was also the case for the individual categories of A and B, and was nearly significant for category C.

We also examined whether assessment of important skills correlates with number of years of working experience. The average working experience for the total sample ($n = 66$) was a mean of 12.5 years, with a standard deviation of 10 years.

The entire sample shows a significant positive correlation for the importance of skills and experience. This correlation is attributed to the data of itinerant professionals, not to the special education teachers. In the group of itinerant professionals, the ones with a teaching degree show a moderately good correlation, but not the itinerant professionals with a degree in speech–language therapy (relationship not significant).

A more qualitative analysis yields the five competencies with the highest percentage E rankings (>90%) and the lowest percentage N rankings, respectively, for special education and itinerant professionals (Table 6.1).

Those competencies ranked as highest are mainly from the B category (*professional skills*); only one competency is from the C category (personal attribute) by special education teachers and one from category A (knowledge and understanding) by the itinerant professionals. Both special education teachers and itinerant professionals ranked three of the same competencies in the top five.

Among the special education teachers and itinerant professionals, the least important competencies were listed in the C category (personal attributes). It is striking that the competencies for maximizing hearing and creating optimal conditions for auditory function scored low. To establish whether this is related to the teaching degree, the person's working position (as a teacher in special education or as an

Table 6.1 Highest and lowest ranked competencies by teachers of the deaf and itinerant professionals in Flanders.

	Highest Ranked Competencies		Lowest Ranked Competencies
IT	Having strong communication, consulting, and training skills (**cat A**)	IT	Acting professionally as a manager or key figure with families and deaf children/young people to ensure proper support; being able to mediate (**cat A**)
SE	Knowing the factors that contribute to an optimal learning environment for all deaf children/teenagers (**cat A**)	IT	Being familiar with the regional, national, and European policies regarding deaf children/teenagers (**cat B**)
SE IT	Understanding how a language problem can affect learning throughout the curriculum (**cat B**)	SE IT	Being able to do and interpret electroacoustic checks on hearing aids and amplification equipment (**cat C**)
SE IT	Understanding the impact of deafness on language acquisition and communication (**cat B**)	SE IT	Developing hearing training programs for individual deaf children/young people and monitoring their implementation (**cat C**)
SE IT	Understanding how auditory and visual information is processed and its impact on education (**cat B**)	SE	Assessing the condition and suitability of the earpiece (**cat C**)
IT	Understanding the extent to which communication problems may affect cognitive, emotional, and social development influences (**cat B**)	SE	Judging the effectiveness and appropriateness of amplification equipment under different listening conditions (**cat C**)
SE	Acquiring a minimum of sign language skills (**cat C**)	SE	Being able to use individual (reinforcing) equipment to support inclusion and learning in certain classes (**cat C**)
		IT	Advising and supporting families in creating a facilitating visual and sound environment (**cat C**)

cat A, knowledge and understanding; cat B, professional skills; cat C, personal attributes; IT, itinerant professional; SE, special education teacher.

itinerant professional), and/or any additional training, those questions related to maximizing hearing and creating optimal conditions for auditory function were analyzed separately. The average rank orders of the scores for hearing were significantly greater for itinerant professionals than for teachers in special education. Itinerant professionals ranked these competencies significantly more as E than teachers in special education. No significant differences were established between itinerant teachers (n = 18) and itinerant SLTs (n = 15).

Competencies and Training as a Sign Language Interpreter

Currently, the sign language interpreter courses are the most important and only additional courses designed specifically for deaf education in Flanders. Therefore, we also examined whether the teachers in special education and the itinerant professionals who took an interpreter training course, which has a strong emphasis on visual communication, rank the importance of the variable maximizing hearing in the same way as special education teachers and itinerant professionals who did not have additional training as sign language interpreters. For the total sample (n = 57), maximizing hearing was rated significantly lower by special education teachers and itinerant professionals who were trained as sign language interpreters (n = 28) compared with those who did not receive this training. In the group of special education teachers, no meaningful distinction was found for the variable maximizing hearing by teachers with (n = 10) or without (n = 18) an interpreter degree; but, as noted earlier, as a group they ranked this variable significantly lower than the itinerant professionals.

Of the itinerant teachers, those with interpreter training (n = 8) ranked maximizing hearing significantly lower than the teachers without interpreter training (n = 7). For the itinerant SLTs, no significant difference was observed, but in that group the number of persons with an interpreter degree (n = 3) was much fewer than those without a degree (n = 11). Similar to the itinerant SLTs, the special education teachers ranked maximizing hearing lower when they were trained additionally as a sign language interpreter than when they were not.

Not only maximizing hearing, but all the competencies presented in this study were ranked significantly lower by the special education teachers and itinerant professionals with an interpreter degree (n = 28) than by those without one (n = 38).

In Sum

The upbringing and education of children and young people with a hearing loss, as well as supporting families with a child with a hearing loss, require specific skills, knowledge, and attitudes. In Flanders, no training exists that covers all the necessary topics (Scheetz & Martin, 2008).

Our survey showed that all respondents agreed that a ToD and other professionals should have specific competencies to work with deaf children, young people, and their families. Most respondents (98%) also believed this should be done through specialized training. The need for specific skills mainly applies to the area of communication, deaf awareness, and didactics.

Perspectives on the number of basic skills and competencies that should be acquired differed, depending on the working position, and the training and additional training received by the respondents. Both groups ranked the competencies within category B (knowledge and understanding) as most essential compared with categories A (professional attributes and ability to work with other professionals and stakeholders) and C (professional skills). Compared with special education teachers, itinerant professionals ranked significantly more competencies as essential. But, within the group of itinerant professionals, the SLTs ranked more skills as essential than the special education teachers. The results suggest this ranking of competencies is related to the person's training rather than his or her working position. Initially, SLTs will have acquired more competencies from their training concerning persons who are deaf. Teachers receive a generic training for children with a disability, which is not aimed specifically at children with a hearing impairment. This they learn "on the job" (depending on their working position) with the target population. Teachers in the group of itinerant professionals also consider more competencies important after they have gained more experience in their job.

It is quite striking that the qualitative analysis of the five highest ranked and five lowest ranked competencies showed that specific skills to optimize auditory skills are ranked low by both the special education teachers and itinerant professionals. Although itinerant professionals ranked these competencies significantly higher than the special education teachers, both groups probably assumed that the more technical aspects (such as frequency modulation systems) will be monitored by other professionals. This suggests that the importance of this competency depends on the working position/function and/or the target population associated with the various functions. As a result of newborn hearing screening and early bilateral implantation in Flanders, an increasing number of children with cochlear implants attend mainstream education, whereas a large group of children with multiple disabilities attend special schools for the deaf (De Raeve & Lichtert, 2012). For the latter children, other competencies are more important than for the former. Presumably, competencies with regard to the auditory function are considered less important, because only interpreter training for Flemish Sign Language is offered in Flanders.

In this study, teachers in the itinerant professional group who had interpreter training ranked the competencies linked with the variable hearing significantly lower than teachers without interpreter training. For the speech–language pathologists, a similar but not significant trend was observed. Of the teachers in schools for the deaf, no difference was observed between those with and without interpreter training, but they ranked these competencies significantly lower than the itinerant professionals. Not only auditory factors, but all 87 competencies were ranked as significantly less essential by special education teachers and itinerant professionals with interpreter training than professionals without interpreter training.

Our findings suggest that, in addition to the responsibilities and target population, training as a sign language interpreter can and will play a role in the validation of competencies. It is reasonable that people will judge the competencies that are learned during (continuing) education as important, and that it is difficult to judge their own lack of knowledge and skills (see Chapter 18). However, to ensure quality care and education to children who are deaf in a changing education landscape, some thought should be given to a balanced curriculum for different functions and target groups, preferably specific to European and other contexts.

THE NEED FOR NEW COMPETENCIES FOR SPEECH–LANGUAGE THERAPISTS WORKING IN AN AGE OF NEWBORN HEARING SCREENING AND EARLY COCHLEAR IMPLANTATION

Cochlear implantation has proved to be a successful intervention that provides significant restoration of hearing and development of spoken language in profoundly deaf children (e.g., Boons et al., 2012; Fagan & Pisoni, 2010; Geers et al., 2003; Nikolopoulos et al., 2006). However, the development of spoken language was a goal long before the development of cochlear implants (CIs) for children who were deaf. Interventions were enacted via the professional collaboration of audiologists, speech–language pathologists, and ToDs (Pollack, 1970) and, interestingly, the same team is in charge today of rehabilitation programs around the globe for children with CIs. The vital role of SLTs, now as then, in the development of the language of deaf children has been described by Carney and Moeller (1998).

Although the same professionals are now involved in interventions with deaf children with CIs, the characteristics of the population have changed as a result of technological advances and because of the newborn screening procedures adopted worldwide (American Academy of Pediatrics, 1999; see also Chapter 2). Consequently, along with audiologists, who had to learn to manage the technological device and the hearing of a child with a CI, speech–language pathologists and educators were called to change their approaches to accommodate very young children with CIs and their developmental cognitive, auditory, and communication schemata (Muma & Perigoe, 2010) as well as the older ones with rapidly growing communication skills who lagged behind.

The full impact of CI technology on the medical, technological, rehabilitation, and educational sectors has not yet been assessed, and this chapter presents several emerging changes in the role of ToDs in the educational/rehabilitation system as well in the provision of services in Europe and the United States. This section of the chapter highlights some of the results of an initial investigation into the knowledge, experience, and practices of SLTs working in Greece with children with CIs conducted by the Hearing Group of the Panhellenic Association of Logopedists (Okalidou et al., 2014).

Although highly specialized speech–language therapy services are needed to support children with CIs both in early intervention and in the classroom, such training is not often offered in the curricula of studies in communication disorders, even in countries with highly sophisticated programs (Ying, 2008). Consequently, there is a scarcity of such services offered by SLTs, as indicated by the Joint Committee on Infant Hearing (2007). On the other hand, an array of specialized continuing education programs and specialized organizations, such as the Ear Foundation in the United Kingdom and the Alexander Graham Bell Association for the Deaf and Hard of Hearing in the United States, serve this purpose by providing seminars and specialized training around the world.

In Greece, most SLTs work privately and get reimbursed by family insurance; a few SLTs work in the public education system and in hospitals. Yet, several CI teams have no SLTs aboard. Moreover, Greece has many islands, and children with CIs often must travel to major cities on the mainland for rehabilitation. Currently, there are three undergraduate programs in speech therapy in Greece (Georgieva, 2010) and one graduate program at the University of Athens that trains graduates from related fields to become SLTs. However, they do not offer systematic training of SLTs in pediatric cochlear implantation.

Few studies have investigated the knowledge and skills of SLTs regarding pediatric cochlear implantation (Cosby, 2009; Watson & Martin,1999). Both Cosby (2009) and Watson and Martin (1999) documented the relative lack of knowledge and skills of SLTs in managing children with CIs and emphasized the need for specialized services. In the following section, some results are reported from a study by Okalidou et al. (2014) regarding the knowledge and skills of SLTs who work with children in Greece who are deaf.

Questionnaire for Speech–Language Therapists

The participants in the study by Okalidou et al. (2014) were SLTs who filled out an online questionnaire, which was addressed to the two largest associations of SLTs in Greece: the Panhellenic Association of Logopedists—Speech Therapists and the Association of Scientists of Speech Pathology—Speech Therapy of Greece.

The construction of material is described in detail in Okalidou et al. (2014). Briefly, the questionnaire consisted of 25 items addressing topics related to CIs, divided into three sections: (a) training and experience, (b) knowledge and professional views, and (c) current practices. A 4-point scale from highly agree to disagree was used for the last two parts of the questionnaire (1 point, strongly agree; 2 points, slightly agree; 3 points, slightly disagree; 4 points, disagree).

Training and Experience of Speech–Language Therapists

The vast majority of SLTs, 108 of 134 (78%), worked with children who were deaf and fitted with CIs. Of these, 38% of the SLTs had a postgraduate degree, 78% attended seminars after they graduated, and 63%, were trained in practicum, primarily during the past 5 years. Interestingly, 60%—that is, more than half—of the experienced SLTs (working experience with children using CIs for 6 years or longer) had received postgraduate training, and almost all of them (92%) had attended related seminars. Of the less experienced SLTs (working experience less than 6 years), only 23% had received postgraduate training, 68% attended seminars, and 48% worked with children using CIs in their practicum. Of the SLTs (22%) who worked with deaf children who wore conventional hearing aids, 30% had postgraduate training, 50% attended seminars on CIs, and 50% worked with children with CIs in their practicum. In sum, the SLTs who worked with deaf children tended to seek specialized training in the field of cochlear implantation, especially via seminars or practicum.

Knowledge and Professional Views

Data analysis was based on central tendencies of responses along the 4-point Likert scale, which were expressed by the weighted average on each response set. All SLTs with experience working with deaf children believed there are differences in therapy among deaf children with CIs and those with conventional hearing aids (weighted average, 1.68–1.86 points). The responses for those SLTs who worked with children who are deaf but do not have a CI indicated some knowledge on aspects of CIs, such as candidacy criteria for implantation (weighted average, 1.90 points) and the developmental stages of listening skills (weighted average, 2.00 points), but not others, such as CI technology (weighted average, 2.47 points). Knowledge of these aspects was greater for SLTs with prior experience with CIs (weighted averages, 1.61, 1.94, and 1.61, respectively) and increased as a function of work experience. All SLTs working with children with deafness with or without CIs, and regardless of the amount of work experience, denoted adequate to strong skills in setting up therapeutic goals for prosody and prelinguistic skills during the early stages of therapy (weighted average, 1.37 points and 1.51 points, respectively). As for their attitudes toward sign language, both SLT groups tended to "slightly agree" (weighted averages, 2.17 points and 2.20 points, respectively) to a statement that sign language is harmful to the development of oral language skills. However, the clinicians more experienced with CIs tended to agree even less (weighted average, 2.43 points).

Furthermore, the need for further training on cochlear implantation was acknowledged by all SLT groups, more so for the SLT group with no CI experience (weighted average, 0.97 point) compared with the one with experience in CI (weighted average, 1.71 points). Last, all groups acknowledged the need for supervision. The first group of SLTs, with no CI experience, felt a stronger need for supervision when working with children with CIs (weighted average, 1.07 points) compared with those with CI experience who, nevertheless, also gave rather strong positive responses (weighted average, 1.58 points).

Practices of Speech–Language Therapists in Greece

This section addresses those SLTs (n = 96) who have been working with children with CIs in their therapy practice. The practice of SLTs in Greece with children with CIs involves a less than adequate collaboration with the medical staff of CI centers (weighted average, 2.51 points), despite their attested adequate skills (weighted average, 2.14 points) to contribute to the CI fitting process. However, a better collaboration is seen between SLTs and special educators (weighted average, 2.16 points), especially school-based special educators (weighted average, 2.02 points). Moreover, most SLTs (68.4%) felt strongly or adequately competent to design and implement specialized therapy programs for children with CIs, but one-third seemed to lag behind on these skills. There is less use of alternative–augmentative communication (weighted average, 2.38 points), such as Makaton, picture exchange communication systems, and sign language, to facilitate the development of communication and spoken language. Use of telepractice, the application of telecommunications technology to the delivery of speech and language professional services at a distance by linking SLTs to client/patient (Houston & Stredler-Brown, 2012) was not a preferred scheme at present (weighted average, 3.81 points). Last, they all valued parental involvement (weighted average, 1.07 points).

Need for Advanced Training and Active Involvement in Interdisciplinary Teams

One of the first observations was that the educational level of SLTs who worked with deaf children—and more so children with CIs—tended to be high, and the trend increased as a function of work experience. However, those who worked with children with CIs for a period of up to 5 years seemed to lag behind in the level of formal education, but compensated with informal training. Data suggested a need for providing opportunities for advanced studies in the field of cochlear implantation.

Knowledge of cochlear implantation by SLTs working in the field of deafness was adequate for candidacy criteria for implantation and for building hierarchical listening skills, but lagged behind on cochlear implantation technology. This is accounted for by the fact that cochlear implantation technology changes constantly, encompassing complex algorithms of speech processing, design innovations, and product updates that are barely understood by nontechnical professionals without considerable effort. Regarding the use of sign language in therapy, it was a less preferred choice among both SLT groups, but it seemed to be an option for more experienced clinicians. A tentative hypothesis is that experienced clinicians have a variety of children with CIs in their caseload. These include (a) children who received their CIs late and had been using signing systems or other communication methods before their implantation, and (b) children with additional disabilities who often need to use supplementary or alternative communication systems. The disparity in preferences of SLTs with respect to signing systems is on a par with literature findings (e.g., Geers, 2006; Giezen et al., 2014; McDonald Connor et al., 2000; Ruffin et al., 2013; Svirsksy et al., 2000). Last, all respondents, even those with the longest amount of work experience, stressed the need for further training and supervised work. This is another indication that the field of cochlear implantation is highly specialized and calls for continuous education services (such as supervision).

The investigation also pointed out that speech and language services for children with CIs in Greece are not based within a formal interdisciplinary network. The lack of established collaboration between medical specialists and SLTs deprives the latter of gaining more hands-on expertise and knowledge about important aspects of CIs, and the former from exploiting the SLT skills for team benefits. Hence, training and expertise of SLTs regarding cochlear implantation can be enriched not only via professional training programs, but also by their active involvement in interdisciplinary CI teams. These service delivery models have been implemented to some extent in Europe and also in the United States (Joint Committee on Infant Hearing, 2007; Nevins & Chute, 1996), and they should be promoted by government policy and professional organizations for other countries in the European Union or elsewhere. A certification for the deaf and hard-of-hearing (DHH) related to cochlear implantation may be a necessary future step to advance professional development and ensure quality of services. Moreover, more modern methods such as telepractice need to be implemented more aggressively to suit the needs of the pediatric population with CIs from remote or rural areas.

THE NEED FOR FAMILY-CENTERED COMPETENCIES FOR TEACHERS OF THE DEAF AND OTHER PROFESSIONALS WORKING AS HOME-BASED SERVICE PROVIDERS

More than half a century ago, the importance of early home-based guidance for families and children with a hearing loss was emphasized by Wendy Galbraith at the Twelfth International Congress on Education of the Deaf in Washington, DC, in 1963 (Brill, 1984). This was the first time, since those congresses were first organized in 1878, that the role of the parents in education for the deaf was addressed at this important international forum. Galbraith, who worked as an educational consultant in London, found that congenitally deaf children diagnosed by the age of 6 to 9 months (the earliest target ages for screening at that time) should, like children who are typically hearing, learn their language and speech at home. She therefore argued that education for these very young children should start with the education of the adults and siblings at home.

Although thinking about how the roles of parents and service providers has changed over time, the idea that parents have to be empowered to raise a child with a significant hearing loss is still gaining importance in this new era of universal newborn hearing screening (Holzinger et al., 2011; Moeller, 2000; see Chapter 2; but see Chapter 18). During the past decade, home-based early intervention has changed dramatically. A paradigm shift occurred from an expert model with the focus on the child to a partnership model with the focus on the whole family context. When a child is diagnosed as deaf shortly after birth, the news affects the parents immediately, not the child (Lichtert & van Wieringen, 2013). By its very nature, deafness is never an isolated phenomenon affecting a single person. It is a communicative issue par excellence, and therefore is always interwoven with the child's entire interactional context. This is especially true for babies. Involving parents as full partners from the beginning during the rehabilitation process also fits in with the modern concept of disability as defined by the International Classification of Functioning model (ICF) of the World Health Organization. The ICF considers functioning and disability as a dynamic interaction between health conditions and contextual factors, both personal and environmental. The better the interaction between the person and his or her "context," the less restricted the disability. This means that limiting rehabilitation programs to individual therapy for children outside the educational context conflicts with the current ICF disability model (Wilcox & Woods, 2011; World Health Organization, 2013).

Family-centered help includes practices that treat families with dignity and respect; it is individualized, flexible, and responsive to family concerns and priorities; it includes information sharing so that families can make informed decisions; it honors family choice regarding any number of aspects of program practices and intervention options; it applies parent–professional collaboration and partnerships as a context for family–practitioner relations; and it promotes families' abilities to obtain and mobilize resources and support necessary for them to care for and raise their children in a competency-strengthening manner (Ingber & Dromi, 2010; Shelton & Stepanek, 1995). This paradigm shift from an expert model (with its focus on the child) to a partnership model (with its focus on the whole family context) requires new competencies of the professionals working with families of deaf children.

In Flanders (Belgium), a variety of professionals work in home-based guidance. Most of them are trained as SLTs, audiologists, special education psychologists, clinical psychologists, or social workers, and only a few have received special training to work with families. Of the 87 competencies formulated in the Leonardo survey, only a few refer to working with families. Because working with families is gaining in importance, a study was done to explore how family-centered competencies (FCCs) for home-based service providers (HBSPs) are evaluated by parents of deaf children and children with language disorders in Flanders. As noted earlier, Flanders is the Dutch-speaking part of Belgium, with about six million inhabitants.

In brief, home-based guidance was defined by a government decree in 1988 as "a form of assistance which aims to provide educational support to families with a disabled child, focused on the acceptance of disability on the handling and/or educating of the person with a disability and on the forward-looking orientation, so development is encouraged and the family situation is supported." In Flanders, five centers for support of DHH individuals are recognized by the Flemish Agency for Persons with a Handicap, one in each province. Access to home guidance is quite straightforward based on a prescription of an ear, nose, and throat specialist. Guidance is mostly provided at home, but it can also be organized at the guidance center itself, in a daycare center, by grandparents, or by a daycare supervisor. An individual family service plan is developed with each family. Home guidance services are allowed to work together with a wide range of other care providers such as medical, audiological, and rehabilitation services as well as parents who are willing to share their experience ("contact parents"), and/or deaf role models.

Evaluating Family-Centered Competencies

Parents of deaf children and children with language disorders ranging from birth to 12 years from all home guidance centers in Flanders were asked to evaluate the FCCs of their HBSP with an adapted version of the Family-Centered Practices Checklist from Wilson and Dunst (2005). To be included in the study, parents must have received home guidance for at least 3 months and not ceased doing so for more than 6 months. At least one parent needed to have a full understanding of written Dutch, the language of the inventory. Of the 125 distributed questionnaires, 65 were returned, but only 53 fulfilled all the criteria to be included (response rate of 42%).

The main objective of the study was to examine how FCCs for professionals working in home-based intervention, with different qualifications and demographic backgrounds, are evaluated by parents of deaf children and children with language disorders. More specifically, we asked whether there is a significant difference between the desired and available FCCs depending on the professional qualifications, years of work experience, different kinds of disorders (deaf, hard of hearing, speech–language impairment), hearing device (CI, hearing aid), school type (inclusive, special), and age of the child.

An adapted version of the Family-Centered Practices Checklist developed by Wilson and Dunst (2005) was used. In this checklist, both *relational* as well as *participatory* components of family-centered practices were evaluated. Each of these components has two clusters of practices. The *relational* component includes practices typically associated with (a) good clinical skills (such as active listening, compassion, empathy, respect, and being nonjudgmental) and (b) professional beliefs about and attitudes toward families, especially those pertaining to parenting capabilities and competencies. The *participatory* component includes practices that (a) are individualized, flexible, and responsive to family concerns and priorities; and (b) provide families with opportunities to be actively involved in decisions and choices (Dunst &Trivette, 1996).

In the original English checklist, 17 statements are scored on a 4-point Likert scale to indicate the extent to which the relevant skill is applied by the HBSP. Also, it is possible to give an example of a specific situation. According to the developers of the checklist, this list can be used for self-reflection to optimize family-oriented practices (Dunst et al., 2007).

In the adapted Flemish version, the 17 statements were translated and accompanied by two examples to illustrate the more general statement. These examples were generated carefully and were selected on the basis of a pilot study with parents and professionals in the field. During the first phase, interviews were conducted with three of the five coordinators of the home guidance centers in Flanders for deaf children and children with speech and language impairments. These interviews were also done with seven HBSPs with different professional qualifications. The aim of these interviews was to control the face validity of the checklists and to gather concrete examples for each statement of the questionnaire. Each interview lasted approximately 1 hour. To illustrate the adapted questionnaire (Table 6.2), one general statement

Table 6.2 Examples in the Flemish Version of the Family-Centered Practices Checklist

Interpersonal Skills	Asset-Based Attitudes	Family Choice & Action	Practitioner Responsiveness
Interact with the family in a warm, caring, and empathetic manner	Focus on individual and family strengths and values	Work in partnership with parents/family members to identify and address family-identified desires	Support and respect family members' decisions.
My HBSP is taking the necessary time to listen to my story and my concerns.	My HBSP looks at my child in a positive way and recognizes his or her talents and interests.	My HBSP always consults us and treats us as equals.	My HBSP respects our choice for an inclusive/or special education.

HBSP, home-based service provider.

is given for every cluster, together with one example to illustrate that particular statement.

For each of the 17 statements, parents had to decide to what extent these statements applied to their HBSP on a Likert scale, with "A" ranging from always (1 point) to mostly (2 points) to sometimes (3 points) to never (4 points). Parents also had to rank how important this skill was for them on a 4-point Likert scale, with B ranging from necessary (1 point) to important (2 points) to less important (3 points) to not important (4 points). A coding scheme was constructed to evaluate the match or mismatch between the observed competencies of the HBSP by the parents and the expectations of the parents. Responses 1–1, 2–2, and 1–2 were considered a positive match, with 1–1 and 2–2 a perfect match. Positive and perfect matches were considered as matches, and any other combinations (3–1, 3–2, 4–1, 4–2) was considered a mismatch. All questionnaires were collected and processed anonymously.

Parents' Experience

As noted, the aim of the study was to examine how parents experienced the FCCs of their HBSP. About 70% of the HBSPs were qualified as SLTs, and 5% of them had additional qualifications in audiology. Another 26% of the HBSPs were qualified as clinical psychologists (13%) or special educational psychologists (13%). Only 4% of the HBSPs had another qualification that was not specified. The number of years of experience as HBSPs of the entire sample ranged from 2 to 25 years (mean, 9.5 years; standard deviation, 5.27 years). These HBSPs supported families with deaf children (47%), children with speech–language impairment (36%) or both (15%), and unknown (2%). Of the deaf children, 45%

wore hearing aids, 32% had CIs, and 3% had both. Nineteen percent of the children did not (yet) have a hearing device.

At the time of the survey, 4% of the children ranged between birth and 1 year, 66% between 1 year and 6 years, and 30% between 6 years and 12 years. Of these children, 28% did not attend a school yet, 43% attended a mainstream school (with 32% relying on itinerant professionals), and 28% attending a special school setting. Most of the surveys (71%) were filled out by mothers, 6% by fathers, and 23% by both parents. Most parents (91%) indicated the survey was easy to fill out, whereas 9% found it rather difficult. For 66% of the parents, the language of the survey was felt to be normal; for 32%, easy; and for one parent, too difficult.

The survey showed that the "match" between expectation and FCC was significantly different for HBSPs with a qualification of SLT than for HBSPs with other qualifications. The perfect match between the FCCs for SLTs and the expectations of the parents was less (69.5% of the measured items) than for the HBSPs with another qualification (77% of the measured items), but SLTs were less frequently mismatched on the measured items of FCCs (0.5% of the measured items) compared with the HBSPs with another qualification (2% of the measured items).

For the total group, no significant differences were observed between matched FCCs realized by HBSPs with more or fewer years of work experience than the average of 9.5 years and the expectations of the parents. Less experienced HBSPs, however, had significantly more mismatches than experienced ones. Of the child-related variables, matches were not significantly different for age, type of disability (deaf or speech–language impairment, or a combination of both) or type of education (mainstream, specific). Surprisingly, of the children who were deaf, parents of children with CIs indicated significantly more mismatches (between expectations and competencies) compared with children with hearing aids. More detailed analyses suggested that result was probably explained by the combination of fewer SLTs and somewhat less experienced HBSPs working in the group of children with CIs.

In general, the balance between reality and the expectation of FCCs seemed to be better for SLTs and audiologists compared with the other professionals. There were significantly fewer mismatches between expectations and competencies. For the whole group of HBSPs, the number of years of experience also seemed to affect the results significantly.

SUMMARY AND CONCLUSIONS

Competencies Are Necessary But Not Guaranteed

According to article 24 of Education, passage 3c of the United Nations Convention on the Rights of Persons with Disabilities, state parties are called to take the necessary steps for "ensuring that the education of persons, and in particular children, who are blind, deaf or deaf–blind, is delivered in the most appropriate languages and modes and means of communication for the individual, and in environments which maximize academic and social development" (http://www.un.org/disabilities/convention/conventionfull.shtml).

In this chapter, several studies that examined different facets of the qualifications and competencies of persons working with children and students in Europe were considered. Although we represent different countries and focus on a variety of settings in which children or students who are deaf are educated, there is one common theme running through all of these studies: the necessity for mandatory competencies that are consistent from country to country for ToDs, SLTs, and other qualified professionals.

In the Flemish (Belgian) study, conducted in the country where specific (mandatory) training for educating deaf children is lacking, professionals working with deaf children ranked different competencies as important, depending on the setting in which they worked. Teachers working in special schools ranked significantly fewer competencies as important compared with itinerant teachers in mainstream schools. This is probably related to the type of student with whom they work. Deaf children in special schools in Flanders have much more complex needs than children in mainstream schools (De Raeve & Lichtert, 2012). Teachers in special schools for the deaf also work more often in teams with SLTs; audiologists; ear, nose, and throat specialists; educational psychologists; and social workers than itinerant teachers. As a result, more competencies are available through the different members of a team compared with an itinerant teacher who has to work more as a single specialist in a mainstream school, where a team of specialists in deaf issues is not present. However, professionals who have learned more about deafness during their initial professional training (such as SLTs) ranked significantly more competencies as important compared with teachers without this knowledge during their training, even when they performed the same job as an itinerant teacher.

Results also made clear that training as a sign interpreter has an important influence on the need for competencies, and probably also on what these professionals expect of a deaf child to learn. Professionals working with deaf children in Flanders, who were trained as sign language interpreters, regardless of whether they worked in a special or mainstream school or had a qualification as a teacher or SLT, ranked competencies regarding auditory competences of the deaf child significantly lower than professionals without the additional training as a sign language interpreter. From the study in Flanders on professionals working in home-based guidance, paradoxically, HBSPs with more specific therapeutic training regarding the problems of the children (such as SLTs) were experienced by parents as being more family centered compared with HBSPs with a more contextual training (such as psychologists). It seems that working in partnership with families first of all requires expertise in the specific problems of the child.

Formal and Postgraduate Training of Teachers of the Deaf

It is commonly accepted that the population of DHH children is a highly heterogeneous one. Hence, the types of services needed to ensure what is described earlier for each child are reflected in the different roles that ToDs and other professionals are called on to play for the academic and social welfare of DHH children.

The fact that the working environments of ToDs and other professionals differ as much as the population of DHH children they serve calls for building a variety of professional skills, including those related to working with other professionals (interdisciplinary collaboration) and parents (via training them to provide home intervention). We argue that a well-balanced curriculum for the additional training of ToDs and other professionals is necessary to guarantee high-quality education and educational support for a diversity of deaf children and their families. We should ask ourselves whether it is still realistic to have only a generic "specific" training for this variety of deaf children. Maybe it is better to develop different curricula, depending on the special needs of the children. Working with deaf children with complex needs, for example, is different from working with typically developing deaf children with good-functioning CIs who received their implants at an early age. Educating deaf children in a bilingual setting is different from educating children in an oral-only setting, and so on. Further specialization is required to make parents and children more conscious of what they can expect from these professionals.

Another requirement is the need for telepractice, which is a promising tool for delivering intervention and for promoting the professional development of ToDs. Telecommunication technologies (telepractice, teleconferencing) need to be incorporated in the service delivery of SLTs working with children with hearing impairment and their families who live in remote and difficult-to-access areas. These skills can be built by changing policies and encouraging the specialization of ToDs and other professionals via formal educational systems in different countries. Because the field is changing dynamically as a result of technological innovations and the types of DHH children being served, along with evolving social and interest groups and the concomitant changes in ethics and rights, one might hope for a tighter collaboration among associations in different countries. This is important: to exchange knowledge and experience to build networks and to advocate for policies that meet more effectively the needs of DHH children and the professionals who serve them.

It became apparent from our studies that the majority of ToDs and other professionals agreed to the need for the development of specific competencies for working with children with deafness, because many of the proposed competencies were ranked as mandatory by the survey participants. This consensus emphasizes that there is a strong professional belief that the field of deafness and deaf education is highly specialized, and therefore it is important that formal educational systems incorporate specialized programs to bridge the gap between formal education and current professional practice. In particular, the professional skills of itinerant teachers, as well as the ones needed to work with children with CIs, and in home intervention, are some of the current areas of practice that call for specialized training of ToDs and other professionals.

ACKNOWLEDGMENTS

We acknowledge the contribution of the key partners in the European Leonardo da Vinci Research project (LDV-PAR-P-407) titled Development of Pan-European Competencies for Teachers of the Deaf through Partnership. The inspiration came from the late Andrew Broughton of Telford and the Wrekin Local Authority in the United Kingdom along with Graham Groves, Dr. Marie Alexander of the University of Malta, Drs. Guido Lichtert and Astrid van Wieringen of the KU Leuven, Sue Lewis and Simon Thompson of the Mary Hare School in liaison with Oxford Brookes University, and Paul Simpson, President, La Fédération Européenne des Associations de Professeurs de Déficients Auditifs.

We thank the coordinators, home-based supervisors, parents of the home guidance centers in Flanders (Belgium), and students of Speech Pathology and Audiology Sciences KU Leuven for their help with collecting data. We also thank the Hearing Group of the Panhellenic Association of Logopedists for granting us permission to discuss their published work in the context of this chapter. Part of the research is supported by the FP7 people programme (Marie Curie Actions), Research Executive Agency grant agreement no. FP7-607139 (Improving Children's Auditory Rehabilitation).

APPENDIX 1: DEVELOPMENT OF PAN-EUROPEAN COMPETENCIES FOR TEACHERS OF THE DEAF THROUGH PARTNERSHIPS

You will be presented with a number of competencies. Please indicate by using a tick (✓) which statement you would agree with for each competency. You may agree with more than one statement.

Statement Number		
1	**Essential** for **all** those working with deaf children and young people (E)	
2	Helpful but not essential (P)	
3	Not important (N)	

COMPETENCE AREA—A			
Personal attributes, professional and interpersonal skills			
Learning, Access and Inclusion	E	H	N
Have a clear commitment to inclusion in society, understanding of what inclusive practice for deaf children and young people looks like and what needs to be in place to secure it			
Use information available about the achievements and well-being of deaf children to measure the success of current approaches, policies and provision			
Make well-founded evaluations of situations upon which they are asked to advise and offer advice that can be acted on			
Understand the range of provision, resources and support available to deaf children, students and their families at different times in their lifelong learning journey and how to access these			
Know the different placement options for deaf children/students in their own country, their criteria for admission, advantages and disadvantages and how to evaluate their potential effectiveness			
Understand the roles and responsibilities of a range of specialist services and agencies that work with deaf children/students and their families. These include the range of communication and learning support workers and technological support services.			
Contribute to reviews of provision and how well it matches needs, recognizing their accountability to parents/caregivers, managers, local authority officers and/or inspectors			

Reflect carefully on the progress of all deaf students they are responsible for, making recommendations as to the effectiveness of services and what needs to change if necessary			
Have advocacy skills and the confidence to use them in support of deaf children/students and their families			
Keep up to date with research and innovations in practice including new technologies			
Working with other professionals and stakeholders			
Have strong communication, advisory and training skills that enable teachers, teaching assistants, families and other professionals to acquire skills and meet the needs of deaf children/students effectively			
Have skills and support skills of others in the use (and modification) of materials and specialist equipment			
Have skills and support skills of others in the identification of deaf children/students' strengths and needs			
Have skills and support skills of others in the identification of targets or next steps for children/students and the devising of programs to meet them			
Act as a lead professional or key worker for families and children where necessary, a) helping families to access services and express their views, b) coordinating the team working with the family so that the child/student's needs are met, c) ensuring that services for deaf children/students continue to improve			
Recognize support staff's strengths and areas of improvement through sensitive and constructive feedback			
Ensure all professionals involved are clear about next steps for child/student and how these will be achieved			
Provide information in ways which take account of family diversity and supports their ability to make informed choices			
Deliver and/or help parents or others deliver the parents' choice of communication			
Model, coach, encourage and work in partnership with the family and others so that the deaf child/student's linguistic development is optimized			
Work collaboratively with colleagues, other specialists and parents/caregivers to assess and support deaf children/students to maximize their opportunities through joint planning, implementation of policies, evaluation of practices and reporting			
Train and advise families and other professionals so that they can check, understand and use amplification equipment effectively			

COMPETENCE AREA B—Knowledge and understanding			
Educational philosophy: education policy, human development, and curriculum theory and the application to deaf education			
Understand the different attitudes to inclusion and deafness including those related to deaf identity and deaf culture			
Understand the potential educational, psychological, social and cultural implications of deafness			
Understand the factors that contribute to securing optimum learning environments for all learners and steps that can be taken to make these more appropriate for deaf children/students at different ages			
Understand the curriculum, including the National Curriculum if in place, and its challenges for deaf children/students			
Understand how language difficulties affect learning across the curriculum			
Be familiar with regional, national and European legislation, policies, procedure and guidelines related to deaf children/students			
Teaching approaches and assessment for learning			
Know about the different teaching approaches that can be used with deaf children/students in order to meet the specific needs of deaf children/students in different educational settings			
Have a detailed understanding of child development and learning and the challenges a hearing loss might present			
Understand the relationship between language and literacy and how different approaches support reading and writing with deaf children/students			
Know about the range of additional needs that deaf children/students might have, including additional learning difficulties and how these may affect their development			
Understand the range of ways in which learning and development (including language and communication) can be assessed and how to identify learning priorities following assessment			
Know about different approaches supporting the well-being of deaf learners, including through personal, social and health education			
Communication and language			
Understand how deaf children/students process auditory and visual information and how this might affect the teaching and learning approach			

Understand the impact of deafness on the process of language acquisition and communication			
Understand how communication difficulties might impact the cognitive, emotional and social development of deaf children/students and the need for urgent intervention			
Know how to support the deaf child's/student's expressive and receptive language to enable him or her to access the curriculum more independently			
Understand the full range of approaches to communication and how they support the development of spoken and/or sign language competence—for example: a) understand the different auditory oral approaches, b) understand the range of sign language systems, including total communication approach and when and how to use them			
Have knowledge of different programs and technologies that can support language acquisition particularly where deaf children/students have additional needs			
Working with parents/caregivers and other stakeholders			
Understand the rationale, principles, objectives, strategies and practices of working in partnership with families, stakeholders and other agencies			
Understand and respect the diversity and uniqueness of each family and deaf child/student including their different challenges and strengths			
Understand the variety of responses of parents following diagnosis of hearing impairment in deaf children and the potential impact that such a diagnosis may have on family life			
Hearing and vision			
Have a detailed understanding of how we hear, the different types and degrees of hearing loss and how we measure these			
Know about the range of different types of amplification devices available to support children's/student's use of residual hearing including hearing aids, cochlear implants, frequency modulation and other systems and how they might be used to meet individual need			
Understand the stages of listening development and how to support and assess these			
Know how to assess the listening and visual environments and make recommendations			
Understand the importance of audiological review especially if there are concerns regarding the child/student's progress			
Understand the role of vision in the communicative and other development of deaf children/students			

COMPETENCE AREA C—Professional skills			
Supporting learning			
Teach a wide range of deaf children/students demonstrating high expectations for their learning and behavior			
Develop, implement and evaluate a range of approaches to help deaf children/students achieve agreed outcomes			
Identify and anticipate the difficulties that particular study areas present for different children/students or groups			
Support deaf children's/student's literacy and numeracy development			
Assessment and assessment for learning			
Use assessments to prioritize learning targets and support next steps, including writing personal learning plans, behavior plans or education plans			
Prepare and write accurate assessment reports, whose findings can be understood and used by teachers, other professionals, and parents/caregivers			
Include deaf children/students and their parents/caregivers in assessment and target-setting processes and procedures, ensuring that they contribute to and understand what targets are set and why			
Language development			
Use a range of appropriate procedures (formal and informal) to assess and evaluate all aspects of children's/student's communication and language development (spoken and/or signed)			
Have skills in observing and promoting very early communicative behavior in deaf babies and young children, including supporting the skills and understandings of families/carers			
Educational development			
Assess, monitor and evaluate the deaf child's/student's progress in all aspects of the curriculum, including the National Curriculum where in place			
Assess, monitor and evaluate the deaf child's/student's learning attitude and thinking skills			
Personal, social and emotional development			
Assess and monitor the social and emotional well-being of deaf children/students, including their behavior			
Assess and monitor the self-help and independence skills of deaf children/students, including their independent learning behavior			

Advise and support families and schools in providing environments and experiences that support the child's emotional well-being			
Provide targeted support on key skills and at key times, such as transition that smooth the child's/student's individual learning journey			
Curriculum access and inclusion			
Differentiate mainstream curriculum and personalize provision to match and develop the abilities of deaf children/students			
Foster perseverance and concentration by structuring tasks and learning so that learners are clear about what is expected of them and why			
Help deaf children/students become independent and take responsibility for their own learning			
Use effective strategies to promote positive behavior, manage difficult situations in accordance with the school's/setting's policy on discipline and the deaf child's/student's needs			
Promote and support knowledge and skills related to personal, social and health education, and sex and relationship education			
Use strategies to overcome barriers created by additional learning needs such as limited cognitive ability and other disabilities in conjunction with hearing loss			
Communication and language			
Design and implement a coherent communication program based on known best practice in relation to the deaf child's/student's language/communication choice and needs			
Provide a wide range of opportunities for the development of receptive and expressive language to age-appropriate levels as swiftly and fully as possible			
Support language acquisition and extension in all lessons regardless of the subject being taught			
Acquire sign language skills to a required minimum level, and beyond this, wherever there are sign language users on their caseload or in their class			
Maximizing use of residual hearing and vision			
Enable deaf children/students to make optimal use of their listening and speech reading skills			
Carry out listening checks of personal hearing aids and other equipment			

Carry out electroacoustic checks of personal hearing aids and other amplification equipment and interpret data related to this			
Make functional checks of ear-mold condition and suitability			
Evaluate the effectiveness and appropriateness of the deaf child's/student's amplification package for the different listening environments in which they are placed			
Use personal amplification and assistive devices to support more fully inclusion and the child's/student's learning in a particular lesson			
Identify and link the most effective technology/devices to support access to auditory and visual information for a specific child/student and environment			
Use a range of educational technology effectively and demonstrate its use to others			
Develop listening programs for individual children/students and monitor their implementation			
Evaluate the deaf child's/student's listening development, making recommendations and referrals to audiology and other professionals where appropriate			
The listening and visual environment			
Assess and recommend adaptations to the physical environment of classrooms and homes in order to meet the needs of deaf children/students			
Evaluate the acoustic (listening) environment and know how to adapt it to support access and inclusion			
Advise and support families in creating a facilitative listening and visual environment			

Also, please feel free to add any competencies that you feel may not have been included.

_____

_____

Source: Leonardo Da Vinci Lifelong Learning Project (2009). *Development of Pan-European Competencies for Teachers of the Deaf Through Partnership*. http://www.europeansharedtreasure.eu/detail.php?id_project_base=2009-1-GB2-LEO04-01424.

REFERENCES

American Academy of Pediatrics. (1999).Task force on newborn and infant hearing: Newborn and infant hearing loss: Detection and intervention. *Pediatrics, 103*(2), 527–530.

British Association of Teachers of the Deaf (January 2005). *Models of Deaf Education*. Association Magazine [entire volume].

Boons, T., Brokx, J., Dhooge, I., Frijns, J., Peeraer, L., Vermeulen, A., Wouters, J., & van Wieringen, A. (2012). Predictors of spoken language development following pediatric cochlear implantation. *Ear & Hearing, 33*(5), 617–639.

Brill, R. G. (1984). *International congresses on education of the deaf. An analytical history 1878–1980*. Washington, DC: Gallaudet College Press.

Calderon, R. (2000). Parental involvement in deaf children's education programs as a predictor of child's language, early reading and socio-emotional development. *Journal of Deaf Studies and Deaf Education, 5*,140–155.

Carney, A. E., & Moeller, M. P. (1998). Treatment efficacy: Hearing loss in children. *Journal of Speech, Language & Hearing Research, 41*(1), S61–S85.

Cosby, J. (2009). Pediatric cochlear implants: Knowledge and skills of speech–language pathologists. *The ASHA Leader, 14*(2), 1–6.

De Raeve, L., & Lichtert, G. (2012). Changing trends within the population of children who are deaf or hard of hearing in Flanders (Belgium): Effects of 12 years of universal newborn hearing screening, early intervention, and early cochlear implantation. *The Volta Review, 112*(2),131–148.

Dunst, C. J., & Trivette, C. M. (1996). Empowerment, effective helping practices and family-centred care. *Pediatric Nursing, 22*, 334–337, 343.

Dunst C. J., Trivette, C. M., & Hamby, D. W. (2007). Meta-analysis of family-centered helpgiving practices research. *Mental Retardation and Developmental Disabilities Research Review, 13*(4), 370–378.

Easterbrooks, S. R. (2008a). Knowledge and skills for teachers of individuals who are deaf and hard of hearing: Advanced set development. *Communication Disorders Quarterly, 30*(1), 37–48.

Easterbrooks, S. R. (2008b). Knowledge and skills for teachers of individuals who are deaf or hard of hearing: Initial set revalidation. *Communication Disorders Quarterly, 30*(1), 12–36.

Easterbrooks, S. R. (2008c). Knowledge and skills for all teachers of children who are deaf or hard of hearing: New standards and their evidence base. *Communication Disorders Quarterly, 30*(1), 3–4.

European Commission, Directorate-General for Education and Culture (2011). *Education and Training 2020 Programme Thematic Working Group Teacher Professional Development; Policy approaches to defining and describing teacher competencies.* http://ec.europa.eu/education/policy/strategic-framework/doc/defining-teacher-competences_en.pdf.

Fagan, M. K., & Pisoni, D. B. (2010). Hearing experience and receptive vocabulary development in deaf children with cochlear implants. *Journal of Deaf Studies and Deaf Education, 15*(2), 149–161.

Geers, A. E. (2006). Factors influencing spoken language outcomes in children following early cochlear implantation. *Advances in Otorhinolaryngology, 64*, 50–65.

Geers, A. E., Nicholas, J. G., & Sedey, A. (2003). Language skills of children with early cochlear implantation. *Ear and Hearing, 24*(1), 46S–58S.

Georgieva, D. (2010). Education of logopedists or speech–language pathologists in Bulgaria, Greece, Macedonia, Poland and Russia. *Folia Phoniatrica et Logopaedica, 62*, 217–222.

Giezen, M. R., Baker, A. E., & Escudero, P. (2014). Relationships between spoken word and sign processing in children with cochlear implants. *Journal of Deaf Studies and Deaf Education, 19*(1), 107–125.

Green, E. (2014). *Building a better teacher: How teaching works.* New York, NY: W.W. Norton.

Holzinger, D., Fellinger, J., & Beitel, C. (2011). Early onset of family centred intervention predicts language outcomes in children with hearing loss. *International Journal of Pediatric Otorhinolaryngology, 75*, 256–260.

Ingber, S., & Dromi, E. (2010). Actual versus desired family-centered practice in early intervention for children with hearing loss. *Journal of Deaf Studies and Deaf Education, 15*(1), 59–71.

Joint Committee on Infant Hearing (2007). 2007 Position statement: Principles and guidelines for early hearing detection and intervention. http://www.asha.org./polcy. Retrieved May 2, 2010.

Leonardo da Vinci Lifelong Learning Project (2011a). *Final report: Guidance from reports approved in 2008.* Lifelong Learning Programme, Development of Pan-European Competencies for Teachers of Deaf Through Partnership, National ID: 2009-LDV-PAR-P-407 [internal document].

Leonardo da Vinci Lifelong Learning Project (2011b). *Survey.* Lifelong Learning Programme, Development of Pan-European Competencies for Teachers of Deaf Through Partnership, National ID: 2009-LDV-PAR-P-407 [internal document].

Lichtert, G., & van Wieringen, A. (2013). The importance of early home-based guidance (EHBG) for hearing-impaired children and their families in Flanders. *B-ENT, 9*(Suppl. 21), 27–36.

Mason-Williams, L. (2014). Unequal opportunities: A profile of the distribution of special education teachers. *Exceptional Children, 81*(2), 247–262.

McDonald Connor, C., Craig, H. K., Raudenbush, S. W., Heavner, K., & Zwolan, T. A. (2000). The age at which young deaf children receive cochlear implants and their vocabulary and speech-production growth: Is there an added value for early implantation? *Ear and Hearing, 27*(6), 628–644.

McLoughlin, M. G. (1987). *A history of education of the deaf in England and Wales.* Liverpool: G.M. McLoughlin.

Meadow-Orlans, K., Mertens, D., & Sass-Lehrer, M. (2003). *Parents and their deaf children.* Washington, DC: Gallaudet University Press.

Moeller, M. P. (2000). Early intervention and language development in children who are deaf and hard of hearing. *Pediatrics, 106*(3), e43.

Muma, J. & Perigoe, C. (2010). Professional preparation: Developing language in children with hearing loss. *The Volta Review, 110*(2), 179–190.

National Council Accreditation of Teacher Education (2006). What makes teachers effective? http://www.ncate.org/dotnetnuke/LinkClick.aspx?fileticket=JFRrmWqa1jU%3D&tabid=361. Retrieved March 11, 2015.

Nevins, M. E., & Chute, P. M. (1996). *Children with cochlear implants in educational settings.* San Diego, CA: Singular Publishing Group.

Nikolopoulos, T. P., O'Donoghue, G. M., & Archbold, S. (2006). Age of implantation: Its importance in pediatric cochlear implantation. *The Laryngoscope, 109*(4), 595–599.

Okalidou, A., Kitsona, M., Anagnostou, F., Tsoukala, M., Santzakli, S., Gouda, S., & Nikolopoulos, P. (2014). Knowledge, experience and practice of SLTs regarding (re)habilitation in deaf children with cochlear implants. *International Journal of Pediatric Otorhinolaryngology, 78,* 1049–1056.

Pollack, D. (1970). *Educational audiology for the limited-hearing infant.* Springfield, IL: Charles C. Thomas.

Ruffin, C. V., Kronenberger, W. G., Colson, B. G., Henning, S. C., & Pisoni, D. B. (2013). Long-term speech and language outcomes in prelingually deaf children, adolescents and young adults who received cochlear implants in childhood. *Audiology Neurootology, 18*(5), 289–296.

Scheetz, N. A., & Martin, D. S. (2008). National study of master teachers in deaf education: Implications for teacher education. *American Annals of the Deaf,153*(3), 328–343.

Shelton, T. L., & Stepanek, J. S. (1995). Excerpts from family-centered care for children needing specialized health and developmental services. *Pediatric Nursing, 21*(4), 362–364.

Svirsksy, M. A., Robbins, A. M., Kirk, K. I., Pisoni, D. B., & Miyamoto, R. T. (2000). Language development in profoundly deaf children with cochlear implants. *Psychological Science, 11*(2), 153–158.

Teaching Development Agency. (2009). *Specification for mandatory qualifications for specialist teachers of children and young people with hearing impairments.* London: Author.

Watson, M. M., & Martin, K. (1999). Providing services to children with cochlear implants in the public schools: Results of a survey of speech–language pathologists. *Journal of Educational Audiology, 7,* 1–7.

Wilcox, M. J., & Woods J. (2011). Participation as a basis for developing early intervention outcomes. *Language, Speech, and Hearing Services in the Schools, 42*(3), 365–378.

Wilson, L. L., & Dunst, C. J. (2005). Checklist for assessing adherence to family-centered practices. *Case Tools, 1*(1),1–6.

World Health Organization (2013). World report on disability. http://whqlibdoc.who.int/publications/2011/9789240685215_eng.pdf.

Ying, E. (2008). Speech/language/auditory management of infants and children with hearing loss. In J. R. Madell, & C. Flexer (Eds.), *Pediatric audiology: Diagnosis, technology, and management* (1st ed., pp. 240–249). New York, NY: Thieme.

Yoshinaga-Itano, C. (2000). Successful outcomes for deaf and hard of hearing children. *Seminars in Hearing, 21,* 309–325.

7

Exploring Signed Language Assessment Tools in Europe and North America

Charlotte Enns, Tobias Haug, Rosalind Herman,
Robert Hoffmeister, Wolfgang Mann,
and Lynn McQuarrie

EDUCATIONAL AND RESEARCH CONTEXTS

The increasing diversity of the cultural and linguistic backgrounds of children in North American and European countries challenges traditional approaches to language testing (Johnston, 2004; Menyuk & Brisk, 2005). This diversity makes it difficult to determine the expected course of language development in bilingual children (Johnston, 2004). Therefore, it is important to develop parallel testing instruments for bilingual and multilingual children to measure their development in all their languages. Cultural influences, attitudes toward testing, and definitions of language proficiency are just a few issues that need to be considered for a fair evaluation of bilingual children's language proficiency (Menyuk & Brisk, 2005). These issues are also of concern for deaf children; increasing heterogeneity within deaf communities has been reported in many countries (Christensen & Delgado, 1993; Gerner de Garcia, 2000).

Education for deaf children has always emphasized measurable outcomes of language and literacy learning, and the focus on bilingual and bimodal education for deaf children has highlighted the need for more information about early signed language development (DeLana et al., 2007). Although assessment is a pivotal component in educational programs serving hearing children, teachers in deaf education have typically relied on informal assessments in the form of naturalistic observations and anecdotal progress monitoring because of the limited tests supporting signed language assessment (Haug, 2005; Herman, 1998a; McQuarrie et al., 2012; Singleton & Supalla, 2011). In the current era of standards, accountability, and achievement testing, there is ever-increasing pressure to document learning outcomes (McQuarrie et al., 2012).

Accurate assessment can serve a variety of purposes, including determining the level of signed language proficiency when children begin school and the need to monitor progress. Children struggling to acquire language skills are often identified by professionals through assessment; therefore, identification of acquisition difficulties and strengths is yet another purpose of assessment. Assessment is also required for reporting purposes to inform parents and administrators of individual or group levels of functioning and rates of progress. These various purposes clearly identify the need for effective signed language assessment tools, and yet such tools are just beginning to be developed. The gap in the area of reliable and valid assessment measures of signed language acquisition, in comparison with the multitude of assessments available for spoken and written languages, leaves professionals working with deaf children without the necessary tools to assess, document, and track children's developing signed language competence. Therefore, another critical purpose for developing accurate signed language assessment measures is to emphasize the value of the role these skills play in deaf children's learning and facilitate teaching approaches that build on their strengths and abilities with visual language.

Common Challenges

The need for assessments notwithstanding, there are legitimate challenges to the development of signed language assessment tools that contribute to the small number of tests currently available in this area. These challenges include the limited amount or lack of information regarding the acquisition of signed languages, the appropriateness of test formats based on spoken language tests, and the process for determining normative samples given the diversity of deaf children.

Signed Language Acquisition Data

Language researchers have defined some key developmental milestones and acquisition patterns in the signed language development of young deaf children (French, 1999; Lillo-Martin, 1999; Newport & Meier, 1985; Schick, 2003). More information is available for some signed languages (for example, American Sign Language [ASL] and British Sign Language [BSL]), and knowledge of the linguistic features of these languages and their relative grammatical complexity have been used to develop guidelines regarding the sequence of acquisition (Neidle et al., 2001; Valli & Lucas, 1992).

In addition to the variability in knowledge of language acquisition among signed languages, there is also variability regarding the knowledge of specific language components (phonology, morphology, semantics, syntax, and pragmatics) of signed languages. Research into these components is primarily motivated by how specific signed language skills can contribute to the development of reading, or literacy in written language. Increasingly, researchers have explored the use of signed languages to promote the acquisition of written languages (Chamberlain & Mayberry, 2008). Although several correlational studies found positive relationships between ASL proficiency and reading proficiency (Hoffmeister, 1994, 2000; McQuarrie & Abbott, 2010; Padden & Ramsey, 2000; Prinz & Strong, 1998; Strong & Prinz, 2000), the exact nature of this relationship is not yet understood. To address this question further, developmental data regarding signed language phonology, vocabulary, and syntax have been used to create assessment measures that provide reliable indicators of these skills in young bilingual deaf children. The connection between signed language acquisition research and the development of practical assessment tools continues to be strengthened and extended across signed languages in the creation of important experimental and formal measures.

Test Formats

In many ways, signed languages function similar to spoken languages; therefore, numerous assessments tasks used with spoken language can also be applied to signed language. A key difference, however, is modality and the need for visual versus auditory stimuli. The increased availability of video formats and the accessibility of technology to play video have reduced the challenge of incorporating visual stimuli—specifically signed language stimuli—within assessment measures.

There are several issues specific to signed languages that need to be taken into consideration when developing test items. The first issue concerns lexical item selection. Published high-frequency word lists or vocabulary lists for signed languages are not readily available, so simply determining appropriate lexical items suitable for young deaf children can be a challenge. In addition, although many spoken language tasks involve visuals—pictures, wordless books, even videos or cartoons—some aspects of these stimuli can be overly distracting and are not designed for visual language users. To overcome the challenges of test format and design, the process of signed language test development should always involve consultation with a panel of experts. These panels would consist of native signed language users who are researchers or specialist teachers in the particular signed language being assessed. The expert review panel, usually over a series of sessions, would conduct a content review of the test items to verify that the target sign stimuli, videos, and/or pictures represent the constructs intended to be measured, and that any distracter items represent the most appropriate potential errors. Consultation with experts is a key component in the development of valid tests of signed language acquisition.

Normative Samples

Identifying developmental problems in the acquisition of minority languages, whether signed or spoken, is challenging because norms for these populations often do not exist (Johnston, 2004). There is a lack of controlled elicited data from representative samples of native users of various natural signed languages on which norms for competency can be established (Schembri et al., 2002). The number of studies of signing deaf children's language development is limited and, in the studies that do exist, the number of subjects is small. This is because only a minority of deaf children (<10% [Mitchell & Karchmer, 2004]) can be considered native signers, with a normal experience of language acquisition from exposure to deaf parents who sign. For this reason, the general procedure for establishing signed language assessment involves initial pilot testing of items with native signers (children of deaf parents), followed by a broader normative testing process to include children with early exposure (before the age of 3 years) to the natural signed language.

To date, there is very little information on age-related knowledge of signed languages and its impact on learning. Studies of the relationship between specific areas of children's signed language abilities and areas of their spoken/written language literacy are important for determining the factors that predict reading ability—a crucial issue for both educators of deaf students and researchers interested in bilingual acquisition issues. Tests of natural signed languages have tremendous practical value. The intent in developing formal assessments of signed language is to assist educators and researchers alike who work with deaf children in identifying children whose language is developing at age-appropriate levels as well as those who are potentially at risk for language delay, language learning difficulties, learning disabilities, and classroom problems.

TEST DESCRIPTIONS

Despite the common challenges of acquisition data, test format, and normative sampling, several effective assessment tools of various signed languages have been established. We present descriptions of several such tests for ASL, BSL, German Sign Language (DGS), and Swiss German Sign Language (DSGS), including those that have been standardized as well as those still in development. This is not an exhaustive list of all available signed language assessments in these four languages, but rather a sample of tests that were presented in 2015 as part of a symposium at the International Congress for Education of the Deaf that we, as authors, have developed in collaboration with each other and our research teams. In addition, the test descriptions are summarized in Table 7.1.

Table 7.1 Summary of Signed Language Tests

Test/Authors	Purpose	Format	Target Population	Normative Sample
ASLAI/Hoffmeister et al., 2014	Comprehensive measure of receptive: (a) ASL vocabulary, (b) reasoning skills, (c) ASL syntax, and (d) ASL text comprehension	Web based: • Sign to sign • Picture to picture • Picture to sign • Drag and drop • Response only • Video event to sign	4–18 years: 4–7 years (7 tasks), 7–12 years (12 tasks), 12–18 years (11 tasks)	All deaf children, DCDP, DCHP
BSL RST/Herman et al., 1999	Comprehension of selected aspects of BSL morphosyntax (number/distribution, noun–verb distinction, negation, spatial verbs, handling classifiers, and size-and-shape classifiers)	Video based (DVD), Web-based version now available	3–12 years	135 deaf children (deaf and hearing families), 3–13 years, no additional needs, normal nonverbal IQ
ASL RST/Enns et al., 2013	Comprehension of ASL morphology and syntax (number/distribution, noun–verb distinction, negation, spatial verbs, handling classifiers, size-and-shape classifiers, conditionals, and role shift)	Video based (DVD), Web-based version being developed	3–13 years	203 deaf children (deaf and hearing families), 3–13 years, no additional needs, normal nonverbal IQ
DGS RST/Haug, 2011a	Comprehension of DGS morphology and syntax (number and distribution, negation, spatial verbs, handling classifiers, and size-and-shape classifiers)	Web based	3–11 years	54 deaf children (deaf and hearing families)

(continued)

Table 7.1 Continued

Test/Authors	Purpose	Format	Target Population	Normative Sample
BSL PT/Herman et al., 2004	Narrative skills and use of BSL grammar based on a narrative recall task (analysis of narrative content, narrative structure, and BSL grammar)	Video (DVD) elicitation and video recording of narrative recall for later analysis using scoring form	4–11 years	71 deaf children (deaf and hearing families), 4–11 years, no additional needs, normal nonverbal IQ
ASL PT/Enns et al., 2014	Narrative skills and use of ASL grammar based on a narrative recall task (analysis of narrative content, narrative structure, and ASL grammar)	Video (DVD) elicitation and video recording of narrative recall for later analysis using scoring form; online elicitation, recording, and scoring procedure being developed	4–12 years	N/A
BSL NSRT/Mann et al., 2010	Ability to repeat nonsense signs of differing phonetic (hand shape and movement) complexity in BSL	Video based; scored for overall correct response, phonological errors, deletion of movements	3–11 years	91 deaf children (deaf and hearing families), hearing control group (n = 46)
BSL VT/Mann et al., 2013	BSL vocabulary—degree of strength between form and meaning for core lexicon	Web-based; 4 tasks: meaning recognition, form recognition, meaning recall, and form recall	4–15 years	67 deaf children (deaf and hearing families), 4–17 years; variable BSL exposure

ASL VT/Mann et al., 2015	Receptive and expressive ASL vocabulary	Web-based; 4 tasks: meaning recognition, form recognition, meaning recall, and form recall	6–10 years	20 DCDP, 6–10 years
ASL PAT/McQuarrie and Spady, 2012	Receptive phonological similarity judgment task to assess knowledge of the sublexical properties of sign formation (hand shape, location, and movement)	Web based; video instructions and test items; online scoring of accuracy (number correct), error analysis, and reaction time	4–8 years	N/A
DSGS SRT/Haug et al., 2015	Sentence repetition task as a global measure of expressive DSGS linguistic skills (phonology, morphology, syntax)	Video based (DVD), responses video-recorded for scoring (scoring tool being developed)	6–12 years	N/A

ASL, American Sign Language; ASLAI, American Sign Language Assessment Instrument; BSL, British Sign Language; DCDP, deaf children of deaf parents; DCHP, deaf children of hearing parents; DGS, German Sign Language; DSGS, Swiss German Sign Language; N/A, not applicable; NSRT, Nonsense Sign Repetition Test; PAT, Phonological Awareness Test; PT, Production Test; RST, Receptive Skills Test; SRT, Sentence Repetition Test; VT, Vocabulary Test.

The American Sign Language Assessment Instrument

History and Purpose

The American Sign Language Assessment Instrument (ASLAI) (Hoffmeister et al., 2014) is reliable and modeled on tests for spoken language development and tests of reading achievement, measuring conversational abilities, academic language knowledge, language comprehension, analogical reasoning, and metalinguistic skills. More specifically, it provides a measure of the relationship between specific areas of children's receptive signed language abilities and comparable areas of their English literacy skills. The results of the ASLAI are critical for determining factors that predict English reading ability. In addition to obtaining age-related norms on the previously mentioned language components, the ASLAI tasks can aid in identifying specific learning and/or language problems, which can lead to improved instruction and classroom settings. The ASLAI is designed to test deaf and hard-of-hearing students between the ages of 4 years and 18 years. There are 12 subtasks in the total battery.

Psychometric Information

Reliability information for the ASLAI tasks comprising the vocabulary, reasoning, comprehension, and syntax domains indicates high reliability for all tasks.

Face validity for the ASLAI was established in two ways. First, the ASLAI tasks were developed by a team of native signers (deaf and hearing) whose first language was ASL. This ensured the tasks used appropriate ASL forms and were suitable for the targeted constructs of the assessment. Second, all questions developed for the tasks were piloted with native deaf signers. Questions that did not have more than 85% agreement were not used in the final version of the ASLAI.

Predictive validity was established for the vocabulary tasks in the ASLAI by determining how much variability on three different English reading and vocabulary assessments (the Stanford Achievement Test Reading Comprehension and Stanford Achievement Test Reading Vocabulary tasks, and the Measures of Academic Progress Reading subtask) could be predicted by each of the ASLAI tasks. All ASLAI tasks predicted a significant amount of variability for the Stanford Achievement Test Reading Comprehension, Stanford Achievement Test Reading Vocabulary, and Measures of Academic Progress Reading tasks. The overall results of the predictive validity of the ASLAI strengthen the use of the ASLAI as an appropriate measure of ASL age-related skills, but also strongly demonstrates the relationship between ASL vocabulary knowledge and English (Hoffmeister et al., 2015).

Format/Platform

The ASLAI is a Web-based assessment application, which allows for multiple participants to take the assessment simultaneously without the need for one-on-one administration. The Web-based approach minimizes the resources necessary to assess large numbers of participants, and allows rapid testing and provision of timely results.

The multiple-choice structure of the ASLAI has an advantage over criterion-based screening tools. Norm-based, multiple-choice assessments such as the ASLAI remove the subjective component of scoring. Responses are either right or wrong, which increases the efficiency of data collection, analysis, and reporting, which is helpful for schools and researchers.

The ASLAI testing platform is a proprietary design, developed from the ground up to ensure the security and confidentiality of all data collected from participants. Three components comprise the fundamental design of the ASLAI task platform: (a) a stimulus window, (b) up to four response windows, and (c) a response review screen. The windows containing videos or images are shown sequentially, starting with the stimulus and followed by each of the responses in turn.

The testing procedure consists of five phases: (a) the login phase, (b) the instruction phase, (c) the practice phase, (d) the task phase, and (e) the review phase. Students log in to the ASLAI task battery using an individualized username and password combination that is maintained in case the participant is tested again in future years. Confidentiality and anonymity are maintained throughout the testing and analysis processes. During the instruction phase of the ASLAI, two types of instructions are presented: (a) a general introduction to the ASLAI and how to interact with the testing platform, and (b) instruction specific to each subtask.

During the third phase of the testing procedure, the practice phase, the instructions provided during the instruction phase are reinforced and participants are given the opportunity to answer up to five different practice questions that reflect the kind of questions used in the task. The design of the practice interface (Figure 7.1) mirrors what is used in the task interface. For example, the practice interface for Vocabulary: Simple has a picture stimulus and four responses. During the practice phase, participants receive feedback regarding whether they have chosen the correct response (correct responses are highlighted in green and incorrect ones are noted in red).

During the task phase of the ASLAI testing process, the actual task is executed. During this phase, participants are not given feedback on whether the selected response is correct; rather, the task advances automatically to the next question after the participants select a response. Tasks in the ASLAI are in one of six formats: (a) picture to sign, (b) sign

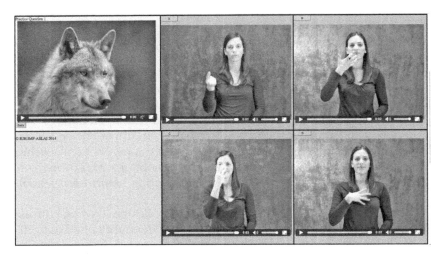

Figure 7.1 American Sign Language Assessment Instrument: Practice question.

to sign, (c) picture to picture, (d) drag-and-drop sorting, (e) response only (grammaticality judgment), and (f) video event to sign. Data collected during the task phase are sent securely to a central database, where performance is scored automatically and compared with other scores in the norming pool.

The review phase (Figure 7.2) is the final phase in which participants are given an opportunity to review the responses they selected and change any answers if they so desire. During this phase, participants view a review screen that shows the stimuli from all task questions as well as the responses they selected. Participants are able to select questions and revise their answers before the final submission of task data.

Content/Design

The tasks in the ASLAI battery can be divided into four categories: (a) tests of vocabulary, (b) tests of reasoning skills, (c) tests of syntax, and (d) tests of ASL text comprehension. This section provides more detail about the tasks that compose the ASLAI test battery.

Tests of Vocabulary
The vocabulary tasks in the ASLAI examine breadth and depth of vocabulary via antonymy, synonymy, and sign/word knowledge. These tasks require some level of metalinguistic judgment. Antonyms and Synonyms require students to make use of metalinguistic knowledge to understand and identify differences and similarities among vocabulary items. The Vocabulary in Sentences task is a higher level vocabulary task; participants must know both the meaning of the vocabulary item as well as its appropriate use in different syntactic environments

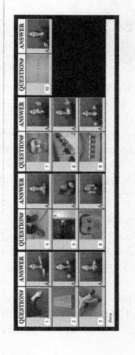

Figure 7.2 American Sign Language Assessment Instrument: Review screen.

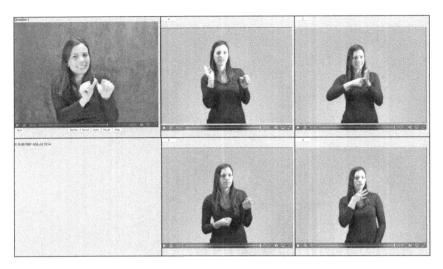

Figure 7.3 American Sign Language Assessment Instrument: Difficult Vocabulary task (sign-to-sign format).

(sentences). In addition, the vocabulary items used as stimuli are taken from a pool of what we refer to as rare ASL vocabulary—that is, in-group vocabulary that is not often encountered unless one is intimate with the deaf community. This task was developed for students age 7.6 to 18 years old (Figure 7.3).

Test of Reasoning Skills: Analogies (24 Questions)
The Analogies task is a test of classic language analogies in the sign-to-sign format. As seen in Figure 7.4, the analogical stimulus sentence (*A is to B, as C is to what?*) is signed. Participants then view four possible signed lexical item responses, from which they are to select the correct one. Analogies contains a total 24 questions divided among six types of relationship categories: (a) causal, (b) purpose, (c) antonym, (d) noun–verb pairs, (e) whole to part/part to whole, and (f) phonology.

Tests of Syntax
The third category of ASLAI tasks contains 27 items that examine knowledge of diverse aspects of ASL syntax. Nine different sentence types are represented: (a) plain, (b) conditionals, (c) topic-comment, (d) complement, (e) relative clause, (f) negation, (g) rhetorical question, (h) wh-question, and (i) subject–object agreement.

The Classifier Category Sorting task uses a drag-and-drop format and is designed to measure knowledge of the ASL classifiers system. Classifier types represented in this task include semantic, handling, and size and shape specifiers.

The Real Objects and Plurals task measures knowledge of verbs of motion, verbs of location, classifiers, and pluralization processes in ASL. Scores indicate age-related knowledge of which classifier represents

Exploring Sign Language Assessment Tools in Europe and North America 183

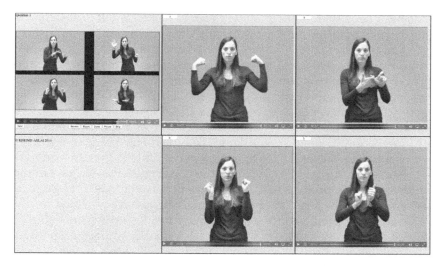

Figure 7.4 American Sign Language Assessment Instrument: Analogies task (sign-to-sign format).

which object(s) (singular or plural) appropriately, and how these classifier forms function in verbs of motion and verbs of location.

Test of ASL Comprehension: ASL Text
Comprehension (10 Questions)
The fourth and final category of tasks in the ASLAI contains one subtask: ASL Text Comprehension. It presents ASL texts (1–1.5 minutes in duration) and then asks five multiple-choice comprehension questions in ASL about that text. This task examines the ability of participants to extract both literal and inferential meaning from ASL texts. Participants view two ASL texts, responding to a multiple-choice selection of 10 questions. This task was designed for students in all age groupings, with age-appropriate texts selected for each group.

Reporting/Data

The ASLAI obtains age-related data from three different norming groups representative of the general population of deaf children: (a) all deaf children; (b) native signers, or deaf children of deaf parents; and (c) nonnative signers, or deaf children of hearing parents. For each ASLAI task, norms were created using the means and standard deviation as they relate to age. Half standard deviations were used to compare ASLAI participants resulting in a more granular analysis of the language abilities relative to their peers. This is important especially at ages when participant language skills are rapidly developing and any small change can cause gaps in language acquisition.

The strength and promise of the ASLAI has led schools to use the ASLAI as part of their yearly standardized testing battery. The ASLAI has been used with more than over 1500 students, and it is designed to support schools and programs serving deaf children to identify those students who are performing as expected and those who are not acquiring or are delayed in achieving ASL proficiency. Preliminary results based on this sample demonstrate that fluency in ASL, including knowledge of breadth and depth of ASL vocabulary, predicts English reading ability (Hoffmeister & Caldwell-Harris, 2014; Novogrodsky et al., 2014a, 2014b). Furthermore, the types of language errors fluent first language (L1) users of ASL make are similar to the types of language errors fluent L1 users of English make (Novogrodsky et al., 2014b). Last, the strength of the relationship between ASL abilities and English that we have found indicates that a positive relationship exists between ASL and English. As a result of the large sampling population we have obtained for the ASLAI, we are confident these preliminary results are generalizable.

Achieving ASL proficiency as an L1 is critically important to learning English via print as a second language (L2) (see Chapter 10 and Chapter 11). The ASLAI provides us with a measure that is able to predict those students who may be having difficulty in learning English (L2). The ASLAI may also serve to separate those students who are having language learning problems displayed in both their L1 and their L2. This information has not been available for schools until now.

British Sign Language Receptive Skills Test

History, Purpose, and Target Population

The BSL Receptive Skills Test (RST) (Herman et al., 1999) was the first standardized measure available for any signed language. The test targets comprehension of selected aspects of BSL morphosyntax and was designed for child signed language users between the ages of 3 years and 12 years. Under certain circumstances, the test can also be used with older children whose sign language skills are delayed or impaired or who have cognitive delays, although in such cases the standard scores do not apply.

Use of the test enables professionals working with deaf children to make baseline assessments, identify language difficulties, and evaluate the outcomes of language therapy programs (Herman, 1998b; Herman et al., 1998). The test provides an overall level of functioning that can be determined as age appropriate or not (above/below, or significantly above/below average) and also a profile of errors to guide instruction about which grammatical structures students are struggling to understand. Children's results on this test can be compared with results for expressive language using the BSL Production Test (PT) (Herman et al., 2004). Both these tests were key measures in a recent United Kingdom research program seeking to identify and characterize language impairment in deaf signing children (Mason et al., 2010).

The BSL RST is used widely in schools throughout the United Kingdom and has been used in its original or adapted form in a number of research studies with deaf children (e.g., Dammeyer, 2010; Davidson et al., 2014; Falkman et al., 2007; Jackson, 2001; MacSweeney et al., 2002; Mason et al., 2010; Sieratzki et al., 2001; Surian et al., 2010; Tomasuolo et al., 2012; Woolfe et al., 2002).

The test has been adapted into many different signed languages including DGS (Haug, 2011b), ASL (Enns & Herman, 2011), Spanish Sign Language (Valmaseda et al., 2013), Italian Sign Language (Meristo et al., 2007), and Polish Sign Language (Kotowicz, pers. comm., April 27, 2013), among others. More recently, the DVD format has been redeveloped into a Web-based format, offering the possibility of updating test norms through use (Haug et al., 2014).

Content/Format

The BSL RST has two components: the vocabulary check and the video-based RST. The original RST was presented on VHS and was later updated to a DVD version. A Web-based version is now available (www.signlanguagetest.com). The main test is presented on video; therefore, minimal BSL skills are required by testers, although some BSL skills are needed to administer the vocabulary check.

The vocabulary check is optional and is designed to ensure children understand the vocabulary used in the RST. It is particularly recommended for very young children, for those who have had late exposure to BSL, or for children with suspected language difficulties. Children complete the vocabulary check live using a simple picture-naming task that identifies signs in their lexicon that vary from those used in the RST. This is particularly important for languages such as BSL, for which there is much regional variation of signs. The vocabulary check takes approximately 5 minutes to administer.

The RST consists of 40 items, organized in order of difficulty. The items in the test assess children's comprehension of BSL morphosyntax in the following areas: negation, number and distribution, verb morphology, noun–verb distinction, size and shape specifiers, and handling classifiers.

The test procedure is explained by a deaf adult on the test video using a child-friendly BSL register. The test includes three practice items to familiarize the child with the test format. Children respond by selecting the most appropriate picture from a choice of four, presented previously in the accompanying color picture booklet and, more currently, displayed on the computer screen. Repetition of test items is permitted for the practice items but not for the main test. An exception is for the very youngest age group (3–4 years), for whom a single repetition is allowed.

The test takes up to 20 minutes, depending on the age and ability of the child. Testing is discontinued after four consecutive failed items.

Scoring is on a pass/fail basis. It is also possible to analyze a child's performance according to the grammatical features tested to identify strengths and weaknesses, and targets for intervention.

Psychometric Information

The BSL RST was initially developed and piloted on 41 children (28 deaf and 13 hearing) age 3.0 to 11.6 years, all from native signing backgrounds. The revised and shortened test was subsequently administered to 135 deaf children within the age range of 3 to 13 years located throughout the United Kingdom to establish test norms. For the standardization phase, children were included from both deaf and hearing families to represent the broader population of children who use BSL. Children previously diagnosed as having additional disabilities were excluded from the standardization sample. In addition, children scoring below one standard deviation on two subtests of the Snijders-Oomen Test of Non-Verbal Abilities (Snijders et al., 1989) were excluded from the sample. All tests were administered by a deaf researcher with fluent BSL and a hearing researcher with good BSL skills.

Test–retest reliability, split-half reliability, and interscorer reliability were all investigated and reported for the revised task, showing the test to be robust psychometrically. Data were collected subsequently from an unselected sample of deaf children throughout the United Kingdom who used BSL for comparison with the standardization sample, as reported by Herman and Roy (2006). The wider sample of children included many with additional learning difficulties and some older than the target test age, although they were excluded for the purpose of comparison with the original sample. Children in the new data set were found to achieve lower levels than those of the standardization sample, highlighting the importance of language monitoring and the need to improve language support provided in schools for deaf signing children.

American Sign Language Receptive Skills Test

History

The ASL RST (Enns et al., 2013) was adapted from the BSL RST through a series of phases, including consultation with experts, development of new test items, videotaping of ASL stimuli, and redrawing of picture responses. Two rounds of pilot testing were administered with native signing children (deaf children of deaf parents) to establish appropriate stimuli and distracter items, and the accurate developmental ordering of test items. Following the first round of pilot testing (with 47 children in Canada and the United States), revisions were needed for 23 of the original 41 pilot test items, including changes to distracter drawings (11 items), signed stimulus sentences (four items), and changes to both drawings and signed sentences (eight items). Four new items were added to assess understanding of the more complex structures of role shift and conditional clauses. Test items were reordered to reflect more accurately the developmental level of difficulty according to the number of children who passed each item.

The second round of pilot testing revealed that modifications to previous test items and the new test items made the test more challenging and distinguished children's skills at different ages more clearly. Analysis comparing age and raw score showed a significant correlation and high r value (r (34) = 0.821, $p < .001$). Final modifications included deleting three test items (considered redundant) and reordering test items to reflect more appropriately the developmental sequence of ASL acquisition (for more detailed information regarding the adaptation process, see Enns and Herman [2011]).

Purpose and Target Population

The purpose and target population are similar to the BSL RST but for ASL—that is, a measure of children's (age, 3–13 years) comprehension of ASL morphology and syntax.

Content/Format

The content and format of the ASL RST is similar to the BSL RST in that a vocabulary check (20 items) precedes the main test of 42 items. In addition to the six grammatical structures (number/distribution, noun–verb distinction, negation, spatial verbs, handling classifiers, and size and shape classifiers) assessed in the BSL RST, the ASL RST also assesses the complex syntactic ASL structures of conditional clauses and role shift. The original test format was revised by digitizing the picture responses and incorporating them into the test DVD (Figure 7.5). This eliminates the need for the picture book, and the child is not required to shift eye gaze between the computer screen and the picture book, thus reducing distractibility errors. A Web-based version is currently in development (www.signlanguagetest.com).

Psychometric Information

The ASL RST was administered to 203 children throughout Canada and the United States for standardization. Deaf children from hearing families were included in the standardization sample, but only if they had been exposed to ASL by age 3 years or younger. All 203 children were deaf and had a nonverbal IQ of 70 or more (or, when formal testing was not available, were determined to be functioning within the average range intellectually by school personnel). There were 77 native signers and 126 nonnative signers (acquired at younger than 3 years), 106 females and 97 males, and the ages ranged from 3 to 13 years. Testing took place in the children's schools and was administered by

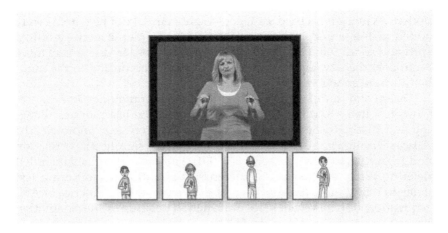

Figure 7.5 Example of American Sign Language Receptive Skills Test test item.

deaf and hearing researchers with fluent ASL skills. We recognize that our sample of 203 children is limited in how accurately it represents the overall population of deaf children, and for this reason future research will involve additional testing and data collection to expand our sample. However, several statistical analyses of the standardization data did reveal that the test was reliable (showed internal consistency) and was a valid measure of developmental changes in ASL skills.

German Sign Language Receptive Skills Test

History

The DGS RST (Haug, 2011a) was adapted in a series of steps from the original BSL RST to DGS (see also Table 7.2). The first revisions included changing some of the images of the BSL test to adapt it to the German context. For example, the British red, round mailbox was replaced by a yellow German mailbox. After reviewing the literature on DGS research, the items were adapted into DGS. Most of the linguistic structures that occur in the BSL test could also be represented in DGS, whereas others are not part of DGS morphology (noun–verb derivation). Ten additional items were created because, potentially, not all items would work equally well in DGS as in BSL. The original adapted items followed the same order as the BSL items, followed by the 10 additional
items. After the pilot study, the test was administered to 54 deaf children age 3 to 10 years.

Purpose and Target Population

The purpose and target population are identical to the BSL and ASL tests—targeting deaf children (ages 3–11 years) to evaluate their comprehension of DGS morphology and syntax.

Table 7.2 Steps in Adapting the British Sign Language Receptive Skills Test to German Sign Language

Steps	Description of Steps
1. Review and revision of test stimuli	Picture materials reviewed and changes made, e.g., replacing the red British mailbox with a yellow German mailbox
2. Pilot 1	Suitability of test items established: check for regional variation in three regions with deaf adults and children
3. Adaptation of items	(1) Order of test items (2) Comparability of BSL and DGS linguistic structures (3) Development of 10 additional items
4. Filming of test	Filming of test instructions and test items
5. Programming test interface	Programming of a user-friendly test interface that runs on a laptop and can store the results automatically
6. Pilot 2	Piloting first test version with: (1) Non-signing hearing children and (2) Deaf adults
7. Revisions of first version	Revision of the first version based on Pilot 2: (1) Changes to the pictures (2) Re-filming of items (3) Changes to the layout
8. Planning of main study	(1) Contacting the schools (2) Development and distribution of educational background questionnaires for children
9. Main study	Conducting the main study at five school sites in Germany

Source: Haug, T. (2012). A review of sign language acquisition studies as the basis for informed decisions for sign language test adaptation: The case of the German Sign Language Receptive Skills Test. *Sign Language and Linguistics, 15*(2), 213–239.

Content/Format

The current version of the DGS RST consists of a vocabulary check (22 items) and 49 test items, representing DGS structures of number and distribution, negation, spatial verbs, handling classifiers, and size and shape classifiers. The first version of the DGS RST was delivered on a laptop using a specially designed stand-alone application. A Web-based version is currently in development (www.signlanguagetest.com).

Psychometric Information

The DGS RST has been tested on 54 deaf children in Germany; 34 of these children had at least one deaf parent and the remaining children had hearing parents (e.g., Haug, 2011a, 2012). Based on an item analysis, 10 of 49 items needed to be removed or revised, and many items were "too easy"; therefore, more difficult items are currently being developed.

Evidence for reliability was established across all 49 items through statistical analysis, and a significant correlation between chronological age and raw score determined the test was sensitive to age differences. These results applied to the sample as a whole as well as to both subsamples separately: deaf children of deaf parents and deaf children of hearing parents. Currently, we are looking into funding for a planned norming study in 2015/2016. Normative data will enable educators to determine whether children are acquiring DGS in an age-appropriate manner and/ or to establish goals and effective teaching strategies for those who are demonstrating delays or disorders in their language development.

British Sign Language Production Test

History, Purpose, and Target Population

The BSL PT (Narrative Skills) (Herman et al., 2004) targets narrative skills and use of BSL grammar based on a narrative recall task. The test is designed for child signed language users between the ages of 4 years and 11 years because narrative skills develop during these years. Using a narrative sample is valid ecologically because the language produced is more naturalistic than that found in other types of assessments (such as sentence repetition). Furthermore, narrative skills are sensitive to language impairments (Norbury & Bishop, 2003) and correlate with literacy development (e.g., Reese et al., 2010) in hearing children.

To use the BSL PT, testers must have advanced fluency in BSL and complete a training course to learn the coding system. The test is used in schools throughout the United Kingdom and has been used in research studies with deaf children to serve effectively as a baseline measure of BSL abilities, to assist in the assessment of language and learning difficulties, and to monitor progress after intervention (e.g., Herman et al., 2014; Kennedy et al., 2006; Mason et al., 2010). To date, the test has been adapted into Australian Sign Language (Hodge et al., 2014) and plans are underway to develop an ASL (see the next section) and Spanish Sign Language version (Perez Martin, pers. comm., October 29, 2014). In addition, a spoken English version of the test (Jones et al., 2015) is currently under development that will enable practitioners and researchers to use the same test to assess a deaf child's spoken and signed narratives.

Content/Format

The BSL PT is a narrative recall task based on children watching a 2-minute language-free video presented on TV/computer. The video features a boy and a girl acting out a series of events without communicating to each other in either signed or spoken language. Children are told they will watch a video and then tell the story to a deaf BSL user who has not seen the video. If the tester is not a fluent BSL user, it is recommended that a fluent BSL user be involved when children tell the story to ensure narratives are delivered in BSL rather than

English-based signing. The child may watch the video a second time if they wish and the child's story is video-recorded for later analysis.

The child then answers questions that target story comprehension and inferencing skills. The questions are prerecorded for presentation on video; however, for some children (such as very young children or those with attention or language processing difficulties), testers may need to present questions live. Responses to questions are video-recorded for later analysis.

Scoring is based on spontaneous recall of the story without prompts and children's responses to questions. Samples are coded for three aspects:

a. *Narrative content*: Children's narratives are coded for the explicit mention of 16 narrative episodes (maximum = 16). The score for responses to questions (maximum = 6) is included in the narrative content score.
b. *Narrative structure*: Based on a high point analysis (Labov & Waltesky, 1967), narratives are coded for orientation, complicating actions, climax, resolution, evaluation and sequence (maximum = 12).
c. *BSL grammar*: Correct use of morphological inflections is coded for spatial verbs including classifiers, agreement verbs, manner inflections, and aspectual inflections (maximum = 30). Narratives are also rated for mastery of role shift (rated 0–4).

The test takes up to 10 minutes to administer, depending on the age and ability of the child. Following the analysis of a child's story and responses to questions, the raw scores obtained can be converted to percentiles. It is also possible to analyze a child's performance according to the narrative and grammatical features tested to identify strengths and weaknesses and identify targets for intervention. The test manual provides details of the aspects of BSL grammar included in the test, and information about the development of narratives in deaf and hearing children, including those with special educational needs.

Psychometric Information

The BSL PT was initially developed and piloted on the same 41 native signers used to develop the BSL RST. After piloting, the test was administered to 75 deaf children (34 boys) from deaf and hearing families within the age range of 4 to 11 years located throughout the United Kingdom to establish test norms. As for the BSL RST, children with additional disabilities or who scored outside the normal range on nonverbal measures were excluded. All tests were administered by a deaf researcher with fluent BSL skills.

Test–retest reliability, split-half reliability, and interscorer reliability were all investigated and found to be good. Concurrent validity, explored by comparing scores on the BSL RST and BSL PT, was found to be high.

American Sign Language Production Test

History, Purpose, and Target Population

The ASL PT (Enns et al., 2014) is an adaptation of the BSL PT. Because the BSL PT involves a narrative elicitation task through the use of a language-free story on video (*Spider Story*), it has good potential for use in any language. Essentially, the analysis and scoring of narrative content (events in the story) and narrative structure (story development) are the same across languages. So the adaptation to ASL focused specifically on the grammar analysis. The BSL grammatical categories of spatial verbs, agreement verbs, aspect, manner, and role shift fit well with ASL grammatical categories; therefore, adapting the scoring to the specific features of how these are marked in ASL was quite straightforward.

The next phase in the project was to create additional versions of the test, or parallel video-based stories that would elicit comparable narratives. Having alternate elicitation videos allows for retesting students without them becoming familiar with the story over repeated viewings. It also allowed for updating the original *Spider Story*, from the BSL test, to incorporate American cultural features and improve video quality. Throughout this process, however, it was essential to keep the narrative content, structure, and grammar similar across all three versions of the test videos. We used the basic narrative structure of the *Spider Story* and aligned the two new stories, *Home Alone* and *Tiffany's Breakfast* to this framework. Each story consists of similar events to the *Spider Story* (a series of back-and-forth interactions between protagonist and antagonist) but with slightly different settings, characters, and consequences. There are also parallels between the objects and actions in each of the stories that allowed for opportunities to elicit the same kinds of grammatical structures (spatial verbs, agreement verbs, aspect, manner, and role shift). In addition, the stories needed to be enjoyable and engaging for children so they would remember them and be interested in retelling them.

The third phase of the adaptation process, pilot testing of the adapted and new test versions with a sample of typically developing native ASL signers age 4 to 12 years, is currently underway. The results will provide valuable feedback regarding the effectiveness and reliability of the scoring guidelines, as well as the equivalency across the three test versions. After the necessary revisions are made based on the results of pilot testing, the final phase of standardization on a larger normative sample will be conducted.

Content/Format

The test content and format is similar to the BSL PT (Herman et. al., 2004), in that the child watches the video elicitation and then retells the story spontaneously and answers three comprehension questions. The child's responses are video-recorded and analyzed according to specific scoring guidelines. The goal for the ASL PT is to create both an online training process (mandatory for all testers) and an online scoring system (to view simultaneously the scoring rubric and the child's narrative). The required training process is needed to ensure all testers have the skills to score the narratives accurately and consistently. As described previously, the ASL PT will also have three possible test versions (language-free video stories) to elicit comparable narratives from children over time.

Psychometric Information

The pilot testing phase is currently being conducted; therefore, test results are not yet available. The reliability of the ASL PT will be investigated using intra- and interscorer comparisons, test–retest analyses, and a measure of internal consistency. Test validity will also be investigated by comparing scores from the same children on both the ASL RST and the ASL PT, as well as other measures of academic skills and performance (nonverbal IQ, reading comprehension). The results of the analyses will determine the final version of the test to be used for larger scale standardization (planned for 2016). Standard scores will be determined through statistical analysis of the collected norms.

British Sign Language Nonsense Sign Repetition Test

History

Research into the development of signed language phonology is often supported only by partial linguistic descriptions of signed languages and far fewer studies of the acquisition of those languages. Because most signs are only one syllable long (Brentari, 1998), it is not possible to manipulate the length of a sign. Therefore, adapting a nonword repetition paradigm for signed language offers the possibility of manipulating signs with regard to their phonological complexity along two parameters: hand shape and movement. This methodology makes it possible to investigate the perception, retention, and production of novel phonological forms in both deaf and hearing children.

Purpose

The Nonsense Sign Repetition Test (NSRT) for BSL (Mann et al., 2010) assesses signing deaf children's ability to repeat nonsense signs of differing phonetic (hand shape and movement) complexity in BSL. The test is based on a pilot by Marshall et al. (2006).

Target Population

The NSRT was developed for signing deaf children ages 3 to 11 years. As part of the norming study, two groups of children were tested: (a) deaf children who acquired BSL as a first language (3–11 years old) and (b) hearing children with no prior experience/exposure to signing (6–11 years old). The first group consisted of 91 deaf children, who were divided into three age groups: 3 to 5 years old (n = 26), 6 to 8 years old (n = 26), and (3) 9 to 11 years old (n = 38). Fourteen of these children had deaf parents, and the remaining children had exposure to BSL from nursery school. The second group consisted of 46 hearing children, divided into two age groups: 6 to 8 years old (n = 23) and 9 to 11 years old (n = 23) (Mann et al., 2010).

Content/Format

The chosen methodology is based on the nonword repetition methodology used in spoken language acquisition research (e.g., Dollaghan & Campbell, 1998; Gallon et al., 2007; Gathercole, 2006). Items of the NSRT for BSL consist of items that are possible phonotactically, but do not carry any meaning in BSL. These items differ with regard to their phonetic complexity along two phonological parameters: hand shape and movement. For each parameter, items are either phonetically "simple" or phonetically "complex." With respect to hand shape, "simple" hand shapes are the four unmarked BSL hand shapes, labeled here as B, 5, G, and A (Sutton-Spence & Woll, 1999); "complex" hand shapes are all marked hand shapes. With respect to movement, the test developers define just one movement, whether internal or path, as "simple" and two movements (internal and path combined) as "complex." The NSRT consists of a total of 40 items distributed equally across different levels of complexity. All items were modeled by a deaf signer and presented via a computer format.

Each child is tested individually and the test takes about 10 to 20 minutes. Before the actual test, instructions are presented on video by a deaf native signer, followed by three practice items. Each item is presented only once. The 40 items are shown in blocks of 10 items, with a short break between each block during which the child is shown a brief cartoon (Figure 7.6).

The responses are coded/scored according to whether the overall response was correct, whether any errors were made on the phonological parameters, and also whether one of the movements in a movement cluster was deleted.

Psychometric Information

The NSRT was developed and piloted on 91 deaf children with exposure to BSL from very early on through nursery school, including

Exploring Signed Language Assessment Tools in Europe and North America 195

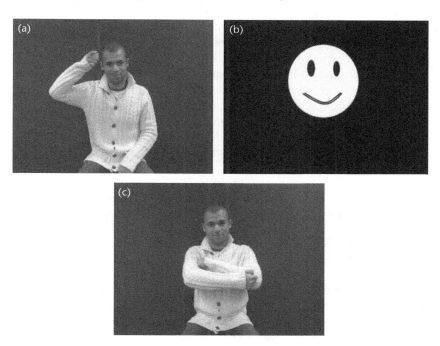

Figure 7.6 (a–c) Example from the Nonsense Sign Repetition Test (© 2006, W. Mann).

14 children with deaf parents. Children with additional disabilities were excluded. All tests were administered by a hearing researcher with fluent BSL skills.

Parallel-forms reliability and interrater reliability were all investigated and found to be good. Content validity in the form of feedback given by three native signers resulted in the removal of any signs that were not suitable. Concurrent validity was explored by comparing test-takers' scores on the NSRT with a hearing control, as well as with their performance on a fine motor skills task. All showed good values (see Mann et al. [2010] for more detailed information).

American Sign Language Phonological Awareness Test

History

The ASL Phonological Awareness Test (ASL-PAT) (McQuarrie & Spady, 2012) represents an adaptation of well-known spoken language psycholinguistic paradigms. It is designed to measure knowledge of the sublexical properties of sign formation: hand shape [H], location [L], and movement [M]. McQuarrie's (2005) receptive-based phonological similarity judgment task (for ages 9 years to adult) was used as a prototype in developing a downward extension of the measure suitable for 4- to 8-year-old children (preschool through second grade) because performance on the earlier measure identified reliably students' awareness of the sign language phonological segments that comprise signs; performance on this sign segmenting task was also correlated with success in English word-reading and reading comprehension (e.g., McQuarrie & Abbott, 2010, 2013; see review in McQuarrie and Parrila [2014]). During the first phase of test development, an initial pool of test items was vetted by a team of native ASL users who were knowledgeable about child language development and were able to suggest representative content. The items were then pilot-tested on a group of 12 deaf children (four children in each of the youngest age categories). The purpose of the pilot test was to evaluate the feasibility, usefulness, and usability of the test items, and to examine the effectiveness of the instructions, items, and item delivery method. Only items that showed at least a 95% agreement among the young deaf respondents were retained in the item pool. After the initial test item pilot and subsequent item revisions, the revised test items were again pilot-tested with an additional group of young deaf children to examine response patterns, difficulty level of items, and how well test items discriminated among various groups of deaf children (early vs. late sign-exposed children). A final round of pilot testing with a sample of typically developing native ASL signers age 4 to 8 years is currently underway. The final version of the ASL-PAT will be optimized by including only the items that best predict phonological awareness in ASL and are most sensitive to developmental differences in phonological awareness (see McQuarrie et al. [2012] for more detailed information regarding test development and design). The final phase of standardization on a larger normative sample will begin in fall 2015.

Purpose and Target Population

The ASL-PAT is being developed for use with signing deaf children ages 4 to 8 years old (preschool through second grade). The aim is to develop a signed language phonological measure that is sensitive enough to discriminate young children's phonological knowledge based on age, and to distinguish native and late-learners of ASL.

Content/Format/Test Platform

The ASL-PAT measures the ability to identify phonological similarity relations in signs under three comparison conditions:

 a. Signs with three shared parameters (H + M + L)
 b. Signs with two shared parameters (H + M, L + M, and H + L)
 c. Signs that share a single parameter (H, M, or L)

The ASL-PAT is a Web-based assessment application. Similar to the ASLAI, multiple individual users can access the assessment at the same time and all individual user responses are uploaded to a central database in real time. The testing procedure consists of five phases: (a) login and background demographic questionnaire, (b) vocabulary check, (c) instruction video, (d) practice trials, and (e) test block. The testing takes about 10 to 15 minutes for each test-taker.

Login
An identification number is assigned to each user on login. A brief questionnaire, including background information (such as date of birth, gender, age of onset, age of exposure/acquisition, use of hearing technologies, age of implantation), is completed online by the tester.

Vocabulary Check
The test begins with a vocabulary check in the form of a picture dictionary presented as a five-by-five grid picture display. Children are required to sign (name) each picture. If a child is uncertain or unable to generate a sign for a picture item, a video prompt of the sign is available by clicking the picture. Prompted items are subsequently added to the end of the picture display and retested without the video prompt before beginning the test. It is essential that children know the vocabulary associated with the test pictures before taking the test.

Instruction Video, Practice Trials, Test Block
Video instructions are presented in ASL by a deaf adult signer (Figure 7.7), followed by 7 practice trials and 28 test items. Feedback is provided on the practice items; no feedback is provided on test items. Each practice and test item consists of a signed cue (video) with three picture items below it that represent the target/phonological match and two distracter items. Test-takers are required to select the picture that matches the cue along the phonological parameter(s) tested (Figure 7.8).

Scoring
The online database records accuracy (correct match, 1 point; incorrect match, 0 point) and error response choice for each test item. Overall test performance scores are determined by the number of correct responses out of 28. Reaction/response time data are also recorded.

Psychometric Information

The ASL-PAT is still in development, and psychometric information is not yet available. Preliminary findings from pilot studies offer support for (a) the plausibility of assessing signed language phonological awareness by targeting key phonological parameters identified in the literature and (b) the potential of Web-based test delivery using a dynamic/video presentation format. In addition, McQuarrie and Enns (2015), using multiple single-case studies incorporating a multiple

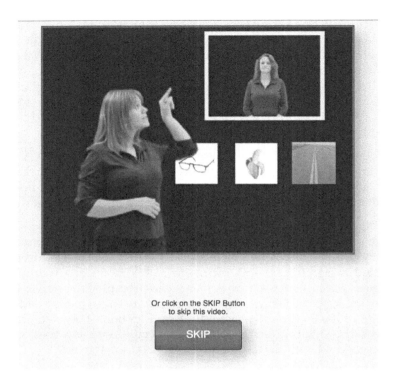

Figure 7.7 Screen shot of American Sign Language–Phonological Awareness Test instructions.

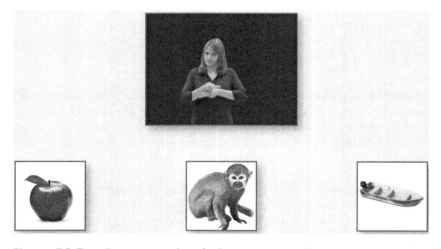

Figure 7.8 Test item example of the American Sign Language (ASL)–Phonological Awareness Test (© 2012, L. McQuarrie). The ASL cue (CAREFUL), the target (BOAT), and two distracters (APPLE and MONKEY) are displayed. The cue and the target share two parameters: location and movement.

probe across skills design, found a clear functional relation between explicit instruction in ASL phonological awareness and increases in sign vocabulary and print vocabulary learning in young, deaf dual-language learners. These results were confirmed by changes on the ASL-PAT administered at the beginning and end of the study. On completion of the test development project and associated validation studies, the ASL-PAT will be available for teachers and clinicians to provide diagnostic information on children's sign phonological development and to identify children who lack explicit sign phonological knowledge. The test is expected to give reliable indicators of the development of ASL phonological awareness in young bilingual deaf children, which may allow educators to establish targeted phonological learning objectives and plan effective sign phonological instructional interventions for bilingual deaf students.

Web-based British Sign Language Vocabulary Test

History

Most standardized assessments of children's vocabulary draw on the mapping between phonological form and meaning. Typically, the task involves presenting the phonological form (word) and requiring the test-taker to select a picture that matches its meaning from a set of three or four (Dunn & Dunn, 1997), or providing a picture and the test-taker must produce the phonological form that matches the meaning (Brownell, 2000). These assessments are limited in that they measure only one level of vocabulary knowledge—for example, meaning recognition or form recall. These task limitations, along with the lack of standardized vocabulary assessments for signed language, motivated the development of a set of vocabulary tasks to assess different levels of deaf children's vocabulary knowledge in BSL. One advantage of having an assessment that provides more detailed information about a child's different levels of vocabulary knowledge is the impact it can have on guiding and improving intervention (Mann et al., 2013). In addition, because the BSL Vocabulary Test (VT) (Mann & Marshall, 2012) enables identical items to be compared across more than one task, it is possible to identify unusual language profiles as demonstrated by Mann et al. (2013). In their study, the BSL VT was administered to a larger, more diverse deaf sample, including deaf children with additional needs such as attention deficit hyperactivity disorder, autism spectrum disorder, and dyslexia. Although there was no significant effect of additional needs on vocabulary performance, an unusual response pattern was noted in one child with autism spectrum disorder that was consistent with reports of autism in spoken languages. This stresses the value of studies that assess vocabulary development in deaf children with a wide range of additional disabilities and might contribute important information about possible effects of disabilities on word learning commonly found within the group of deaf language users (Mann et al., 2013). In this context, the BSL VT is particularly valuable because of its unique format.

Purpose

The purpose of the Web-based BSL VT is to assess deaf children's vocabulary knowledge in BSL "by specifically measuring the degree of strength of the mappings between form and meaning for items in the core lexicon" (Mann & Marshall, 2012, p. 1031). One particular aim for developing it was to investigate whether there is a hierarchy of difficulty for these tasks, and therefore whether BSL vocabulary acquisition proceeds incrementally, as is the case for spoken languages.

Target Population

The target population for this test is signing deaf children between the ages of 4 years and 15 years. At this point, data have been collected from 67 children. Twenty-four deaf children from five programs that use BSL as the language of instruction participated in the pilot study (Mann & Marshall, 2012). Of these 24 children, 12 were boys and their average age was 11 years. All the participants had a hearing loss of more than 70 dB in their better ear. They were either native signers or strong signers who all used BSL as their preferred language/means of communication.

In a follow-up study, an additional 43 children were assessed, resulting in a total of 67 deaf children (37 boys, 30 girls) age 4 to 17 years (Mann et al., 2013). One difference from the pilot study was that the newly added participants had more variable BSL skills and also included children from diverse language learning backgrounds and children with additional needs. The goal of this study was to investigate whether some key variables in deaf signing children, such as parental hearing loss and additional needs, affect deaf children's vocabulary knowledge in BSL (Mann et al., 2013). Average scores for three of the four tasks were reported.

Content/Format

The Web-based BSL VT consists of four tasks to assess different degrees of vocabulary knowledge: (a) meaning recognition (test-taker sees a prerecorded BSL sign followed by four pictures and must select the picture that corresponds to the meaning of the signed prompt), (b) form recognition (test-taker sees a picture followed by four prerecorded BSL signs and must select the sign that matches the meaning of the picture prompt), (c) meaning recall (test-taker sees a prerecorded BSL sign and must generate another BSL sign with an associated meaning), and (d) form recall (test-taker sees a picture and must produce the corresponding BSL sign). Each task consists of 120 items. The test draws on a model for second language learning (Laufer & Goldstein, 2004; Laufer et al., 2004) in which the same items are used across all tasks. The test includes two receptive and two production tasks. The two receptive tasks (meaning recognition, form recognition) use a multiple-choice format and can be self-administered. The two production tasks (meaning recall, form recall) require an administrator, who scores each response based on four options and also documents the given response in a text box on the computer screen, using English glosses.

The items for the test were selected from several sources: (a) a BSL norming study (Vinson et al., 2008); (b) a receptive vocabulary test for DGS (Bizer & Karl, 2002a, 2002b); (c) commonly used, standardized, English vocabulary tests; and (d) feedback from deaf and hearing researchers and teachers who collaborated with us during the item development (Mann & Marshall, 2012).

The order of the items in each set is randomized every time someone takes the test. The items of the test belong to the grammatical categories of nouns, verbs, and adjectives. Signs known to have regional variations (including colors and numbers) were excluded from the test. It was important to develop effective distracters for the two receptive skills tasks involving multiple-choice responses. These tasks include four types of responses that are presented randomly for each item: (a) the target, (b) a phonological distracter, (c) a semantic distracter, and (d) a visual or unrelated distracter. Signs that are known to be iconic (such as body parts, animals, and numbers) were excluded as much as possible, although they are commonly used in spoken English vocabulary tests (Mann & Marshall, 2012).

Procedure
The test is presented individually for each child by a signing tester, preferably a deaf native signer (Figure 7.9). Both receptive tasks can be self-administered by the test-taker, depending on age and familiarity with a computer and mouse. For the two production tasks, the test-taker produces responses in BSL and the tester enters the answer as English gloss during test administration. All results are saved automatically in the database on the Web server. The four tasks are completed in two sessions, and each session includes two tasks. There should be at least 1 week between the first and second session to minimize learning. Each session takes about 30 minutes. Before the tasks start, the test-taker sees prerecorded instructions in BSL, which can be elaborated on by the tester for younger children, and is given the chance to practice on two items.

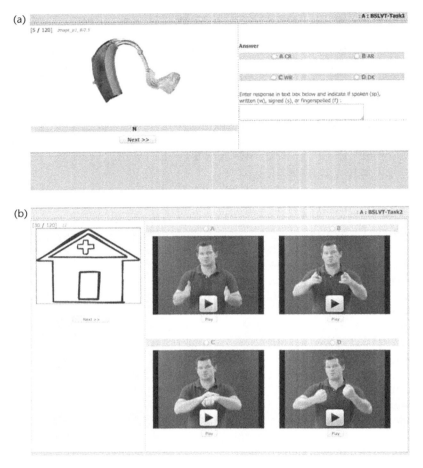

Figure 7.9 (a–d) Example from the Web-based British Sign Language–Vocabulary Test (© 2008, W. Mann).

Scoring
The responses for the two receptive skills tasks are scored as 1 for correct and 0 for incorrect. For the production tasks, four answer choices are provided for the tester to code answers live. For the form recall task, these scoring choices are (a) correct sign (scored as 1), (b) partially correct sign (scored as 0.5), (c) wrong sign/different sign (scored as 0), and (d) do not know (scored as 0). For the meaning recall task, they are (a) categorical response (scored as 1), (b) noncategorical response (scored as 0.5), (c) different/unrelated response (scored as 0), and (d) do not know (scored as 0). These scores are presented in codes (for example, CS means correct sign) so as not to affect the test-taker's motivation. In addition, the English gloss is entered in a textbox below the

Exploring Signed Language Assessment Tools in Europe and North America   203

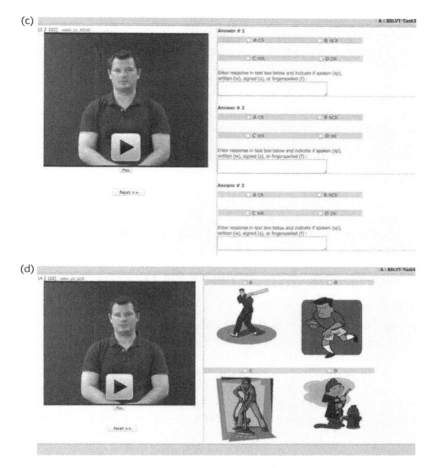

Figure 7.9 Continued

coded answer as an added measure of reliability and in lieu of video-recording the responses, which would render the task less time efficient for practitioners.

Psychometric Information

The Web-based BSL VT was developed and pilot-tested on 24 deaf children, including deaf children with deaf parents and those recommended by teachers as strong signers. After piloting, the test was administered to 43 deaf children from deaf and hearing families within the age range of 4 to 17 years located throughout the United Kingdom, including children with additional needs. All tests were administered by a hearing researcher with fluent BSL skills.

Reliability was established in the form of interrater reliability and was found to be good. Content validity was established based on feedback from a panel of deaf and hearing experts. Construct validity, explored by correlating test-takers' performance on each of the four tasks and age, was found to be high. Concurrent validity was explored by comparing scores on the Web-based BSL VT with nonverbal IQ (Raven's Progressive Matrices) and controlling for age. Findings showed moderate correlations for all tasks (for more detailed information, see Mann et al. [2013]).

Web-Based American Sign Language Vocabulary Test

History

There are currently no standardized ASL vocabulary tests available that measure strength of vocabulary knowledge. The Web-based ASL VT (Mann et al., 2015) was adapted from the Web-based BSL VT. It was developed as a baseline measure for a larger study investigating how deaf children respond to mediated learning in ASL, in addition to investigating the reliability and validity of the adapted measure.

Purpose and Target Population

The purpose of the Web-based ASL VT is to assess receptive and expressive vocabulary knowledge of signing deaf children in the United States (and other countries using ASL). The target population is deaf children age 6 to 10 years. At this point, data have been collected from 37 children, including deaf children with deaf parents, deaf children with hearing parents, and deaf children with additional needs. The findings, to date, indicate a similar hierarchy regarding level of difficulty for the four tasks as found in the BSL study. Specifically, deaf children perform best on the meaning recognition task, followed by the form recognition task, and experience more difficulties with the two recall tasks—form recall and meaning recall. Our work on the Web-based ASL VT is still in progress and awaits standardization on a larger sample.

Content/Format

The test uses the same format as the Web-based BSL VT, including two receptive (multiple-choice) tasks and two production tasks (Figure 7.10). Sixty-six items were translated directly from the Web-based BSL VT and 14 revised or new items were added for a total of 80 items (this is fewer than the Web-based BSL VT because of the smaller age range of participants in U.S. pilot).

Psychometric Information

The Web-based ASL VT was developed and pilot-tested on 20 deaf children, age 6 to 10 years, all of whom came from deaf families. All tests were administered by a deaf native signer with fluent ASL skills.

Exploring Signed Language Assessment Tools in Europe and North America   205

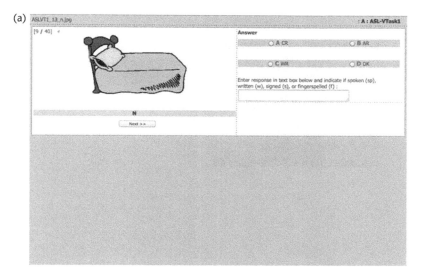

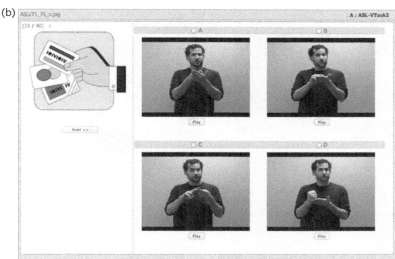

Figure 7.10 (a–d) Example from the Web-based American Sign Language–Vocabulary Test (© 2011, W. Mann).

Reliability was established in the forms of internal consistency, interrater agreement, and item analysis. Content validity was established based on feedback from an expert panel, which included deaf native signers and rating scores from teachers. Construct validity was explored by correlating test-takers' performance on each of the four tasks and age, analysis of differences between participants'

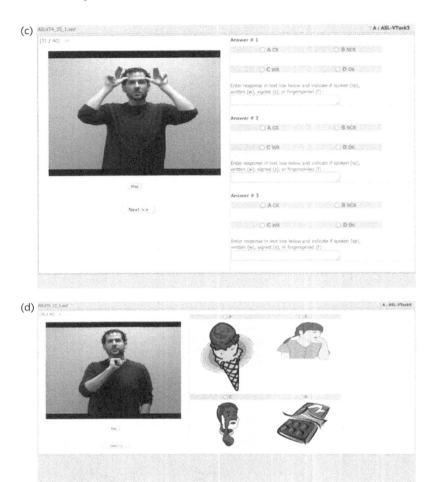

Figure 7.10 Continued

performances across tasks, and comparison of deaf children's performance on the two receptive tasks with age-matched hearing children with no previous knowledge of sign. Concurrent validity was explored by comparison of Web-based ASL VT scores with performance on the ASL Receptive Skills Test (Enns et al., 2013); for more detailed information, see Mann et al., 2015.

Our similar findings for ASL and BSL suggest the underlying construct—that is, vocabulary knowledge has different degrees of strength based on the mapping between form and meaning of signs—holds true for these two sign languages and indicates the tasks would be applicable to other signed languages as well.

Swiss German Sign Language Sentence Repetition Test

History

A survey among schools for the deaf in German Switzerland (Audeoud & Haug, 2008) confirmed the need for an educational assessment of signed language—a need that has also been confirmed in other international studies (e.g., in Germany [Haug & Hintermair, 2003], in the United Kingdom [Herman, 1998a], and in the United States [Mann & Prinz, 2006]). In German Switzerland, where one of the three Swiss signed languages is used (Boyes Braem et al., 2012), no standardized and normed test of DSGS exists. To meet this need, a research team at the University of Applied Sciences of Special Needs in Zurich applied for funding to develop a sentence repetition test (SRT) for DSGS (Haug et al., 2015). The test was developed by a team of deaf and hearing researchers in cooperation with deaf signed language instructors experienced in working within a school context.

Purpose and Target Population

The purpose of the DSGS SRT is to develop a global measure of DSGS development that is easy to administer and score. The DSGS SRT provides information on different linguistic levels, such as phonology, morphology, and syntax. Because only one study of DSGS acquisition (Fosshaug, 2010) is available, creating a test for DSGS development posed a methodological challenge. It was necessary to rely on available adult data to develop the reference measure.

The target population for the DSGS SRT is signing deaf children between 6 years and 12 years of age, with either deaf or hearing parents.

Content/Format

SRTs from other signed languages—such as American (Hauser et al., 2008); German (Kubus & Rathmann, 2012); British, children's version (Cormier et al., 2012); Swedish; and Italian Sign Language—served as templates for DSGS SRT development. In addition, sentences from "e-kids," an online portal with DSGS teaching materials for children from the Swiss Deaf Federation (http://ekids.sgb-fss.ch) were used and new sentences were developed.

Because the ASL and the DGS versions target adult signers, the sentences adapted for DSGS were changed in regard (a) to avoiding lexical variations, (b) to adapting the signing style to be more child appropriate, and (c) to matching children's experiences (for example, "The last time I was on vacation was 7 years ago" does not match the experience of a 6-year-old child). Lengthy sentences more appropriate for adults were removed, and specific DSGS linguistic features were added. The

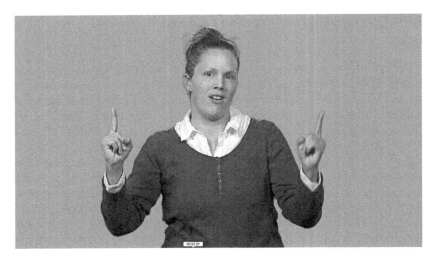

Figure 7.11 Example from the Swiss German Sign Language Sentence Repetition Test (© HfH, 2015).

first version of the DSGS SRT consisted of 76 sentences of increasing length and complexity. The panel of experts provided feedback on the initial version of the test, which resulted in removal and revision of some sentences. This process reduced the number of sentences to 60. The panel of experts met regularly during the life of the project to provide ongoing feedback.

The DSGS SRT is presented on video, embedded in PowerPoint, and administered with a laptop computer. After prerecorded instructions in DSGS, three practice sentences are presented, followed by the test sentences (Figure 7.11). The test participants watch a sentence and then repeat it as accurately as possible. The test participants were video-recorded with the built-in webcam of the laptop on which the test was presented. The tester was sitting opposite and slightly to the right side of the test participants.

After training two deaf testers, a pilot study was conducted with three deaf adults and three children (ages 7–11 years old). Besides feedback on the test procedure (test instructions), 20 additional sentences were removed when they were either mastered/not mastered at all by the pilot test participants. Also, based on feedback from the deaf adult participants and testers, some sentences were revised.

The 40 remaining sentences were video-recorded in a professional video studio. For the main study, 45 deaf children (6–16 years old) and 15 deaf adults were tested. The results are currently scored with a newly developed scoring tool, which is similar to that developed for the BSL SRT for children (Marshall et al., 2014).

Psychometric Information

The investigation of the test's psychometric properties is currently underway.

DISCUSSION

The primary purpose of assessment is to inform educational decisions and instruction. With accurate tools to assess signed language competence, educators are able to establish baseline measurements and determine progress, identify students with language delays or disorders, and evaluate the outcomes of classroom or individual therapy programs. Researchers also have the tools to compare populations and provide consistency across studies. It is important that practitioners and researchers work together to develop signed language interventions based on valid and reliable test results to improve deaf children's language proficiency. The assessment tools described here clearly demonstrate that significant gains are being made toward establishing effective measures to enhance deaf children's acquisition of signed languages. Throughout the discussion of test development, two issues arose repeatedly and require further mention. These issues are adapting tests for use in other signed languages and implementing new technologies for test presentation.

Test Adaptation

The process of adapting tests from one signed language to another requires careful consideration of the linguistic differences that exist between the two languages; however, limited cross-linguistic research related to signed languages can make this a challenging task (Mason, 2005). These challenges are illustrated by Haug and Mann (2008) through examples involving differences in the categorization of linguistic features, lexical differences, and morphosyntactic issues. Cultural issues also play a part in test adaptation. This can be as simple as pictures depicting the size, color, and shape of a British mailbox versus a German mailbox or as complex as a story involving the experience of obtaining a driver's license, which is common in America but not in Switzerland (Haug & Mann, 2008).

The decision of whether it is advantageous to adapt an existing instrument that has already been tested and standardized must be considered within the framework of evaluating the linguistic and cultural differences between the original and target languages. If test developers determine these differences can be overcome by modifications to pictures, distracter items, or stimuli, then the adaptation process is considered worthwhile because important test development decisions have already been evaluated. For example, the BSL RST was based on what was known about signed language acquisition and it highlights grammatical features identified in the research as important indicators of proficiency, such as verb morphology and use of space (Herman et al., 1998). Considering that many signed languages share these important grammatical features, numerous test items are relevant in signed languages other than BSL, as evidenced by the ASL and DGS versions. Another advantage of test adaptation is that clear guidelines for the assessment format have also been validated. Decisions regarding using picture stimuli to keep attention, the number of test items to reduce fatigue effects, and the incorporation of videos to standardize presentation have already been determined for test developers.

It is important to clarify the distinction between "translation," defined as a one-to-one transfer without consideration of linguistic differences, and "adaptation," which involves developing a parallel test that "acknowledges the linguistic, cultural, and social conditions of those taking the adapted test while retaining the measurement of the constructs found in the original" (Oakland & Lane, 2004, p. 239). In the examples described earlier, the new tests were developed to resemble closely the existing tests, but incorporated the specific needs of the target language; therefore, *adaptation* is the appropriate term to use to describe the process.

New Technologies

As has been mentioned by several test developers in the previous descriptions, test delivery through a Web-based format is highly conducive to signed language assessment (Mann & Haug, 2015). This format incorporates multiple picture/video stimuli and response options easily, and can also record video data (signing) expressed by test-takers. A Web-based system allows for multiple people to take the test simultaneously, making the testing process much more efficient. The test results are also recorded and analyzed automatically, and can be entered immediately into a database for further comparison and psychometric evaluation. The potential of such a database is that it can also generate reports for test administrators, parents, and schools, as is the case for the online version of the Sign Language RST that incorporates three signed language formats (ASL, BSL, and DGS) (Haug et al., 2015). Another benefit to Web-based test formats is increased mobility and accessibility; the assessments can be accessed on a variety of different devices. The Sign Language RST online version has a responsive design that enables test participants to take the test on a tablet or smartphone (Figure 7.12).

In summary, the lack of standardized, norm-referenced assessment instruments to measure the acquisition of natural signed languages in children has been an enormous gap in both research and education concerning young deaf children and their development. In comparison, standardized assessment measures of speech and language skills

Exploring Signed Language Assessment Tools in Europe and North America 211

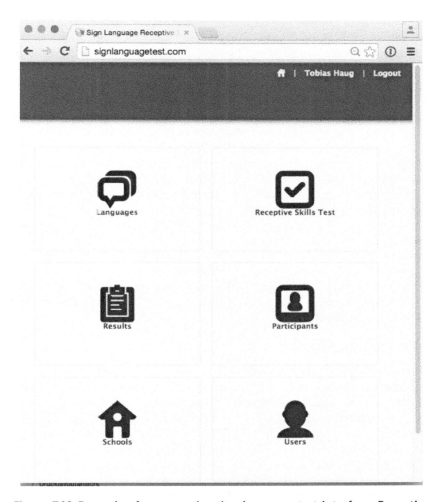

Figure 7.12 Example of a responsive sign language test interface: Receptive Skills Test (© 2015, T. Haug, Sign Language Assessment Services).

of most spoken languages (English, German, French, and so on) are extremely numerous and are constantly being revised and updated (Owens, 2004). Standardized tests of spoken languages allow researchers to communicate more precisely and build on one another's findings with ease. Research in signed language development lags significantly behind with respect to standardized testing. Accurate measurement of signed language skills is particularly critical for children acquiring such languages as their first language, because delays in first-language acquisition have a detrimental impact on later learning and literacy development. Valid and reliable measures of signed language development are needed to understand diversity among deaf children in various areas of development and performance, including behavior, social interaction, cognition, spoken language skills, and literacy levels (for example, see Chapter 12). The assessment tools described in this chapter begin to fill the void and can meet the needs of teachers and researchers in providing appropriate educational programming, monitoring, and reporting. More important, valid and reliable measures enhance the credibility of signed languages, promote strategies that build on deaf children's visual strengths (Herman & Roy, 2006; Hoffmeister & Caldwell-Harris, 2014; Marshall et al., 2006; Mason et. al., 2010; McQuarrie & Parrila, 2014), and value sign languages as equal and legitimate languages of instruction in schools.

During the past several years significant progress has been made toward developing tests to assess the acquisition of natural signed languages. Because many of these tests are still works in progress, the need for valid and reliable assessment tools of signed languages for both practical and theoretical purposes continues to be important. The purpose of this chapter was to provide state-of-the-art descriptions of several currently available tests assessing the acquisition of signed languages and to outline the ongoing need for and challenges to the test development process.

ACKNOWLEDGMENTS

Test development requires teamwork, and the work we report in this chapter would not have been possible without significant assistance from our colleagues, graduate students, research assistants, and technicians, as well as the support we received from schools, parents, and children to complete the testing. We thank our colleagues who were kind enough to share their SRT materials for our project: Peter Hauser (United States), Kate Rowley (United Kingdom), Christian Rathmann (Germany), Krister Schönström (Sweden), and Pasquale Rinaldi (Italy).

We also acknowledge the funding support we have received to conduct our research studies in signed language assessment.

REFERENCES

Audeoud, M., & Haug, T. (2008). "Grundsätzlich wollen wir Tests, die alle sprachlichen Ebenen überprüfen!": Eine Pilot-Studie zum Bedarf an Gebärdensprachtests für hörgeschädigte Kinder an Deutschschweizer Hörgeschädigtenschulen. *Hörgeschädigtenpädagogik, 62*(1),15–20.

Bizer, S., & Karl, A.-K. (2002a). Entwicklung eines Wortschatztests fuer gehoerlose Kinder im Grundschulalter in Gebaerden-, Schrift-, und Lautsprache. Unpublished PhD dissertation, Fachbereich Erziehungswissenschaften, Universitaet Hamburg.

Bizer, S., & Karl, A.-K. (2002b). *Perlesko: Pruefverfahren zur Erfassung lexikalisch-semantischer Kompetenz gehoerloser Kinder im Grundschulalter.* Hamburg: Fachbereich Erziehungswissenschaften, Universitaet Hamburg.

Boyes Braem, P., Haug, T., & Shores, P. (2012). Gebardenspracharbeit in der Schwiez: Ruckblick und Ausblick. *Das Zeichen, 90,* 58–74.

Brentari, D. (1998). *A prosodic model of sign language phonology.* Cambridge, MA: MIT Press.

Brownell, R. (2000). *Expressive one-word picture vocabulary test.* Novato, CA: Academic Therapy Publications.

Chamberlain, C., & R. I. Mayberry. 2008 American Sign Language syntactic and narrative comprehension in skilled and less skilled readers: Bilingual and bimodal evidence for the linguistic basis of reading. *Applied Psycholinguistics, 29,* 367–388.

Christensen, K. M., & Delgado, G. L. (Eds.) (1993). *Multicultural issues in deafness.* White Plains, NY: Longman.

Cormier, K., Adam, R., Rowley, K., Woll, B., & Atkinson, J. (2012). The BSL Sentence Reproduction Test: Exploring age-of-acquisition effects in British deaf adults. Paper presented at the 34th annual meeting of the German Association of Linguistics, March 7–9, 2012. Frankfurt, Germany.

Dammeyer, J. (2010) Psychosocial development in a Danish population of children with cochlear implants and deaf and hard-of-hearing children. *Journal of Deaf Studies and Deaf Education, 15*(1), 50–58.

Davidson, K., Lillo-Martin, D., & Chen-Pichler, D. (2014) Spoken English language development in native signing children with cochlear implants. *Journal of Deaf Studies and Deaf Education, 19,* 238–250

DeLana, M., Gentry, M.A., & Andrews, J. (2007). The efficacy of ASL/English bilingual education: Considering public schools. *American Annals of the Deaf, 152*(1), 73–87.

Dollaghan, C., & Campbell, T. (1998). Nonword repetition and child language impairment. *Journal of Speech, Language and Hearing Research, 41,* 1136–1146.

Dunn, L. M., & Dunn, D. M. (1997). *Peabody picture vocabulary test* (3rd ed.). Circle Pines, MN: American Guidance Services.

Enns, C., Boudreault, P., Zimmer, K., Broszeit, C., & Goertzen, D. (February 2014). Assessing children's expressive skills in American Sign Language. Paper presented at the annual meeting of the Association of College Educators—Deaf/Hard of Hearing. Washington, DC.

Enns, C. J., Zimmer, K., Boudreault, P., Rabu, S., & Broszeit, C. (2013). *American Sign Language: Receptive Skills Test.* Winnipeg, MB: Northern Signs Research.

Enns, C., & Herman, R. (2011) Adapting the Assessing British Sign Language Development: Receptive Skills Test into American Sign Language. *Journal of Deaf Studies and Deaf Education, 16,* 362–374.

Falkman, K. W., Roos, C., & Hjelmquist, E. (2007). Mentalizing skills of non-native, early signers: A longitudinal perspective. *European Journal of Developmental Psychology, 4*(2), 178–197.

Fosshaug, S. (2010). *Entwicklung der gebärdensprachlichen Kompetenz eines gehörlosen Kindes in einer bilingual geführten Schulklasse: eine Logitudinalstudie.* VUGS Informationsheft no. 47. Zurich: VUGS.

French, M. (1999). *Starting with assessment toolkit.* Washington, DC: Gallaudet University Press.

Gallon, N., Harris, J., & van der Lely, H. (2007). Nonsense word repetition: An investigation of phonological complexity in children with grammatical SLI. *Clinical Linguistics and Phonetics, 21,* 435–455.

Gathercole, S. E. (2006). Nonsense word repetition and word learning: The nature of the relationship. *Applied Psycholinguistics, 27,* 513–543.

Gerner de Garcia, B. (2000). Meeting the needs of Hispano/Latino deaf students. In K. M. Christensen & G. L. Deldago (Eds.), *Deaf plus. A multi-cultural perspective* (pp. 149–198). San Diego, CA: Dawn Sign Press.

Haug, T. (2005). Review of sign language assessment instruments. *Sign Language & Linguistics, 8,* 61–98.

Haug, T. (2011a). Approaching sign language test construction: Adaptation of the German Sign Language Receptive Skills Test. *Journal of Deaf Studies and Deaf Education, 16*(3), 343–361.

Haug, T. (2011b). Methodological and theoretical issues in the adaptation of sign language tests: An example from the adaptation of a test to German Sign Language. *Language Testing, 29*(2),181–201.

Haug, T. (2012). A review of sign language acquisition studies as the basis for informed decisions for sign language test adaptation: The case of the German Sign Language Receptive Skills Test. *Sign Language and Linguistics, 15*(2), 213–239.

Haug, T., Herman, R., & Woll, B. (2015). Constructing an online test framework, using the example of a sign language receptive skills test. *Deafness & Education International, 17*(1), 3–7.

Haug, T., & Hintermair, M. (2003). Ermittlung des Bedarfs von Gebärdensprachtests für gehörlose Kinder: Ergebnisse einer Pilotstudie. *Das Zeichen, 64,* 220–229.

Haug, T., Notter, C., Girard, S., & Audeoud, M. (2015). Sentence Repetition Test für die Deutschschweizerische Gebärdensprache (DSGS-SRT). Unpublished test, Hochschule für Heilpädagogik, Zurich.

Haug, T., & Mann, W. (2008). Adapting tests of sign language assessment for other sign languages: A review of linguistic, cultural, and psychometric problems. *Journal of Deaf Studies and Deaf Education, 13*(1), 138–147.

Hauser, P. C., Paludnevičienė, R., Supalla, T., & Bavelier, D. (2008). American Sign Language-Sentence Reproduction Test. In R. M. de Quadros (Eds.), *Sign languages: Spinning and unraveling the past, present and future* (pp. 160–172). Florianopolis, Brazil: Editora Arara Azul.

Herman, R. (1998a). Issues in designing an assessment of British Sign Language development. *International Journal of Language and Communication Disorders, 33* (SI), 332–337.

Herman, R. (1998b). The need for an assessment of deaf children's signing skills. *Deafness and Education: Journal of the British Association of the Teachers of the Deaf, 22*(3), 3–8.

Herman, R., Grove, N., Holmes, S., Morgan, G., Sutherland, H., & Woll, B. (2004). *Assessing BSL development: Production Test (Narrative Skills).* London: City University.

Herman, R., Holmes, S., & Woll, B. (1998). *Design and standardization of an assessment of British Sign Language development for use with deaf children: Final report, 1998.* London: Department of Language & Communication Science, City University.

Herman, R., Holmes, S., & Woll, B. (1999). *Assessing BSL development: Receptive Skills Test.* Coleford, UK: Forest Bookshop.

Herman, R., & Roy, P. (2006). Evidence from the wider use of the BSL Receptive Skills Test. *Deafness and Education International, 8*(1), 33–47.

Herman, R., Rowley, K., Mason, K., & Morgan, G. (2014). Deficits in narrative abilities in child British Sign Language users with specific language impairment. *International Journal of Language & Communication Disorders, 49*(3), 343–353.

Hodge, G., Schembri, A., & Rogers, I. (July 2014). The Auslan (Australian Sign Language) Production Skills Test: Responding to challenges in the assessment of deaf children's signed language proficiency. Paper presented at Disability Studies in Education. Melbourne, Australia.

Hoffmeister, R. J. (1994). Metalinguistic skills in deaf children: Knowledge of synonyms and antonyms in ASL. In J. Mann (Ed.), *Proceedings of the Post Milan: ASL and English Literacy Conference* (pp. 151–175). Washington, DC: Gallaudet University Press.

Hoffmeister, R. J. (2000). A piece of the puzzle: ASL and reading comprehension in deaf children. In C. Chamberlain, J. P. Morford, & R. Mayberry (Eds.), *Language acquisition by eye* (pp. 143–163). Mahwah, NJ: Erlbaum.

Hoffmeister, R. J., & Caldwell-Harris, C. L. (2014). Acquiring English as a second language via print: The task for deaf children. *Cognition, 132*(2), 229–242.

Hoffmeister, R. J., Caldwell-Harris, C. L., Henner, J., Benedict, R., Fish, S., Rosenburg, P., Conlin-Luippold, F., & Novogrodsky, R. (2014). *The American Sign Language Assessment Instrument (ASLAI): Progress report and preliminary findings*. Working paper. Boston, MA: Center for the Study of Communication and the Deaf.

Hoffmeister, R. J., Henner, J., & Caldwell-Harris, C. L. (2015). *The psychometric properties of the American Sign Language Assessment Instrument*. Working paper. Boston, MA: Center for the Study of Communication and the Deaf, Boston University.

Jackson A. L. (2001). Language facility and theory of mind development in deaf children. *Journal of Deaf Studies and Deaf Education, 6*, 161–176

Jones, A., Herman, R., Botting, N., Marshall, C., Toscano, E., & Morgan, G. (March 2015). Narrative skills in deaf children: Assessing signed and spoken modalities with the same test. Paper presentation at SRCD Preconference: Development of Deaf Children. Philadelphia, PA.

Johnston, T. (2004). The assessment and achievement of proficiency in a native sign language within a sign bilingual program: The pilot Auslan Receptive Skills Test. *Deafness and Education International, 6*(2), 57–81.

Kennedy, C. R., McCann, D. C., Campbell, M. J., Law, C. M., Mullee, M., Petrou, S., Watkin, P., Worsfold, S., Yuen, H. M., & Stevenson, J. (2006). Language ability after early detection of permanent childhood hearing impairment. *New England Journal of Medicine, 354*(20), 2131–2141.

Kubus, O., & Rathmann, C. (2012). Degrees of difficulty in the L2 acquisition of morphology in German Sign Language. Paper presented at the 34th annual meeting of the German Association of Linguistics. March 7–9, 2012. Frankfurt, Germany.

Labov, W., & Waltesky, J. (1967). Oral versions of personal experiences. In J. Helm (Ed.), *Essays on the verbal and visual arts* (pp. 12–44). Seattle, WA: University of Washington Press.

Laufer, B., Elder, C., Hill, K., & Congdon, P. (2004). Size and strength: Do we need both to measure vocabulary knowledge? *Language Testing, 21*, 202–226.

Laufer, B., & Goldstein, Z. (2004). Testing vocabulary knowledge: Size, strength, and computer adaptiveness. *Language Learning, 54*, 469–523.

Lillo-Martin, D. (1999). Modality effects and modularity in language acquisition: The acquisition of America Sign Language, pp. 531–567. In W. Ritchie & T. Bhatia (Eds.). *Handbook of child language acquisition*. San Diego, CA: Academic Press.

MacSweeney, M., Woll, B., Campbell, R., McGuire, P. K., David, A., Williams, S. C. R., Suckling, J., Calvert, G. A., & Brammer, M. J. (2002). Neural systems underlying British Sign Language and audio-visual English processing in native users. *Brain*, 125(7),1583–1593.

Mann, W., & Haug, T. (2015). New directions in sign language assessment. In M. Marschark & P. E. Spencer (Eds.), *The Oxford handbook of deaf studies in language* (pp. 412–421). New York, NY: Oxford University Press.

Mann, W., & Marshall, C. (2012). Investigating deaf children's vocabulary knowledge in British Sign Language. *Language Learning*, 62(4), 1024–1051.

Mann W., Marshall C. R., Mason K., Morgan G. (2010). The acquisition of sign language: The impact of phonetic complexity on phonology. *Language, Learning, and Development*, 6, 60–86.

Mann, W., & Prinz, P. (2006). The perception of sign language assessment by professionals in deaf education. *American Annals of the Deaf*, 151(3), 356–370.

Mann, W., Roy, P., & Marshall, C. (2013). A look at the other 90 per cent: Investigating British Sign Language vocabulary knowledge in deaf children from different language learning backgrounds. *Deafness & Education International*, 15(2), 91–116.

Mann, W., Roy, P., & Morgan, G. (2015). Adaptation of a vocabulary test from British Sign Language to American Sign Language. *Language Testing*, 31, 1–20.

Marshall, C. R., Denmark, T., & Morgan, G. (2006). Investigating the underlying causes of SLI: A non-sign repetition test in British Sign Language. *International Journal of Speech–Language Pathology*, 8(4), 47–355.

Marshall, C., Mason, K., Rowley, K., Herman, R., Atkinson, J., Woll, B., & Morgan, G. (2014). Sentence repetition in deaf children with specific language impairment in British Sign Language. *Language Learning and Development*, 10(1), 1–15.

Mason, T. C. (2005). Cross-cultural instrument translation: Assessment, translation, and statistical application. *American Annals of the Deaf*, 151, 356–370.

Mason, K., Rowley, K., Marshall, C., Atkinson, J., Herman, R., Woll, B., & Morgan, G. (2010). Identifying specific language impairment in deaf children acquiring British Sign Language: Implications for theory and practice. *British Journal of Developmental Psychology*, 28, 33–49.

McQuarrie, L. M. (2005). *Deaf children's Awareness of Phonological Structure: Syllable, Rhyme, and Phoneme*. Doctoral dissertation, University of Alberta, Edmonton, Alberta, Canada. Available from ProQuest Dissertations and Theses. (UMI No. 305384757).

McQuarrie, L., & Abbott, M. (2010). Does ASL phonology underlie the ASL–reading link? Poster presented at the 21st International Congress on the Education of the Deaf (ICED). Vancouver, British Columbia.

McQuarrie, L., & Abbott, M. (2013). Bilingual deaf students' phonological awareness in ASL and reading skills in English. *Sign Language Studies*, 14(1), 80–100 [special issue on assessment].

McQuarrie, L., Abbott, M., & Spady, S. (2012). American Sign Language phonological awareness: Test development and design. In *Proceedings of the 10th Annual Hawaii International Conference on Education* (pp. 1–17).

McQuarrie, L., & Enns, C. (2015). Bridging the gap: Investigating the effects of a signed language phonological awareness intervention on language and literacy outcomes in bilingual deaf children. Paper presented at the 22nd International Congress on the Education of the Deaf (ICED). Athens, Greece.

McQuarrie, L., & Parrila, R. (2014). Literacy and linguistic development in bilingual deaf children: Implications of the "and: for phonological processing. *American Annals of the Deaf, 159*(4), 372–384 [special literacy issue].

McQuarrie, L., & Spady, S.(2012). The American Sign Language Phonological Awareness Test (ASL-PAT). Unpublished test. University of Alberta, Edmonton, Canada.

Menyuk, P., & Brisk, M. E. (2005). *Language development and education: Children with varying language experience.* New York, NY: Palgrave Macmillan.

Meristo, M., Falkman, K. W., Hjelmquist, E., Tedoldi, M., Surian, L., & Siegal, M. (2007). Language and theory of mind reasoning: Evidence from deaf children in bilingual and oralist environments. *Developmental Psychology, 43*, 1156–1169.

Mitchell, R., & Karchmer, M. (2004). Chasing the mythical ten percent: Parental hearing status of deaf and hard of hearing students in the United States. *Sign Language Studies, 4,*138–163.

Neidle, C., Kegl, J., MacLaughlin, D., Bahan, B., & Lee, R. G. (2001). *The syntax of American Sign Language: Functional categories and hierarchical structure.* Cambridge, MA: MIT Press.

Newport, E., & Meier, R. (1985). The acquisition of American Sing Language. In D. I. Slobin (Ed.), *The crosslinguistic study of language acquisition* (Vol. 1, pp. 881–938). Hillsdale, NJ: Lawrence Erlbaum Associates.

Norbury, C. F., & Bishop, D. V. M. (2003). Narrative skills of children with communication impairments. *International Journal of Language and Communication Disorders, 38,* 287–313.

Novogrodsky, R., Caldwell-Harris, C., Fish, S., & Hoffmeister, R. J. (2014a). The development of antonym knowledge in American Sign Language (ASL) and its relationship to reading comprehension in English. *Language Learning, 64*(December), 749–770.

Novogrodsky, R., Fish, S., & Hoffmeister, R. (2014b). The acquisition of synonyms in American Sign Language (ASL): Toward a further understanding of the components of ASL vocabulary knowledge. *Sign Language Studies, 14*(2), 225–249.

Oakland, T., & Lane, H. (2004). Language, reading and readability formulas: Implication for developing and adapting tests. *International Journal of Testing, 4,* 239–252.

Owens, R. (2004). *Language development: An introduction.* Needham Heights, MA: Allyn & Bacon.

Padden, C., & Ramsey, C. (2000). American Sign Language and reading ability in deaf children. In C. Chamberlain, J. Morford, & R. Mayberry (Eds.), *Language acquisition by eye* (pp. 165–189). Mahwah, NJ: Lawrence Erlbaum Associates.

Prinz, P., & Strong, M. (1998). A study of the relationship between American Sign Language and English literacy. *Journal of Deaf Studies and Deaf Education, 2*(1), 37–46.

Reese, R., Suggate, S., Long, J., & Schaughency, E. (2010). Children's oral narrative and reading skills in the first 3 years of reading instruction. *Reading and Writing, 23*(6), 627–644.

Schembri, A., Wigglesworth, G., Johnston, T., Leigh, G., Adam, R., & Barker, R. (2002). Issues in development of the test battery for Australian Sign Language morphology and syntax. *Journal of Deaf Studies and Deaf Education, 7,* 1, 18–40.

Schick, B. (2010). The development of American Sign Language and manually coded English systems. In M. Marschark & P. E. Spencer (Eds.), *Oxford Handbook of Deaf Studies* (pp. 229–240). New York, NY: Oxford University Press.

Sieratzki, J. S., Calvert, G., Brammer, A. M., David, A., & Woll, B. (2001) Accessibility of spoken, written, and sign language in Landau-Kleffner syndrome: A linguistic and functional MRI study. *Epileptic Disorders, 3*(2), 79–89.

Singleton, J. L., & Supalla, S. J. (2011). Assessing children's proficiency in natural signed languages. In M. Marschark & P. E. Spencer (Eds.), *The Oxford handbook of deaf studies, language, and education* (2nd ed., Vol. 1, pp. 289–302). New York, NY: Oxford University Press.

Snijders, J. T., Tellegen, P. J., & Laros, J. A. (1989). *Snijders-Oomen Non-verbal Intelligence Test: Manual & Research Report*. Groningen: Wolters-Noordhoff.

Strong, M., & Prinz, P. (2000). Is American Sign Language skill related to English literacy? In C. Chamberlain, J. P. Morford & R. Mayberry (Eds.), *Language acquisition by eye* (pp. 131–142). Mahwah, NJ: Lawrence Erlbaum Associates.

Surian, L., Tedoldi, M., & Siegal, M. (2010). Sensitivity to conversational maxims in deaf and hearing children. *Journal of Child Language, 37,* 929–943.

Sutton-Spence, R., & Woll, B. (1999). *The linguistics of British Sign Language: An introduction*. Cambridge, UK: Cambridge University Press.

Tomasuolo, E., Valeri, G., Di Renzo, A., Pasqualetti, P., & Volterra, V. (2012). Deaf children attending different school environments: Sign language abilities and theory of mind. *Journal of Deaf Studies and Deaf Education, 18,* 12–29.

Valli, C., & Lucas, C. (1992). *A resource text for ASL users*. Washington, DC: Gallaudet University Press.

Valmaseda, M., Pérez, M., Herman, R., Ramírez, N., & Montero, I. (2013). Evaluación de la competencia gramatical en LSE: Proceso de adaptación del BSL Receptive Skill Test (test de habilidades receptivas). www.cnlse.es/sites/default/files/Evaluacion%20de%20la%20competencia%20gramatical%20en%20LSE.pdf. Accessed March 11, 2016.

Vinson, D., Cormier, K., Denmark, T., Schembri, A., & Vigliocco, G. (2008). The British Sign Language (BSL) norms for age of acquisition, familiarity and iconicity. *Behavior Research Methods, 40,* 1079–1087.

Woolfe, T., Want, S. C., & Siegal, M. (2002). Signposts to development: Theory of mind in deaf children. *Child Development, 73*(3), 768–778.

8

Language Use in the Classroom: Accommodating the Needs of Diverse Deaf and Hard-of-Hearing Learners

Harry Knoors

LANGUAGE USE AND LEARNING

Any discussion about language use in the classroom is closely connected to thinking about learning. That is why children and adolescents are in classrooms in the first place: for learning. Learning is the result of education, both formal and informal; formal education is still predominantly constituted in schools, and thus in classrooms.

In this age of globalization and informatization, education has become more important than ever before. According to the American futurist Alvin Toffler, "tomorrow's illiterate will not be the man who can't read; he will be the man who has not learned how to learn" (Toffler, 1973, p. 414). Toffler thought of the illiterate of the 21st century as those who cannot learn, unlearn, and relearn. The challenges created by globalization and informatization with respect to participation of specific groups of citizens—among those people with less than sufficient language, literacy, and learning skills—may only be tackled through education. If education fails, globalization and informatization may lead easily to social exclusion, to the inability to participate in today's and tomorrow's society (Knoors & Marschark, 2015).

Learning results from complex interactions between characteristics of the learner, the topic of learning, and the learning environment (Knoors & Marschark, 2014). According to Alexander et al. (2009, p. 176), "one cannot begin to understand the true nature of learning without embracing its interactional complexity." Thus, learning is an ecological process (Bronfenbrenner, 1979) shaped by the learner and by the context in which the learner is being taught and, hopefully, learns.

The contexts for learning among deaf and hard-of-hearing (DHH) students in many countries have changed considerably during the past few decades. Historically, deaf students were educated only with other deaf students in special schools for the deaf, residential ones at first and, later on, more and more day schools. Currently, a considerable proportion of DHH students, in many countries even the vast majority, are taught together with hearing peers in regular schools. This is a consequence of changes in DHH students' characteristics (especially the increase in access to spoken language through early cochlear implantation) as well as of changes in educational policy, with the latter promoting the inclusion of students with disabilities (Archbold, 2015; Knoors & Marschark, 2014). DHH students may be placed in regular schools on an individual basis, in co-enrollment programs in which small groups of DHH students are included in classrooms with hearing peers and are being taught by regular teachers and (sometimes deaf) teachers of the deaf, or in special units located in or near a regular school. In the last case, all or part of the curriculum is still taught to groups of DHH students separated from their hearing peers, similar to the situation in those special schools for the deaf that still exist. In other words, teaching and learning of DHH students is situated in a variety of contexts characterized by different school and classroom dynamics. Still, the effect of the school setting alone is relatively limited. Variation in academic achievement, as a result, seems to be more related to what happens in the classroom, to the way in which classroom instruction and interaction are constructed (Knoors & Hermans, 2010; Stinson & Kluwin, 2011).

This is easy to understand, because learning is both a social and a cognitive activity. Learning as a cognitive process is embedded in social contexts. Because, in school, students are grouped in classrooms, classrooms become a dominant environment for learning. Social interactions between teachers and students in the classroom and among students themselves, with language as the main vehicle, constitute the context in which cognitive processes lead to the construction of meaning in learners (Knoors & Marschark, 2014; Swanwick, 2015). The cognitive processes are constrained to a varying extent by accessibility of the language input, by social interaction and didactic skills of the teachers, and by learner characteristics such as prior knowledge, memory, and executive functioning.

FUNCTIONS OF LANGUAGE IN THE CLASSROOM

Language may serve various functions in the classroom. On the one hand, a first language may be a subject for the students to study, most certainly in primary and secondary education. Increasing vocabulary, learning more complex grammatical structures, using language more formally in cognitively more challenging and contextually more reduced tasks and settings—these are all aspects of studying one's first language as a subject in school. Learning to use a language in other forms than the spoken (or signed) one is another goal of language teaching, implying teaching children to read and write (see Chapter 10). And of course second (and third and fourth) language teaching may become another important aspect of teaching language as a subject, often somewhat later in one's educational career.

But language is more than a subject to teach. Language serves thinking. It is a cognitive tool for students. It helps them to form concepts, to solve problems, and to communicate (Blank, 1974; Vygotski, 1998). Language also serves important purposes in computer-assisted learning, because language is instrumental for information seeking, information presentation, knowledge organization, knowledge integration, and knowledge generation (Robertson et al., 2007)—all skills essential to 21st-century learning.

And last, as noted earlier, language is the vehicle of interaction and communication in the classroom. Language transmits ideas, ideas from teachers to students and vice versa, but language also allows the exchange of ideas among students themselves. Language in the form of classroom talk is thus one of the foundations for learning to read and write, and thus for becoming literate (Fisher et al., 2008). Language in class also has important social dimensions. It plays a crucial role in social interactions in the classroom, again, between a teacher and the students, but also among students themselves. It mediates these interactions as a sort of social vehicle that enables exchanges of meaning through discourse in specific contexts between learners (Kumpulainen & Wray, 1999). Asking questions, transmitting information, clarifying new information, and reflecting on what has been learned are all supported by language use in the classroom.

In traditional classrooms, these interactions, and thus language use, often are asymmetric. The right to speak is controlled by the teacher. And it is the teacher who nominates which student is allowed to talk, because teachers have the right to speak at whatever moment in time and with whom they want, but students usually are not in this position (Cazden, 2001). This teacher-dominated discourse, consisting of initiation, followed by response and feedback, is not very supportive for fruitful classroom discussions, and neither is the fast pace of most communication exchanges. Teachers often hardly wait more than one second before students are supposed to respond and, immediately after a student has replied, the teacher follows up either by giving feedback or by asking the next question. The absence of time for reflection and consolidation may even be a more prominent problem in teacher–student interactions in schools for the deaf, especially if teachers and students do not really share an accessible language for all (Wood et al., 1986).

DEAF AND HARD-OF-HEARING STUDENTS: LINGUISTIC DIVERSITY AS A KEY CHARACTERISTIC

If access to language is restricted, as is often the case with spoken language for DHH students, not only does teaching language as a subject become more complicated, but also classroom interaction may become endangered. Restricted access to communication will, first of all, limit the richness and fluency of communication in the family and, as a result, may lead to limitations in spoken or sign language proficiency in DHH children. Rightfully, much effort is being put into early detection of a hearing loss in children and in subsequently early intervention. Increasing access through amplification, cochlear implantation, the use of sign language or a sign system and coaching parents in their interaction styles are all part of evidence-based early intervention (Moeller et al., 2013; see also Knoors, 2015; and Chapter 2). The mix of early intervention strategies very much depends on the needs of DHH children and the strengths, weaknesses, and desires of parents, most of them being hearing themselves.

Considerable progress has been made in increasing access to spoken language by DHH children through digital hearing aids and cochlear implants (Archbold, 2015). Access to language also may be established successfully through the use of the sign language of the deaf community in those families in which parents opt for bilingual upbringing of their DHH child, although for many hearing parents this is a considerable challenge (Marschark et al., 2014). But whatever route has been taken in early intervention, success in terms of age-appropriate language proficiency will not be achieved in all DHH children, and most definitely not in all DHH children to the same extent. In addition, just like many hearing children, a considerable proportion of DHH children is born in hearing families who speak a language different from the nation's dominant one (Leigh & Crowe, 2015).

So, in actual practice, and acknowledging all the efforts made by parents and by professionals of early-intervention programs, language proficiency in DHH children varies widely when they enter school and, in many cases, it is not or not fully age appropriate (Marschark & Wauters, 2008). Linguistic diversity thus is the norm for DHH children on entrance into school; it is a key characteristic. This diversity is not only reflected in variations in language proficiency, but also is shown in language choice: in the home language and in the preferred modality (signed or spoken). Just as important are the individual language profiles of DHH students. These profiles indicate strengths and weaknesses in various linguistic domains, but also shed light on the use of multiple languages and modalities by students and their families according to specific situations or contexts. Swanwick (2015) has applied Bronfenbrenner's (1979) ecological learning theory to the description of language and learning profiles in real practice, including individual student characteristics, but also the micro-, meso-, exo-, and macrosystems in which these students function, to the roles teachers of DHH students may adopt.

Lederberg et al. (2013) clearly illustrated linguistic diversity in their review of research into language trajectories and language proficiency of DHH children. One may model language learning environments for these children into three distinct categories: spoken communication only, simultaneous communication in which spoken language is supported with manual signs, and bilingual education in which communication takes place in both sign and spoken language, but separately. In actual practice, however, there is much more variation, because these models "are idealized and oversimplify variations in individuals' experiences. Programs, teachers, parents, and others demonstrate a wide range of fidelity to the target model, and children are exposed to more than one model over time and in different contexts" (Lederberg et al., 2013, p. 17). And, in part as a result of this, but also because of differences in characteristics of DHH children themselves, rates and patterns of language acquisition differ considerably among these children, leading to diversity in the languages being used, in the access to and availability of these languages, and in the ultimate proficiency in these languages. Therefore, teaching DHH students, in essence, is teaching communicatively and linguistically diverse students, no matter whether this teaching takes place in regular or in special schools. This, of course, has considerable impact on classroom interaction.

THE IMPORTANCE OF CLASSROOM INTERACTION

According to Cazden (2001, p. 2), "the basic purpose of school [learning] is achieved through communication." Or, as Ellis (2000, p. 209) put it, "learning arises not through interaction, but in interaction." In the context of the classroom, this attaches much importance to classroom interaction and thus to the role of the teacher in establishing and maintaining fruitful classroom discourses during instruction and during cooperative and collaborative learning.

There are several variables that determine the quality and effectiveness of education, one of the most important ones being the quality of the teacher (Hanushek, 2004; Hattie, 2013; Knoors & Marschark, 2014; Marzano, 2003). Teachers exert their influence on the learning of students, hearing and deaf alike, to a large extent through classroom interaction. What is it in those interactions that promotes learning in students? Hamre et al. (2013) conceptualized the key factors in one of the more influential explanatory frameworks, the "Teaching through Interaction model," building on the finding that interactions between teachers and their students are one of the most important aspects of teachers' jobs.

The Teaching through Interactions model is a three-factor model. Interactions in the domains emotional support, classroom organization, and instructional support are thought to promote learning and social development of students. Emotional support aids learning because students will take more risks in their explorations if they know that adults—in this case, teachers—will help them when needed. At the same time, teachers will encourage students to feel competent, to learn autonomously, but also to cooperate with others. The organization of classrooms helps students in their learning because well-structured classrooms provide students with clear and consistent opportunities for appropriate behavior and effective time use. Instructional support aims to help students in constructing rich and cohesive knowledge instead of learning simple facts only. This form of support builds on the linguistic and conceptual knowledge students bring to the classroom. Scaffolding and providing feedback by teachers are important in this respect, as is explicitly connecting new and prior information, which is something of considerable difficulty for many DHH students (Marschark & Wauters, 2008).

The basic line of thinking in this model is that "emotional supports promote social development, classroom management and organization promote positive behavior and attention, and instructional supports enhance learning" (Hamre et al., 2013, p. 480). In a study covering 4326 preschool to sixth-grade classrooms in the United States, the model was shown to fit observational data about classroom interaction and learning very adequately. Initial evidence suggests the model also holds explanatory power for understanding the contributions of classroom interactions in secondary education and across cultures (Hamre et al., 2013). Data from systematic observations of classroom interactions in combination with student feedback and student achievement gains further predict, to a considerable extent, the future effectiveness of teachers in bringing about rich learning in their students (Kane & Staiger, 2012).

Cross-validation of various aspects of the three factors in the Teaching through Interactions model comes from the work of John Hattie. He performed an immense meta-analysis covering more than 800 separate meta-analyses, addressing more than 50,000 scientific studies, and including more than 200 million students (Hattie, 2013). The aim was to identify what works and what does not with respect to effective teaching by focusing on effect sizes (the strength of the relationship between two variables) among a large number of potential contributing factors. Classroom interaction in itself, and also the provision of feedback, the clarity of explanations, reciprocal teaching (instructional support), teacher–student relationships (emotional support), and classroom behavior (classroom organization) were among the 15 factors that influenced student learning most (see, for comparative accounts, Marzano [2003] and American Psychological Association, Coalition for Psychology in Schools and Education [2015]).

Thus, interaction does not influence learning directly; the effect of interaction on learning is mediated by emotional support, instructional support, and classroom management. Again, one therefore should not overemphasize the role of language for learning. It is an indirect one, and there are other factors that influence learning, too.

Unfortunately, large-scale studies like the one by Hattie (2013) do not exist when it comes to the education of DHH students. Reviews that focused on the evidence base of practices in deaf education have led researchers to conclude that this evidence base is rather weak (Knoors & Marschark, 2014; Spencer & Marschark, 2010; see Chapter 18). Given the importance of classroom interactions for learning, it may come as a surprise that classroom interaction with DHH students has been the topic of relatively few studies, most of them dating from the 1980s or 1990s. Research that focuses on mediators of classroom interaction for learning of DHH students as conceptualized in the Teaching through Interaction model is relatively recent and not yet very comprehensive. Much more effort is put into the never-ending discussion of which language best serves communication and interaction, language development, and learning of DHH students, in the quest for the one-size-fits-all solution. Whether this is the best way to address the linguistic diversity of DHH children in the classroom is an issue addressed later in this chapter. First, let us explore what is known about classroom interaction with DHH students and what is known about mediators of interaction for learning in class.

CLASSROOM INTERACTION AND LEARNING OF DEAF AND HARD-OF-HEARING STUDENTS

What about the impact and implications of the Teaching through Interaction model for education of DHH students? What information do we have about classroom interaction and its influence on learning through provision of emotional and instructional support to DHH learners and effective classroom management in educating DHH students? Some research is available, but it allows only for a sketchy picture.

Classroom Interaction and Language Use

Studying interactions between teachers and DHH students is intimately connected with the work of David and Heather Wood in the United Kingdom, and Des Power in Australia. In teaching profoundly deaf students in settings emphasizing spoken language use, teachers of the deaf showed a teaching style characterized by much control, an overload of questions, and much communication repair because of frequent misunderstandings between them and their students (Wood et al., 1986). These orally educated, profoundly deaf students had hardly any auditory access to spoken language, because digital hearing aids and cochlear implants were not available at the time. The teaching style incorporating much interaction control was associated negatively with students' initiatives in classroom interaction.

In an earlier study, Wood and Wood (1984) were able to show that, through intervention, it was possible to make three teachers of the deaf in oral settings change their interactional teaching style to a less controlling one, resulting in an increase in students' initiatives and in mean length of conversational turns. Before the intervention started, the teachers interacted in the way they were taught in teacher training: "Our teachers, however, were merely asked to ask a lot of questions and the ensuing conversations were ones where misunderstandings abounded on both sides. Repair was a frequent outcome of these incidences and teachers tended to chase after answers to their questions at great length. Rarely did they relent to follow up on what their children offered them" (Wood & Wood, 1984, p. 57).

The study by Wood and Wood (1984) was replicated in Australia by Power et al. (1990), and involved teachers of the deaf who either used signed English (six teachers), cued speech (four teachers), or spoken English only (three teachers). Again, an association was found between the amount of teacher control over turns in classroom interaction and student contributions. More control was associated with fewer DHH student initiatives. Frequent misunderstandings between teachers and DHH students contributed significantly to this pattern. And again, if through intervention teachers' power over interaction was lessened (by increasing phatic remarks and personal contributions by the teachers), this resulted in an increase in students' contributions. There were no significant differences between teacher conversational styles or DHH students' contributions related to the mode of communication, either in the frequency of misunderstanding or in the frequency of repairs. If there were (nonsignificant) results to be found, they tended to be in favor of teachers and students who used manual support (signs or cues) in their spoken communication. To conclude, Wood (1991) wrapped up results of this classroom interaction research in the following remark: "I think it is possible to summarize in one phrase one of the main problems hearing people face in communicating with deaf children, whether that communication takes place in speech, sign supported English, or Signed English. The phrase is 'too much control'" (p. 249).

The main cause of this control problem is the difficulty that teachers and DHH students in these studies experienced in understanding each other, resulting in frequent misunderstandings and equally frequent repairs. So, what if classroom language becomes more accessible, because it is either visual by nature (a sign language) or because technology enhances auditory access through digital hearing aids or cochlear implants in combination with Frequency Modulation (FM) equipment?

What if sign language is used in the classroom? Will teachers exert less control if they use sign language and/or if they are deaf themselves? Will DHH students take more initiatives under these conditions? Will teachers and students understand each other better? The answer is that we do not know. Unfortunately, studies such as those carried out by Wood and Power have not been replicated in bilingual deaf education. We might speculate that using an accessible sign language will increase the chance of fluent, rich classroom interaction and reduce the frequency of misunderstandings (and thus the need for repairs), certainly if all those involved in this interaction are really proficient in sign language. Theoretically, we should observe this most prominently in classrooms with deaf teachers and DHH students raised in deaf families. Whether this also translates into practice, we do not know, because research is lacking. But, many DHH students are not fully proficient in sign language, not even after years of bilingual deaf education, especially if they are brought up in hearing families (Herman et al., 2009). So, teaching DHH students in sign language in bilingual schools for the deaf often might also come down to teaching linguistically diverse students. And the teachers may not be completely fluent in sign language themselves, not even when they are deaf, because many deaf teachers were born in hearing families just like their students, implying that their sign language proficiency might be limited to some extent because of relatively late input.

On the other hand, there is some small-scale qualitative research that suggests deaf teachers are better able to direct attention in visually oriented classroom interactions. To regulate turn-taking effectively in a class of signing DHH students, systematic application of both individual and group-wise eye gaze seems very helpful (Mather, 1987). Mather (1987) found that one deaf teacher outperformed a hearing teacher in this respect, but it remains unclear whether this was a result of hearing status, sign language proficiency, or individual conversation style. Another study showed how difficult it is for DHH students in visually oriented classroom interactions to sustain and to split visual attention effectively (Matthews & Reich, 1993). Classroom interactions among profoundly deaf students 13 to 15 years of age and their teachers were videotaped in two classes at a school for the deaf. The students and teachers used multimodal communication (signs and speech). An overall percentage of 44% of the signing of the teachers to all students was actually attended to by them, indicating they missed 56% of all their teachers' communication. If the signing of a teacher was targeted to an individual student, the percentage of utterances seen by the student involved ranged from 40% to 66%. The higher percentages were probably a result of more effective use of eye gaze by the teacher, in line with the study by Mather (1987). In these two classes, students signed more utterances than teachers, indicating that teacher control was not much of an issue. Unfortunately, much of the signing of students was missed by fellow students. Signing by peers was attended to in 30% of all instances; student-to-student signing was attended to by the target 48% of the time. Matthews and Reich (1993) concluded: "Stated simply, the data indicate that line-of-sight communication places a profound constraint on classroom communication. Even with well-trained teachers and relatively sophisticated students, the level of possible reception of transmitted messages is disappointingly low, somewhat below 50%" (p. 16). Mather (2009, as cited in Mather and Clark [2012]) designed a five-day course to improve didactic skills of teachers focusing on effective handling of the need for their DHH students to split their visual attention. According to Mather, "On the fifth day, the instructors were able to integrate their signing along with props more effectively" (p. 24), but unfortunately no data about course effectiveness were provided.

How about classroom interaction with DHH students who received cochlear implants early in their lives and, most of the time, were educated in mainstream settings? Again, research into classroom interaction in mainstream settings involving DHH students is lacking. Given the fact that, increasingly, these DHH students have relatively good access to spoken language because of early (often bilateral) cochlear implantation and use of digital hearing aids, one might expect that classroom interaction most often would be in spoken language only. The spoken language proficiency of these students has increased considerably (Boons et al., 2012), and speech perception is relatively good (Blamey et al., 2015). One thus might argue, on one hand, that DHH students have more chances than ever before in perceiving of and participating in speech-dominated classroom interaction. On the other hand, as De Raeve (2015) explained at length, classrooms and schools are very noisy environments, with much background noise and considerable reverberation of sound. So, even if speech perception in quiet is relatively intact, speech perception in the classroom may be difficult because of the tough listening conditions, resulting in the necessity to speech-read much more and to rely more on the context. Participation in group discussion remains difficult, because entering a group is more difficult than dyadic conversations, at least for young DHH children (Martin et al., 2010). Using FM systems certainly helps for instructional purposes, mainly for teacher-dominated interactions. The extent to which these DHH students may participate fruitfully in classroom interactions remains to be determined, as does the impact of missed conversations on academic achievement and well-being. Taking successful classroom interaction for granted in the case of DHH students with implants or digital hearing aids thus does not seem very wise. And the same goes for thinking that one and only one language and language modality will enhance classroom interaction with all DHH learners in all situations.

To summarize, there are simply too few studies carried out to draw any firm conclusions about whether classroom interaction with DHH students proceeds smoothly, and which communication modality and language supports this interaction best. And the studies that have been carried out are limited to special deaf education settings decades ago. If we can conclude anything at all, it is, first of all, the urgency to conduct much more studies in this domain. Second, we may assume that problems in classroom interaction will always arise more frequently with DHH students, no matter what language or modality is used in class. Or, to put it differently, each language or modality used in class will create its own challenges; the nature of these challenges depends not only on the language in use, but also on those who use it—teachers and students alike—and the situation in which language is used (see Chapter 18).

CLASSROOM INTERACTION WITH DHH STUDENTS: CLASSROOM MANAGEMENT, INSTRUCTIONAL, AND EMOTIONAL SUPPORT

As explained earlier, the influence of interaction, and thus of classroom talk, on learning is an indirect one. Teachers are thought to exert their influence on student learning through classroom interactions in which they provide emotional and instructional support and through which they manage classroom organization. How does this proceed in classrooms with DHH students? It is only recently that research started to shed some light on these factors of the Teaching through Interaction model with respect to DHH learners.

Classroom management influences student learning in the sense that effective management will lead to more opportunities for learning. The few studies that have been carried out on classroom management (summarized in Knoors and Marschark [2014], Chapter 11) all point to challenges in this respect when it comes to teaching DHH students, particularly with regard to pulling out students from class for therapy or other support services. This is likely to have negative consequences for student engagement and for the relatively limited time for important curriculum topics such as reading and mathematics. What we do know is that it is possible to influence aspects of classroom management in ways that will lead to improvements that subsequently influence learning positively (see, for example, Guardiano and Antia [2012]). What we do not know is whether the relatively few studies reflect educational practices that may be generalized more widely to deaf education.

Hermans et al. (2014) studied Dutch DHH and hearing students' perceptions about instructional support of their teachers. Their study included 145 DHH students from bilingual schools for the deaf and 355 hearing students, all between 8 years and 12 years of age. Hermans et al. (2014) concluded: "Focusing on the classroom as instruction environment, DHH students experienced less time for tasks, more classroom management but less support and less effective explanations by their teachers, and thus they rated achievement pressure higher than hearing students" (p. 286).

The quality of emotional support, and to some extent instructional support as well, is reflected in the quality of teacher–student relationships. Knoors and Marschark (2014, Chapter 11) summarized research in the domain of teacher–student relationships. The quality of teacher–student relationships turns out to be an important predictor of school adaptation in toddlers (Pianta & Steinberg, 1992) and of success in school in older students (Hamre & Pianta, 2001). Two dimensions of teacher behavior are considered to be particularly important for student–teacher relationships: influence (ranging from dominance to submission) and closeness (ranging from opposition to cooperation) (Wubbels & Brekelmans, 2005).

The impression students have of their relationships with their teachers is closely related to their academic and social achievements. High scores on the dimensions of closeness (helping, being friendly, being understanding) and influence (directive, authoritative, and tolerant) are associated with high student achievement. The association between a student's impression and achievement seems to be mediated by specific learning activities. For example, during group classroom instruction, students seem to value the leadership of teachers particularly. Nonverbal teacher behavior is very important in this respect: looking at the students while speaking with a loud and clear voice adds to a positive image of the teacher by the students (Wubbels & Brekelmans, 2005). Regardless of ethnic background, better contact and more closeness between students and teachers influence student motivation positively. But, positive relationships with teachers prove to be even more important for students from ethic minority backgrounds (den Brok et al., 2010).

Student–teacher relationships are particularly important for the well-being of students with disabilities. Many of these students in special education run an elevated risk of mental health problems (Murray & Paint, 2007) (for DHH students see, for example, Hindley [2005] and Van Gent et al., 2007). Positive student–relationships may be seen as a protective factor in the context of such problems. Unfortunately, students with disabilities often are less satisfied about the quality of their relationships with teachers compared with peers without disabilities (Eisenhower et al., 2007; Lapointe et al., 2005; Murray & Greenberg, 2001).

In the Netherlands, teacher–DHH student relationships have been studied in special schools and in mainstream education. Wolters et al. (2012) used the Dutch School Questionnaire to study teacher–student relationships cross-sectionally in 759 grade 6 (672 hearing, 87 DHH) and 840 grade 7 (736 hearing, 104 DHH) students. Thirty-five of the 87 DHH students in grade 6 were in special education settings; in grade 7, 42 of the 104 students were educated in schools for the deaf. DHH and hearing students in mainstream settings valued teacher support more than the students in special (bilingual deaf) education.

Hermans et al. (2014) studied not only instructional support (discussed earlier), but also teacher–student relationships in 145 DHH and 355 hearing students in primary education. All DHH students were enrolled in bilingual schools for the deaf; they reported their relationships with hearing teachers of the deaf. Again, the DHH students in bilingual schools for the deaf were significantly less satisfied about the relationship with their teachers than their hearing peers in mainstream education. According to Hermans et al. (2014): "It is tempting to conclude that this is all about mismatches in hearing status and lack of sensitivity and responsiveness due to communication difficulties, the implication being that results would be more positive in the case of teachers of the deaf. However, alternative interpretations should not be overlooked" (p. 286).

The assumption that it is the quality of interpersonal communication that affects the quality of DHH student's relationships with their teachers, at first, seems not implausible. According to Korthagen et al. (2014), contact is fundamental to teacher–student relationships. These researchers explored the meaning of contact in two small-scale studies, using data from teacher interviews and from classroom observations involving hearing students and their teachers. Contact is certainly related to communication, because contact between students and teachers results in part from communication skills that are used to develop and maintain friendships. Use of these skills by teachers was related to motivation and learning in students (Frymier & Houser, 2000). But there is more to contact than communication only. Korthagen et al. (2014) concluded that "contact seems a two-way interactive process in which all three dimensions of thinking, feeling, and wanting, as well as doing (behavior) are important" (p. 30). Personal aspects such as empathy, ideals, and values thus are important too. Contact occurs in moments; good contact during momentary encounters reinforces more fruitful contacts—a kind of resonance in interaction is triggered. Experiencing good contact contributes to the perception and validation of the relationship between teacher and students. The relationship between teachers and students thus may be seen as "the accumulation of their momentary contact experiences" (Korthagen et al., 2014, p. 30).

That qualitatively good teacher–student relationships are determined by factors other than just good communication may be illustrated by the results from a recent study by Knoors and Hermans (manuscript in preparation). Teacher–student relationships were studied in relation to the quality of classroom communication as measured by the Classroom Participation Questionnaire (Antia et al., 2007). Forty DHH students took part, 27 girls and 13 boys, all placed in schools for the deaf in the Netherlands. They varied in age between 10 years and 18 years. These students were taught by deaf and by hearing teachers. Seven deaf teachers participated in the study; they selected to participate with them seven hearing teachers who could communicate equally well with the students as they themselves (as deaf teachers) could. In this way, the question of whether teacher–student relationships are more influenced by a match or mismatch in hearing status or by the quality of communication was explored. In the latter case, there should be no difference in teacher–student relationship quality because the deaf teachers judged the communication skills of their hearing colleagues as equally good as their own. The results, however, showed that the deaf teachers judged the quality of their relations with their DHH students greater than the hearing teachers. Similarly, the DHH students judged the quality of their relationships with their deaf teachers greater than with their hearing teachers. There were no differences in their judgments of the communication skills of their deaf and hearing teachers, thus validating the selection deaf teachers made in selecting communicatively equally skilled hearing colleagues. These results seem to point to the contribution of sharing a hearing status (sameness) to the quality of teacher–student relationships, just as (at least in hearing students) sharing ethnic status or gender contributes to these relationships. Interestingly, hearing teachers valued the quality of communication skills of their DHH students higher than deaf teachers. Either one group of teachers was better in making judgments than the other group or the hearing teachers overestimated the communication skills of their students. Finally, a strong correlation was found between judgments of the quality of communication and the quality of relationships in pairs of deaf teachers and DHH students, but no (teachers) or only a modest (students) correlation in pairs of hearing teachers and DHH students.

In summary, there are indications that teachers' relationships with DHH students are less valued, reciprocally, than would be desirable, at least if hearing teachers are concerned. This may influence student motivation and subsequent learning negatively. Although it cannot be excluded that problems in access to classroom and teacher talk contribute to these less than optimal relationships, it seems that this is only one factor, and may be not even the most important one. In other words, learning as a result of effective classroom interactions may be mediated in DHH students by emotional support, as reflected in their relationships with their teachers, but these relationships are not completely dependent on sharing a language in class. So, again, language use in classroom interactions to provide emotional support is important, but should not be overemphasized.

ACCOMMODATING THE NEEDS OF DIVERSE DEAF AND HARD-OF-HEARING LEARNERS

Knowing that, on the one hand, classroom interaction and thus language use in these interactions is important for learning, but on the other hand that it influences learning rather indirectly, how do we handle the apparent communicative and linguistic diversity among DHH students generally in class and in classroom interactions? Which language and communication modality should we choose? This question has been debated healthily ever since formal education of deaf students started. Trying to answer this question outside the specific context in which the language is used and apart from the purpose for which language is used has been proved unfruitful, not only for teaching deaf learners, but also for teaching culturally and linguistically hearing diverse students. As Calderón et al. (2011) stated in their analysis of effective teaching of linguistically diverse students who were, in their words, "English learners": "Among researchers, the debate between advocates of bilingual and English-only reading instruction has been fierce, and ideology has often trumped evidence on both sides of the debate. Based on the findings from recent studies ... what matters most in educating English learners is the quality of instruction" (p. 107). In various publications, Knoors and Marschark have emphasized the same line of thinking if we want to be able to teach all DHH students more effectively than before (e.g., Knoors & Marschark, 2012, 2014). If we discuss the language and modality we use in teaching DHH students, we have to take the context (the classroom) and the actual purpose (learning) into account. In which context will which language and modality result in the most optimal learning of DHH students? This is the essential question teachers have to ask themselves. And then it becomes obvious that there is not one answer to that question, because characteristics of contexts vary and DHH students are so diverse.

As illustrated earlier, each language and modality creates its own specific challenges in classroom interaction involving DHH students. This extends to contexts in which interaction is unidirectional, from teacher to students, serving the purpose of instruction. Several studies have looked into the relation between language use in teacher instruction and learning gain in DHH students (see Chapter 18). Since the scientific recognition of sign languages as full-fledged languages and the subsequent advent of bilingual deaf education, the assumption of many advocates of this type of education has been that DHH students learn the most if classroom instruction proceeds in sign language. This seems not odd at all, given the accessibility of a sign language for DHH students. But, contrary to this assumption, the advantage of sign language over written language (captioning) or simultaneous communication for classroom learning by groups of students has not been demonstrated.

Several experiments have shown that from middle school through college, students learn as much from instruction in sign language as from captioning (see, for example, Borgna et al., 2011; Marschark, et al., 2006, 2009; Stinson et al., 2009). It also has been demonstrated that students may learn as much from instruction provided directly by teachers fluent in sign language as from spoken language instruction mediated by very skilled sign language interpreters (Marschark et al., 2008). This result was also found in experiments involving DHH students in secondary education (Marschark et al., 2006).

Other experiments with DHH college students in the United States have failed to provide evidence for an advantage of sign language over simultaneous communication or vice versa for learning from instruction (Marschark et al., 2004, 2008). In a meta-analysis of 10 experiments involving DHH students in mainstream classrooms in secondary education, Convertino et al. (2009) found that only receptive skills in simultaneous communication (and not signed or spoken language proficiency) predicted learning gain, even if simultaneous communication was not used as a medium of instruction in the experiments. Probably, these receptive skills are a proxy for language flexibility. The researchers concluded: "At least by the time they get to college, neither sign language nor spoken language skills are definitive predictors of academic performance for DHH students, performance that is, on average, consistently below the level of their hearing peers" (Convertino et al., 2009; p. 335).

In a recent study, Blom and Marschark (2015) compared learning from instruction in either spoken English or sign-supported English in 40 DHH college students using cochlear implants. Learning gain was larger if sign-supported English was used, but only in situations when the instructional material was difficult, and thus cognitively more challenging. It might be that in those situations, combining speech with signs adds to redundancy in instruction, preventing cognitive overload from happening in students. Further research is needed to explore whether this hypothesis holds for younger DHH students with implants and in which learning contexts.

A study comparing learning gain in Sign Language of the Netherlands and sign-supported Dutch in 26 DHH students in primary deaf education (Hermans et al., 2014) showed that these students learned as much from sign-supported Dutch as from Sign Language of the Netherlands. Remarkably, the students learned as much in the preferred as in the nonpreferred mode of communication (as indicated by their teachers or by institutional files), a finding also obtained with college-age students (Marschark et al., 2005).

How should we interpret these findings? There is, so far, no evidence to support the preference for one communication modality and one language as a vehicle in instruction focusing on accomplishing learning gain in all DHH students. However, the fact that this could not be demonstrated for groups of DHH students as a whole does not mean that for individual DHH students a specific modality or language choice might not be needed to enhance learning; the direction of this choice may vary among students and, possibly, contexts. Because the directions of individual choices differ, for the group as a whole often no effect of one language or modality over another is found. Thus, all seems to point to the need of handling communicative and linguistic diversity in a different way, promoting flexibility in communication and language choice by, in this case, classroom teachers (Knoors & Marschark, 2012) and thus differentiating in language choice for learning.

DIFFERENTIATION AND LANGUAGE USE

Promoting flexibility in language use in the classroom to encourage rich and effective classroom interaction implies differentiation in classroom teaching depending on the teaching situation, the number and the characteristics of DHH and hearing students, and thus also the educational setting. In other words, differentiation of language use in the classroom is situated in a specific context. Thus, it makes sense that we must take the goal of language use in interaction into account: learning. So, if learning progress requires it, teachers really need to provide differentiated instructions for their students. And if language use causes limited progress in learning, only then should differentiation in language use be contemplated—or, in other words, differentiation in teaching because of diversity of DHH students focuses on accommodating variation in learning progress among DHH students. This differential teaching make take many forms—for example, more time on task, adapted instruction, adapted content. Differential teaching through adaptation of language use is but one form, and is required only if the modality or language in the classroom causes less than sufficient learning for one or more DHH students.

How might differentiation of language use in the classroom be constituted effectively in these cases? What forms may it take? Because not much is known from research involving DHH students, we should build on studies teaching linguistically or cognitively diverse hearing students. Using a multitier approach in interaction and instruction has been supported empirically in studies among linguistically diverse learners (Success for All; see Calderón et al. [2011]) and in studies focusing on teaching reading skills effectively to students with and without special educational needs in one classroom (Response to Intervention; see, for example, Fletcher and Vaughn [2009] and Fuchs and Fuchs [2006]). Multitier approaches start with whole-class instruction (first tier), followed by (temporarily) small-group interventions for those whose learning progresses less than envisaged (second tier), then by intensive, often individual instruction (third tier; see, for example, Solis et al., 2014) for those students who have failed to progress enough in the small-group interventions. Intensive monitoring of learning progress is a crucial element in all multitier approaches. The precise structuring of the respective tiers allows for some flexibility, depending on the student's needs and the educational context, but this approach has admittedly been carried out most often in regular school settings, because multitier approaches have been developed to tackle diversity in mainstream education. However, a multitier approach seems just as feasible for special education, certainly for teaching DHH students, because the variation in strengths and weaknesses among these students is considerable in schools for the deaf.

What would the first tier in a multitier approach look like in regular school classrooms that contain one or more DHH students? What language would we want to use for learning in such an inclusive classroom, given that most students are hearing? What language and mode of communication might act as a sort of lingua franca through which all students would be able to participate in classroom discourse and learning? To promote whole-group learning, in this case a spoken language for interaction and for direct instruction would seem to fit best. Access to interaction and instruction for the DHH students included could be optimized by FM systems, by using text interpretation or sign support, and by incorporating sign language interpretation. Note that none of these measures changes the language used for whole-class interaction and instruction. Only if monitoring shows insufficient progress in learning a specific topic (such as vocabulary learning, reading, mathematics) by specific students, would differentiation in second or third tiers for these students take place. In what ways could instruction in these second and third tiers be adapted to enhance learning and accomplish reentering of the students in whole-class interaction and instruction? Only part of the answer to this question lies in adapting the language for interaction and instruction (for example, using a sign language in direct instruction), because language influences learning only indirectly, and others factors are important to consider in differentiation too. Or, to state it differently, differentiation in second or third tiers may include various measures, ranging from including more time for practice, using a special instruction method, applying specific didactics, to adapting the language of instruction.

The same line of reasoning applies to teaching a classroom of DHH students in a school for the deaf. The first question to be answered for whole-class instruction (the first tier) is which language would serve learning of a specific topic best for the entire DHH group? In the Netherlands, in many classes with DHH students this would probably mean using sign-supported Dutch as the best communicative compromise, given the considerable differences in proficiency in Sign Language of the Netherlands and in spoken Dutch, but of course these latter languages should be possible too, if that would lead to optimal learning of the whole group given a particular subject. Whichever approach teachers choose, monitoring often will show that some DHH students' progress is insufficient, and these DHH students need to be instructed, preferably temporarily, in small groups (second tier) or individually (third tier). Adapting the language of instruction in these situations is one of the possible ways to differentiate and to enhance learning, just as in mainstream education, if analysis shows the language used in whole-group teaching is the (or at least a) cause of lack of progress in learning.

Multitier approaches to classroom interaction and classroom learning involving DHH students will only succeed if progress is monitored carefully. Thus, handling linguistic diversity in the classroom includes thorough assessment of linguistic, cognitive, and social strengths and weaknesses of DHH learners compared with other DHH and/or hearing peers in class (Herman, 2015; Knoors & Marschark, 2014; Leigh & Crowe, 2015). To relate assessments to decisions regarding classroom interaction, specific attention should be paid to assessment of pragmatic functions and social skills (see Chapter 9).

Handling linguistic diversity of DHH learners through differentiation is not only facilitated by a multitier approach. The effects of applying a multitier approach may be enhanced even more if it is combined with adequately grouping students and proper timing of strategies for differentiation.

Student Grouping

Student grouping is one of the most studied ways of differentiation in teaching students with different abilities. There are various ways to group students. One may either opt for homogeneous ability grouping or for heterogeneous grouping of students in classrooms. If one chooses to group students with heterogeneous abilities in one class, teachers may either adapt their instruction, the learning content, and/or the time for mastery. Teachers may strive for convergence in achievement, focusing on a minimum level that all students have to attain, subsequently helping low-achieving students to progress more. Alternatively, a divergent strategy may be used, helping all students to reach their own maximum potential (Bosker, 2005). In reality, most teachers use a combination of convergent and divergent strategies.

Between 1982 and 1996, several meta-analyses were conducted of the effects of various forms of student grouping on achievement, with contradictory results. One recent meta-analysis, focusing on the effects of student grouping in preschool, primary, and secondary education was carried out by Deunk et al. (2015). Their meta-analysis clearly showed that it is hard to reach any general conclusions if ability grouping is not studied in the context of the specific teaching strategies teachers use in adapting their instruction to diverse learners. This is in line with a conclusion from one of the earlier meta-analyses, the results of which were not replicated this time: "It appears that the positive effects of within-class grouping are maximized when the physical placement of students into groups for learning is accompanied by modifications to teaching methods and instructional materials. Merely placing students together is not sufficient for promoting substantive gains in achievement" (Lou et al., 1996, p. 448). According to Deunk et al. (2015), the real question is

> "how teachers take into account differences between students in daily classroom practice and how they can be supported in doing so. Sensible ability grouping (both homogeneous and heterogeneous) and sensible application of other differentiation practices, like adaptive questioning during whole class activities, assume two things: teachers need to have an accurate view of students' level of understanding and teachers need to know which instruction and learning activity is appropriate for children at different levels, given the goals they strive for. (p. 52)

Timing of Differentiation: Reactive or Proactive?

Teacher expectations color their perceptions of differences among students. Of course, these perceptions of differences are also based on student characteristics (learning potential, gender, ethnicity, language proficiency). Teacher perceptions of student differences form the foundation for differentiated teaching. The goal of differentiated teaching is to match individual proficiencies and motives of students on the one hand and educational demands on the other. If teachers adapt their teaching to match individual differences among students, this will enhance student achievement (Lou et al., 1996; Reis et al., 2011).

The timing of didactic adaptations as a consequence of student differences may be proactive or reactive (Tomlinson et al., 2003). Proactive differentiation takes place during the preparation of lessons. In the design of lessons, of a course, or of the curriculum (for the latter, see de Klerk et al. [2015]), the teacher takes individual student differences into account. Proactive differentiation is a conscious activity. Reactive differentiation occurs when a teacher adapts his teaching during the actual course of it (McKown & Weinstein, 2008). Reactive differentiation may lead to adaptations in the pedagogical climate, the type of feedback, the quality and quantity of instruction, and in interaction style. Reactive differentiation may happen both consciously and unconsciously. According to Tomlinson et al. (2003), proactive differentiation is much more effective than reactive differentiation in addressing differences among students.

Earlier studies with hearing students have shown that most didactic adaptations are rather reactive and improvised (Hootstein, 1998; McIntosh et al., 1994; Tomlinson, 1999). Although teachers state that proactive differentiation is desirable, many of them think it is not feasible in actual practice (Berndsen, 2012; Schumm & Vaughn, 1991). Hermans et al. (2013) studied expectations of teachers in terms of their perceptions about differences and similarities among the students they teach and the way they address student differences in their teaching. The study involved 11 teachers of DHH children and children with specific language impairment (SLI) in a special school in the Netherlands. Nine teachers were classroom teachers, one was a sign language teacher, and one, a teacher of gymnastics. Six teachers (the sign language teacher and five classroom teachers) taught DHH students in primary special education, the remaining five teachers taught children with SLI. All teachers were asked to make mental class maps (MCMs), which were used in interviews. An MCM is a graphical representation of teacher perceptions of differences and similarities among students. Teachers group photographs of their students. If photographs are placed distant from each other in space, the differences among the students involved are perceived as rather large. If photographs are grouped close to each other, the students seem, according to the teacher, more alike. Each MCM addressed a specific aspect of the functioning of students.

Teachers in this special school indicated relevant differences between their students on a similar number of domains as teachers of hearing students in mainstream education. However, the number of differences as a proportion of the number of students in a classroom was considerably greater in the special school. This may indicate that the diversity of students in a special school for DHH students and students with SLI is larger than in mainstream education. A smaller class size in special education therefore does not imply that teachers need to differentiate less. The perceptions of differences among DHH students by teachers result from their observations and, to a lesser extent, from results of assessments as well, as noted in students' files. Asked about the way they accommodate diversity among DHH learners or SLI learners, the teachers in this study stated most frequently that they use a combination of proactive and reactive differentiation, followed in frequency by reactive differentiation alone. Exclusively proactive differentiation took place much less frequently. Almost 92% of all examples of reactive differentiation were indeed visible in the classroom during classroom observations by the researchers, validating the responses in teacher interviews.

All teachers seemed to make conscious choices in differentiation. At the same time, the interviews provided evidence of the inability of teachers always to match individual profiles of their DHH or SLI students. Relatively often, didactic adaptations were made for the whole class, whereas only one or two students really needed them. In quite a number of cases, teachers said that one should adapt the level of instruction to the weakest students in class. The study by Hermans et al. (2013) did not show evidence for general lower expectations of DHH students and students with SLI by their teachers. Adapting instruction to the weakest students in class thus seemed not so much caused by a general negative bias in teacher expectations, but the effect may nevertheless be the same: underachievement of more competent students because of relatively limited exposure to complex information.

Of course, this small-scale study needs to be replicated; more schools, teachers, and students should be included. Still, the picture this study provided does not seem gloomy. Teachers do recognize individual differences among DHH students or among students with SLI—differences that may be relevant for learning. Teachers subsequently do differentiate their teaching. However, the timing of differentiation could be improved; the frequency of proactive differentiation should be increased. At the same time, the frequency of collective classroom adaptations needs to be limited, because this may result in understimulation of more competent DHH students and students with SLI in class. Using a multitier approach would be one way to reduce whole-group adaptations in favor of adaptation for only those who need them, carried out either in small groups or individually.

CONCLUSION

One of the most important functions of language in the classroom is acting as a vehicle in classroom interaction. Classroom interaction is one of the most important processes through which teachers exert their influence on learning. And learning is what students are in classrooms for in the first place.

DHH students are linguistically diverse learners. Accommodating their needs in the classroom is, in essence, accommodating their needs with respect to learning. In this context, accommodating needs takes place trough differential teaching. Differential teaching may imply adapting the language used in classroom interaction, but only if language is the fact that causes variation in learning progress. Applying a multitier approach to accommodating the needs of diverse DHH students seems most effective, in combination with adequate student grouping and proper timing of differentiation.

In short, given the linguistic diversity of DHH students as a key characteristic from the very start of their educations, a narrow focus on language use in the classroom of DHH students should be avoided. The quest for identification of the sole language that will tackle all challenges in teaching and learning of DHH students is a waste of energy, because one size fits none. The ecological nature of learning in combination with the variation in DHH student's strengths and weaknesses in the linguistic, cognitive, and social domains require teachers and researchers to focus on comprehensive modeling and to take into account multiple factors that may optimize language-mediated classroom interactions situated in various classroom contexts and educational settings to enhance learning of all DHH students.

REFERENCES

Alexander, P. A., Schallert, D. L., & Reynolds, R. E. (2009). What is learning anyway? A topographical perspective considered. *Educational Psychologist, 44*(3), 176–192.

American Psychological Association, Coalition for Psychology in Schools and Education (2015). Top 20 principles from psychology for preK–12 teaching and learning. http://www.apa.org/ed/schools/cpse/top-twenty-principles.pdf.

Antia, S. D., Sabers, D. L., & Stinson, M. S. (2007). Validity and reliability of the Classroom Participation Questionnaire with deaf and hard of hearing students in public schools. *Journal of Deaf Studies and Deaf Education, 12*(2), 158–171.

Archbold, S. (2015). Being a deaf student: Changes in characteristics and needs. In H. Knoors & M. Marschark (Eds.), *Educating deaf learners: Creating a global evidence base* (pp. 23–46). New York: Oxford University Press.

Berndsen, M. (2012). Percepties van VO docenten van verschillen tussen leerlingen in hun klas. Master's thesis, Radboud Universiteit Nijmegen.

Blamey, P. J., Maat, B., Başkent, D., Mawman, D., Burke, E., Dillier, N., Beynon, N., Kleine-Punte, A., Govaerts, P. J., Skarzynski, P. H., Huber, A. M., Sterkers-Artières, F., van de Heyning, P., O'Leary, S., Fraysse, B., Green, K., Sterkers, O., Venail, F., Skarzynski, H., Vincent, C., Truy, E., Dowell, R., Bergeron, F., & Lazard, D. S. (2015). A retrospective multicenter study comparing speech perception outcomes for bilateral implantation and bimodal rehabilitation. *Ear & Hearing, 36*(4), 408–416.

Blank, M. (1974). Cognitive functions of language in the preschool years. *Developmental Psychology, 10*(2), 229–245.

Blom, H., & Marschark, M. (2015). Simultaneous communication and cochlear implants in the classroom? *Deafness and Education International, 17*, 123–131.

Boons, T., Brokx, J. P., Frijns, J. H., Peeraer, L., Philips, B., Vermeulen, A., Wouters, J., & van Wieringen, A. (2012). Effect of pediatric bilateral cochlear implantation on language development. *Archives of Pediatrics & Adolescent Medicine, 166*(1), 28–34.

Borgna G., Convertino, C., Marschark, M., Morrison, C., & Rizzolo, K. (2011). Enhancing deaf students' learning from sign language and text: Metacognition, modality, and the effectiveness of content scaffolding. *Journal of Deaf Studies and Deaf Education, 16*, 79–100.

Bosker, R. J. (2005). *De grenzen van gedifferentieerd onderwijs* [The limits of differentiated education]. Groningen: Rijksuniversiteit Groningen [inaugural address].

Bronfenbrenner, U. (1979). *The ecology of human development.* Cambridge, MA: Harvard University Press.

Calderón, M., Slavin, R., & Sánchez, M. (2011). Effective instruction for English learners. *The Future of Children, 21*(1), 103–127.

Cazden, C. B. (2001). *The language of learning and teaching* (2nd ed.). Portsmouth, NH: Heinemann.

Convertino, C. M., Marschark, M., Sapere, P., Sarchet, T., & Zupan, M. (2009). Predicting academic success among deaf college students. *Journal of Deaf Studies and Deaf Education, 14*(3), 24–343.

de Klerk, A., Fortgens, C., & Van der Eijk, A. (2015). Curriculum design in Dutch deaf education. In H. Knoors & M. Marschark (Eds.), *Educating deaf learners: Creating a global evidence base* (pp. 573–594). New York: Oxford University Press.

den Brok, P., Tartwijk, J., Wubbels, T., & Veldman, I. (2010). The differential effect of the teacher–student interpersonal relationship on student outcomes for students with different ethnic backgrounds. *British Journal of Educational Psychology, 80*(2), 199–221.

De Raeve, L. (2015). Classroom adaptations for effective learning by deaf students. In H. Knoors & M. Marschark (Eds.), *Educating deaf learners: Creating a global evidence base* (pp. 547–572). New York: Oxford University Press.

Deunk, M., Doolaard, S., Smale-Jacobse, A., & Bosker, R. (2015). *Differentiation within and across classrooms: A systematic review of studies into the cognitive effects of differentiation practices.* Groningen: Rijksuniversiteit Groningen, GION onderwijs/onderzoek.

Eisenhower, A. S., Baker, B. L., & Blacher, J. (2007). Early student–teacher relationships of children with and without intellectual disability: Contributions of behavioral, social, and self-regulatory competence. *Journal of School Psychology, 45*(4), 363–383.

Ellis, R. (2000). Task-based research and language pedagogy. *Language Teaching Research, 4*(3), 193–220.

Fisher, D., Frey, N., & Rothenberg, C. (2008). *Content-area conversations: How to plan discussion-based lessons for diverse language learners.* Alexandria, VA: ASCD.

Fletcher, J. M., & Vaughn, S. (2009). Response to intervention: Preventing and remediating academic difficulties. *Child Development Perspectives, 3*(1), 30–37.

Frymier, A. B., & Houser, M. L. (2000). The teacher–student relationship as an interpersonal relationship. *Communication Education, 49*(3), 207–219.

Fuchs, D., & Fuchs, L. S. (2006). Introduction to response to intervention: What, why, and how valid is it? *Reading Research Quarterly, 41*(1), 93–99.

Guardino, C., & Antia, S. D. (2012). Modifying the classroom environment to increase engagement and decrease disruption with students who are deaf or hard of hearing. *Journal of Deaf Studies and Deaf Education, 17*(4), 518–533.

Hamre, B. K., & Pianta, R. C. (2001). Early teacher–child relationships and the trajectory of children's school outcomes through eighth grade. *Child Development*, 72(2), 625–638.

Hamre, B. H., Pianta, R. C., Downer, T., DeCoster, J., Mashburn, A. J., Jones, S. M., Brown, J. L., Cappella, E., Atkins, M., Rivers, S. E., Brackett, M. A., & Hamagami, A. (2013). Teaching through interactions: Testing a developmental framework of teacher effectiveness in over 4,000 classrooms. *The Elementary School Journal*, 113(4), 461–487.

Hanushek, E. A. (2004). Some simple analytics of school quality. NBR working paper 10229. National Bureau of Economic Research. http://www.nber.org/papers/w10229.

Hattie, J. (2013). *Visible learning: A synthesis of over 800 meta-analyses relating to achievement*. London: Routledge.

Herman, R. (2015). Language assessment of deaf learners. In H. Knoors & M. Marschark (Eds.), *Educating deaf learners: Creating a global evidence base* (pp. 197–212). New York: Oxford University Press.

Hermans, D., Knoors, H., & Verhoeven, L. (2009). Assessment of sign language development: The case of deaf children in the Netherlands. *Journal of Deaf Studies and Deaf Education*, 15(2), 107–119.

Hermans, D., Wauters, L., & de Klerk, A. (2013). *Het verwachtingspatroon van de leerkracht: Halen we eruit wat erin zit?* Sint-Michielsgestel: Kentalis Expertise & Innovatie.

Hermans, D., Wauters, L., de Klerk, A., & Knoors, H. (2014). Quality of instruction in bilingual schools for deaf children. In M. Marschark, G. Tang, & H. Knoors (Eds.), *Bilingualism and bilingual deaf education* (pp. 272–291). New York: Oxford University Press.

Hindley, P. A. (2005). Mental health problems in deaf children. *Current Paediatrics*, 15(2), 114–119.

Hootstein, E. (1998). *Differentiation of instructional methodologies in subject-based curricula at the secondary level*. Research brief no. 38. Richmond, VA: Metropolitan Educational Research Consortium.

Kane, T. J., & Staiger, D. O. (2012). Gathering feedback for teaching: Combining high-quality observations with student surveys and achievement gains. Research paper. MET Project. Bill & Melinda Gates Foundation.

Knoors, H. (2015). Foundations for language development in deaf children and the consequences for communication choices. In M. Marschark & P. E. Spencer (Eds.), *Oxford handbook of deaf studies in language* (pp. 19–31). New York: Oxford University Press.

Knoors, H., & Hermans, D. (2010). Effective instruction for deaf and hard-of-hearing students: Teaching strategies, school settings, and student characteristics. In M. Marschark & P. Spencer (Eds.), *The Oxford handbook of deaf studies, language, and education* (Vol. 2, pp. 57–71). New York: Oxford University Press.

Knoors, H., & Marschark, M. (2012). Language planning for the 21st century: Revisiting bilingual language policy for deaf children. *Journal of Deaf Studies and Deaf Education*, 17(3), 291–305.

Knoors, H., & Marschark, M. (2014). *Teaching deaf learners: Psychological and developmental foundations*. New York: Oxford University Press.

Knoors, H., & Marschark, M. (2015). Educating deaf students in a global context. In H. Knoors & M. Marschark (Eds.), *Educating deaf learners: Creating a global evidence base* (pp. 1–22). New York: Oxford University Press.

Korthagen, F. A., Attema-Noordewier, S., & Zwart, R. C. (2014). Teacher–student contact: Exploring a basic but complicated concept. *Teaching and Teacher Education, 40,* 22–32.

Kumpulainen, K., & Mutanen, M. (1999). The situated dynamics of peer group interaction: An introduction to an analytic framework. *Learning and Instruction, 9*(5), 449–473.

Lapointe, J. M., Legault, F., & Batiste, S. J. (2005). Teacher interpersonal behavior and adolescents' motivation in mathematics: A comparison of learning disabled, average, and talented students. *International Journal of Educational Research, 43*(1), 39–54.

Lederberg, A. R., Schick, B., & Spencer, P. E. (2013). Language and literacy development of deaf and hard-of-hearing children: Successes and challenges. *Developmental Psychology, 49*(1), 15–30.

Leigh, G., & Crowe, K. (2015). Responding to cultural and linguistic diversity among deaf and hard-of-hearing learners. In H. Knoors & M. Marschark (Eds.), *Educating deaf learners: Creating a global evidence base* (pp. 69–92). New York: Oxford University Press.

Lou, Y., Abrami, P. C., Spence, J. C., Poulsen, C., Chambers, B., & d'Appolonia, S. (1996). Within-class grouping: A meta-analysis. *Review of Educational Research, 66*(4), 423–458.

Marschark, M., Leigh, G., Sapere, P., Burnham, D., Convertino, C., Stinson, M., Knoors, H., Vervloed, M. P. J., & Noble, W. (2006). Benefits of sign language interpreting and text alternatives for deaf students' classroom learning. *Journal of Deaf Studies and Deaf Education, 11*(4), 421–437.

Marschark, M., Sapere, P., Convertino, C., & Pelz, J. (2008). Learning via direct and mediated instruction by deaf students. *Journal of Deaf Studies and Deaf Education, 13*(4), 546–561.

Marschark, M., Sapere, P., Convertino, C. M., Mayer, C., Wauters, L., & Sarchet, T. (2009). Are deaf students' reading challenges really about reading? *American Annals of the Deaf, 154*(4), 357–370.

Marschark, M., Sapere, P., Convertino, C., & Seewagen, R. (2005). Access to postsecondary education through sign language interpreting. *Journal of Deaf Studies and Deaf Education, 10*(1), 38–50.

Marschark, M., Sapere, P., Convertino, C., Seewagen, R., & Maltzen, H. (2004). Comprehension of sign language interpreting: Deciphering a complex task situation. *Sign Language Studies, 4*(4), 345–368.

Marschark, M., Tang, G., & Knoors, H. (Eds.) (2014). *Bilingualism and bilingual deaf education.* New York: Oxford University Press.

Marschark, M., & Wauters, L. (2008). Language comprehension and learning by deaf students. In M. Marschark & P. Hauser (Eds.), *Deaf cognition: Foundations and outcomes* (pp. 309–350). New York: Oxford University Press.

Martin, D., Bat-Chava, Y., Lalwani, A., & Waltzman, S. B. (2010). Peer relationships of deaf children with cochlear implants: Predictors of peer entry and peer interaction success. *Journal of Deaf Studies and Deaf Education, 16*(1), 108–120.

Marzano, R. J. (2003). *What works in schools: Translating research into action.* Alexandria, VA: ASCD.

Mather, S. A. (1987). Eye gaze & communication in a deaf classroom. *Sign Language Studies, 54*(1), 11–30.
Mather, S., & Clark, M. D. (2012). An issue of learning the effect of visual split attention in classes for deaf and hard of hearing students. *Odyssey, 13,* 20–24.
Matthews, T. J., & Reich, C. F. (1993). Constraints on communication in classrooms for the deaf. *American Annals of the Deaf, 138*(1), 14–18.
McIntosh, R., Vaughn, S., Schumm, J., Haager, D., & Lee, O. (1994). Observations of students with learning disabilities in general education classrooms. *Exceptional Children, 60,* 249–261.
McKown, C., & Weinstein, R. S. (2008). Teacher expectations, classroom context, and the achievement gap. *Journal of School Psychology, 46,* 235–261.
Moeller, M. P., Carr, G., Seaver, L., Stredler-Brown, A., & Holzinger, D. (2013). Best practices in family-centered early intervention for children who are deaf or hard of hearing: An international consensus statement. *Journal of Deaf Studies and Deaf Education, 18*(4), 429–445.
Murray, C., & Greenberg, M. T. (2001). Relationships with teachers and bonds with school: Social emotional adjustment correlates for children with and without disabilities. *Psychology in the Schools, 38*(1), 25–41.
Murray, C., & Pianta, R. C. (2007). The importance of teacher-student relationships for adolescents with high incidence disabilities. *Theory Into Practice, 46*(2), 105–112.
Pianta, R. C., & Steinberg, M. (1992). Teacher–child relationships and the process of adjusting to school. In R. C. Pianta (Ed.), *Beyond the Parent: The role of other adults in children's lives: New directions for child development* (pp. 61–80). San Francisco, CA: Jossey-Bass.
Power, D. J., Wood, D. J., & Wood, H. A. (1990). Conversational strategies of teachers using three methods of communication with deaf children. *American Annals of the Deaf, 135*(1), 9–13.
Reis, S. M., McCoach, D. B., Little, C. A., Muller, L. M., & Kaniskan, R. B. (2011). The effects of differentiated instruction and enrichment pedagogy on reading achievement in five elementary schools. *American Educational Research Journal, 48*(2), 462–501.
Robertson, B., Elliot, L., & Robinson, D. (2007). Cognitive tools. In M. Orey (Ed.), *Emerging perspectives on learning, teaching, and technology.* https://www.textbookequity.org.
Schumm, J. S., & Vaughn, S. (1991). Making adaptations for mainstreamed students general classroom teachers' perspectives. *Remedial and Special Education, 12*(4), 18–27.
Solis, M., Miciak, J., Vaughn, S., & Fletcher, J. M. (2014). Why intensive interventions matter longitudinal studies of adolescents with reading disabilities and poor reading comprehension. *Learning Disability Quarterly, 37*(4), 218–229.
Spencer, P. E., & Marschark, M. (2010). *Evidence-based practice in educating deaf and hard-of-hearing students.* New York: Oxford University Press.
Stinson, M. S., Elliot, L. B., Kelly, R. R., & Liu, Y. (2009). Deaf and hard-of-hearing students' memory of lectures with speech-to-text and interpreting/note taking services. *The Journal of Special Education, 43*(1), 52–64.
Stinson, M., & Kluwin, T. (2011). Educational consequences of alternative school placements. In M. Marschark & P. Spencer (Eds.), *The Oxford handbook of deaf studies, language, and education* (Vol. 2, pp. 47–62). New York: Oxford University Press.

Swanwick, R. (2015). Re-envisioning learning and teaching in deaf education: Toward new transactions between research and practice. In H. Knoors & M. Marschark (Eds.), *Educating deaf learners: Creating a global evidence base* (pp. 595–616). New York: Oxford University Press.

Toffler, A. (1973). *Future shock.* New York: Bantam Books.

Tomlinson, C. A. (1999). Mapping a route toward differentiated instruction. *Educational Leadership, 57,* 12–17.

Tomlinson, C. A., Brighton, C., Hertberg, H., Callahan, C. M., Moon, T. R., Brimijoin, K., Conover, L.A., & Reynolds, T. (2003). Differentiating instruction in response to student readiness, interest, and learning profile in academically diverse classrooms: A review of literature. *Journal for the Education of the Gifted, 27*(2–3), 119–145.

Van Gent, T., Goedhart, A. W., Hindley, P. A., & Treffers, P. D. (2007). Prevalence and correlates of psychopathology in a sample of deaf adolescents. *Journal of Child Psychology and Psychiatry, 48*(9), 950–958.

Vygotsky, L. S. (1998). *The collected works of L.S. Vygotsky* (Vol. 2). New York: Plenum Press.

Wolters, N., Knoors, H., Cillessen, A. H., & Verhoeven, L. (2012). Impact of peer and teacher relations on deaf early adolescents' well-being: Comparisons before and after a major school transition. *Journal of Deaf Studies and Deaf Education, 17*(4), 463–482.

Wood, D. (1991). Communication and cognition: How the communication styles of hearing adults may hinder—rather than help—deaf learners. *American Annals of the Deaf, 136*(3), 247–251.

Wood, H. A., & Wood, D. J. (1984). An experimental evaluation of the effects of five styles of teacher conversation on the language of hearing-impaired children. *Journal of Child Psychology and Psychiatry, 25*(1), 45–62.

Wood, D., Wood, H., Griffiths, A. J., & Howarth, I. (1986). *Teaching and talking with deaf children.* London: Wiley.

Wubbels, T., & Brekelmans, M. (2005). Two decades of research on teacher–student relationships in class. *International Journal of Educational Research, 43*(1), 6–24.

9

The Development of Pragmatic Skills in Children and Young People Who Are Deaf and Hard of Hearing

Dianne Toe, Pasquale Rinaldi, Maria Cristina Caselli, Louise Paatsch, and Amelia Church

The acquisition of language is often described in terms of its subsystems. Language subsystems relate to the form (syntax, phonology, and morphology), content (semantics) and use (pragmatics). Pragmatics pertains to the social use of language and includes skills such as turn taking, topic initiation, and topic maintenance. Speakers and listeners must integrate both their verbal and nonverbal communication skills to become competent communication partners. Conversational partners work together to coconstruct a conversation. Pragmatic skills are closely linked to social skills and significantly impact a child's opportunities to interact with others and to build social relationships (Cutting & Dunn, 2006). Children with normal hearing develop skills such as turn taking in infancy and are thought to acquire foundational pragmatic skills by the age of 8 years (Owens, 1996; Paul, 2007). To develop pragmatic skills, young children need to engage in many interactions with their carers. Infants learn much about turn taking during the rich and plentiful interactions that occur between them and their caregivers, practicing to use nonverbal cues such as the use of eye gaze and gesture to engage with their interactive partners. As they develop, they use vocalizations and eventually words to gain attention and maintain interactions (Owens, 1996). These interactions provide both access to strong adult models and numerous opportunities for practicing all aspects of conversation. During these early years of development, young children who are deaf or hard-of-hearing (DHH) may exhibit a wide range of pragmatic language skills influenced by their access to language via either a sensory device or sign language, their opportunities for interactions with a range of partners, and the quality of the language input they receive (Lederberg & Everhart, 2000; Nicholas et al., 1994; Spencer, 1993).

During primary school, children continue to interact with family members but also engage with a wide range of peers and other adults, providing them with opportunities to practice and refine their pragmatic skills. This language subsystem develops alongside the other subsystems so that growing sophistication in syntactic and semantic knowledge can be used for more sophisticated and sustained conversations. School-age students extend the number of turns taken in a communicative exchange, learning how to maintain and extend conversational topics. They also increase their repertoire of conversational moves, asking questions, making comments, seeking affirmation, and providing extended responses to questions from others (Paatsch & Toe, 2014).

During adolescence, young people add additional layers of sophistication to their language and their interactions, interweaving humor and learning to read their communicative partners in more sophisticated ways (Nippold, 2000). Face-to-face interactions at this age are rarely mediated by concrete objects such as toys, and much of the talk is rapid, frequently decontextualized, idiosyncratic, and abstract.

Adolescents are reported to spend more time talking to peers rather than family where they use figurative language, jokes, rapid topic shifts, interruptions, and verbal mazes (Larson & McKinley, 1998). Young people use their conversational skills to facilitate the development of friendships (Berndt, 1982; Cutting & Dunn, 2006; Stinson & Foster 2000; Yont et al., 2002). The link between pragmatic skills and social skills becomes more acute during adolescence, and individuals with poor skills in this aspect of language may find themselves increasingly frustrated and potentially isolated (Conti-Ramsden & Botting, 2004). Pragmatic skills develop through rich and varied interactions. As with literacy development, the "Matthew effect" applies so that children and young people with well-developed pragmatic skills who can communicate with relative ease "get richer" with a range of communicative partners whereas those who struggle with turn taking and topic initiation or contingency may find themselves with fewer and fewer communication partners and less opportunity to learn.

Since the 1980s, researchers have investigated pragmatic skills with a wide range of participants who are DHH at various developmental levels (e.g., Jeanes et al., 2000; Lederberg & Everhart, 2000; Nicholas et al., 1994; Spencer, 1993; Wood et al., 1982). Early studies of young children have shown that pragmatic skills were delayed severely compared with children with normal hearing (Nicholas et al., 1994), and that this delay appeared to relate to overall delays in language development. Interestingly, Spencer (1993) found few differences in how frequently deaf and hearing infants of hearing parents communicated with their mothers. Both groups showed equivalent intentions to communicate and also increased their communications from 12 to 18 months.

However, hearing toddlers were more likely to use language whereas toddlers who were DHH continued to use nonlinguistic methods of communication.

Lederberg and Everhart (2000) monitored language and communication competence of hearing and DHH toddlers age 22 months to 3 years old. Although few differences were observed at 22 months, by age 3 years the hearing toddlers displayed more sophisticated interactions. In their study, DHH toddlers used more directives and displayed less varied communicative functions. Their study indicated that, even at this early age, young children with hearing loss have more difficulty with maintaining a topic of conversation and with using their language to comment and ask questions compared with their hearing peers. Much technological development has taken place since these studies with young children. Cochlear implants (CIs) have been developed and refined during the past 25 years, and hearing aids have also become much more sophisticated. The majority of children in developed countries now have access to early cochlear implantation. As an example, most profoundly deaf children in Australia now receive bilateral CIs. This technology affords young children greater access to hearing for the purpose of improving language and communication development. This chapter presents three recent studies that provide insight into how pragmatic skills develop in DHH children today. It presents snapshots of the most recent pragmatic research at three developmental stages: in toddlers, school age children from age 8 to 13 years, and finally in adolescents. These studies provide an excellent opportunity to explore the way pragmatic skills develop in children who are DHH. Previous studies have explored pragmatic skills in both sign language and spoken language users. This chapter focuses on the development of pragmatic skills in children and young people who use spoken language for communication.

THE DEVELOPMENT OF PRAGMATIC SKILLS IN TODDLERS WITH COCHLEAR IMPLANTS

An increasing number of DHH children have received CIs during the first years of life. Several studies have found that the increased access to sound provided by CIs can help children to develop language skills in both comprehension and production; however, early CI implantation in itself does not ensure a child will develop facility with spoken language, and that language abilities will be within normal limits, even with up to 6 years of CI experience (Caselli et al., 2012; Duchesne et al., 2009; Rinaldi et al., 2013).

Data collected after cochlear implantation have shown contrasting results and large individual variability. These outcomes can be attributed to diverse factors, including age at diagnosis of deafness, age at

CI activation, family environment, and the language or languages the child is acquiring. Furthermore, the percentage of children with CIs who are within normal limits for language development varies from less than 20% to more than 80% depending on the specific linguistic domain. For a very recent review on these aspects, see Caselli et al. (2015).

Few studies have focused on pragmatic skills in children with a CI (Duchesne et al., 2009; Lichtig et al., 2011; Most et al., 2010; Paatsch & Toe, 2014). Even fewer studies have evaluated the relationship between pragmatic and linguistic skills in children with a CI who are younger than 3 years of age.

Deafness is not only a clear risk factor for difficulties in spoken language acquisition and development, but it can also cause difficulties in early social experiences and interactions mediated by language, especially when a DHH child is born to parents with normal hearing (Knoors & Marschark, 2014; Vaccari & Marschark, 1997). More than 95% of parents who have a DHH child have normal hearing, and the vast majority of people in the child's environment are also normally hearing and use spoken language as their mode of communication. Children who are DHH may struggle to communicate with their hearing parents, resulting in frustration on the part of both the parents and the child (Barker et al., 2009). In theory, a CI could improve the access to spoken language and facilitate parent–child communication, limiting the difficulties experienced by DHH children in acquiring pragmatic skills. However, according to a study in which pragmatic skills were evaluated in children with a CI who were at least 6 years of age, there was still a significant delay when compared with their age-matched hearing peers (Most et al., 2010).

In this section of the chapter, the results of a study on linguistic and pragmatic skills of Italian DHH children with CIs are reported. Data were collected on 12 profoundly deaf children between 24 months and 34 months of age (mean age, 29 months) without other reported disabilities, with CIs activated between 9 months and 26 months of age, and with a mean length of CI use of 14 months (range, 7–21 months). All children had participated in auditory–verbal therapy both before and after implantation, and none had been exposed to sign language, simultaneous communication, or baby signs at home.

To evaluate lexical production, the "Vocabulary" section of the Words and Sentences short form of the Italian version of the MacArthur–Bates Communicative Development Inventories (Caselli et al., 2007) was used. This form has already been used in a study of Italian DHH children with hearing aids (Rinaldi & Caselli, 2009). Parents of 11 children who are DHH filled in this questionnaire.

To evaluate pragmatic skills, the Social Conversational Skills Rating Scale (referred to as the *ASCB*, or *Abilità Socio-conversazionali del Bambino*)

(Bonifacio & Girolametto, 2007) was administered. This parent report questionnaire is used for evaluating assertive and responsive conversational skills in children from 12 to 36 months of age in everyday dyadic contexts. Items belong to two different scales: the Assertiveness Scale, with 15 items on the child's ability to ask questions, make requests, and make suggestions; and the Responsiveness Scale, with 10 items on the ability to respond to questions, respond to requests, and maintain turn taking in conversation. For each of the items, which are listed in random order, the parents are asked to assign a rating from 1 to 5 based on the frequency with which the child exhibits the behavior (1, never; 2, almost never; 3, sometimes; 4, often; 5, always). Parents of all 12 DHH children filled in this questionnaire. The scores obtained by children in these two questionnaires were transformed into z scores.

Findings from this study showed that the mean z scores were very low, with lexical production = –1.35; assertiveness = –2.41, and responsiveness = –2.61. Only four children had z scores in the normal range (more than –1) for lexical production. Five children exhibited z scores in the normal range for assertiveness, and four children had a z score within the normal range for responsiveness.

Eleven of the 12 children had negative z scores for both the ASCB subscales, three children had z scores within the normal limit (from 1 to –1) for both subscales, and two children had z scores within the normal limit for both (ASCB subscales as well as for lexical production). Significant correlations were found between the two subscales of the ASCB: between lexical production and assertiveness, and between lexical production and responsiveness.

This group of children with CIs showed delayed lexical and pragmatic skills with respect to same-age hearing children. In fact, fewer than one-third of the children who participated in this study were within the normal range for lexical production and/or for pragmatic skills, and even children within the normal range displayed skills close to the lower limits of the normal range. This weakness in lexical production, which was demonstrated previously for older Italian deaf children and adolescents with hearing aids (Rinaldi & Caselli, 2009; Volterra et al., 2001), and in older Italian preschoolers with a CI (Caselli et al., 2012), is already evident in the earliest stages of language acquisition.

The significant correlations between vocabulary size and pragmatic skills might be understood by considering parent–child interactions. Some studies have reported that, very often, hearing parents of DHH children tend to be more controlling in their interactions with their children compared with deaf parents of deaf children or hearing parents of hearing children (Barker et al., 2009; Capirci et al., 2007), resulting in environments that do not adequately scaffold language acquisition and language development. These data suggest that, even after cochlear implantation, children still have difficulties in early social experiences and interactions mediated by language that could have negative cascading effects on subsequent development of linguistic and social skills.

Early cochlear implantation may provide DHH children with a good opportunity to develop language skills, but difficulties in early social experiences and interaction mediated by language can still be observed in a high percentage of children. For this reason, early intervention for children who are DHH continues to be vital after implantation. Moreover, these interventions should not be limited to the development of spoken language skills, but should aim at scaffolding communicative and social experiences within the context of the family in which acquired language skills may be applied effectively and developed further (see Chapter 2). Further research focused on this family communicative context would provide rich data to support well-targeted interventions. The transition to school and the demands placed on pragmatic skills as young children extend their circle of communicative partners is also underresearched and would support the development of inclusive practice during the early years of schooling.

MAINTAINING MUTUAL ENGAGEMENT DURING CONVERSATIONS: A COMPARISON OF PRAGMATIC SKILLS BETWEEN SCHOOL-AGE CHILDREN WITH COCHLEAR IMPLANTS AND THEIR HEARING PEERS

In contrast to the previous study with toddlers, in which parents provided an evaluation of their children's language and pragmatic skills, much of the research that has investigated the pragmatic skills of school-age children with hearing loss has observed and measured these skills during interactions with adult partners using spoken language (Lloyd et al., 2001, 2005; Most, 2002). Typically, these interactions occur within the contexts of structured tasks, such as barrier games, or during conversations with parents, teachers, or clinicians (Most et al., 2010; Toe et al., 2007; Wood et al., 1982). Research investigating DHH children's pragmatic skills during interactions with their peers has also predominantly used structured tasks as a way to stimulate communication (Ibertsson et al., 2009a, 2009b). There are fewer studies, however, that have specifically investigated school-age children's pragmatic skills during informal, spontaneous conversations within familiar environments.

The task of setting up contexts that replicate naturalistic peer-to-peer interactions is often challenging as a result of the contrived environment in which the conversation takes place. Often these environments include clinics or classrooms within schools where, typically, conversations between peers do not take place. However, given these constraints, these contexts still enable a close examination of some of the pragmatic skills evident in school-age children with hearing loss. Results from these studies show these children are active communicators and demonstrate a range of well-developed pragmatic skills, including turn taking, requests for clarification, provision of personal comments, topic initiation, questioning, and providing responses (Lloyd et al., 2001; Most et al., 2010; Paatsch & Toe, 2014; Toe & Paatsch, 2013; Tye-Murray, 2003; Wood et al., 1982). However, there also appears to be reported differences in the pragmatic behaviors of these children when compared with their hearing peers (Most et al., 2010; Paatsch & Toe, 2014; Toe & Paatsch, 2013).

Findings from a recent study by Paatsch and Toe (2014) of 93 children (57 girls and 36 boys) between 7 years 7 months and 12 years 9 months of age showed significant differences between 31 pairs of DHH and hearing (D/H) children when compared with aged-matched pairs of hearing children (H/H). Pragmatic skills were measured against broad categories, including conversation turns, conversational balance, conversational turn type, and conversational maintenance. Results showed that, within the pairs of D/H children, deaf children appeared to take longer turns and initiate more topics whereas the pairs of H/H conversations were well balanced. Furthermore, deaf children tended to ask more questions and make more personal contributions, whereas the hearing children in the D/H pair used more conversational devices (such as, "Uh huh" and "Really") and responded with more minimal answers. In contrast, the hearing children in the H/H pairs used similar numbers and types of turns, engaging in a more balanced conversation. These findings showed that the DHH children appeared to be more dominant, suggesting that it may be a deliberate strategy used by these children as a way of avoiding communication breakdown.

In a subsequent analysis of the conversational interactions from the study by Paatsch and Toe (2014), a number of interesting findings were reported in relation to the subtle differences evident between the D/H pairs and the H/H pairs (Paatsch & Toe, 2016). Paatsch and Toe (2016) reported there were other disfluencies apparent in the deaf children's talk that were not attributable to the broad categories measured in the earlier study. Such disfluencies appeared to be a barrier to the conversational fluency between students with hearing loss and their age-matched peers. For example, the children with hearing loss were able to use a range of questions, but the talk-in-interaction was often characterized by uncomfortable, drawn-out sequences of questions and minimal answers, followed by lengthy pauses. The investigators also reported evidence of the lack of conversational contingency during which both partners appeared not to share and extend the topics by adding information to the prior utterances.

Paatsch and Toe (2016) also suggested there were limitations to their broad approach to their analysis in accounting for the subtle features of the talk, and recommended that a different approach to the data was necessary. As a result, conversation analysis (CA) was used as a method to analyze the more subtle differences in the talk in 10 of the 31 pairs of DHH and hearing school-age children. CA is an approach that aims to describe, analyze, and understand the sequential organization of the talk, and enables observations of how each speaker coconstructs the talk and how he or she interprets the prior turn (Hayashi et al., 2002; Sacks et al., 1974). Preliminary analysis showed that many of the children with hearing loss in the study by Paatsch and Toe (2014) experienced difficulties with providing feedback throughout the talk by offering listener tokens such as "Yeah" to maintain topics or to show sensitivity to the uptake of the topic. The data also revealed atypical eye gaze, with infrequent mutual gaze to signal a change of speaker or to invite an opportunity for their feedback, and limited extension of topics. The most striking feature of the data, however, was occasional, but problematic, failure to repair misunderstanding.

The main aim of the study presented in this section is to build on the previous investigation by Paatsch and Toe (2016) to explore how children with hearing loss and their hearing peers go about resolving trouble sources in their interactions. Data reported here were taken from the same interactions between the 10 D/H pairs of school-age children age 7 years 7 months and 12 years 9 months (Paatsch & Toe, 2016). Ten H/H pairs, matched by age and year level, also participated in spontaneous conversations. All children were selected from three primary schools in Melbourne, Australia, ranging from year 3 (7- to 8-year-olds) to year 6 (11- to 12-year-olds). The children with hearing loss were fully mainstreamed in these schools, where they had access to specialized facilities or units for students with hearing loss with support from teachers of the deaf either in mainstream classroom activities or in individual sessions. All 10 children with hearing loss were CI users, used spoken language as their main mode of communication, and were rated as having intelligible speech using the Speech Intelligibility Rating Scale (Wilkinson & Brinton, 2003).

Each child with hearing loss was invited to nominate a friend with normal hearing from their class. This hearing child was also invited to choose another hearing friend from their class to participate in a conversation. Each D/H and H/H pair was asked to talk to each other about any topic of interest. Topics ranged from favorite movies, sports, television shows, to weekend activities. These 6- to 10-minute conversations took place in a classroom and were videotaped for later transcription and analysis.

CA was used as a method of analysis to explore the sequential organization of the children's talk (Sidnell, 2010). There were some noticeable phenomena that only appeared in the talk-in-interaction between the D/H pairs that were not observed in the H/H pairs. The focus of this section is to present the atypical practices of repair, including the absence of repair, that were evident in the D/H pairs. In typical conversations, speakers encounter troubles with hearing, speaking, and understanding (Schegloff et al., 1977; Sidnell, 2010). Troubles in speaking usually occur when a speaker uses the wrong word, whereas troubles in listening occur when the listener does not understand what the speaker has said, or when a listener misunderstands what a speaker has said. When such troubles occur in conversations, both speakers and listeners use a number of "repair mechanisms" to resolve the problems (Sidnell, 2010, p. 110). These mechanisms are used to ensure "the interaction does not freeze in its place and when troubles arise, that intersubjectivity is maintained or restored, and that the turn and sequence and activity can progress to possible completion" (Schegloff [2007] as cited in Kitzinger [2013, p. 229]).

Transcriptions of these conversations showed that the school-age children with CIs used several examples of open-class other-initiated repair whereby the listener used devices such as "What?," "Pardon," and "Sorry" to indicate there were difficulties with the prior turn as a whole (Drew, 1997). Often these devices are used to indicate the listener did not hear, or when there is a challenge to some unspecified content of the prior turn. Open-initiated repair usually involves the listener of the troublesome talk initiating the repair but leaving it to the speaker to resolve the trouble in the ensuing turns (Schegloff, 1997). There were some examples of typical examples of repair within the D/H pairs. For example, in the following extract Kate (hearing) and Zara (CI user) have been talking about the upcoming holidays. Kate asks Zara whether she receives Easter eggs from the Easter bunny. This is followed by a pause. Zara then asks for repair through the use of an unspecified initiator of repair ("What?"). It appears that Kate treats this other-initiator device as Zara's inability to hear her question as evidenced by Kate's verbatim repeat of the initial question and the extra emphasis on the word "Easter" through elongation of the vowel (line 68). Please note that CA conventions have been retained in this transcript:

```
63   KATE:   do you get easter eggs;= from easter bunny?
64           (1.8)
65   ZARA:   wha?
67           (0.3)
68   KATE:   do you get ea:ster eggs;=from ea:ster bunny?
69           (1.0)
70   ZARA:   °(yeah).°
```

In the data set, however, there were unusual cases where there was an apparent absence of repair, or delayed repair, resulting in a marked problem for enabling smooth progress within the conversations.

256   Diversity in Deaf Education

Before the following transcript Pina (CI user) and Rebecca (hearing) were talking about a movie they had both seen during the past couple of weeks. Pina explains that because the movie was so long she had to keep leaving the theater to buy more popcorn and that "it was so busy that time" (line 69). Rebecca acknowledges her contribution with "Yeah" (line 70). This is then followed immediately by Pina introducing a new, unrelated topic with the question, "What's your favorite band?" (line 72). Such an abrupt unannounced shift in topic causes a trouble source in the conversation marked by a lengthy pause, a nod, a listener token "Oh," another pause before Rebecca then attempts to fix the problem with a partial repeat of the question. Pina's response consisting of an enthusiastic "Yeah" accompanied by a smile, suggesting she was relieved the source of the trouble was resolved by the listener rather than what should typically be resolved by the speaker.

```
69  PINA:     it was [sO busy; that time.
70  REBECCA:  [y:eah.
71  REBECCA:  °ye:ah°=
72  PINA:     =what's your favourite band.
73            (1.2)
74  REBECCA:  ((nods))
75  REBECCA:  mm.
76            (0.6)
77  REBECCA:  >OH. (.) my favourite band.<
78  PINA:     =>YEH<
79  REBECCA:  >yeh um< (.) black eyed peas¿=hh °↑ha.° .h yours?
80            (0.6)
81  PINA:     ah w'll.
82            (0.7)
83  PINA:     i don't really have one;=but highschool °musical.°
84  REBECCA:  yeah.[=hahaha. .hh
```

A further example of the absence of repair is presented in the following transcript. Harry (CI user) and Paul (hearing) are talking about two Australian Rules football teams (Essendon and St. Kilda) that they support. They discuss that neither of the teams did very well in the previous football season, particularly in the finals. Harry continues the conversation by indicating there were "two reasons why" his team, St. Kilda, were not in the finals. This was accompanied by Harry banging his hand on the table, emphasizing "two" with his fingers. This is followed by Paul's disconnection to Harry's contribution with a short pause, a delayed "Yeah" followed by another pause, then a generic assessment "It's a shame you got beaten" (line 71). Harry's nonverbal behaviors indicate there is a problem in the interactions, but there is no attempt to repair the source of trouble and the conversation continues.

```
60   HARRY:   if (0.2) s'Nt kIlda had beated collingwood. ↓which
61            they lost by nine points? (.) we'd be in
             the grand
62           final.>if adelaide< had lo:st, (0.6) they'd-
63           (0.4) we'd be in the °grand final.°
64           (0.3)
65   HARRY:   two reasons [why.
66   HARRY:   [((bangs hand on table while holding out
                67 two fingers))
68           (0.5)
69   PAUL:    (.hh) yeah.
70           (1.6)
71   PAUL:    °(it's/.hh)° shame you got beaten.
72           (0.8)
73   HARRY:   what about you?
74           (0.4)
75   HARRY:   >where did< essendon finish on the ladder.
76           (0.8)
77   PAUL:    think abo:ut, (1.9) tenth?
```

Both these transcripts show that repair was required but was not taken up, resulting in marked problems in the talk. These examples also show that the children with CIs did not have the necessary skills to repair the talk when their hearing partner did not follow their topic or attend to their prior talk. Both children with hearing loss (Pina and Harry) were aware of the awkwardness in the conversation, as displayed through their nonverbal behaviors, but waited for their hearing partners to repair or to move on to the next utterance. It is not clear from these occurrences of awkwardness whether the absence of repair was the result of both partners showing a degree of sensitivity about drawing attention to the hearing loss itself or whether they just displayed sensitivity around seeking clarification during these conversations. It appears these children would benefit from developing strategies for repair and that there may also be a need to highlight that repair in itself is a mechanism used in typical, everyday interactions between hearing peers.

These difficulties in social interactions attributed to pragmatic competencies echo the findings outlined earlier in the study with young Italian children with CIs. Although the causes of these pragmatic differences are multifaceted, the challenges of atypical opportunities for collaboration and coconstruction of talk are evident in the data reported throughout the chapter. What is highlighted is the role that conversational partners play in building pragmatic skills. Parents of toddlers may need additional support and guidance to increase opportunities for balanced interactions when children who are DHH can take a less passive role. Similarly, with school-age children with CIs, we cannot look at their pragmatic skills in isolation. It is the way they interact with their peers, and in this case negotiate or fail to negotiate issues with repair, that has significant implications for building productive conversation skills.

Findings from this study highlight the benefit of using CA as a method of providing more in depth and precise ways of understanding how children with hearing loss interact with their hearing peers. In addition, it highlights the need to refine the methods used for assessing pragmatic skills to do justice to the collaborative, coconstructed nature of interactions (Egbert & Deppermann, 2012). CA can reveal both successful negotiations as well as difficulties within interactions. The ethnological–methodological approach of CA, with its focus on behaviors to which speakers themselves pay attention, provides evidence to inform strategies for intervention. Primary school-age students might be aware of the awkwardness of interactions but may not be able to pinpoint the source of the difficulties. By reflecting on the results of CA, teachers can help young people learning together in inclusive settings to be more proactive in identifying when repair is needed and whether it is the task of the speaker or the listener. These insights can guide young people toward more satisfying and successful interactions that ultimately lead to increased social acceptance and the formation of strong friendships. By solving some of the issues with the ways young people with CIs converse with their hearing peers during the upper primary years, it may be possible to enhance the transition to secondary school and the communicatively challenging adolescent years.

DEVELOPING PRAGMATIC SKILLS FROM CHILDHOOD TO ADOLESCENCE

The adolescent years are often characterized as a period of rapid change during which young people develop their identity and move away from the influence of parents (Erikson, 1994). Peer interactions are seen as critical for this process, and the nature of these interactions has been the focus of a number of studies (Ibertsson, 2009b; Larson & McKinley, 1998, Nippold, 2000). Larson and McKinley (1998) conducted a longitudinal study of conversations between adolescents and their peers and compared these conversations with those that took place between adolescents and an adult partner. The peer-to-peer interactions between adolescents were characterized by more occurrences of figurative language, more questions, new and abrupt topic shifts, more verbal mazes, and the use of nonspecific language. Previous studies have identified a sequence of development in pragmatic skills (Paatsch & Toe, 2014; Toe & Paatsch, 2013; Toe et al., 2007). Younger students have less balanced conversations that are characterized by many pauses and repeated question-and-answer sequences. As both DHH and hearing young people reach the end of primary school, their conversation is more likely to overlap, and speakers and listeners become more contingent, although young DHH people still have challenges with contingency (Most et al., 2010; Paatsch & Toe, 2014). Given that exchanges between normally hearing adolescents have been identified as quite demanding, adolescents with hearing loss might be significantly challenged by social interactions in inclusive secondary settings.

Researchers have explored the impact of deafness on adolescent interactions and on pragmatic skills during these critical years. Early studies focused primarily on the repair strategies adopted by adolescents, either while interacting with a peer or with an adult. Several studies have used referential communication tasks in which students work in pairs to identify a specific card from a selection of cards placed on either side of a barrier on a table. The nature of this task ensures participants use a range of clarification strategies to help identify the card they are seeking with maximum efficiency. Jeanes et al. (2000) showed that DHH children and young people age 8, 11, 14, and 17 years used fewer specific requests for clarification and less appropriate responses to their partners' clarification than hearing pairs; however, these skills did appear to improve with age. Most (2002) found that adolescents age 11 to 17 years with age-appropriate expressive grammar used quite a limited repertoire of repair strategies, relying predominantly on repetition.

More recent studies have reported improving pragmatic skills in teenagers who are DHH. Ibertsson et al. (2009b) reported that "deaf teenagers with cochlear implants were equally collaborative and responsible conversational partners as the hearing teenagers" (p. 320). Using a referential communication task, they found few differences between pairs of hearing teens and pairs in which one adolescent was DHH and the other hearing (mean age, 15 years 9 months). They exhibited similar numbers of turns and length of turns, and very few breakdowns occurred; however, some more subtle differences in the use of clarifications were still seen in the teenagers with CIs. This finding is in stark contrast to the findings reported in the earlier sections of this chapter relating to delayed pragmatic skills in DHH toddlers and to the difficulties encountered with repair with pairs of hearing and DHH school-age children.

The study presented in this section of the chapter compared new conversational data collected with pairs of adolescents (13–16 years) with earlier findings of peer-to-peer conversational interactions in middle and upper primary students. The earlier study (Paatsch & Toe, 2014) collected data with 31 D/H pairs and 31 H/H pairs of middle and upper primary students. Each pair was invited to come to a quiet room in the school to have a chat. The H/H pair conversations took place 1 week after the D/H pairs. One hearing partner was common to both pairs. Each pair was invited to converse for approximately 10 minutes about any topic of interest and was provided with picture prompts of movies, pets, sports, and so on, if required. All conversations were videotaped then transcribed into the Systematic Analysis of Language Transcripts software program (research version, 2012) for analysis.

All conversations were coded for each of the D/H pairs and H/H pairs according to conversational turns, balance, and turn type (see Paatsch and Toe [2014] for further details of the coding scheme). Conversational turn is defined as one or more utterances or nonverbal communicative acts preceded, and followed by, a change of speaker or a pause of two or more seconds (Caissie & Rockwell, 1993). Conversational balance included measures of the number of turns per partner, number of topic initiations per conversational partner, and mean length of turns in words per partner. Conversational maintenance was coded according to four broad measures: (a) the number of topics per conversation, (b) the number of turns per topic, (c) the number of pauses between turns, and (d) the average pause time between turns. Turn type was coded using five turn-type categories drawn from a study by Lloyd et al. (2001). The five categories comprised questions, personal contributions, conversational devices (for example, phatics such as "Oh," "Ah," "Yeah," and "Cool"), minimal answers, and extended answers.

New data were collected with D/H and H/H pairs of adolescent students in years 7 to 10 attending mainstream secondary schools (age range, 13 years 5 months–16 years 3 months). All participants used spoken language for communication and all the participants with hearing loss had attended both a mainstream primary and secondary school. One student used a CI and three students were hearing-aid users. Each of the deaf participants selected a hearing friend with whom to converse in the study. Pairs of hearing friends attending the same school and in the same year levels were also invited to participate in the adolescent study. This is an ongoing project and, to date, data have been collected for four pairs of H/H students and four D/H pairs. The data have been transcribed using the Systematic Analysis of Language Transcripts software program and coded according to the scheme outlined earlier.

To explore the development of conversational skills from primary school to the adolescent years, the original group of 31 sets of students was reanalyzed in two groups: year 3 and 4 students (middle primary, n = 15) and year 5 and 6 students (upper primary, n = 16). These two groups were then compared with the adolescent pairs (n = 4). Table 9.1 presents the findings for conversational balance and maintenance and Table 9.2 presents the findings for conversational turn type

Table 9.1 Conversational Balance and Conversational Maintenance for Conversational Partners According to School Year Level

Year Level	Years 3 and 4 (n = 15)					Years 5 and 6 (n = 16)					Years 7–10 (n = 4)				
Conversational pair	Deaf/hearing pair		Hearing pair			Deaf/hearing pair		Hearing pair			Deaf/hearing pair		Hearing pair		
Hearing status	D	H	H1	H2		D	H	H1	H2		D	H	H1	H2	
Mean total turns for pair	75		77			74		98			155		145		
Mean turns for each partner	37	36	39	38		37	37	49	49		76.5	76	86	86	
Mean no. of topics for pair	6.7		6.6			5.3		6.9			5.75		5.5		
Mean turns per topic	15.3		18.8			17		22			15.7		16.8		
Mean turn length	9.5	6.4	8.02	9.95		11.2	8.2	7.7	8.1		11.13	12.3	12.6	14.5	
Mean percentage of topics initiated	62.3	38.7	49.7	50.1		56.2	45	51.6	48.0		50.95	48.9	48.13	51.8	

D, deaf; H, hearing; H1, first hearing partner; H2, second hearing partner.

In Table 9.1, some important developmental changes in patterns of interaction that occur between peers can be seen, regardless of hearing status, as children move from middle to upper primary and then on to the adolescent years. The 10-minute conversations are characterized by an increasing number of turns as well as an increase in turn length. Comparing the adolescents with the middle primary students we see double the number of turns. Although turn length does not change substantially from middle primary to upper primary, the small group of adolescents in this study took substantially longer turns than the primary school-age participants. This paints a picture of rapid adolescent conversational exchange with few pauses and substantial potential for overlapping turns. Less change is observed in some of the other measures; for example, the mean number of topics covered in each conversation and the number of turns for each topic remains relatively stable through the primary and junior secondary school years.

The conversational balance and maintenance measures in Table 9.1 also highlight some differences in the conversations observed between D/H pairs and H/H pairs of participants. In the youngest pairs, grade 3 to 4, there appears to be a conversational imbalance, with the DHH partners initiating more topics and taking longer turns than their hearing partners. In contrast, the H/H pairs of middle primary students appear to have more evenly balanced conversations, with an equal share of topics initiated and a similar mean turn length. By the time they are in grades 5 and 6, the balance is beginning to shift and, although the participants who are DHH still initiate more topics and take longer turns than their hearing partners, the mean differences are less marked. No differences can be observed between the D/H adolescent pairs and the H/H adolescents. Turn length is very similar and, for both sets of pairs, the number of topics initiated is very evenly balanced. This finding suggests that, by adolescence, young people who are DHH who use spoken language and attend mainstream schools are, at least according to these broad measures, conversing in a very similar way to their hearing peers.

Table 9.2 reports the distribution of conversational turn type for the three age groups of participants. Some developmental changes in conversational structure can be observed easily in Table 9.2. These changes appear to occur, regardless of the hearing status of the participants. Younger students ask more questions and provide a larger percentage of minimal answers. By adolescence, conversations are substantially made up of personal comments, and the proportion of questions and answers have decreased dramatically. On their journey to adult conversational exchange, adolescents appear to spend a lot of time telling each other things, describing their experiences, and giving their opinions on a wide range of topics. Conversational devices appeared to make up a consistent proportion of turns through the three year-level groups, but may serve a different purpose with younger and older students.

Table 9.2 Turn Type for Conversational Partners, Grouped According to School Year Level

Year level	Years 3 and 4 (n = 15)				Years 5 and 6 (n = 16)				Years 7–10 (n = 4)			
Conversational pair	Deaf/hearing pair		Hearing pair		Deaf/hearing pair		Hearing pair		Deaf/hearing pair		Hearing pair	
Hearing status	D	H	H1	H2	D	H	H1	H2	D	H	H1	H2
Mean percentage questions	40.9	12.4	28.7	28.0	27.7	25.9	33.8	24.1	6.73	15.08	15.8	16.13
Mean percentage personal comments	28.0	19.1	28.9	35.8	36.4	32.5	33.6	32.2	51.6	66.4	55.15	53.95
Mean percentage conversational devices	10.1	18.4	17.2	9.5	14.6	20.6	12	15.5	24.65	9.98	12.2	12.95
Mean percentage minimal answers	13.0	26.1	17.6	15.7	11.1	13.5	10.4	15.7	8.15	3.3	7.78	5.3
Mean percentage extended answers	6.7	6.9	6.1	10.6	8.9	6.9	8.1	11.4	6.05	2.7	8.4	9.5

D, deaf; H, hearing; H1, first hearing partner; H2, second hearing partner.

Table 9.2 also highlights the impact of hearing status on conversations in primary school-age students and adolescents. A striking difference can be observed in the youngest group, with the D/H pairs exhibiting a substantial difference from the H/H pairs. For these participants, conversations were characterized by a much larger percentage of questions asked by the DHH participants than the hearing participants (40.9% vs. 12.4%, respectively). Consistent with this finding was the observation of the hearing partners of the DHH students who exhibited a greater proportion of minimal answers and conversational devices. In these pairs, it appeared the participants who were DHH were doing a lot of the work to keep the conversation going and received limited assistance from their hearing friends. In contrast, the conversations between H/H pairs of grade 3 and 4 students were much more balanced, with similar numbers of questions, and minimal answers in each conversational partner. In stark contrast, there are very few differences to observe between the D/H and H/H pairs of adolescent participants. Both pairs exhibited similar mean percentages of personal comments, conversational devices, and both minimal and extended answers. The DHH participants in the D/H pairs do appear to contribute a smaller percentage of questions to the conversations, but because questions make up such a reduced proportion of the conversations, and the number of participants is small, this might reflect small numbers of question instances rather than a genuine trend.

Some of the differences in conversational skills between the pairs are further illustrated by some brief conversational samples. In the following transcript, we see a conversation between two 9-year-old grade-3 girls, Dana (DHH) and Poppy (hearing). Note the interview style initially adopted by the DHH conversational partner and the way the two participants struggle to build common ground.

```
55   DANA:    okay, (um) (what's your favourite hol), what's
              your favourite holidays?
56   POPPY:   (um)when I went to Sydney for three days.
57   DANA:    okay so
58   POPPY:   and also at Sydney we saw the Sydney Harbour
59            Bridge.
60            (2.0)
61   POPPY:   do you know the Sydney Harbour Bridge?
62   DANA:    yeah.
63   POPPY:   and the Sydney Opera House.
64            and
65            (2.0)
66            the Three Sisters in the Blue Mountains.
```

In contrast, the conversation between two 13-year-old year-7 girls, one hearing (Harriet) and one CI user (Imogen), in their first year of secondary school highlights the development that has taken place. These friends coconstruct the conversation, building on each other's comments to create a shared story, each adding humor and, during the process, demonstrating a significant level of contingency.

```
91   IMOGEN:   Yeah, so we don't get the wrong food and they
               eat it and then someone dies or something
               like that.
92   HARRIET:  But like if they
93   IMOGEN:   It's not funny.
94   HARRIET:  If they were real allergic then (um) they
               wouldn't eat the food.
95   IMOGEN:   Yeah but like sometimes like they have pies
               and like for example they're (um) allergic
               to herbs and sometimes there could be
               chicken pies that had herbs in it like,
               I had a pie and it had herbs in it.
96   IMOGEN:   It could have that and then if what if someone
               eat it and you know it's invisible and they
               eat it and they die that's very sad.
97   HARRIET:  We'll just clean the body away.
```

Not all D/H pairs demonstrate such a high level of contingency. The following conversation follows a typical adolescent pattern with a high percentage of personal comments, however, these 14-year-old year-7 girls, Molly (DHH) and Sarah (hearing), do not build the conversation as effectively as the adolescents in the previous sample.

```
22   SARAH:   What are you doing on the holidays?
23   MOLLY:   Well I'm going down to New South Wales pretty much
24            for a week when my Mum finishes work.
25   SARAH:   What are you doing down there - like camping or-?
26   MOLLY:   Well we're seeing family down there, like I've got
27            family down in Forster,
28            and all that so yeah.
29   SARAH:   Last time I was in New South Wales we went down to
30            the Murray River like camping right next to it and-
31   MOLLY:   Yep.
32   SARAH:   We were in Yarrawonga and were on kind of like the
33            right side of the River and we went down to the like
34            river nearly every day and swum.
35   MOLLY:   Yep. Well last time I went down to the - New South
36            Wales - I was camping at the Murray River and it
               was really low.
```

This interaction has a parallel quality. Although the girls stay on topic and add information about their own experiences, using consecutive personal comments, it lacks the high level of contingency seen in the previous conversation. This suggests that, although the quantitative analysis of the conversations presented in Tables 9.1 and 9.2 show some remarkable development of pragmatic skills in both H/H and D/H pairs of adolescents, with few observable differences based on hearing status, there may still be more subtle differences in contingency that merit further analysis. The affordances of rich, qualitative ethnographic tools such as CA could provide additional windows into the nuances of adolescent pragmatic skills.

IT TAKES TWO TO TANGO

The three studies reported in this chapter highlight the changes that occur in pragmatic skills from infancy to adolescence in both hearing children, and children and young people who are DHH (Caselli et al., 2012; Paatsch & Toe, 2014; Toe & Paatsch, 2013). Although there may be significant delays in pragmatic skills in toddlers with CIs as judged by their parents, it was evident in these studies that by middle to upper primary school, children who are DHH can engage in meaningful, sustained conversation with their hearing peers. They exhibit a useful repertoire of turn-taking skills, but also tend to adopt strategies to take control of the conversation. By adolescence, conversations between pairs of H/H students and D/H pairs appear very similar, when broad measures are applied.

All three studies reported in this chapter draw focus to the role of conversational partners in building pragmatic skills and supporting children with hearing loss to refine their social use of language. It is possible that parents of young DHH children may tend to control interactions with their children rather than foster more equally shared interactions. Further investigation of parent interactions with children with CIs may help to understand the way these interactions impact young children's pragmatic skill development.

CA has identified the less effective ways that pairs of hearing and DHH friends negotiate conversational repair. This analytic tool facilitated a much deeper understanding of the more subtle challenges and roadblocks that children who are DHH can experience when conversing with hearing friends. Understanding where such roadblocks occur can give teachers and parents real direction for intervention and support. These findings guide teachers and parents in the way they can support the development of pragmatic skills in children and young people who are DHH by alerting them to the importance of self-repair and to the signals that listeners and speakers use to facilitate smooth communication. This focused intervention needs to take place in the context of real conversations, working with both hearing and DHH children and young people. This work highlights the shared nature of conversational development. We cannot focus on the pragmatic skills of children and young people who are DHH in isolation. Supporting this critical area of language development will be effective only if it takes place in the context of collaboration with the wide range of hearing partners with whom children and young people play and learn.

REFERENCES

Barker, D. H., Quittner, A. L., Fink, N. E., Eisenberg, L. S., Tobey, E. A., Niparko, J. K., & the CDACI investigative team (2009). Predicting behavior problems in deaf and hearing children: the influences of language, attention, and parent–child communication. *Development and Psychopathology, 21*, 373–392.

Berndt, T. J. (1982). The features and effects of friendship in early adolescence. *Child Development, 53*(6), 1447–1460.

Bonifacio, S., & Girolametto, L. (2007). *Questionario ASCB: Le abilità socioconversazionali del bambino* [ASCB Questionnaire: Socioconversational Skills of the Child]. Tirrenia: Del Cerro.

Caissie, R., & Rockwell, E. (1993). A videotape analysis procedure for assessing conversational fluency in hearing impaired adults. *Ear & Hearing, 14*, 201–209.

Capirci, O., Pirchio, S., & Soldani, R. (2007). Interazioni fra genitori e figli sordi in una situazione di gioco: analisi delle modalità e delle funzioni communicative [Interactions among parents and deaf children: analysis of communicative functions and modalities]. *Psicologia Clinica dello Sviluppo, 3*, 407–428.

Caselli, M. C., Pasqualetti, P., & Stefanini, S. (2007). *Parole e frasi nel "Primo Vocabolario del Bambino": Nuovi dati normative fra 18 e 36 mesi e forma breve del questionario* [Words and Sentences in "The First Vocabulary of the Child": New Normative Data from 18 to 36 Months and Short Form of the Questionnaire]. Milan: Franco Angeli.

Caselli, M. C., Rinaldi, P., Onofrio, D., & Tomasuolo, E. (2015). Language skills and literacy of deaf children in the era of cochlear implantation: Suggestions for teaching through E-learning visual environments. In H. Knoors & M. Marschark (Eds.), *Educating deaf learners: Creating a global evidence base* (pp. 443–460). New York, NY: University Press.

Caselli, M. C., Rinaldi, P., Varuzza, C., Giuliani, A., & Burdo, S. (2012). Cochlear implant in the second year of life: lexical and grammatical outcomes. *Journal of Speech, Language, and Hearing Research, 55*, 382–394.

Conti-Ramsden, G. M., & Botting, N. F. (2004). Social difficulties and victimization in children with SLI at 11 years of age. *Journal of Speech, Language and Hearing Research, 47*(1), 145–161.

Cutting, A., & Dunn, J. (2006). Conversations with siblings and with friends: Links between relationship quality and social understanding *British Journal of Developmental Psychology, 24*(1), 73–87.

Drew, P. (1997). 'Open' class repair initiators in response to sequential sources of trouble in conversation. *Journal of Pragmatics, 28*, 69–101.

Duchesne, L., Sutton, A., & Bergeron, F. (2009). Language achievement in children who received cochlear implants between 1 and 2 years of age: group

trends and individual patterns. *Journal of Deaf Studies and Deaf Education, 14,* 465–485.
Egbert, M., & Deppermann, A. (2012). Introduction to conversation analysis with examples from audiology. In M. Egbert and A. Deppermann (Eds.), *Hearing aids communication* (pp. 40–47). Mannheim, Germany: Verlag für Gesprächsforschung.
Erikson, E. H. (1994). *Identity and the life cycle.* New York, NY: W. W. Norton.
Hayashi, M., Mori, J., & Takagi, T. (2002). Contingent achievement of co-tellership in a Japanese conversation: An analysis of talk, gaze and gesture. In C. Ford, B. Fox, and S. Thompson (Eds.), *The language of turn and sequence* (pp. 81–122). Oxford: Oxford University Press.
Ibertsson, T., Hansson, K., Asker-Arnason, L., & Sahlen, B. (2009). Speech recognition, working memory and conversation in children with cochlear implants. *Deafness and Education International, 1*(3), 132–151.
Ibertson, T., Hansson, K., Maki-Torkko, E., Willstedt-Svensson, U., and Sahlen, B. (2009). Deaf teenagers with cochlear implants in conversation with hearing peers. *International Journal of Language and Communication Disorders, 44*(3), 319–337.
Jeanes, R. C., Nienhuys, T. G., & Rickards, F. W. (2000). The pragmatic skills of profoundly deaf children. *Journal of Deaf Studies and Deaf Education, 5*(3), 237–247.
Kitzinger, C. (2013). Repair. In . J. Sidnell and T. Stivers (Eds.), *The handbook of conversation analysis* (pp. 229–256). Malden, MA: Wiley-Blackwell.
Knoors, H., & Marschark, M. (2014). *Teaching deaf learners: Psychological and developmental foundations.* New York, NY: Oxford University Press.
Larson V., & McKinley, N. L. (1998) Characteristics of adolescents conversations: A longitudinal study. *Clinical Linguistics and Phonetics, 12*(3), 183–203.
Lederberg, A., & Everhart, V. S. (2000). Conversations between deaf children and their hearing m Mothers: Pragmatic and Dialogic Characteristics. *Journal of Deaf Studies and Deaf Education, 5,* 303–322.
Lichtig, I., Vieira Couto, M. I., Mecca, F. F. D. N., Hartley, S., Wirz, S., & Woll, B. (2011). Assessing deaf and hearing children's communication in Brazil. *Journal of Communication Disorders, 44,* 223–235.
Lloyd, J., Lieven, E., & Arnold, P. (2001). Oral conversations between hearing-impaired children and their normally hearing peers and teachers. *First Language, 21,* 83–107.
Lloyd, J., Lieven, E., & Arnold, P. (2005). The oral referential communication skills of hearing-impaired children. *Deafness and Education International, 7*(1), 22–42.
Most, T (2002). The use of repair strategies by children with and without hearing impairment. *Language, Speech, and Hearing Services in Schools, 33,*112–123.
Most, T., Shina-August, E., & Meilijson, S. (2010). Pragmatic abilities of children with hearing loss using cochlear implants or hearing aids compared to hearing children. *Journal of Deaf Studies and Deaf Education, 15,* 422–437.
Nicholas, J. G., Geers, A. E., & Kodak, V. (1994). Development of communicative function in young hearing-impaired and normally hearing children. *Volta Review, 96,* 113–135
Nippold, M. A. (2000). Language development during the adolescent years: Aspects of pragmatics, syntax, and semantics. *Topics in Language Disorders, 20*(2), 15–28.

Owens, E. R., Jr. (1996). *Language development: An introduction* (4th ed.). Needham Heights, MA: Allyn & Bacon.
Paatsch, L., & Toe, D. (2014). A comparison of pragmatic abilities of children who are deaf or hard of hearing and their hearing peers. *Journal of Deaf Studies and Deaf Education, 19*(1), 1–19.
Paatsch, L., & Toe, D. (2016). The fine art of conversation: The pragmatic skills of school-aged children with hearing loss. In M. Marschark & P. E. Spencer (Eds.), *The Oxford handbook of deaf studies in language: Research, policy and practice* (pp. 94–112) New York, NY: Oxford University Press.
Paul, R. (2007). *Language disorders from infancy through adolescence: Assessment and Intervention* (3rd ed.). Mosby Elsevier: St. Louis, Missouri.
Rinaldi, P., Baruffaldi, F., Burdo, S., & Caselli, M. C. (2013). Linguistic and pragmatic skills in toddlers with cochlear implant. *International Journal of Language & Communication Disorders, 48*, 715–725.
Rinaldi, P. & Caselli, M. C. (2009). Lexical and grammatical abilities in deaf Italian preschoolers: The role of duration of formal language experience. *Journal of Deaf Studies and Deaf Education, 14*, 63–75.
Sacks, H., Schegloff, E. A., & Jefferson, G. (1974). A simplest systematics for the organization of turn-taking for conversation. *Language, 50*(4), 696–735.
Schegloff, E. A. (1997). Whose text? Whose context? *Discourse & Society, 8*, 165–187.
Schegloff, E. A., Jefferson, G., & Sacks, H. (1977). The preference for self-correction in the organisation of repair in conversation. *Language, 53*, 361–382.
Sidnell, J. (2010) *Conversation analysis: An introduction*. West Sussex: Wiley.
Spencer, P. E. (1993). Communication behaviors of infants with hearing loss and their hearing mothers. *Journal of Speech and Hearing Research, 36*, 311–321.
Stinson, M. S., & Foster, S. (2000). Socialization of deaf children and youths in school. In P. E. Spencer, C. J. Erting, & M. Marschark (Eds.),*The deaf child in the family at school* (pp. 191–209). Mahwah, NJ: Lawrence Erlbaum Associates.
Toe, D., Beattie, R., & Barr, M. (2007). The development of pragmatic skills in children who are severely and profoundly deaf. *Deafness and Education International, 9*(2), 101–117.
Toe, D. M., & Paatsch, L. E. (2013). The conversational skills of school-aged children with cochlear implants. *Cochlear Implants International, 14*(2), 67–79.
Tye-Murray, N. (2003). Conversational fluency of children who use cochlear implants. *Ear and Hearing, 24*(1 Suppl.), 82S–89S.
Vaccari, C., & Marschark, M. (1997). Communication between parents and deaf children: implications for social-emotional development. *Journal of Child Psychology and Psychiatry, 38*, 793–801.
Volterra, V., Capirci, O., & Caselli, M. C. (2001). What atypical populations can reveal about language development: the contrast between deafness and Williams syndrome. *Language and Cognitive Processes, 16*, 219–239.
Wilkinson, A., & Brinton, J. (2003). Speech intelligibility rating of cochlear implant children: Inter-rater reliability. *Cochlear Implant International, 4*(1), 22–30.
Wood, D. J., Wood, H. A., Griffiths, A. J., Howarth, S. P., & Howarth, C. I. (1982). The structure of conversations with 6- to 10-year-old deaf children. *Journal of Child Psychology, Psychiatry, and Allied Disciplines, 23*, 295–308.
Yont, K. M., Hewitt, L. E., & Miccio, A. W. (2002). What did you say? Understanding conversational breakdowns in children with speech and language impairments. *Clinical Linguistics and Phonetics, 16*(4), 265–285.

10

Addressing Diversity in Teaching Deaf Learners to Write

Connie Mayer

TEACHING WRITING

In keeping with the theme of this volume, the focus of this chapter is on diversity—specifically, on how to take diversity into account when teaching deaf learners to write. The emphasis is on how educators can develop a program for teaching writing that is flexible enough to meet the needs of an increasingly wide range of deaf learners. To that end, diversity is examined as it exists in the population of deaf learners and has been realized in their writing outcomes. Such a consideration is necessary, because planning for diversity in writing programs and interventions requires taking into account the characteristics of the learner beyond the audiogram, as well as the intended goals for these learners—goals that will be as varied as the learners themselves. In other words, there is no one deaf learner who represents the group, and no one outcome to which they can all be directed—beyond a very general notion of "improved writing" or "realized potential."

Such a focus on writing and questions of diversity is especially timely for a number of reasons. First, it could be argued that at no period in the history of the field has there been greater diversity in the cohort of deaf learners and in the range of literacy outcomes they might achieve (Archbold, 2015; Mayer & Leigh, 2010), even in the area of writing in which the research has historically been less robust (Mayer, 2010; Williams & Mayer, 2015). In addition, it would reasonable to suggest that writing is playing an increasingly diverse and critical role for deaf learners in the context of the communication technologies available in the current environment. Although deaf individuals have always depended on writing as a means for communication, its utility was limited by the nature of the available technologies in which writing played a role (such as TTYs). With the introduction and proliferation of a growing range of communication technologies and social media (texting, e-mail, and Facebook, for example), the ability to write effectively is assuming a role in the lives of deaf individuals greater than at any time in the past (see Chapter 17). These text-driven technologies afford deaf learners access to the hearing world, and to unfettered communication in ways that are equal to that of their hearing peers, provided they have the writing ability to use these tools effectively.

A focus on writing is also important because this is the area of literacy education that has received less attention historically than reading for both deaf and hearing children (Kress, 1994; Marschark et al., 2002; Mayer, 2010; Moores, 1987). This lack of pedagogical attention is perplexing given that most individuals would characterize writing as more difficult than reading, and that it is one of the most demanding cognitive activities in which most learners engage (Singer & Bashir, 2004). Therefore, concentrating on the status of writing instruction and any associated research should be a priority for the field of literacy education more broadly (Troia, 2007), and deaf education in particular (Mayer, 2010).

In this chapter, a model for teaching writing to deaf learners is presented—a model that can be implemented flexibly to meet a wide spectrum of student needs from the early years to high school, even into college and university. An argument is made that this model is grounded in a sound theoretical framework, is based on what constitutes effective practice in teaching writing to hearing learners, and can be effective in addressing questions of diversity—in learners and in outcomes—in teaching deaf learners to write. Although English is the language referenced most often in this chapter, the discussion is applicable to other alphabetic languages and, with some adaptation, to syllabic and logographic languages as well.

THEORETICAL UNDERPINNINGS

The model for teaching writing that is being argued for in this chapter is grounded in two understandings. The first is that a well-established theoretical framework and solid research evidence inform the pedagogical approach, and that it be based on a consideration of what all skilled writers do, and what is critical in the process of learning to write and writing effectively. The second is the contention that deaf learners are not different than hearing learners in what it is they need to know and do in the process of writing and learning to write, and they must gain control of the same foundational requisites as their hearing peers if they are, ultimately, to become competent writers (Mayer, 2007; Mayer & Trezek, 2011; Paul & Lee, 2010; Trezek et al., 2010). These two understandings are examined in more detail in the sections that follow.

A Model of the Writing Process

Prior to the 1970s, the focus in writing instruction and research was on product (Nystrand, 2006), and this played out in practice via an emphasis on form and correctness (such as spelling, punctuation, and grammar). This emphasis shifted in the latter third of the 20th century with a move from focusing mainly on the product to also attending to the process (Bereiter & Scardamalia, 1987; Berninger & Swanson, 1994; Flower & Hayes, 1980). This shift was characterized by a rethinking of writing as a recursive rather than a linear process—a process that encompasses planning, organizing, generating, and revising a text. In contrast to earlier notions of learning to write that tended to privilege the quality of the written product, in a process model all aspects of the composing process are attended to and valued, highlighting the tensions writers face as they go about organizing their thoughts into the grammatically bound, linear sequence of a written text (Collins & Gentner, 1980).

The composing model proposed by Bereiter and Scardamalia (1987) captures the essence of this shift and is informative in thinking about what effective writers do, and thus also provides direction for what needs to be taught (Figure 10.1).

In their model, Bereiter and Scardamalia (1987) proposed a tension between two problem spaces in the writing process that they have described as the content space and the rhetorical space. The content space is tied up with what the writer wants to say. This content knowledge—the writer's meanings and understandings—are conceptualized intramentally in the language of everyday discourse, in the abbreviated inner language of cognition (Mayer & Wells, 1996; Vygotsky, 1978).

The rhetorical space is concerned with how to say what is meant, in how to move ideas from the content to the rhetorical space so that the intended meaning is captured as clearly as possible in the written form. The challenge for all writers is to rearticulate their intramental meanings in the language of the text, taking into account the constraints of text production during the process. These constraints include making meaning with an absent interlocutor, without the benefit of the auditory and visual aspects of face-to-face communication, necessitating

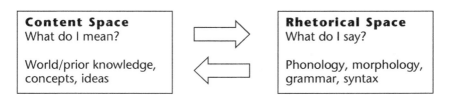

Figure 10.1 Model of the composing process.
Source: Bereiter, C., & M. Scardamalia. 1987. *The psychology of written composition*. Hillsdale, NJ: Lawrence Erlbaum Associates. From *The Psychology of Written Composition* by Carl Bereiter and Marlene Scardamalia. Reproduced by permission of Taylor and Francis Group, LLC, a division of Informa plc.

greater precision in the use of language, and providing more expansion and elaboration of thought than is required when speaking or signing (Halliday, 1989, 1993; Olson, 1977, 1993).

A fundamental requisite for this reformulation of meaning in the rhetorical space is a threshold level of competence in a primary form of the language to be written. Although meaning in the content space can be made in any language (signed or spoken), capturing this meaning in print requires that the writer construct this meaning in the language of the text (Mayer, 1999). In this way, the spoken language provides the foundation for the morphosyntactic and semantic understandings, and the development of the phonological awareness and other code-related abilities needed for learning to write (Whitehurst & Lonigan, 1998; but see also Dickinson et al. [2003] for a review). Singer and Bashir (2004) referred to this as being able to encode implicitly in the process of text generation, relying on the intuitive knowledge of the language that is an outcome of having acquired it.

Beginning writers rely on this foundation and compose as they speak, trying to capture in text what they can already say, while simultaneously sorting out encoding challenges such as spelling and letter formation. More experienced writers have generally mastered these encoding skills and the mechanics of writing, but continue to wrestle with the central challenge of composition, capturing what is meant in what is said. It is in this process that writing becomes a recursive activity, one in which skilled writers view the text as a malleable object that needs to be reread and revised as many times as needed, anticipating where an intended reader might need more clarification or explanation and then making changes accordingly. This requires that the writer have adequate control, not only of the language of the text, but also of the lower frequency vocabulary, greater morphosyntactic complexity, and textual coherence that writing demands. The claim being made in this chapter is that an understanding of this writing process must be taken into account when developing a model for teaching writing if the approach is going to be effective.

Diversity Not Difference

There is no theoretical argument or research evidence base to suggest that this model of the composing process does not apply to deaf learners, nor that deaf learners would differ from their hearing counterparts with respect to what it is they need to know and master if they are going to become skilled writers (Mayer & Trezek, 2015). Evidence from other diverse groups of writers (such as language-minority learners, those with low socioeconomic status, and those with learning disabilities) supports this contention (see Ehri [2009] for a discussion). In other words, to become competent writers, deaf learners are not different in terms of what they need to know and master, because the process of learning to write is essentially the same across populations. The differences rest in the nature of what the learners bring to the activity and how these differences can be accommodated during the teaching and learning process.

As noted earlier, language proficiency is fundamental to learning to write, and there is general agreement that learners who present with deficiencies in the language system have concomitant struggles with text generation (Pugh et al., 2006; Singer & Bashir, 2004). Given the difficulties that deaf learners have traditionally faced in acquiring the spoken language of the text, it is not surprising that learning to write would present a singular set of challenges (Geers, 2006). "In the absence of this language foundation, deaf writers are put in the untenable position of learning to write when they have minimal control of the language that has to be committed to paper" (Mayer, 2016, p. 360).

Arguments have been made that bilingual deaf learners who are proficient in a signed first language (L1) (such as American Sign Language) can rely on this L1 in the composing process, bypassing the need for face-to-face proficiency in the second language (L2) (such as English). However, this contention runs counter to the available evidence from other bilingual contexts in which it is well established that L2 proficiency is necessary to construct meaning effectively and readily in text in L2 (Berman, 1994; Bialystok, 2011; Cummins, 2000; Freedman et al., 1983; Yau, 1991). And although there is scant evidence in this area to consider with respect to deaf bilinguals, the available research indicates difficulties in learning to write, even when writers have relatively strong signed language abilities (e.g., Singleton et al., 2004), often being unable to capture in print what is intended in their own signed productions (Marschark, 1993).

Although L1 proficiency can be supportive during this process as a consequence of some interdependence, or cross-linguistic transfer, this association between languages is not straightforward—sometimes yielding benefits, sometimes deficits, and sometimes no consequences at all—resulting in effects that can be characterized as positive, negative, or neutral (Bialystok, 2011). Therefore it seems reasonable to suggest that developing proficiency in a face-to-face form of the language of the text is necessary for all deaf learners, just as it is for their hearing counterparts, even for those who have another first language in place, whether L1 is signed or spoken (see Mayer and Akamatsu [2011], Mayer and Leigh [2010], Mayer and Wells [1996], and Mayer and Trezek [2015] for discussions).

With respect to the learning and teaching of writing, there can be no diversity on this point: a threshold level of face-to-face proficiency *in the language that is to be read and written* is the price of admission. That being said, diversity does come in to play with respect to the ways in which this language foundation can be developed. For some deaf learners, the spoken language of the text is acquired primarily via audition and the use of hearing technologies. For others, this auditory input is supplemented to varying degrees by visual modalities (such as speech-reading, sign support, and cued speech). The key issue is that proficiency in the language is established—the modality (spoken or signed) is extraneous to this fundamental point (see Mayer 2015 for a discussion). This understanding backgrounds all further discussion of teaching writing presented in this chapter.

DIVERSITY IN THE POPULATION OF LEARNERS

The population of deaf learners has always been a heterogeneous one, and it was never possible to identify a "typical" deaf learner. Although this was ever the case, it would be fair to say that the current cohort of deaf learners has become increasingly diverse given the changing context in the field. As Archbold (2015) argues, advances in hearing technologies including improved hearing aids, cochlear implants (CIs), middle ear implants, and bone conduction hearing implants have rendered audiological definitions of hearing loss as rather arbitrary, and designing educational programs on the basis of hearing loss may not be appropriate. In other words, although deaf learners may still be described as being deaf or hard of hearing—or having a loss that is mild, moderate, severe, or profound—the educational implications of these "labels" are increasingly difficult to predict.

This is particularly the case with respect to learners with more profound hearing losses. In the past, this was the group of deaf learners who had minimal meaningful access to spoken language given the limits of the hearing technologies that were available, who were most often educated in schools for the deaf, and who faced the most significant obstacles in developing language and literacy. Although some in this cohort did develop spoken language, they represented the minority. Rather, these were the deaf learners who were most likely to have used a signed language as their primary means of communication.

In contrast, in the current climate, the majority of profoundly deaf learners (where the technology is available) now receive CIs, bilaterally and at increasingly younger ages, even in the presence of additional needs. This has allowed for the development of age-appropriate spoken language for many learners with profound hearing losses, allowing them to function as well as (or even better than) learners who are not as "audiologically deaf." In fact, recent indications are that learners with moderate to severe losses are now emerging as the group who face more challenges educationally and in the development of language and literacy.

It is also important to emphasize that even learners with mild and unilateral losses can experience difficulties achieving age-appropriate communication, language, and educational outcomes (Delage & Teller, 2007; Lieu et al., 2010; Moeller et al., 2007). In the past, these were seen as the students who would have "less trouble" developing language and learning to read and write because they could "hear more," representing the often overlooked deaf cohort in the mainstream. In the past, such a perspective (although not grounded in research evidence) was understandable, given the stark disparity between these deaf learners and those with more profound losses. But as has been pointed out, in the current context these characterizations are no longer tenable, and level of hearing loss has become a very poor predictor of whether a learner will face challenges in developing language and literacy, including learning to write.

Beyond diversity as it relates to hearing loss, there are growing numbers of students with additional or complex needs. It has always been the case that there was a relatively greater number of deaf learners presenting with multiple needs than in the hearing population, given the etiologies of hearing loss that are often associated with concurrent disabilities (such as rubella, meningitis, and numerous syndromes) (van Dijk et al., 2010). However, medical and surgical advances have served to alter this landscape and increase this number. Children born at extremely early gestational ages, who would not have survived in the past, are now being saved through intensive medical interventions. They are presenting not only as deaf students, but also as those with more complex needs (Akamatsu et al., 2008; Mulla et al., 2013). Estimates of this cohort with additional needs ranges from 25% to 35% (Bruce et al., 2008; Luckner & Ayantoye, 2013; Power & Hyde, 2002) to 40% or more (Blackorby & Knokey, 2006; Mitchell, 2004; Mitchell & Karchmer, 2006), with Hauser and Marschark (2008) concluding there is an abundant evidence base indicating that learning disabilities and other neurological, physical or psychological issues affect a significant proportion of deaf learners.

The implications for practice are that educators will need to design writing programs and instruction to accommodate a diverse range of deaf learners, including those with complex needs, those who come from other countries, those who had a late start in schooling, those with a weak foundation in the language of the text, and those who use a range of first languages (spoken and/or signed). Imagining that there will be one goal or set of outcomes that could be identified for such a diverse cohort seems ill-advised. Rather, it could be argued that the range of learning goals will be as varied as the population itself. In practice, this means determining appropriate goals for individual learners through effective assessment, and then evaluating the extent to which these individual goals have been met by examining outcomes. (Assessment plays a critical role in planning any writing program, but it is beyond the scope of this chapter to provide a comprehensive overview of this topic. See Mayer [2016] for further discussion.) It would be foolhardy to imagine that any writing program or intervention, no matter how well implemented, could serve to bring all students to the same outcome (age-appropriate writing development, for example) when there is so much diversity in the cohort of learners.

DIVERSITY OF OUTCOMES: ACHIEVED AND ACHIEVABLE

Although there has always been wide diversity in the population of deaf learners, it could be argued that, at least historically, there was much less diversity evident in terms of literacy outcomes—an observation not worthy of celebration given that, overall, the performance of deaf learners has been poor. In reviewing the literature from the early 20th century onward, a consistent finding is evident with respect to writing outcomes: deaf individuals have struggled with all aspects of writing and learning to write, rarely attaining levels commensurate with their hearing age peers (see Mayer [2010] for a discussion and overview). They have faced difficulties with text production that include phonology, morphology, lexicon, grammar, syntax, conceptual coherence, and text and discourse structures (e.g., Conte et al., 1996; Musselman & Szanto, 1998; Taeschner, 1988; Yoshinaga-Itano et al., 1996), and with the composing process itself (e.g., Albertini et al., 1994; Kelly, 1988; Mayer, 1999). The examples in Box 10.1a and Box 10.1b illustrate how these challenges are evident in the writing of both younger and older deaf writers.

It would be worth noting that this characterization of deaf writers may be underestimating, or at the very least misrepresenting, the writing outcomes of deaf students in mainstream settings, because they are often not included in the study sampling (Antia et al., 2009). This is not to say that all deaf writers in general education classrooms are working at age-appropriate levels, but rather to suggest their writing evidences issues that are markedly different from those described earlier, and may have less to do with their hearing loss specifically, than with more generic issues that apply to all learners (such as the nature of the instruction) (Antia et al., 2005).

Recent studies of writers with CIs are showing a shift in writing outcomes, with evidence of improved performance being realized as

---

Box 10.1a Text Written by an 8-Year-Old Deaf Student

Boy walk see to cat say "Meow" he pet to cat.
Boy walk to but balloon said help
me boy hear to balloon boy climb
he got to balloon

> **Box 10.1b Text Written by a College-Age Deaf Student**
>
> Two smarts men have the equipment to the depth of ocean with bowl head and heavy outfit, impossible to go there but it is successful.

a consequence of using this hearing technology (e.g., Geers & Hayes, 2011; Spencer et al., 2003) (see the examples in Box 10.2a and Box 10.2b). From this nascent evidence, it seems there has been a pronounced, positive shift in the writing outcomes for deaf learners so that many more are performing at age-appropriate levels.

And even when learners with CIs are not working at grade level, their writing does not evidence the same weaknesses in morphology, syntax, and so on, that typified the writing of deaf learners in the past (see Figure 10.2). This is not to propose that learners with CIs do not face challenges in learning to write, but rather that they may differ from the challenges deaf learners faced in the past, and perhaps have more in common with the those of deaf learners in general education settings as described by Antia et al. (2009).

Clearly there has been (and continues to be) a range of outcomes across the diverse population of deaf writers—some of which are closer to the goal of age-appropriate performance than others. This raises the question of what "one goal" means in terms of teaching the individual deaf learner to write. It would not be reasonable for the benchmark to be age-appropriate outcomes for all deaf learners, any more than it would be the expectation for all hearing learners. Rather, it would be more reasonable and realistic to argue for setting writing goals that are matched to the needs and potential of the learner. The end game is not the same for everyone, and diversity in outcomes is inevitable, with success being measured differently given such a heterogeneous deaf population. This is the inherent messiness that diversity engenders, that educators need to contend with, and that must be addressed in practice.

> **Box 10.2a Text Written by a 10-Year-Old Deaf Student, Implanted Unilaterally at 4;7 Years**
>
> *My Dog*
>
> Over the summer we got a dog named Teddy. He is a rascal. We don't know what to do with his biting, though. We still love him though! He has a tennis ball that he goes after like crazy! One time me and my dad were playing monkey-in-the-middle with him and the tennis ball. It went on for hours! When we first got him, he was as red as a fox. Now he is getting lighter.

> **Box 10.2b Text Written by a 16-Year-Old Deaf Student, Implanted Unilaterally at 4;5 Years**
>
> *Ableism Around the World [an excerpt from a longer text]*
> In a novel, events occur that sometimes may mirror those that occur in reality, including those in the past, present or even the future. "The View From a Kite" is about a teenaged girl, Gwen MacIntyre who has Tuberculosis. Due to the nature of the content of this novel, it can relate to the past as well as to the current idea of the social justice issue ableism.
>
> In the past, when an epidemic struck the world, those who had the illness in question were often hurried off to emergency, or makeshift, hospitals to prevent the spread of said illness. Such diseases include the Spanish Flu and the Bubonic Plague; when these struck years ago, extreme measures were made to ensure that patients would be isolated from civilization to prevent further contamination of the general healthier populations.

ADDRESSING DIVERSITY IN PRACTICE

In what may appear to be a departure from the theme of this volume—that of diverse pathways to one goal—an argument is made for a single model or conceptualization of what constitutes effective practice in teaching deaf learners to write. This should not be taken as an argument for a single prescriptive curriculum or program, but rather as a way of thinking about what is fundamental in teaching writing that provides a framework or set of principles to inform practice. The instructional approach that is proposed here is grounded in the theoretical underpinnings described earlier, and has proven efficacy when it has been implemented with hearing learners from a range of backgrounds. This pedagogical model is most usually referred to as the *process writing model* (Graves, 1983), and in its implementation it reflects what is known about the composing process and what skilled writers do. This includes the integration of reading and writing instruction (Clay, 1982, 1983), and an emphasis on using writing purposefully for authentic purposes, viewing accuracy and correctness as subordinate to meaning making.

A Process Writing Model

A process approach to teaching writing is the most prevalent and widespread pedagogical model used with hearing learners, and although research into its efficacy has been uneven (for example, the extent to which explicit teaching plays a role), it remains the preferred approach for teaching writing across a range of contexts, with general

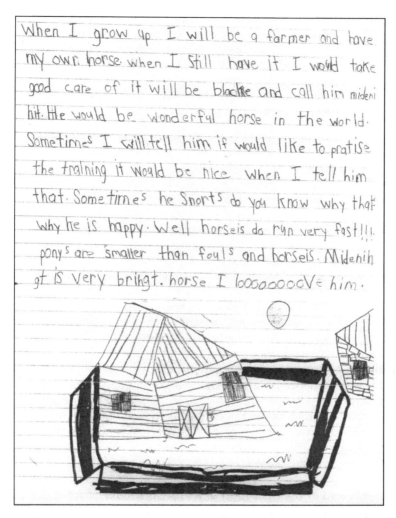

Figure 10.2 Text written by 7-year-old deaf student, implanted unilaterally at 2 years.

agreement that there is no compelling evidence to desert the model (see Pritchard and Honeycutt [2006] for discussion). Although a process approach to teaching writing may be realized in practice in different ways (such as Writer's Workshop) (Calkins, 1994), the defining feature at the core of this approach is that it reflects the process in which proficient writers engage—that of planning, independently composing, writing multiple drafts, then reviewing and revising numerous times based on feedback from others along the way (Wong & Berninger, 2004).

The writing process has its weaknesses; it is poorly implemented in many instances; it is not a panacea. But it is a better candidate for improving writing performance than the traditional approach ... we must listen to the critics; we must be willing to rethink and adjust our theories, procedures and practices. But there is not sufficient evidence to cause us to abandon the writing process. (Cramer [2001], as cited in Pritchard and Honeycutt [2006], p. 282)

Given the scant evidence that any previous approaches or interventions for teaching writing have been generally successful with deaf learners (only three intervention studies in 20 years for emerging deaf writers) (Williams & Mayer, 2015), there would be no reason to think that a process approach would not also be appropriate for deaf learners, and it might actually target those areas of difficulty—regulating the processes underlying proficient composing, especially planning and revising—that most struggling writers face (see Troia [2007] for a discussion). There is some history of the use of process approaches with deaf learners (e.g., Conway, 1985; Ewoldt, 1985; Mayer, 1994; Williams, 1993, 2011; Wolbers, 2008; Wolbers et al., 2012), and the evidence from these studies suggests that students were able to engage in the process and came to see writing as meaningful, purposeful, and a tool for communication (in other words, the content space). But despite these positive shifts, weaknesses remained with respect to linguistic form, including grammar and syntax (the rhetorical space). This should not be taken as evidence for giving up on a process approach, but rather an indication that without face-to-face to facility in the language of the text in place as a precondition, the outcomes that can be realized in a process approach are constrained. As has been noted earlier, the expectation that any writing program can also serve as the vehicle for teaching the language, is misplaced.

Elements and Implementation of a Process Model

A process approach to the teaching of writing can be implemented flexibly to meet the needs of both beginning writers and those who are more experienced, those who are skilled or less able, whether they are educated in a school for the deaf or a mainstream setting, taught one-to-one or in group, or whether they use signed or spoken communication. The key understandings driving the implementation of this approach are that writing is a messy process that involves the planning, generating, and revising of texts; that the process has as much value as the product; and that writing is always done for a purpose (Collins & Gentner, 1980). One of main differences when working with more skilled, more mature writers, compared with more beginning or less able writers, is not in the nature of the process itself or the reasons for writing, but in the length and sophistication of the texts produced and the time spent revising a single piece of writing. Although there is not a single way to implement a process writing approach, there are a number of elements that are fundamental to putting this approach into practice that apply across a diverse range of learners and teaching goals.

Time on Task

The first and most basic element is that sufficient time in the schedule be devoted to writing. It is ironic that although writing is an area of relative difficulty for all learners, and arguably more so for those with hearing loss, research indicates that very few programs meet the threshold of 90 minutes per week that has been deemed necessary to implement a process approach effectively (Troia, 2007). Admittedly, devoting this much time to writing can be challenging even in classroom settings, and even more so when working as an itinerant or visiting teacher when the weekly contact hours with a student may be less than 90 minutes in total. As in everything, there is no easy answer, but process writing time can do "double duty" (such as applying the process model to working on assignments from other subject areas—an essay required for history class—or developing the writing skills needed across the curriculum, such as a writing a summary) or can be used as the opportunity to develop language abilities more broadly (vocabulary development, for example).

Engaging in an Authentic Process

Beyond devoting enough time to writing, it is important that writers engage in the activity of writing authentically with respect to both process (learning to do what skilled writers do) and product (writing to serve a meaningful purpose). This stands in marked contrast to the writing instruction that has often typified the field, in which the emphasis is inordinately on the correctness of the final product, with minimal attention paid to the process of text creation. Many traditional writing programs feature strictly sequenced curricula with an emphasis on direct instruction and activities such as cloze or sentence completion (for example, the Appletree curriculum for developing written language) (Anderson et al., 2010). Although there is a place for this type of explicit intervention, it is not a model that addresses what is really important in developing as a writer, nor is there any evidence that these sorts of programs have been efficacious for deaf learners.

Therefore, the second element critical to a process approach is that the process of planning, generating, and revising a text is privileged and made explicit. To accomplish this, the teacher can (a) design a writing program with a focus on process (such as Writer's Workshop), (b) model the process overtly, and (c) provide learners with the metalanguage to talk about the process (for example, using terms such as *writing a first draft, editing,* and so on). In addition to modeling the steps of the writing process, the teacher can also model the strategies that can be used in planning, creating, and editing a text (see Mayer [2016] for a detailed discussion of strategies and examples).

An effective way that modeling can be done is via "think-alouds"—a strategy by which a teacher (or more expert writer) verbalizes his or her covert mental processes aloud—affording the learner insights into what more skilled writers do (for example, I need to add a word there to make the meaning clearer, I should start a new paragraph here, I should separate these ideas with a comma, I need a better opening sentence). In turn, these become strategies the developing writer can take onboard to use as self-regulation strategies as they compose (Zimmerman, 2002). This explicit modeling has been shown to be a critical pedagogical element for all writers, but especially for those who have difficulty, keeping in mind there will be great variability in what is taught directly and in the adaptations made for writers who struggle (Graham et al., 2003; Troia, 2007).

The instructional strategy at the heart of a process approach is the student–teacher conference, because it is during these interactions that the teacher works individually with writers to assist them in developing and revising their texts, and in identifying those strategies that can be supportive during the process. These conferences should not be thought of as lessons with a predetermined goal, but rather as generative sessions in which the teaching focus arises as a consequence of the interactions with the writers and the discussion about their text. This allows the teacher to be responsive to the needs of the individual learner, setting goals and proposing strategies that can be tailored to the individual, and that can focus on aspects of meaning (such as adding more information for clarification), and/or form (the use of quotation marks, for example). The intention is these strategies will be applied not only to the current piece of writing, but also, with practice, to future work as well. Because these conferences are not lengthy, they can happen frequently even in a classroom setting, and there can be multiple conferences about a single piece of writing (during the planning stage and again during the revising stage). This is especially easy to manage when working one-to-one in itinerant settings.

A general rule to follow in the process approach is that the focus should be on meaning first (the content space), asking the writer, "tell me what you wrote about" and then asking the writer to read the text aloud. Approaching the conference in this way allows writers an opportunity to say more than they may have written down, include this additional information in a revised version of the text, and/or reorganize the information to make the meaning clearer. This focus is critical, because a central challenge of the revising process is to rework the content of the text so that it is coherent, and any mismatches between the intended meaning and the text can be resolved. This runs counter to the tendency to focus first (or primarily) on the surface features of form that can be addressed more easily (such as putting capital letters at the beginning of sentences, using correct spelling), and that are more typical of what all struggling writers attend to during the revising process.

This focus on content is possible even when the writer has a relatively poor command of the language of the text. In Figure 10.3, we see that, after conferencing with the teacher, this 7-year-old deaf writer was able to add information to clarify and expand the meaning of the text.

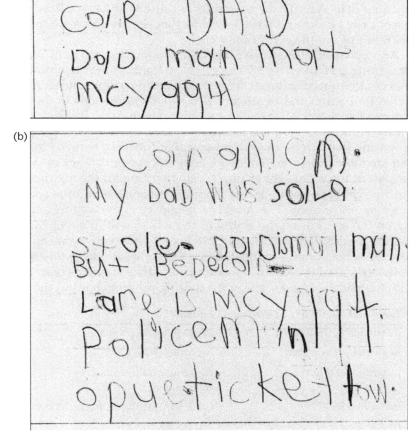

Figure 10.3 (a) First draft of a text written by a 7-year-old deaf student: "Dad was in the car. Dad was mad at the man. The license was MCY 994." (b) Second, revised draft of a text written by a 7-year-old deaf student: "My Dad was near the store. Dad was mad at the man because he smashed the car. The license number is MCY 994. The policeman gave the man two tickets."

Now attention can be turned to matters of form that for this student are significant, illustrative of a writer who is limited in learning to write by her lack of implicit control of the language of the text (and perhaps the language of instruction).

Writing for Authentic Purposes

In addition to engaging in an authentic process, it is equally important that writing be seen as a tool for meaningful communication, for achieving a genuine goal. In the absence of such purpose, learners are often reluctant to write, are disengaged, and see writing as an academic exercise—a concern that teachers often raise with respect to deaf writers. Therefore, during the planning stage of any piece of writing, the first step is to identify the reason for writing in the first place. These reasons can be as varied as the writers themselves, and apply regardless of the age or the skill of the writer.

An expedient framework for thinking about the range of reasons for writing is Halliday's (1975) hierarchical framework that outlines the uses of face-to-face language from the earliest developing instrumental (What do I want) and regulatory (Do as I say) functions to the more complex heuristic (Tell me why) and informative (I've got something to tell you) functions (see Table 10.1). Across the hierarchy there are genres of writing that can be used to achieve that function, realized in ways that are more or less sophisticated, accommodating a range of skill on the part of the writer. For example, using writing for the instrumental function could be as simple as a shopping list or a memo, or as complex as a persuasive essay. This level of complexity in the writing depends not on the age, but on the ability of the writer, and in either case the writing is serving the same purpose (to get what you want), and can be seen as meaningful by the learner. This is what makes this framework particularly valuable in working with diverse groups of learners, and in broadening the scope of the writing program beyond the more

Table 10.1 Functions of Written Language

Instrumental (I want)	Request, cajole, persuade
Regulatory (Do as I say)	Direct behavior
Interactional (Me and you)	Disagree, promise, criticize, compliment
Personal (I feel)	Complain, justify, express emotions
Imaginative (Let's pretend)	Tell stories, role play
Heuristic (Tell me why)	Clarify, predict, probe
Informative (I've got something to tell you)	Describe, compare, discuss, suggest

Source: Adapted from Halliday, M. A. K. (1975). *Learning how to mean*. London: Edward Arnold.

typical assignments seen in writing classrooms (such as a daily diary or writing on an assigned topic [e.g., Albertini & Shannon, 1996]).

Within this framework it is also easy to see a role for both narrative and expository texts. Although narratives predominate in the writing that students do during the early years of schooling (Cutler & Graham, 2008; Duke, 2000), it is the expository texts that constitute the bulk of the writing they do in later grades and in work (report writing and essays, for example). In general, these expository texts are more challenging to write because they are more removed from the everyday discourse of face-to-face communication, and are typified by the use of lower frequency vocabulary and the complex grammar and syntax of written discourse.

To reflect a better balance, it would be important to provide learners with more opportunities to develop expository writing. To this end, the writing of expository texts should be introduced during the early years to accomplish those functions that require this type of text (such as writing instructions for playing a game, as an instance of the regulatory function). For all learners, it can be useful to read expository texts (summaries, essays, newspaper articles, and so on) aloud (in spoken and/or signed language) as part of the writing program. This strategy exposes students to the language and structure of these written forms—forms that are often unfamiliar, because learners have had much less experience with them. Consider the fact that most students are asked to write some of these genres, such as an essay, before they have read one or had one read to them, thus having little sense of what constitutes a well-written paper. Contrast this with the number of narratives in which students have engaged before they are ever expected to write one.

Although an argument has been made for writing for a purpose and on a topic of interest to the learner, this does not rule out teachers introducing particular genres or assigning topics to ensure all aspects of the writing curriculum are attended to, and to make the links between writing and other subject areas as part of the process writing program (writing a summary of an article or a book chapter, for example).

Developing a Sense of Audience

In conjunction with having a reason for writing, developing a sense of audience is key to a process model. This is tied up with understanding that what is written has to stand alone in making meaning. In other words, learners must develop the ability to write and revise a text, anticipating where the reader may misunderstand or misconstrue what has been written, and be able to address this in the absence of any immediate feedback from the reader.

One of the best ways to develop this sense of audience is to read texts aloud to a group, to the teacher, or to a peer. For example, "Author's

Chair," a feature of Writer's Workshop, provides a student author with the opportunity to read a piece of writing aloud to the class. Classmates provide feedback by asking questions and making comments, thus providing the writer with insights into how the text has been understood and perceived by others, and where revisions need to be made to achieve the best intended meaning. Conversely, it can also be useful to a read a text to the author of that text, because it puts writers in the position of being the audience for their own composition, and requires they identify any deficiencies in what has been written. Ultimately, these opportunities for reading texts aloud provide writers with the input that informs the editing and revising process, modeling how to "read like a writer," and externalizing a process that, in a skilled writer, has become internalized.

Rethinking the Role for Direct Instruction

It was noted earlier that prescriptive curricula have proved to be less than effective in teaching deaf learners to write, and lack the flexibility to address the needs of diverse learners. That said, there is a role for explicit instruction within a process approach (such as mini lessons in Writer's Workshop), with the proviso that this instruction is directed at goals that have been identified as a consequence of assessment or have arisen out of the conferencing process, and that they are elements that lend themselves to direct teaching. For example, it is possible to model the elements of the composing process or teach a strategy such as joining two independent clauses with a conjunction.

However, other grammatical aspects of writing (such as using articles correctly and word order) are not very amenable to explicit instruction, especially to younger learners in the elementary years (Graham et al., 2012). These elements of text generation rely in great measure on the intuitive knowledge of the language of the text, harkening back to the argument made earlier that it is not possible to write competently in the absence of language proficiency. Even for older learners for whom some explicit instruction can be effective, it is not possible to teach writing simply by presenting a set of rules to be followed. As Markman and Dietrich (1998) pointed out, although many systems can be described by rules, this is not the same thing as using the rules to carry out a process. Most learners of a second language can relate to the fact that it is easier to talk about the rules for how a language works (such as conjugating German verbs) than to put these rules into practice.

A PEDAGOGICAL MODEL TO ADDRESS DIVERSITY

An argument has been made in this chapter that the most effective approach to teaching writing to deaf learners is a process model, a position that is in line with both the theoretical and research evidence, and is grounded in an understanding of what skilled writers do. But more important, from the perspective of addressing issues of diversity, this is an approach that allows teachers to work with deaf students at their level of functioning regardless of age, grade, or educational setting. It is a flexible model that can be implemented to accommodate a diverse range of deaf students, moving each and every learner forward from where they started, to a writing goal that is attainable, meaningful, and appropriate. Although there is an emphasis in this approach on maintaining a balance between both meaning (what I want to say) and form (how do I say it), as there should be in all well-designed literacy programs (Pressley, 2006; Stanovich, 2000), it is always with the understanding that, at its core, writing should be viewed as a tool for communication, and for accomplishing authentic purposes.

Although implementing this approach with fidelity dictates that writing be taught as a creative, recursive process of planning, generation and revision, it is also possible to differentiate instruction within the model, particularly with respect to the reasons for writing, the length and complexity of the text produced, the focus for any revisions, and the relative emphasis on meaning and form (Xue & Meisels, 2004). These are determined not by the age, but by the ability of the writer, and in this way the model can be adapted to meet the needs of a diverse deaf cohort.

Given that there is a role for direct instruction, the process approach can be supplemented by more structured curricula or interventions as appropriate to address any identified gaps. For example, if a student is demonstrating weaknesses in vocabulary, there are discrete programs that can be implemented to work on this area (such as the Words Their Way series; for a description see http://www.pearsonhighered.com/educator/series/Words-Their-Way-Series/10888.page), or a system such as Visual Phonics that can be taught to support the encoding process (Trezek & Wang, 2006; Trezek et al., 2007). It should never be the case that teaching writing is reduced to the teaching of a set of skills, but there is a place for explicit, targeted instruction in a process model.

The one area that is not amenable to direct instruction is developing facility in the language sustaining the text. Although it is certainly the case that learning to write can provide unique insights into one's spoken language (Olson, 1977, 1994), and that reading and writing can support language development after a threshold level of competence is achieved, it is asking too much of any writing program to expect that it can be the vehicle for teaching the language—just as it is too much to expect any deaf student to acquire a language while simultaneously learning to write it. This far exceeds what is demanded of any hearing student in the process of writing and learning to write.

Instances when process approaches have been implemented with deaf students, but when outcomes have fallen short (e.g., Conway, 1985;

Ewoldt, 1985; Mayer, 1994; Williams, 1993, 2011; Wolbers, 2008; Wolbers et al., 2012), are illustrative of what happens when this dual learning is expected as an outcome of a writing program. This should not be construed as an indictment of the process model, and it should be noted that some gains were realized in their implementation, but rather it should be seen as an acknowledgment that a process model was never intended to be the vehicle for teaching language. It is a pedagogical approach for writing instruction that assumes a level of language proficiency as the entry point, and therefore the first order of business would be to develop this language base with those learners who have not yet acquired it. The good news in the current climate in the field is that greater numbers of deaf children are developing this language at age-appropriate or near-age-appropriate levels, allowing them to benefit from instruction via a process approach in a manner comparable with their hearing peers. Tracking the outcomes of this new cohort of deaf learners, with all their diversity, would make for a very worthwhile research agenda to provide evidence regarding the efficacy of this approach for this population of students.

Although there have been writing programs developed specifically for deaf learners, they have not proved to be particularly efficacious, or are limited in their scope. To broaden the focus, the emphasis in this chapter has been on applying what is known about effective writing instruction for all learners to the context of deaf education, and to propose a process model. The strength of this pedagogical approach in a time of increasing diversity is that it can be adapted and differentiated to accommodate the needs of a range of learners, and to target an array of learner outcomes. In this way, it can be viewed as an approach that has the best chance of improving the writing outcomes of all deaf learners—an aspect of literacy learning that has, historically, been the most difficult to achieve, but one that has ever-more currency in the diverse lives of deaf learners.

REFERENCES

Akamatsu, C. T., Mayer, C., & Hardy-Braz, S. (2008). Why considerations of verbal aptitude are important in educating deaf and hard-of-hearing students. In M. Marschark & P. Hauser (Eds.). *Deaf cognition: Foundations and outcomes* (pp. 131–169). New York, NY: Oxford University Press.

Albertini, J., Meath-Lang, B., & Harris, D. P. (1994). Voice as muse, message, and medium: The views of deaf college students. In K. B. Yancey (Ed.), *Voices on voice* (pp.172–190). Urbana, IL: National Council of Teachers of English.

Albertini, J., & Shannon, N. (1996). Kitchen notes, "the Grapevine," and other writing in childhood. *Journal of Deaf Studies and Deaf Education, 1,* 64–74.

Anderson, M., Boren, N. J., Kilgore, J., Howard, W., & Krohn, E. (2010). *The Appletree curriculum for developing written language* (2nd ed.). Austin, TX: Pro-Ed.

Antia, S. D., Jones, P. B., Reed, S., & Kreimeyer, K. H. (2009). Academic status and progress of deaf and hard-of-hearing students in general education classrooms. *Journal of Deaf Studies and Deaf Education, 14*(3), 293–311.

Antia, S., Reed, S., & Kreimeyer, K. (2005). The written language of deaf and hard-of-hearing students in public schools. *Journal of Deaf Studies and Deaf Education, 10*(3), 244–255.

Archbold, S. (2015). Being a deaf student: Changes in characteristics and needs. In H. Knoors & M. Marschark (Eds.), *Educating deaf learners: Creating a global evidence base* (pp. 23–46). New York, NY: Oxford University Press.

Bereiter, C., & Scardamalia, M. (1987). *The psychology of written composition.* Hillsdale, NJ: Lawrence Erlbaum Associates.

Berman, R. (1994). Learners' transfer of writing skills between languages. *TESL Canada Journal. 12,* 29–41.

Berninger, V. W., & Swanson, H. L. (1994). Modifying Hayes and Flower's model of skilled writing to explain beginning and developing writing. In J. S. Carlson & E. C. Butterfield (Eds.), *Advances in cognition and educational practice, Volume 2: Children's writing: Toward a process theory of the development of skilled writing* (pp. 57–81). Greenwich, CT: JAI Press.

Bialystok, E. (2011). Language proficiency and its implications for monolingual and bilingual children. In A. Y. Durgunnoğlu & C. Goldenberg (Eds.), *Language and literacy development in bilingual settings* (pp. 121–138). New York, NY: Guilford Press.

Blackorby, J., & Knokey, A. M. (2006). *A national profile of students with hearing impairments in elementary and middle school: A special topic report from the Special Education Elementary Longitudinal Study.* Menlo Park, CA: SRI International.

Bruce, S., Dinatale, P., & Ford, J. (2008). Meeting the needs of deaf and hard of hearing students with additional disabilities through professional teacher development. *American Annals of the Deaf, 153*(4), 368–375.

Calkins, L. (1994). *The art of teaching writing.* Portsmouth, NH: Heinneman.

Clay, M. (1982). Research update: Learning and teaching writing: A developmental perspective. *Language Arts, 59,* 65–70.

Clay, M. (1983). Getting a theory of writing. In B. Kroll & G. Wells (Eds.), *Explorations in the development of writing* (pp. 259–284). London: Wiley.

Collins, A. M., & Gentner, D. (1980). A framework for a cognitive theory of writing. In L. W. Gregg & E. Steinberg (Eds.), *Cognitive processes in writing* (pp. 51–72). Mahwah, NJ: Lawrence Erlbaum Associates.

Conte, M. P., Rampelli, L. P., & Volterra, V. (1996). Deaf children and the construction of written texts. In C. Pontecorvo & M. Orsolini (Eds.), *Children's early text construction* (pp. 303–319). Hillsdale, NJ: Lawrence Erlbaum Associates.

Conway, D. (1985). Children (re)creating writing: A preliminary look at the purpose of free choice writing of hearing impaired kindergarteners. *The Volta Review, 87,* 910126.

Cummins, J. (2000). *Language, power and pedagogy: Bilingual children in the crossfire.* Clevedon, UK: Multilingual Matters.

Cutler, L., & Graham, S. (2008). Primary grade writing instruction: A national survey. *Journal of Educational Psychology, 100*(4), 907–919.

Delage, H., & Teller, L. (2007). Language development and mild-to-moderate hearing loss: Does language normalize with age? *Journal of Speech, Language and Hearing Research, 50*(5), 1300–1313.

Dickinson, D. K., McCabe, A., Anastasopoulos, L., Peisner-Feinberg, E., & Poe, M. D. (2003). The comprehensive language approach to early literacy: The interrelationships among vocabulary, phonological sensitivity, and print knowledge among preschool-aged children. *Journal of Educational Psychology, 95*(3), 465–481.

Duke, N. K. (2000). 3.6 Minutes per day: The scarcity of informational texts in first grade. *Reading Research Quarterly, 35,* 202–224.

Ehri, L. (2009). Learning to read in English: Teaching phonics to beginning readers from diverse backgrounds. In L. M. Morrow, R. Rueda, & D. Lapp (Eds.), *Handbook of research on literacy and diversity* (pp. 292–319). New York, NY: Guilford Press.

Ewoldt, C. (1985). A descriptive study of the developing literacy of young hearing-impaired children. *Volta Review, 87,* 109–126.

Flower, L. S., & Hayes, J.R. (1980). The dynamics of composing: Making plans and juggling constraints. In L.W. Gregg & E. Steinberg (Eds.), *Cognitive processes in writing* (pp. 31–50). Mahwah, NJ: Lawrence Erlbaum Associates.

Freedman, A., Pringle, I., & Yalden, J. (1983). The writing process: Three orientations. In A. Freedman, I. Pringle, & J. Yalden (Eds.), *Learning to write: First language/second language.* London: Longman.

Geers, A. (2006). Spoken language in children with cochlear implants. In P. Spencer & M. Marschark (Eds.), *Advances in spoken language development of deaf and hard of hearing children* (pp. 244–270). New York, NY: Oxford University Press.

Geers, A., & Hayes, H. (2011). Reading, writing, and phonological processing skills of adolescents with 10 or more years of cochlear implants experience. *Ear and Hearing, 32,* 49S–59S.

Graham, S., Harris, K. R., Fink, B., & MacArthur, C. A. (2003). Primary grade teacher's instructional adaptations for struggling writers: A national survey. *Journal of Educational Psychology, 95,* 279–292.

Graham, S., McKeown, D., Kiuhara, S., & Harris, K. R. (2012). A meta-analysis of writing instruction for students in the elementary grades. *Journal of Educational Psychology, 104*(4), 879–896.

Graves, D. H. (1983). *Writing: Teachers and children at work.* Portsmouth, NH: Heinemann.

Halliday, M. A. K. (1975). *Learning how to mean.* London: Edward Arnold.

Halliday, M. A. K. (1989). *Spoken and written language.* Oxford: Oxford University Press.

Halliday, M. A. K. (1993). Towards a language-based theory of learning. *Linguistics and Education, 5,* 93–116.

Hauser, P., & Marschark, M. (2008). What we know and what we don't know about cognition and deaf learners. In M. Marschark & P. Hauser (Eds.), *Deaf cognition: Foundations and outcomes* (pp. 439–457). New York, NY: Oxford University Press.

Kelly, L. P. (1988). Relative automaticity without mastery: The grammatical decision making of deaf students. *Written Communication, 5*(3), 325–351.

Kress, G. (1994). *Learning to write* (2nd ed.). New York, NY: Routledge.

Lieu, J. E. C., Tye-Murray, N., Karzon, R. K., & Piccirillo, J. S. (2010). Unilateral hearing loss is associated with worse speech and language scores in children. *Pediatrics.*

Luckner, J., & Ayantoye, C. (2013). Itinerant teachers of students who are deaf or hard of hearing: Practices and preparation. *Journal of Deaf Studies and Deaf Education, 18*(3), 409–423.

Markman, A., & Dietrich, E. (1998). In defense of representation as mediation. *Psycoloquy, 9*(48).

Marschark, M. (1993). *Psychological development of deaf children.* New York, NY: Oxford University Press.

Marschark, M., Lang, H., & Albertini, J. (2002). *Educating deaf students: From research to practice.* New York, NY: Oxford University Press.

Mayer, C. (1994). Action research: The story of a partnership. In G. Wells (Ed.), *Changing schools from within: Creating communities of inquiry* (pp. 151–170). Portsmouth, NH: Heinemann.

Mayer, C. (1999). Shaping at the point of utterance: An investigation of the composing processes of the deaf student writer. *Journal of Deaf Studies and Deaf Education, 4*, 37–49.

Mayer, C. (2007). What matters in the early literacy development of deaf children. *Journal of Deaf Studies and Deaf Education, 12*, 411–431.

Mayer, C. (2010). The demands of writing and the deaf writer. In M. Marschark & P. Spencer (Eds.), *Oxford handbook of deaf studies, language, and education* (Vol. 2, pp. 144–155). New York, NY: Oxford University Press.

Mayer, C. (2015). Total communication: Looking back, moving forward. In M. Marschark & P. Spencer (Eds.), *The Oxford handbook of deaf studies in language: Research, policy, and practice* (pp. 31–44). New York, NY: Oxford University Press.

Mayer, C. (2016). Teaching writing: Principles into practice. In P. Moeller, D. Ertmer, & G. Stoel-Gammon (Eds.), *Promoting language, and literacy in children who are deaf or hard of hearing* (pp. 359–382). Baltimore, MD: Brookes Publishing.

Mayer, C., & Akamatsu, C. T. (2011). Bilingualism and literacy. In M. Marschark & P. Spencer (Eds.), *Oxford handbook of deaf studies, language and education* (2nd ed., Vol. 1, pp. 144–155). New York, NY: Oxford University Press.

Mayer, C., & Leigh, G. (2010). The changing context for sign bilingual education programs: Issues in language and the development of literacy. *International Journal of Bilingualism and Bilingual Education, 13*(2), 175–186.

Mayer, C., & Trezek, B. J. (2011). New (?) answers to old questions: Literacy development in D/HH learners. In *Partners in education: Issues and trends from the 21st International Congress on the Education of the Deaf* (pp. 62–74). Washington, DC: Gallaudet University Press.

Mayer, C., & Trezek, B. J. (2015). *Early literacy development in deaf children.* New York, NY: Oxford University Press.

Mayer, C., & Wells, G. (1996). Can the linguistic interdependence theory support a bilingual model of literacy education for deaf students? *Journal of Deaf Studies and Deaf Education, 1*(2), 93–107.

Mitchell. R. (2004). National profile of deaf and hard of hearing students in special education from weighted survey results. *American Annals of the Deaf, 149*(4), 336–349.

Mitchell. R., & Karchmer, M. A. (2006). Demographics of deaf education: More students in more places. *American Annals of the Deaf, 151*(2), 95–104.

Moeller, M. P., Tomblin, B., Connor C. M., & Jerger, S. (2007). Current state of knowledge, language and literacy of children with hearing impairment. *Ear & Hearing, 28*, 740–753.

Moores, D. (1987). *Educating the deaf: Psychology, principles and practices*. Boston, MA: Houghton Mifflin.

Musselman, C., & Szanto, G. (1998). The written language of deaf adolescents: Patterns of performance. *Journal of Deaf Studies and Deaf Education, 3,* 245–257.

Mulla I., Harrigan S., Gregory S., & Archbold, S. (2013). Children with complex needs and cochlear implants: The parents' perspective. *Deafness and Education International, 124,* 38–41.

Nystrand, M. (2006). The social and historical context of writing research. In C. A. Arthur, S. Graham, & J. Fitzgerald (Eds.), *Handbook of writing research* (pp. 11–27). New York, NY: Guilford Press.

Olson, D. (1977). From utterance to text: The bias of language in speech and writing. *Harvard Educational Review, 47,* 257–281.

Olson, D. (1993). Thinking about thinking: Learning how to take statements and hold beliefs. *Educational Psychologist, 28,* 7–23.

Olson, D. (1994). *The world on paper*. Cambridge, UK: Cambridge University Press.

Paul, P., & Lee, C. (2010). Qualitative-similarity hypothesis. *American Annals of the Deaf, 154*(5), 456–462.

Power, D., & Hyde, M. (2002). The characteristics and extent of participation of deaf and hard-of-hearing students in regular schools in Australia. *Journal of Deaf Studies and Deaf Education, 7*(4), 302–311.

Pressley, M. (2006). *Reading instruction that works: The case for balanced teaching* (3rd ed.). New York, NY: Guilford Press.

Pritchard, R. J., & Honeycutt, R. L. (2006). The process approach to writing instruction: Examining its effectiveness. In C. A. MacArthur, S. Graham, & J. Fitzgerald (Eds.), *Handbook of writing research* (pp. 275–290). New York, NY: Guilford Press.

Pugh, K. R., Sandak, R., Frost, S. J., Moore, D. L., & Mencl, W. E. (2006). Neurobiological investigations of skilled and impaired reading. In D. Dickinson & S. Neuman (Eds.), *Handbook of early literacy research* (Vol. 2, pp. 64–74). New York, NY: Guilford Press.

Singer, B. D., & Bashir, A. S. (2004). Developmental variation in writing composition skills. In C. Stone, E. Silliman, B. J. Ehren, & K. Apel (Eds.), *Handbook of language and literacy: Development and disorders* (pp. 559–582). New York, NY: Guilford Press.

Singleton, J. L., Morgan, D., DiGello, E., Wiles, J., & Rivers, R. (2004). Vocabulary use by low, moderate and high ASL-proficient writers compared to hearing ESL and monolingual speakers. *Journal of Deaf Studies and Deaf Education, 9*(1), 86–103.

Spencer, L., Barker, B. A., & Tomblin, J. B. (2003). Exploring the language and literacy outcomes of pediatric cochlear implant users. *Ear and Hearing, 24,* 236–24.

Stanovich, K. (2000). *Progress in understanding reading: Scientific foundations and new frontiers*. New York, NY: Guilford Press.

Taeschner, T. (1988). Affixes and function words in the written language of deaf children. *Applied Psycholinguistics, 9,* 385–401.

Trezek, B. J., & Wang, Y. (2006). Implications of utilizing a phonics-based reading curriculum with children who are deaf or hard of hearing. *Journal of Deaf Studies and Deaf Education, 10*(2), 202–213.

Trezek, B. J., Wang, Y., & Paul, P. V. (2010). *Reading and deafness: Theory, research and practice*. Clifton Park, NY: Cengage Learning.

Trezek, B. J., Wang, Y., Woods, D. G., Gampp, T. L., & Paul, P. (2007). Using Visual Phonics to supplement beginning reading instruction for students who are deaf or hard of hearing. *Journal of Deaf Studies and Deaf Education, 12*(3), 373–384.

Troia, G. (2007). Research in writing instruction: What we know and what we need to know. In M. Pressley, A. K Billman, K. H. Perry, K. E. Reffitt, & J. Moorehead-Reynolds (Eds.), *Shaping literacy achievement: Research we have, research we need* (pp. 129–156). New York, NY: Guilford Press.

van Dijk, J., Nelson, C., Postma, A., & van Dijk, R. (2010). Deaf children with severe multiple disabilities: Etiologies, intervention and assessment. In M. Marschark & P. Spencer (Eds.), *Oxford handbook of deaf studies, language, and education* (Vol. 2, pp. 172–191). New York, NY: Oxford University Press.

Vygotsky. (1978). *Mind in society: The development of higher psychological processes*. Cambridge, MA: Harvard University Press.

Whitehurst, G., & Lonigan, C. (1998). Child development and emergent literacy. *Child Development, 68*, 848–872.

Williams, C. (1993). Learning to write: Social interaction among preschool auditory/oral and total communication children. *Sign Language Studies, 80*, 267–284.

Williams, C. (2011). Adapted interactive writing instruction with kindergarten children who are deaf or hard of hearing. *American Annals of the Deaf, 156*, 23–34.

Williams, C., & Mayer, C. (2015). Writing in young deaf children. *Review of Educational Research*.

Wolbers, K. (2008). Strategic and interactive writing instruction (SIWI): Apprenticing deaf students in the construction of English text. *International Journal of Applied Linguistics, 156*, 299–326.

Wolbers, K., Dostal, H., & Bowers, L. (2012). "I was born full deaf." Written language outcomes after one year of strategic and interactive writing instruction (SIWI). *Journal of Deaf Studies and Deaf Education, 17*(1), 19–38.

Wong, B. Y. L., & Berninger, V. W. (2004). Cognitive processes of teachers in implementing composition research in elementary, middle and high school classrooms. In C. Addison-Stone, E. R. Silliman, B. J. Ehren, & K. Apel (Eds.), *Handbook of language and literacy: Development and disorders* (pp. 600–624). New York, NY: Guilford Press.

Xue, Y., & Meisels, S. (2004). Early literacy instruction and learning in kindergarten: Evidence from the early childhood longitudinal study: Kindergarten class of 1998–1999. *American Educational Research Journal, 41*,191–229.

Yau, M. (1991). The role of language factors in second language writing. In L. Malave & G. Duquette (Eds.), *Language, culture and cognition* (pp. 266–283). Clevedon, UK: Multilingual Matters.

Yoshinaga-Itano, C., Snyder, L. S., & Mayberry, R. (1996). How deaf and normally hearing students convey meaning within and between sentences. *The Volta Review, 98*, 9–38.

Zimmerman, B. J. (2002). Becoming a self-regulated learner: An overview. *Theory into Practice, 41*(2), 64–70.

11

Many Languages, One Goal: Interventions for Language Mastery by School-Age Deaf and Hard-of-Hearing Learners

Susan R. Easterbrooks, Joanna E. Cannon, and Jessica W. Trussell

As with all educational interventions, good language instruction requires ongoing research to establish, maintain, and renew the pool of best educational practice. Unfortunately the research pool to date offers education practitioners little advice on how to improve language outcomes for school-age students who are deaf and hard of hearing (DHH). This chapter summarizes the literature on aspects of grammar that are difficult for DHH learners to master, the school-based language instruction of DHH students, and newly emerging areas in the evidence base that require renewed efforts. We suggest the need for a concerted and collaborative research effort to take us into the next decade. Last, we describe research from The Radical Middle, a grassroots effort to guide the development of prudent research questions that will help all educators to promote achievement among their students in that most important goal of all: the ability to communicate.

LANGUAGE INTERVENTION IN THE SCHOOL YEARS

Why study interventions in the school years when the research of the past two decades has demonstrated incontrovertibly that early identification and early intervention are keys to the successful attainment of (or at least greatly improved) communication (Moeller, 2000; Yoshinaga-Itano, 2003)? Researchers in the field of deaf education need to study school-based intervention because two intractable issues prevent us from drawing the conclusion that the job is done: (a) not all DHH children have easy access to early intervention either in the United States (Harrison et al., 2003) or elsewhere (Swanepoel et al., 2009), and (b) we have not yet ensured that all children who are DHH have acquired the underlying language base to be successful with that primary metric of language competence, which is the ability to read, or at least to pass reading tests to a degree commensurate with typically hearing children (Traxler, 2000). There is a clear correlation between illiteracy and poverty (Adiseshiah, 1990) reported locally, regionally, nationally, and internationally. The ability to read predicts one's educational attainment (Miller & Warren, 2011); poor literacy limits employability and, therefore, quality of life (Reder, 2010). For children to learn to read, at a minimum they must have a language (Tomblin, 2010) and books (see Chapter 10), neither of which is readily accessible to all DHH children.

We propose that significant research efforts need to be brought to bear on the development of language interventions for school-age children. Although we are making strides with younger children (Moeller, 2000), a significant portion of DHH children are still entering their school years with language skills insufficient to support adequate instruction. In addition, assuming DHH children enter school at least by the preschool years (age, 3 years), educators may have access to them for up to 15 years, and so *school* is the most likely place that children who have not yet mastered language and literacy will have the opportunity to do so.

Students who are DHH have been a source of interest to researchers from diverse fields for many years. However, what we most *need* to know is simply this: When a child is struggling to acquire a language, what evidence-based ways do teachers have to address language in the classroom? Sadly, the answer at this juncture in history is that we have precious few.

HOW DID WE GET OFF-TRACK IN DESIGNING EVIDENCE-BASED LANGUAGE INTERVENTIONS?

Easterbrooks and Maiorana-Basas (2015) summarized the major debates in the field that led historically to deaf education researchers' diversion from developing effective language interventions. These included, but are not limited to, debates over structured versus natural approaches, bottom-up versus top-down/whole-language approaches, mainstream versus separate school education, the place of cochlear implants in the population, bilingualism and the place of created sign systems, and the relative importance of different pieces of the literacy puzzle (see Easterbrooks & Maiorana-Basas [2015] for further explanation). These debates distracted the research community from creating school-based language interventions for teachers and their students. We also learned that the pool of literacy interventions is shockingly poor (Easterbrooks & Stephenson, 2012; Luckner & Cooke, 2010; Luckner & Handley, 2008; Luckner et al., 2005/2006; Luckner & Urbach, 2012; Tucci et al., 2014).

Thus, it is of no surprise that we find the pool of language instructional interventions with a clear evidence base to be shockingly poor as well.

Although there was a clarion call from various forces that led to the focus of research and funding on literacy acquisition around 2000, we saw no similar call in the area of language. In the next section of this chapter, we provide a glimpse into the evidence base in language intervention with the hope of spurring action in language intervention research. We examined the literature from the 1980s onward in the areas of syntax, morphology, and function words (closed-class lexical items), searching for empirical evidence of school-based instructional interventions known to improve language. We used standard online search engines found in the libraries of our different institutions, cross-listing the keywords *intervention* or *deaf* with keywords common to our different topics (such as syntax, grammar, morphemes, morphology, function words, lexical, open-class, closed-class, and others) to get a snapshot of available interventions. After reviewing 80 to 150 articles in each area, we considered this to be a snapshot of the literature, if not a comprehensive review, primarily because there were so few options that presented themselves within our searched keywords.

A VIEW OF THE LITERATURE ON THE NATURE OF MORPHOLOGY AND EVIDENCE-BASED PRACTICES IN MORPHOLOGICAL DEVELOPMENT

What Is Morphology?

Morphology is the study of the internal structure of words and how words are formed (Aronoff & Fudeman, 2011). A meaning-based examination of words at the sublexical level (units within a word) begins with the study of morphemes. Morphemes are the smallest unit of a language that retain meaning. They are categorized in several ways: by how they are combined (unbound or bound) and by their function (inflectional or derivational). Unbound morphemes can stand alone as a word (such as look) or be combined with another unbound morpheme to create a compound word (such as butterfly, eardrum [van Hoogmoed et al., 2011]). Bound morphemes hold meaning but must be combined with other words (such as the *-ed* in *looked* [Reed, 2008]). Inflectional morphemes, such as *-ing* and *-ed*, provide information about the grammatical category, number, or gender of the base word (Verhoeven & Perfetti, 2003). Derivational morphemes, such as *un-* and *-able*, are combined to create words (happy and unhappy) or to change the grammatical class and meaning of a word (agree [verb] and agreeable [adjective] [Reed 2008]). We combine inflectional and derivational morphemes with root words based on a system of rules (Chomsky, 2005). Morphological knowledge requires an understanding of the meaning of affixes, roots, and base words; learning this knowledge may involve deconstructing words into their component morphemes and reconstructing them when children are of school age. Children with typical hearing gain the rule-based possibilities for each morpheme through analyzing and processing innumerable language experiences (Glackin, 2010).

Universals in Morphology

Morphology is found in most of the world's languages. A study of more than 300 languages revealed there are inherent restrictions of a morpheme's possible meanings. Being able to combine morphemes creates rich word meanings and word structures (Bobaljik, 2012). For instance, the superlative -*est,* found in English, thought typically as an indicator of some level of superiority, is actually more complex, implying comparison as well as superiority. However, morphology does not always manifest as bound or unbound morphemes. In the northwestern Mandarin dialect known as *Nanzhuang*, the tonal quality produced along with the word indicates tense and functions as a morpheme (Chen, 2000). Similarly, sign languages have morphology constructions that are focused on meaningful units such as subject–verb agreement, time, facial markers that act as an adverbial, and classifier constructs (Aronoff et al., 2005).

DHH children struggle to achieve competence with morphology (McGuckian & Henry, 2007). Children who use listening and spoken language do not hear many of the quieter or higher frequency morphemes (Guo et al., 2013). DHH children who use American Sign Language (ASL) or signed English do not see English morphemes in face-to-face communication (Gaustad et al., 2002). Children need many exposures to inflectional and derivational morphemes to use these morphological structures in their own expressive language (Dixon et al., 2012). To increase DHH children's morphological knowledge, morphological instruction or interventions are needed (Bow et al., 2004).

Successful Interventions for Typically Hearing Children Struggling to Learn Morphology

Children with specific language impairment (SLI) have difficulty with inflectional morphology (Rice et al., 1995). Several interventions have been developed for children with SLI that may have potential for use with DHH students. These include story-based interventions, computer-based interventions, and dialogic reading.

Story-Based Interventions

Several types of story-based interventions have been studied. One such intervention includes telling the children a story, ensuring the use of the third-person singular -*s* (such as, She runs.) multiples times, providing grammatical contrasts (such as, She runs. They run.), recasting the children's responses to expose them to the correct forms, and self-correcting to indicate the form was required (such as, He walk. Oops, I should have said "He walks." Can you say "He walks?"). Preschool-age children with SLI have made significant gains on the targeted forms following the preceding strategies (Ionin & Wexler, 2002; Leonard et al., 2004, 2006) and these gains were maintained over time (Leonard et al., 2004, 2006, 2008). Other researchers have included explicit instruction of bound morpheme rules within stories, with some of the 4- to 6-year-old participants receiving explicit instruction in usage and others receiving exposure only, or implicit instruction. Children in the implicit intervention were able to generalize the rule that was embedded in the story better than children in the explicit rule condition (Swisher et al., 1995).

Computer-Based Interventions

Educational computer games are popular forms of intervention. When these games include morphology instruction, they should require the student to produce the computer model's target morpheme. Connell (1992) developed two computer games to teach morphological structures to 32 5- to 7-year-old students with SLI. One game required the student to produce the modeled morphological structure. For example, when teaching the plural -s the character would say, "You tell Bobby to move the cars; say Bobby, move the cars." On the other hand, one game did not require the students to produce the target morpheme ("You tell Bobby to move the cars; say, Bobby move it."). The students who practiced saying the target morpheme during the intervention outperformed those who were exposed to the morpheme only on a production task. However, the children's comprehension of the morphemes' meanings did not improve in either condition (Connell, 1992). Although computerized instruction is popular, these inconclusive results indicate that computer games should be implemented with caution until we have conclusive evidence of their success.

Dialogic Reading

Dialogic reading is an active book-sharing activity between an adult and a child during which the adult asks the child questions about the book, evaluates the language in the child's answer, and provides modeling to increase the length or complexity of the child's language (Whitehurst et al., 1988). Dialogic reading has been used successfully to teach the morphological structures past tense -*ed* and possessive -*s* to elementary-age students with SLI (Maul & Ambler, 2014). Similar to the previously discussed story interventions, when three 5- to 8-year-old children with SLI engaged in dialogic reading with recasts, models of the targeted morphemes, and questions intended to encourage the child to imitate the targeted form, their use of the past tense -*ed* or the possessive -*s* generalized to novel storybooks. Although storybook and dialogic reading appear to be promising, most interventions were implemented with preschool-age students, not school-age students with some exceptions. Having an adult provide multiple opportunities for a child to process the target inflectional morphological structure receptively was an effective intervention for school-age children (Maul & Ambler, 2014), as was requiring a child to produce the targeted morphological structure (Connell, 1992).

Explicit Instruction

Instructional strategies have also been developed for children who are English-language learners (ELLs). These tend to focus on derivational morphology (Carlo et al., 2004; Kieffer & Lesaux, 2012) in fifth and sixth graders. Instruction in derivational morphology focuses on helping children learn the meaning of a target root word and the target affix, then understand how to deconstruct words into their component morphemes. In one study, intervention was implemented weekly, whereas in the other study, instruction was implemented during unspecified times across several weeks of academic language instruction. Both interventions embedded derivational morphology instruction within an academic language intervention, and the ELLs improved their derivational morphology knowledge. However, the students who received instruction on a more frequent basis experienced a clinically significant improvement in their derivational morphology knowledge as a result of the intervention (Kieffer & Lesaux, 2012) whereas those who received instruction infrequently only experienced a marginal improvement (Carlo et al., 2004). Thus, dosage of intervention is an important feature that has been underinvestigated in the literature in general.

Successful Interventions for DHH Children Struggling to Learn Morphology

DHH children struggle with inflectional morphology such as third person singular -*s* and past tense -*ed*. These morphemes may be difficult for some DHH children to hear, and therefore the children do not use them in their expressive language (Guo et al., 2013). Tense and number in ASL also pose problems for learners of that language (Breadmore et al., 2014). There is little intervention research on teaching these morphological structures (Bennett et al., 2014; Bow et al., 2004; Cannon et al., 2011). ASL morphology is often represented through the classifier system, and direct instruction increases DHH learners' classifier use (Easterbrooks & Beal-Alvarez, 2014). Researchers have addressed teaching morphological structures in two different ways: (a) as a standalone intervention (Bow et al., 2004) and (b) as part of a package intervention (Bennett et al., 2014; Cannon et al., 2011).

Stand-alone Interventions

Identifying and producing target morphemes may be a successful way to increase the morphological knowledge of elementary-age DHH children. Children can look for the target morphemes in games, stories, worksheets, and puzzles. At the same time, the teacher or parent could use the same materials as an appropriate context to encourage the child to produce the target morpheme. Following a 20-minutes-a-day, 9-week intervention using the activities just described, DHH students were able to determine more accurately if a sentence that contained the third person singular -s or past tense -ed was correct grammatically (Bow et al., 2004).

Package Interventions

Package interventions are implemented to develop more than one language skill over time. Morphological instruction can be one part of a larger lesson. Using readily available language interventions developed typically for hearing children may help DHH children develop inflectional morphological knowledge (Bennett et al., 2014; Cannon et al., 2011). However, readily available packaged interventions may need to be modified before being used with DHH children. Adding sign language or visual supports is one way to make these types of materials more accessible (Bennett et al., 2014). Some package interventions are in the form of computer- or technology-based applications. These multimedia interventions provide personalized and targeted instruction; however, adult support was recommended for some DHH children while interacting with the software to use them successfully (Cannon et al., 2011).

Metalinguistic Interventions

Syntax and morphology interventions often are addressed together in the literature (see the discussion in "Morphology"). Although metalinguistic practices were popular in the late 1970s (Blackwell et al., 1978), they were never placed under the research microscope and so there are no experimental studies with DHH students to support or refute their use. Metalinguistic instruction often accompanies work on written language interventions (such as strategic and interactive writing instruction [Wolbers et al., 2012, 2014; see also Chapter 10), which are designed to increase English structures in writing, thus influencing the linguistic competence necessary for improved language and reading comprehension. Another written intervention with a promising evidence base is teacher-led explicit morphology instruction. Teaching DHH students the meanings of root words and affixes as well as how to deconstruct words that have multiple morphemes into smaller known word parts has the potential to increase their vocabulary knowledge. Furthermore, morphology instruction may provide students with a tool to generate their own vocabulary knowledge when attacking unfamiliar words (Trussell & Easterbrooks, 2015).

A VIEW OF THE LITERATURE ON THE NATURE OF SYNTAX AND EVIDENCE-BASED PRACTICES IN SYNTACTIC DEVELOPMENT

What Is Syntax?

Syntax describes the rules for combining words to form the phrases, clauses, and sentences of a language needed to convey meaning (Chomsky, 2005). Several categories of words comprise the building blocks of language (such as nouns, verbs, adjectives, adverbs, pronouns, prepositions, conjunctions, and interjections) that are combined to express meaning. Syntactic functions work together with vocabulary knowledge in a reciprocal relationship among DHH readers (Kelly, 1993; Moores & Sweet, 1990). As vocabulary knowledge increases, so does the possible "movement" of words within a sentence (such as clause and question formation) that learners can use to receive or express language. Form and function may be acquired at different times and may require scaffolding of one another throughout the process of language acquisition. Students who are DHH experience delays in syntax acquisition relative to their hearing peers (Schirmer, 1985).

When DHH learners do not have a foundational level of syntactic confidence or ability, they struggle to combine words in a manner that conveys meaning (Kelly, 1996). DHH learners' receptive and expressive syntax skills correlate with hearing level, age, educational setting, communication modality, and use of assistive listening technology (Johnson & de Villiers, 2009). Parental use of sign language is associated with increases in syntax comprehension (Dolman, 1983), and the number of word types parents use, paired with higher level facilitative language techniques (such as parallel talk, open-ended questions, expansion, expatiation, and recast), increases receptive language skills in DHH toddlers (Cruz et al., 2013). Age correlates with differing syntactic patterns, constructions, and processing abilities for older DHH students when compared with their hearing peers, but the groups do not differ in the processing of semantic patterns (Sarachan-Deily, 1982).

Deficits in reading comprehension are associated with face-to-face semantic and syntactic processing deficits (Johnson & Goswani, 2010). Students have difficulty mapping known vocabulary onto their corresponding syntactic structures to convey meaning (Miller, 2010). Working memory plays a role in this linguistic mapping process, with a central executive using "slave" systems to retain short-term information (phonological loop, visuospatial sketchpad, and the episodic buffer [Baddeley, 2000]). These systems can be used during the processing of semantic and syntactic information during the writing process.

For example, writing pauses may indicate that DHH learners' storage capacity and processing are overwhelmed during a writing task, and the working memory is unable to complete simultaneous operations involved in written expression (Alamargot et al., 2007). Interesting new research using functional magnetic resonance imaging technology shows that word order activates the lexical and working memory areas of the human brain, and scaffolding of instruction may build capacity of the "cognitive resources required to process specific types of linguistic cues" (Newman et al., 2010, p. 7539). Additional research on the complex interrelationship of syntax, vocabulary, and memory is needed.

The Form of English Syntax

Most of the literature on DHH students' understanding and use of specific grammatical patterns of English (such as simple, compound, and complex sentence types) was conducted during the 1980s (see Cannon and Kirby [2013] for a review). English syntax has been described as comprising five basic sentence patterns (Chomsky, 1957): Sentence Pattern 1 (SP1), Noun Phrase (NP) + Intransitive Verb +/– Adverbial clause (Adv); SP2, NP1 + Transitive Verb + NP2; SP3, NP1 + Linking Verb (LV) + Adjective; SP4, NP1 + LV + NP1; and SP5, NP1 + LV + Adv. These patterns were thought of historically as "kernel" sentences, or building blocks on which to scaffold more complex structures. Newer theories question the genesis of these structures (Londahl, 2014), yet they may still provide teachers with an understanding of how the three verb types (transitive, intransitive, and linking) are used within basic sentences. Basic sentence patterns provide a foundation on which users create ever-increasingly complex language. For example, language users first learn sentences in which a noun precedes a verb (She made John happy.) before learning sentences in which a noun clause precedes a verb (That she won the debate made John happy.). DHH students tend to make distinctive error patterns in their basic sentence construction and comprehension (Berent et al., 2013; Kluwin, 1982; Quigley & King, 1980), the effects of which carry into more complex language.

The verbal system of English provides a challenge for DHH students (Berent, 1996; Cannon & Kirby, 2013; White, 2002), likely because verbs carry a certain semantic primacy in determining overall meaning of a sentence. There are three verb types in English: (a) intransitive verbs, which take no direct object; (b) transitive verbs, which require a direct object; and (c) linking, or "be," verbs, which tie the subject to the predicate either by renaming the predicate nominative using a noun phrase, describing the predicate using an adjective phrase, or telling the location with the predicate using an adverbial phrase. Forms of -wh questions also present a challenge; even after years of exposure to questions, many college-age DHH students continue to struggle with their comprehension and production (Berent, 1996; LaSasso, 1990).

DHH students are typically delayed in their use of universal quantifiers (such as each, every, and all [Berent et al., 2008]) and numerical quantifiers (such as some and several) (Kelly & Berent, 2011), thus influencing comprehension of math and science word problems (Wilbur & Goodhart, 1985). Some have suggested this processing deficit as the underlying difficulty (Lillo-Martin, 1992) not only with quantifiers, but also with relative clauses (Traxler et al., 2014). Similarly, researchers have noted DHH students' inefficient understanding of other sentences structures (active-voice sentences, passive-voice sentences, and sentences incorporating subject and reflexive pronouns); when placed into two groups based on their ASL proficiency (low vs. high), participants with greater ASL skills exhibited better comprehension of word order during reading comprehension activities than low-proficient ASL users (Andrew et al., 2014). Skill in a learner's first language (L1) assists in the development of the learner's second language (L2), even across communication modalities. ASL proficiency also predicts vocabulary recognition and comprehension of English syntax. Without sufficient understanding of the basic building blocks of language, DHH students' acquisition of more complex structures (such as causal clauses and passive voice) may be delayed in their writing (Traxler et al., 2014), resulting in overuse of fragmented narratives (Arfé & Boscolo, 2006).

Universals in Syntax

The delay in acquisition of syntactic structures can be seen across languages. For example, Chinese DHH students exhibit difficulty with complex sentences and dative movement (Shimizu, 1988), passive voice, and double-negative sentences (Man-shu & Jing-zhe, 1984), similar to DHH students whose first language is English (Cannon & Kirby, 2013). Italian DHH students who had cochlear implants demonstrated fewer problems repeating sentences when they were given print support as a scaffold for verbally presented simple sentences (Caselli et al., 2012).

School-age DHH children in many countries and most languages struggle with the syntax of their language. Japanese children who are DHH had trouble with relative and passive clauses both in written and spoken language tasks, and they did not acquire mastery of spoken language until age 12 (Fujiyoshi et al., 2012; Ryuzaki & Ito, 1999). Younger DHH Japanese students tended to overuse and repeat errors of simple sentences in their written expression, whereas older high school students repeatedly produced errors in complex sentences. Written scaffolding of simple and complex language structures appears to provide support (Omori & Sawa, 2008). Dutch DHH students also struggle with relative clauses and prenominal structures in their writing (van Beijsterveldt & van Hell, 2009), and DHH students who use

German Sign Language exhibit similar syntactic processing to hearing L2 students, demonstrating that L1 can promote the development of L2, even across sensory modalities of sign and speech (Skotara et al., 2011). Dutch DHH students also experience difficulties with syntax rules during spoken language assessments (Boons et al., 2013), with similar findings in reading comprehension among those DHH students whose L1 is Hebrew and Arabic (Miller et al., 2012). Students who use Hebrew exhibit difficulties comprehending relative clauses and basic sentence patterns when completing a sentence-to-picture matching task (Friedmann & Szterman, 2006) as well as errors in -wh movement (Friedmann & Szterman, 2011). Iranian DHH students exhibit difficulties during sentence recognition and completion tasks with Persian verb inflections, prepositions, and word order; researchers in the Iranian study concluded that early acquisition is vital if educators are to expect learners to reach proficiency (Gheitury et al., 2014). Miller (2000) found that Israeli DHH children paid more attention to semantic rather than syntactic clues during a reading comprehension task, resulting in deficit skills in comprehension of simple and relative clauses when compared with their hearing peers. DHH students who use Turkish experience delays in reading skills, even after years of instruction; researchers determined that the main barrier was poor retrieval of syntax and prior knowledge during reading tasks (Miller et al., 2013). Table 11.1 provides a list of syntactic structures known to be difficult for DHH students across many languages.

Successful Interventions for Typically Hearing Children Struggling to Learn Syntax

There are surprisingly few interventions specifically designed for school-age children struggling to learn syntax. Most available interventions

Table 11.1 Challenging Syntactic Structures for Deaf and Hard-of-Hearing Learners across Languages

Structures	Functions	Movements
Pronouns (reflexive, reciprocal, and indefinite)	Demonstratives	-wh questions
	Quantifiers (universal, numerical)	Comparatives
Prepositions (nonlocative)		Conditionals
Verbs (irregular, transitive, intransitive, modals)	Aspects of tense (active, passive)	SVO errors
		Complementizers
Prenominal structures	Semantics/pragmatics	Dative movement
	Sentence patterns	Complex sentences
Prepositions	Word order	Overuse of simple sentences
		Relative clauses

-wh questions, who, what, when, where, why, how questions; SVO, subject–verb–object sequences.

have been designed for typically hearing children with SLI or who are new learners of English. For example, Cirrin and Gillam (2008) reviewed the literature on language interventions and found only two studies related to syntax, concluding that the evidence base for syntax interventions is quite poor. We summarize the interventions revealed in our keyword search in the following sections.

Metalinguistic Interventions

Metalinguistic interventions require learners to think about the structure of the syntax they are learning. One metalinguistic intervention with an evidence base is *metasyntactic therapy* (Ebbels & van der Lely, 2001). Designed for SLI students, this approach uses visual codes such as shapes, colors, and arrows to teach the rules of grammar. Ebbels and van der Lely (2001) found visual codes to be effective in supporting mastery of the rules of passive voice and –wh questions by 27 learners with SLI, ages 11 to 16 years.

Modeling and Modeling with Evoked Production and Feedback

Staples in the language intervention arsenal—modeling, elicited production, and feedback—are frequently described but their success is infrequently validated. One study with an evidence base is described by Weismer and Murray-Branch (1989). In this intervention, four participants (ages 5 and 6 years) were provided either with a model of accurate grammar production or a model followed by evoked production and feedback, both during play. The authors found that both types of intervention worked equally well in increasing the participants' use of the target syntax objective when the participants had expressive language problems only. However, neither condition was successful in eliciting target objectives when children had both receptive and expressive language problems. These results were also found when the form of speech (slower or modified) was manipulated by a computerized language program (Bishop et al., 2006).

Other Best Practices

Other best practices reported as effective for ELLs include use of multimodal support (such as auditory, visual, and kinesthetic presentations of content) and explicit and direct instruction paired with experiential language activities (Cannon & Guardino, 2012; French, 1992).

Successful Interventions for DHH Children Struggling to Learn Syntax

Because they lack exposure to incidental vocabulary and language models, DHH students often need instruction that is explicit, scaffolded, and systematic to influence their acquisition of syntax. Because DHH students worldwide appear to have difficulty with syntax, there is a need worldwide for more research and instruction on syntactic structures. The notable lack of face-to-face syntax interventions for school-age children who are DHH is incontrovertible. Herein we summarize the evidence from the literature on interventions that have been found to be effective in helping DHH students to master syntax.

Metalinguistic Interventions

Syntax and morphology interventions often are addressed together in the literature (see the discussion in "Morphology"). DHH writers tend to focus less on grammar during composition than their hearing peers (Kelly, 1988), and so the relationship between face-to-face syntax and written syntax deserves increased attention. Metalinguistic interventions traditionally combine visual, systematic instruction with an environmental approach using the learner's native language and interests.

One successful metalinguistic approach involves helping the student focus on strategies to repair conversations. Moeller (1986) investigated clarification techniques using a repair strategies checklist paired with a hierarchy of question prompts to increase comprehension during conversations with a 12-year-old student with a profound hearing loss. Ongoing task analysis by a clinician conducting the one-on-one sessions began with simple, concrete question prompts that became increasingly more complex over time, with the more abstract questions incorporating visual representation to enhance understanding. Generalization to other conversations with parents and teachers was also incorporated into the strategy.

Another metalinguistic strategy, visually highlighting both good and poor examples of writing within a student's own product, provides clarifying and corrective feedback (Berent et al., 2009). Pre- and postintervention samples were coded for use of specific structures (+PRES or –PRES, for presence or absence of present tense, respectively) and shared with DHH students who also had SLI in a 10-week intervention. Participants in this study not only improved their syntax, but also maintained their new skills at least 6 months after the intervention.

Visual Supports

Visual organizers, such as graphic organizers and concept maps, are a routinely recommended tool in deaf education. DHH students using visual organizers increased the number of adjectives and decreased the number of action words in their writing (Easterbrooks & Stoner, 2006). This strategy provided students with the visual support they needed to expand from overreliance on simple sentences to greater variation in their written products. Graphic organizers might also be used for other aspects of syntax (such as increasing use of prepositional phrases, use of appropriate reflexive pronouns, and so on).

Other Best Practices

Because of the reciprocal relationship between vocabulary and syntax (Kelly, 1996), teaching strategies focused solely on one will not increase the other, so a balanced approach is needed if we are to help students improve their receptive language. Students need explicit instruction with visual and scaffolded support to move them from their overuse of simple sentences to mastery and use of increasingly complex sentences (Channon & Sayers, 2007). Teachers might consider pairing syntax, semantic, and pragmatic instruction (de Villiers, 1983) using explicit and environmental techniques to foster face-to-face and in-print syntax comprehension and use.

A VIEW OF THE LITERATURE ON THE NATURE OF FUNCTION WORDS AND EVIDENCE-BASED PRACTICES IN FUNCTION WORD DEVELOPMENT

Much has been written of the importance of early vocabulary acquisition in face-to-face communication whether spoken or signed (Hayes et al., 2009), its relation to literacy (Johnson & Goswani, 2010), its predictive capacity to suggest trajectory of development (Yoshinaga-Itano et al., 2010), its acquisition in children who are new learners of a language (Nelson et al., 2011), its explicit and incidental exposure (Biemiller, 2001), its relationship to academic success (Convertino et al., 2009), and the interrelationship of lexicons when children are learning more than one language (Hermans et al., 2008). In this section, we address vocabulary from the perspective of function words (closed-set words) and attempt to build the case that phrase-learning surrounding function and lexical combinations provides a clear bridge between meaning (vocabulary) and grammar (morphology and syntax). This may be a fertile ground of study when designing school-based instructional strategies that will improve children's face-to-face and print use of their languages.

What Are Lexical and Function Words?

Function words are those words that have no meaning in and of themselves but have meaning only in relation to the lexical item or items they surround. Function words are also called *closed-class words* in that they are finite, and it is highly unlikely that we will ever add new examples to our lexicon. For example, we can say "dog and cat," "dog or cat," "dog but not cat," and that is about the sum total of how we combine individual nouns. It is unlikely that we will ever invent new examples of conjoining words. Examples of function words are *of, to, on, a, and, either, by, for, while, with, but, so, that, which, other,* and *after*. There are only a couple hundred function words in the English language, and typical readers experience fewer than 100 on a routine basis. Typical categories of function words include articles, possessives, pronouns (subject, object, reflexive, indefinite, and relative) auxiliary and modal verbs, prepositions, connectors, and subordinators. Teachers have been encouraged to treat function words as if they were sight words to be memorized. Yet, relegating function words to sight word mastery belies the fact that they are the glue that holds all other lexical and functional items together in a manner that is both grammatical (syntactic) and meaningful (semantic). Ehri (1976) studied word learning in kindergarten and first-grade learners and determined they learned content (lexical) items relatively easily but had substantial difficulty with context-free function words. Ehri and Wilce (1980) studied first graders further and found they learned function words better in context than in lists. Taken together, these two studies raised concerns about the effectiveness of using flash cards as a means to teach sight word mastery of this word class. Unfortunately, in the decades since that work, little has been done to provide an alternative intervention to assist DHH students in mastering function words.

Lexical words, on the other hand, are also called *content* or *open-class words* in that we are always adding examples to the list. One needs only to think of the latest technology craze to find new vocabulary that has entered our lexicons (such as *trending, selfie,* and *google it*). Lexical or content words include nouns, verbs, adjectives, and adverbs. Children learn thousands of lexical words during their early years, and in general master tens of thousands of words by the end of the elementary years. We continue to learn new words throughout our lifetime.

Universals in Function Words

In most countries around the world, students who are DHH are known to have diminished lexicons relative to their hearing peers (Coppens et al., 2013, Isaka, 2011; Kiese-Himmel & Reeh, 2006; Mann et al., 2013). In most languages, and in the large samples of children's utterances in the MacWhinney (2000) database, function words have a low type count (different number of function words) but a very high token, or frequency, count (they appear with high frequency). Because of their ubiquitous appearance in all verbal interactions, they are of great importance in the generation of communication.

Successful Interventions for Any Student Struggling to Learn Lexical and Function Words

The *What Works Clearinghouse* of the U.S. Institute of Education Sciences (http://ies.ed.gov/ncee/wwc) reports the availability of several evidence-based vocabulary interventions to improve vocabulary in children with typical hearing, such *Kindergarten PAVEd for Success* (Goodson et al., 2010; Schwanenflugel et al., 2010) and *Vocabulary Improvement Program for English Language Learners and Their Classmates*

(Carlo et al., 2004; Lively et al., 2003). We found no vocabulary interventions in the *What Works Clearinghouse*, whether for vocabulary broadly or for function words specifically, designed with DHH school-age students in mind, although much has been written about the importance of vocabulary. Although reviews of the research in vocabulary instruction for DHH students (Luckner & Cooke, 2010) point to clear strategies associated with vocabulary acquisition (such as explicit instruction, repeated viewings, and sufficient practice), there are no interventions created specifically for DHH students' acquisition of either content or function words that have a robust evidence base. Cannon et al. (2009) described one promising technique in the use of signed storybooks as an effective tool in improving vocabulary. Similarly, we see limited literature that would provide advice to teachers of DHH students on how to increase their students' face-to-face and in-print use of function words. Much has been written about the brain's response to open- and closed-word classes (Diaz & McCarthy, 2009; Weber-Fox & Neville, 2001) and the struggles that those with clinical speech disorders and bilinguals experience (Hustad et al., 2007; Weber-Fox & Neville, 2001), but little is written about intervention. Researchers suggest that function/closed-set words are more difficult to acquire because, unlike nouns, verbs, and adjectives, they lack imageability (Bird et al., 2001; Paivio et al., 1968); it is difficult to form a mental image of a lone function word. With no evidence-based interventions readily available for teachers, where must they turn for advice?

TYING IT ALL TOGETHER

The relative importance of semantics and syntax has been debated through the years. Syntacticians have focused on the structure of language without much attention to whether the sentences generated made sense (note the classically referenced sentence, "Curious green colors sleep furiously"). Semanticists, on the other hand, focused on making meaning without much attention to structure. This begs the question: On what theoretical basis can we create language interventions that work? Newer theories suggest that an answer to this question lies in the juxtaposition of linguistic phrase structure (syntax, morphology, and function words) and argument structure (semantics). Although we have spent a considerable amount of recent research on the implications of sound and meaning for syntax (often identified by a measure of reading comprehension), an answer to the syntax-versus-semantics relation lies within phrase structure, at least in those languages that are organized into phrase units. Chomsky's (2005) newer theory, according to Lohndal (2014), suggests that syntactic structure should be mapped directly onto the semantic component; thus, there is "no intermediate level of representation" (p. 5). Logical form does not happen at the level of the sentence but at the level of the phrase (p. 94). Young, typically hearing children show sensitivity to function words and use them to build grammatical categories (Hicks, 2006). What this means for deaf educators and deaf education researchers is that the likely relationship between syntax and semantics, or between structure and meaning, is not occurring at the level of the individual word or at the level of the sentence, but at the supralexical level of the phrase unit, where words are chunked supralexically into meaningful units. We are suggesting that syntax and semantics align supralexically at the phrase level by means of the interrelationship among closed-set (function words), open-set (lexical words), and morphemic items (free and bound morphemes) to form logical and grammatical chunks or units. For example, the supralexical unit, *at a moment's notice,* represents a complete thought that supersedes the sum of the meaning of each of its individual parts (at + a + moment + 's + notice) and promotes imageability (Bird et al., 2001).

The synergistic relationship generated by certain combinations of closed- and open-set words yields meaning, and that meaning can be represented from one language to another, no matter what the specific grammar of that language is, and without a specific one-to-one correspondence. For example, in English, one can say "the three of us." In Spanish, one can say "los tres de notrous"; in Italian, one can say "i tre di noi"; and in ASL, one can represent the same meaning by holding the thumb and first two fingers palm up and circulating this configuration to incorporate the location of all three persons indicated. All four ways of conveying this one thought hold the same meaning, although by different forms. Thus, phrase-reading ability is a language-based skill associated with reading comprehension (Klauda & Guthrie, 2008) that permits us to address both meaning and form without getting bogged down in underresearched metalinguistic strategies that decades of teachers have applied unsuccessfully (e.g., Anderson et al., 1999) to teach the morphology and syntax necessary to support reading comprehension.

READING IN THE RADICAL MIDDLE

Easterbrooks and Maiorana-Basas (2015) proposed that research in deaf education should be conducted from the Radical Middle, a term referring to an effort to "encourage scholars from a wide range of educational, cultural, and linguistic perspectives to develop collaborative research agendas and efforts toward a common goal of affecting positive academic change for all DHH children" (p. 46). We propose that the study of supralexical unitization, whether face-to-face or in print, with the intent of creating language and reading interventions that will improve learning outcomes for students who are DHH, is a radical middle idea. Many languages hold meaning at the phrase level, whether spoken or signed. Struggling readers with typical hearing are known to have difficulty with syntax (Leikin & Assayag-Bouskila, 2004; Nation & Snowling, 2000). Grouping of words into phrases may be the way in which grammar links to reading comprehension in older readers (Mokhtari & Thompson, 2006) and deserves study in younger readers, including DHH readers. Phrase reading is a proxy for syntax in measures relating grammar to text comprehension in the struggling reader population (Nomvete, 2014) and might also be so in the DHH population.

SUMMARY AND CONCLUSIONS

Somewhere along the way in all the wonderful research the world has been doing since the 1970s, when the English-speaking world learned from Quigley et al. (see Cannon and Kirby [2013] for a summary) that DHH children were not mastering the basics of the language they would need to read, we took a wide arc around the topic and looked at reading from every angle except the angle of classroom instruction in language. Perhaps this was because other issues such as bilingualism were more provocative, or because technology was more tantalizing, or because, in our attempts to ensure that our DHH children had equal access to all the same experiences as their hearing counterparts, we forgot that language was at the heart of their every challenge. In this view of the literature, we searched for interventions with an evidence base that were specific to DHH learners. We found several categories of interventions for morphology, syntax, and function words (metalinguistic, visual, computerized, individual and package, and print based), but none with incontrovertible evidence of their success with school-age DHH learners and none verifying which strategy was more productive for an individual language structure. We proposed a hypothesis (gleaned from research on struggling readers) that linguistic structure and argument structure coexist at the phrase-structure level (also referred to herein as *supralexical unitization*). Research on language-based reading comprehension interventions that build around face-to-face and in-print understanding might be a useful line of research because phrase-level language and reading are Radical Middle concepts crossing languages, modes, and other areas of research interest. We hope that the brief review of available interventions summarized in this chapter serves as a call to action. We do not need more research that divides the field. We do not need more research for the purpose of supporting a belief. We do need a consistent, persistent, aggressive, and forward-thinking research plan to imagine, create, develop, implement, research, revise, and then disseminate efficient and effective strategies and interventions that will ensure that all DHH children master the language reflected in the words and phrases they read in whatever print form is used to convey that language.

REFERENCES

Adiseshiah, M. S. (1990). *Illiteracy and Poverty. Literacy Lessons*. Geneva, Switzerland: International Bureau of Education.

Alamargot, D., Lambert, E., Thebault, C., & Dansac, C. (2007). Text composition by deaf and hearing middle-school students: The role of working memory. *Reading and Writing: An Interdisciplinary Journal, 20*(4), 333–360.

Anderson, M., Boren, N., Kilgore, J., Howard, W., & Krohn, E. (1999). *Appletree* (2nd ed.). Austin, TX: Pro-Ed.

Andrew, K. N., Hoshooley, J., & Joanisse, M. F. (2014). Sign language ability in young deaf signers predicts comprehension of written sentences in English. *PLoS One, 9*(2), 1–8.

Arfé, B., & Boscolo, P. (2006). Causal coherence in deaf and hearing students' written narratives. *Discourse Processes, 42*(3), 271–300.

Aronoff, M., & Fudeman, K. (2011). *Thinking about morphology and morphological analysis. What is morphology?* Malden, MS: Wiley.

Aronoff, M., Meir, I., & Sandler, W. (2005). The paradox of sign language morphology. *Language, 81*(2), 301–344.

Baddeley, A. D. (2000). The episodic buffer: a new component of working memory? *Trends in Cognitive Sciences, 4*(11), 417–423.

Beal-Alvarez, J. S., & Easterbrooks, S. R. (2014). Increasing children's ASL classifier production: A multicomponent intervention. *American Annals of the Deaf, 158*(3), 311–333.

Bennett, J. G., Gardner, R., Leighner, R., Clancy, S., & Garner, J. (2014). Explicitly teaching English through the air to students who are deaf or hard of hearing. *American Annals of the Deaf, 159*(1), 45–58.

Berent, G. P. (1996). Learnability constraints on deaf learners' acquisition of English wh-questions. *Journal of Speech & Hearing Research, 39*(3), 625–642.

Berent, G. P., Kelly, R. R., Albertini, J. A., & Toscano, R. M. (2013). Deaf students' knowledge of subtle lexical properties of transitive and intransitive English verbs. *American Annals of the Deaf, 158*(3), 344–362.

Berent, G. P., Kelly, R. R., Porter, J. E., & Fonzi, J. (2008). Deaf learners' knowledge of English universal quantifiers. *Language Learning, 58*(2), 401–437.

Berent, G. P., Kelly, R. R., Schmitz, K. L., & Kenney, P. (2009). Visual input enhancement via essay coding results in deaf learners' long-term retention of improved English grammatical knowledge. *Journal of Deaf Studies and Deaf Education, 14*(2), 190–204.

Biemiller, A. (2001). Teaching vocabulary: Early, direct, and sequential. *American Educator, 24*, 28–47.

Bird, H., Franklin, S., & Howard, D. (2001). Age of acquisition and imageability ratings for a large set of words, including verbs and function words. *Behavior Research Methods, Instruments, & Computers, 33*(1), 73–79.

Bishop, D. V. M., Adams, C. V., & Rosen, S. (2006). Resistance of grammatical impairment to computerized comprehension training in children with specific and non-specific language impairments. *International Journal of Language and Communication Disorders, 41*(1), 19–40.

Blackwell, P., Engen, E., Fischgrund, J., Zarcadoolas, C. (1978). *Sentences and Other Systems*. Washington, DC: A. G. Bell Association for the Deaf.

Bobaljik, J. D. (2012). *Universals in comparative morphology: Suppletion, superlatives, and the structure of words*. Cambridge, MA: MIT Press.

Boons, T., de Raeve, L., Langereis, M., Peeraer, L., Wouters, J., & van Wieringen, A. (2013). Expressive vocabulary, morphology, syntax and narrative skills in profoundly deaf children after early cochlear implantation. *Research in Developmental Disabilities*, 34(6), 2008–2022.

Bow, C. P., Blamey, P. J., Paatsch, L. E., & Sarant, J. Z. (2004). The effects of phonological and morphological training on speech perception scores and grammatical judgments in deaf and hard-of-hearing children. *Journal of Deaf Studies and Deaf Education*, 9(3), 305–314.

Breadmore, H. L., Krott, A., & Olson, A. C. (2014). Agreeing to disagree: Deaf and hearing children's awareness of subject–verb number agreement. *The Quarterly Journal of Experimental Psychology*, 67(3), 474–498.

Cannon, J., Easterbrooks, S. R., Gagné, P., & Beal-Alvarez, J. (2011). Improving DHH students' grammar through an individualized software program. *Journal of Deaf Studies and Deaf Education*, 16(4), 437–457.

Cannon, J., Fredrick, L., & Easterbrooks, S. (2009). Vocabulary instruction through books read in American Sign Language for English-language learners. *Communication Disorders Quarterly*, 31(2), 98–112.

Cannon, J. E., & Guardino, C. (2012). Literacy strategies for deaf/hard of hearing ELLs: Where do we begin? *Deafness and Education International*, 14(2), 78–99.

Cannon, J. E., & Kirby, S. (2013). Grammar structures and deaf and hard of hearing students: A review of past performance and a report of new findings. *American Annals of the Deaf*, 158(3), 292–310.

Carlo, M. S., August, D., McLaughlin, B., Snow, C. E., Dressler, C., Lippman, D. N., Lively, T., & White, C. E. (2004). Closing the gap: Addressing the vocabulary needs of English-language learners in bilingual and mainstream classrooms. *Reading Research Quarterly*, 39, 188–215.

Caselli, M. C., Rinaldi, P., Varuzza, C., Giuliani, A., & Burdo, S. (2012). Cochlear implant in the second year of life: Lexical and grammatical outcomes. *Journal of Speech, Language, and Hearing Research*, 55(2), 382–394.

Channon, R., & Sayers, E. E. (2007). Toward a description of deaf college students' written English: Overuse, avoidance, and mastery of function words. *American Annals of the Deaf*, 152(2), 91–103.

Chen, M. Y. (2000). *Tone sandhi: Patterns across Chinese dialects*. New York, NY: Cambridge University Press.

Chomsky, N. (1957). *Syntactic structures*. The Hague/Paris: Mouton.

Chomsky, N. (2005). Three factors in language design. *Linguistic Inquiry*, 36(1), 1–22.

Cirrin, F. M., & Gillam, R. B. (2008). Language intervention practices for school-age children with spoken language disorders: A systemic review. *Language, Speech, and Hearing Services in Schools*, 39, 110–137.

Connell, P. (1992). Morpheme learning of children with specific language impairment under controlled instructional conditions. *Journal of Speech and Hearing Research*, 35(4), 844–853.

Convertino, C. M., Marschark, M., Sapere, P., Sarchet, T., & Zupan, M. (2009). Predicting academic success among deaf college students. *Journal of Deaf Studies and Deaf Education*, 14(3), 324–343.

Coppens, K.M., Tellings, A., Verhoeven, L., & Schreuder, R. (2013). Reading vocabulary in children with and without hearing loss: The roles of task and word type. *Journal of Speech, Language, and Hearing Research, 56*, 654–666.

Cruz, I., Quittner, A. L., Marker, C., & DesJardin, J. L. (2013). Identification of effective strategies to promote language in deaf children with cochlear implants. *Child Development, 84*(2), 543–559.

de Villiers, P. A. (1983). Semantic and pragmatic factors in the acquisition of syntax. *The Volta Review, 85*(5), 10–28.

Diaz, M. T., & McCarthy, G. (2009). A comparison of brain activity evoked by single content and function words: An fMRI investigation of implicit word processing. *Brain Research, 1282*, 38–49.

Dixon, L. Q., Zhao, J., & Joshi, R. M. (2012). One dress, two dress: Dialectal influence on spelling of English words among kindergarten children in Singapore. *System, 40*(2), 214–225.

Dolman, D. (1983). A study of the relationship between syntactic development and concrete operations in deaf children. *American Annals of the Deaf, 128*(6), 813–819.

Easterbrooks, S., & Maiorana-Basas, M. (2015). Literacy acquisition in deaf and hard-of-hearing children. In H. Knoors & M. Marschark (Eds.), *Educating deaf learners* (pp. 149–172). New York, NY: Oxford University Press.

Easterbrooks, S. R., & Stephenson, B. H. (2012). Clues from research: Effective instructional strategies leading to positive outcomes for students who are deaf or hard of hearing. *Odyssey Magazine, 13*, 44–49.

Easterbrooks, S. R., & Stoner, M. (2006). Using a visual tool to increase adjectives in the written language of students who are deaf or hard of hearing. *Communication Disorders Quarterly, 27*(2), 95–109.

Ebbels, S., & van der Lely, H. (2001). Meta-syntactic therapy using visual coding for children with severe persistent SLI. *International Journal of Language & Communication Disorders, 36*, 345–350.

Ehri, L. (1976). Word learning in beginning readers and prereaders: Effects of form class and defining contexts. *Journal of Educational Psychology, 68*(6), 832–842.

Ehri, L., & Wilce, L. S. (1980). Do beginners learn to read function words better in sentences or in lists? Paper presented at the Annual Meeting of the American Educational Research Association. Boston, MA, April 7–11.

French, M. (1992). Grammar and meaning in a whole language framework. *Perspectives in Education and Deafness, 10*(3), 19–21, 24.

Friedmann, N., & Szterman, R. (2006). Syntactic movement in orally trained children with hearing impairment. *Journal of Deaf Studies and Deaf Education, 11*(1), 56–75.

Friedmann, N., & Szterman, R. (2011). The comprehension and production of wh-questions in deaf and hard-of-hearing children. *Journal of Deaf Studies & Deaf Education, 16*(2), 212–235.

Fujiyoshi, A., Fukushima, K., Taguchi, T., Omori, K., Kasai, N., Noshio, S., Sugaya, A., Nagayasu, R., Konishi, T., Sugishita, S., Fujita, J., Nishkizaki, K., & Shiroma, M. (2012). Syntactic development in Japanese hearing-impaired children. *Annals of Otology, Rhinology & Laryngology, 121*(4), 28–34.

Gaustad, M., Kelly, R., Payne, J., & Lylak, E. (2002). Deaf and hearing students' morphological knowledge applied to printed English. *American Annals of the Deaf, 147*(5), 5–21.

Gheitury, A., Ashraf, V., & Hashemi, R. (2014). Investigating deaf students' knowledge of Persian syntax: Further evidence for a critical period hypothesis. *Neurocase, 20*(3), 346–354.

Glackin, S. (2010). Universal grammar and the Baldwin effect: A hypothesis and some philosophical consequences. *Biology & Philosophy, 26*(2), 201–222.

Goodson, B., Wolf, A., Bell, S., Turner, H., & Finney, P. B. (2010). *The effectiveness of a program to accelerate vocabulary development in kindergarten (VOCAB)* (NCEE 2010-4014). Washington, DC: National Center for Education Evaluation and Regional Assistance, Institute of Education Sciences, U.S. Department of Education.

Gough, P. B., Hoover, W. A., & Peterson, C. L. (1996). Some observations on a simple view of reading. In C. Cornoldi & J. Oakhill (Eds.), *Reading comprehension difficulties: Processes and interventions* (pp. 1–13). Mahwah, NJ: Lawrence Erlbaum Associates.

Guo, L., Spencer, L. J., & Tomblin, J. B. (2013). Acquisition of tense marking in English-speaking children with cochlear implants: A longitudinal study. *Journal of Deaf Studies and Deaf Education, 18*(2), 187–205.

Harrison, M., Roush, J., & Wallace, J. (2003). Trends in age of identification and intervention in infants with hearing loss. *Ear and Hearing, 24*(1), 89–95.

Hayes, H., Geers, A. E., Treiman, R., & Moog, J. S. (2009). Receptive vocabulary development in deaf children with cochlear implants: Achievement in an intensive auditory-oral educational setting. *Ear and hearing, 30*(1), 128–135.

Hermans, D., Knoors, H., Ormel, E., & Verhoeven, L. (2008). The relationship between the reading and signing skills of deaf children in bilingual education programs. *Journal of Deaf Studies and Deaf Education, 13*(4), 518–530.

Hicks, J. (2006). The impact of function words on the processing and acquisition of syntax. PhD dissertation, Northwestern University.

Hustad, K. C., Da rdis, C. M., & Mccourt, K. A. (2007). Effects of visual information on intelligibility of open and closed class words in predictable sentences produced by speakers with dysarthria. *Clinical Linguistics & Phonetics, 21*(5), 353–367.

Ionin, T., & Wexler, K. (2002). Why is "is" easier than "-s"?: Acquisition of tense/agreement morphology by child second language learners of English. *Second Language Research, 18*(2), 195–136.

Isaka, Y. (2011). Changes in vocabulary size of pupils at a school for the deaf: As measured by the Picture Vocabulary Test. *Japanese Journal of Special Education, 49*(1), 11–19.

Johnson, V. E., & de Villiers, J. G. (2009). Syntactic frames in fast mapping verbs: Effects of age, dialect, and clinical status. *Journal of Speech, Language, and Hearing Research, 52*(3), 610–622.

Johnson, C. & Goswami, U. (2010). Phonological awareness, vocabulary, and reading in deaf children with cochlear implants. *Journal of Speech, Language, and Hearing Research, 53*, 237–261.

Kelly, L. P. (1988). Relative automaticity without mastery: The grammatical decision making of deaf students. *Written Communication, 5*(3), 325–351.

Kelly, L. P. (1993). Recall of English function words and inflections by skilled and average deaf readers. *American Annals of the Deaf, 138*(3), 288–296.

Kelly, L. (1996). The interaction of syntactic competence and vocabulary during reading by deaf students. *Journal of Deaf Studies and Deaf Education, 1*(1), 75–90.

Kelly, R. R., & Berent, G. P. (2011). Semantic and pragmatic factors influencing deaf and hearing students' comprehension of English sentences containing numeral quantifiers. *Journal of Deaf Studies and Deaf Education, 16*(4), 419–436.

Kieffer, M. J., & Lesaux, N. K. (2012). Effects of academic language instruction on relational and syntactic aspects of morphological awareness for sixth graders from linguistically diverse backgrounds. *The Elementary School Journal, 112*(3), 519–545.

Kiese-Himmel, C., & Reeh, M. (2006). Assessment of expressive vocabulary outcomes in hearing-impaired children with hearing aids: Do bilaterally hearing-impaired children catch up? *The Journal of Laryngology and Otology, 120*(8), 619–626.

Klauda, S. L., & Guthrie, J. T. (2008). Relationship of three components of reading fluency to reading comprehension. *Journal of Educational Psychology, 100*, 310–321.

Kluwin, T. N. (1982). Deaf adolescents' comprehension of English prepositions. *American Annals of the Deaf, 127*(7), 852–859.

LaSasso, C. J. (1990). Developing the ability of hearing-impaired students to comprehend and generate question forms. *American Annals of the Deaf, 135*(5), 409–412.

Leikin, M., & Assayag-Bouskila, O. (2004). Expression of syntactic complexity in sentence comprehension: A comparison between dyslexic and regular readers. *Reading and Writing, 17*, 801–822.

Leonard, L. B., Camarata, S. M., Brown, B., & Camarata, M. N. (2004). Tense and agreement in the speech of children with specific language impairment: Patterns of generalization through intervention. *Journal of Speech, Language & Hearing Research, 47*, 1363–1379.

Leonard, L., Camarata, S. M., Pawłowska, M., Brown, B., & Camarata, M. (2006). Tense and agreement morphemes in the speech of children with specific language impairment during intervention: Phase 2. *Journal of Speech, Language and Hearing Research, 49*, 749–770.

Leonard, L. B., Camarata, S. M., Pawlowska, M., Brown, B., & Camarata, M. N. (2008). The acquisition of tense and agreement morphemes by children with specific language impairment during intervention: Phase 3. *Journal of Speech and Hearing Research, 51*, 120–125.

Lillo-Martin, D. C. (1992). Deaf readers' comprehension of relative clause structure. *Applied Psycholinguistics, 13*(1), 13–30.

Lively, T., August, D., Carlo, M. S., & Snow, C. E. (2003). *Vocabulary improvement program for English language learners and their classmates*. Baltimore, MD: Brookes Publishing.

Lohndal, T. (2014). *Phrase structure and argument structure: A case study of the syntax–semantics interface*. New York, NY: Oxford University Press.

Luckner, J. L., & Cooke, C. (2010). A summary of the vocabulary research with students who are deaf or hard of hearing. *American Annals of the Deaf, 155*(1), 38–67.

Luckner, J. L., & Handley, C. M. (2008). A summary of the reading comprehension research undertaken with students who are deaf or hard of hearing. *American Annals of the Deaf, 153*, 6–36.

Luckner, J. L., Sebald, A. M., Cooney, J., Young J., III, & Muir S. G. (2005/2006). An examination of the evidence-based literacy research in deaf education. *American Annals of the Deaf, 150*, 443–456.

Luckner, J. L., & Urbach, J. E. (2012). Reading fluency and students who are deaf or hard of hearing: Synthesis of the research. *Communication Disorders Quarterly, 33*(4), 230–241.

MacWhinney, B. (2000). *The CHILDES project: Tools for analyzing talk* (3rd ed., Vol. 2). Mahwah, NJ: Lawrence Erlbaum Associates.

Mann, W., Roy, P., & Marshall, C. (2013) A look at the other 90 per cent: investigating British sign language vocabulary knowledge in deaf children from different language learning backgrounds. *Deafness & Education International, 15*(2), 91–116.

Man-shu, Z., & Jing-zhe, W. (1984). Chinese children's comprehension and production of passive voice and double negative sentences. *International Journal of Behavioral Development, 7*(1), 67–76.

Maul, C. A., & Ambler, K. L. (2014). Embedding language therapy in dialogic reading to teach morphologic structures to children with language disorders. *Communication Disorders Quarterly, 35*(4), 237–247.

McGuckian, M., & Henry, A. (2007). The grammatical morpheme deficit in moderate hearing impairment. *International Journal of Language and Communication Disorders, 42*(S1), 17–36.

Miller, P. F. (2000). Syntactic and semantic processing in Hebrew readers with prelingual deafness. *American Annals of the Deaf, 145*(5), 436–451.

Miller, P. (2010). Phonological, orthographic, and syntactic awareness and their relation to reading comprehension in prelingually deaf individuals: What can we learn from skilled readers? *Journal of Developmental & Physical Disabilities, 22*(6), 549–580.

Miller, P., Kargin, T., & Guldenoglu, B. (2013). The reading comprehension failure of Turkish prelingually deaf readers: Evidence from semantic and syntactic processing. *Journal of Developmental and Physical Disabilities, 25*(2), 221–239.

Miller, P., Kargin, T., Guldenoglu, B., Rathmann, C., Kubus, O., Hauser, P., & Spurgeon, E. (2012). Factors distinguishing skilled and less skilled deaf readers: Evidence from four orthographies. *Journal of Deaf Studies and Deaf Education, 17*(4), 439–462.

Miller, D. C., & Warren, L. K. (2011). *Comparative indicators of education in the United States and other G-8 Countries: 2011.* Washington, DC: National Center for Education Statistics.

Moeller, M. P. (1986). Cognitively based strategies for use with hearing-impaired students with comprehension deficits. *Topics in Language Disorders, 6*(4), 37–50.

Moeller, M. P. (2000). Early intervention and language development in children who are deaf and hard of hearing. *Pediatrics, 106*(3), e43.

Mokhtari, K., & Thompson, H. B. (2006). How problems of reading fluency and comprehension are related to difficulties in syntactic awareness skills among fifth graders. *Reading Research and Instruction, 46*, 73–93.

Moores, D. F., & Sweet, C. (1990). Relationships of English grammar and communicative fluency to reading in deaf adolescents. *Exceptionality, 1*(2), 97–106.

Nation, K., & Snowling, M. J. (2000). Factors influencing syntactic awareness skills in normal readers and poor comprehenders. *Applied Psycholinguistics, 21*, 229–241.

Nelson, J. R., Vadasy, P. F., & Sanders, E. A. (2011). Efficacy of tier 2 supplemental root word vocabulary and decoding intervention with kindergarten Spanish-speaking English learners. *Journal of Literacy Research, 43*(2), 184–211.

Newman, A. J., Supalla, T., Hauser, P., Newport, E. L., & Bavelier, D. (2010). Dissociating neural subsystems for grammar by contrasting word order and inflection. *Proceedings of the National Academy of Sciences of the United States of America, 107*(16), 7539–7544.
Nomvete, P. (2014). Effects of phrase-reading ability, syntactic awareness, and reading rate on reading comprehension of adolescent readers in an alternative setting. PhD dissertation, Georgia State University. http://scholarworks.gsu.edu/epse_diss/96.
Omori, R., & Sawa, T. (2008). Development of linguistic complexity and accuracy in sentences written by students who are deaf. *Japanese Journal of Special Education, 46*(4), 205–214.
Paivio, A., Yuille, J. C., & Madigan, S. A. (1968). Concreteness, imagery and meaningfulness values for 925 nouns. *Journal of Experimental Psychology, 76*, 1–25.
Quigley, S. P., & King, C. M. (1980). Syntactic performance of hearing impaired and normal hearing individuals. *Applied Psycholinguistics, 1*(4), 329–356.
Reder, S. (2010). *Adult literacy development and economic growth*. Washington, DC: National Institute for Literacy.
Reed, D. K. (2008). A synthesis of morphology interventions and effects on reading outcome for students in grade k-12. *Learning Disabilities Research & Practice, 23*(1), 36–49.
Rice, M. L., Wexler, K., & Cleave, P. L. (1995). Specific language impairment as a period of extended optional infinitive. *Journal of Speech, Language, and Hearing Research, 38*(4), 850–863.
Robbins, N. L., & Hatcher, C. W. (1981). The effects of syntax on the reading comprehension of hearing-impaired children. *The Volta Review, 83*(2), 105–115.
Ryuzaki, M., & Ito, T. (1999). Knowledge of the argument and phrase structure of passives in children with hearing impairments. *Japanese Journal of Special Education, 36*(4), 23–30.
Sarachan-Deily, A. (1982). Hearing-impaired and hearing readers' sentence processing errors. *The Volta Review, 84*(2), 81–95.
Schirmer, B. R. (1985). An analysis of the language of young hearing-impaired children in terms of syntax, semantics, and use. *American Annals of the Deaf, 130*(1), 15–19.
Schwanenflugel, P. J., Hamilton, C. E., Neuharth-Pritchett, S., Restrepo, M. A., Bradley, B. A., & Webb, M. Y. (2010). PAVEd for Success: An evaluation of a comprehensive preliteracy program for four-year-old children. *Journal of Literacy Research, 42*(3), 227–275.
Shimizu, Y. (1988). The development of sentence comprehension in hearing-impaired children. *Japanese Journal of Special Education, 25*(4), 21–28.
Skotara, N., Kügow, M., Salden, U., Hänel-Faulhaber, B., & Röder, B. (2011). ERP correlates of intramodal and crossmodal L2 acquisition. *BMC Neuroscience, 12*(1), 48.
Swanepoel, D., Störbeck, C., & Friedland, P. (2009). Early hearing detection and intervention in South Africa. *International Journal of Pediatric Otorhinolaryngology, 73*(6), 783–786.
Swisher, L., Restrepo, M. A., Plante, E., & Lowell, S. (1995). Effect of implicit and explicit "rule" presentation on bound-morpheme generalization in specific language impairment. *Journal of Speech and Hearing Research, 38*(1), 168–173.

Tomblin, B. (2010). Literacy as an outcome of language development and its impact on children's psychosocial and emotional development. *Encyclopedia of Early Childhood Development*. Retrieved from: http://www.child-encyclopedia.com/sites/default/files/textes-experts/en/622/literacy-as-an-outcome-of-language-development-and-its-impact-on-childrens-psychosocial-and-emotional-development.pdf. Accessed January 25, 2016.

Traxler, C. B. (2000). The Stanford Achievement Test, 9th edition: National norming and performance standards for deaf and hard-of-hearing students. *Journal of Deaf Studies and Deaf Education, 5*(4), 337–348.

Traxler, M., Corina, D., Morford, J., Hafer, S., & Hoversten, L. (2014). Deaf readers' response to syntactic complexity: Evidence from self-paced reading. *Memory & Cognition, 42*(1), 97–111.

Trussell, J. W., & Easterbrooks, S. R. (2015). Effects of morphographic instruction on the morphographic analysis skills of deaf and hard-of-hearing students. *Journal of Deaf Studies and Deaf Education, 20*(3), 229–241.

Tucci, S., Trussell, J., & Easterbrooks, S. R. (2014). A review of the evidence on strategies for teaching children who are DHH grapheme-phoneme correspondence. *Communication Disorders Quarterly, 35*(4), 191–203.

van Beijsterveldt, L. M., & van Hell, J. G. (2009). Structural priming of adjective-noun structures in hearing and deaf children. *Journal of Experimental Child Psychology, 104*(2), 179–196.

van Hoogmoed, A. H., Verhoeven, L., Schreuder, R., & Knoors, H. (2011). Morphological sensitivity in deaf readers of Dutch. *Applied Psycholinguistics, 32*, 619–634.

Verhoeven, L., & Perfetti, C. (2003). Introduction to this special issue: The role of morphology in learning to read. *Scientific Studies of Reading, 7*(3), 209–217.

Weber-Fox, C., & Neville, H. J. (2001). Sensitive periods differentiate processing of open- and closed-class words. *Journal of Speech, Language, and Hearing Research, 44*, 1338–1353.

Weismer, S., & Murray-Branch, J. (1989). Modeling versus modeling plus evoked production training: A comparison of two language intervention methods. *Journal of Speech and Hearing Disorders, 54*, 269–281.

White, A. H. (2002). Assessing semantic-syntactic features of verbs from thirteen verb subsets. *American Annals of the Deaf, 147*(1), 65–77.

Whitehurst, G., Falco, F., Lonigan, C., Fischel, J., Debarsyhe, B., & Caulfield, M. (1988). Accelerating language development through picture book reading. *Developmental Psychology, 24*(4), 552–559.

Wilbur, R. B., & Goodhart, W. C. (1985). Comprehension of indefinite pronouns and quantifiers by hearing-impaired students. *Applied Psycholinguistics, 6*(4), 417–434.

Wilbur, R., Goodhart, W., & Montandon, E. (1983). Comprehension of nine syntactic structures by hearing-impaired students. *The Volta Review, 85*(7), 328–345.

Wolbers, K. A., Bowers, L. M., Dostal, H. M., & Graham, S. C. (2014). Deaf writers' application of American Sign Language knowledge to English. *International Journal of Bilingual Education & Bilingualism, 17*(4), 410–428.

Wolbers, K. A., Dostal, H. M., & Bowers, L. M. (2012). "I was born full deaf." written language outcomes after 1 year of strategic and interactive writing instruction. *Journal of Deaf Studies and Deaf Education, 17*(1), 19–38.

Yoshinaga-Itano, C. (2003). From screening to early identification and intervention: Discovering predictors to successful outcomes for children with significant hearing loss. *Journal of Deaf Studies and Deaf Education, 8*(1), 11–30.

12

From Social Periphery to Social Centrality: Building Social Capital for Deaf and Hard-of-Hearing Students in the 21st Century

Gina A. Oliva, Linda Risser Lytle, Mindy Hopper, and Joan M. Ostrove

Spoken conversation is everywhere and occurs constantly—"24/7," as Americans say colloquially. This is a simple fact of life; most people never give it a second thought. Theories about human development take for granted that young people will have continuous and easy access to spoken language, but for individuals who grow up unable to hear or struggling to hear, a virtual glass wall separates them from the ongoing airborne information exchange, which affects their development every single moment of every single day. The goal of this chapter is to call attention to the impact of this "glass wall" on the educational and social–emotional development of young deaf and hard-of-hearing students in public school settings. Their capacity to engage their full humanity—indeed, everyone's capacity to do this—depends on language, social interactions, and the conversations that take place during social interactions.

People talk in homes, schools, workplaces, stores, neighborhoods, and playgrounds—everywhere. People also talk on radio and television and, of course, computers and cell phones. What does it really mean when an individual's ears transmit this never-ceasing exchange of language to the brain? What is missed when this information does not reach the brain? In all the efforts throughout centuries to educate the hearing world about the lives of deaf and hard-of-hearing individuals, 90% of the attention has been focused on how missing all of this ambient talking affects language acquisition. Of course, this is important and, yes, it is ultimately the crux of the matter. But, if you talk to deaf or hard-of-hearing adults, they will tell you not so much about the struggles they had (and likely still have) with reading. They will talk to you about the impact of the "glass wall" that prevented their full access to and inclusion in everyday conversation with their social connections, or lack thereof. Thus, it is critical to address this elusive but important experience of not having access to 24/7 language input. The question posed in this chapter, therefore, is not "Will Janie be able to read?" but "Will Janie be able to make friends?" "Does Billy know that all the kids in school are talking about that new TV program?" More profoundly, "What will happen to Billy when he grows up? Who will be his friends, his support network, his partner?"

Children born into deaf families where members use a sign language absorb that language through their eyes. It goes without saying now that such children will have a natural language, and this language base will serve them well as they learn to read and write. Most likely, they will also have rich social involvements because their parents already have well-developed social relationships and resources within their Deaf community. But for the great majority of deaf children born to hearing parents, visual access to conversation is significantly limited. These children often will be fitted with cochlear implants, or with hearing aids, and an attempt will be made to train them in spoken language. How successful they will be at acquiring natural-enough language, and how successful they will be at picking up all that conversation effortlessly around them, remains controversial and quite variable. It is important to keep in mind that most children with cochlear implants are still deaf and functionally hard-of-hearing. It is these children of hearing parents, and the adults they become, that this chapter addresses primarily.

SOCIAL CAPITAL AND HUMAN DEVELOPMENT

Social capital is a useful term for describing the relationships and connections deaf and hard-of-hearing schoolchildren have (or do not have) with peers and adults in their schools and neighborhood environs. Briefly, social capital encompasses the connections one has with social networks such as family, friends, school, religious organizations or institutions, and community (Putnam, 2000). Stronger and more vital social capital results in greater trust, cooperation, information flow, and reciprocity. In his landmark book *Bowling Alone*, sociologist Robert Putnam (2000) described two kinds of social capital. "Bonding social capital" is built between people who are similar to one another in certain elements (race, social class, and so forth). We can assume bonding social capital is the kind that develops when isolated deaf and hard-of-hearing individuals find others like themselves—the commonality of hearing status becomes a basis for bonding social capital.

Putnam (2000) describes the other form of social capital as "bridging social capital." This form of capital is what develops between individuals who are different from each other in significant ways. Both forms of social capital are vital because they help to build strong connections to communities and to individuals within the communities. These connections serve to enhance life experience in many ways.

When the concept of social capital is applied to deaf and hard-of-hearing students in general-education settings, serious gaps become evident. Many deaf and hard-of-hearing students in these settings are isolated socially. Although some have cochlear implants and/or classroom interpreters, neither the implants nor the interpreters provide full access to all or even most of the conversations that take place beyond direct teacher–student discourse. As a result, there is much information being exchanged—every single day—that deaf and hard-of-hearing students are missing. The loss of information and connections is profound; Hopper's (2011) study, described later, illustrates just how profound.

Impoverished Social Capital in General-Education Settings

For the most part, individual deaf and hard-of-hearing students, their families, and their school personnel do not have the knowledge, willingness, or resources to improve communication access (Drolsbaugh, 2013; Hopper, 2011; Lane et al., 1996; Oliva, 2004; Oliva & Lytle, 2014). This is despite the fact that numerous scholars have been aware of these issues for decades. This awareness has prompted researchers to explore characteristics or elements of the mainstream experience that can make a positive difference for deaf and hard-of-hearing students. For example, studies have shown the positive effects their participation in school, club activities, and sports can have on school success and self-esteem (Kluwin et al., 1992; Stewart & Ellis, 2005; Stinson & Antia, 1999).

In contrast, there are also studies showing that extracurricular participation is limited and comes at a considerable cost to these students. Deaf adults looking back on their school experiences reported they were included and valued only as long as the sport season lasted, then they once again became unwelcome and unseen (Oliva & Lytle, 2014). Also reported are feelings of being left out of the camaraderie that occurs outside the actual sport arenas (bus trips, dinner outings, parties, and so on) that leaves them feeling lonelier when they are with their teammates than when they are truly alone (Dorminy, 2013; Drolsbaugh, 2013; Hopper, 2011; Oliva, 2004; Oliva & Lytle, 2014). These reports are important because they remind us that social capital is not so much built from merely participating in activities with others (such as playing a game of soccer), but from the conversations, connections, and companionship that comes from being part of a group.

Deaf and hard-of-hearing children and youth report they are frequently not able to access the ubiquitous conversations that take place in groups, and they are typically on the periphery of things as observers or bystanders (Drolsbaugh, 2013; Hopper, 2011; Oliva, 2004; Oliva & Lytle, 2014). Although being active in extracurricular activities is beneficial, it is not the same as having a sense of deep belonging, acceptance, and friendship (Dorminy, 2013; Drolsbaugh, 2013; Hopper, 2011; Oliva, 2004; Oliva & Lytle, 2014). Oliva (2004) coined the word "solitaires" to describe deaf and hard-of-hearing individuals who are the only such individual in their school or social world. This word conveys the strong sense of both isolation and loneliness that is expressed so frequently, including when solitaires are active in sports and other extracurricular activities.

In formal classroom settings, deaf and hard-of-hearing students possibly fare a bit better, particularly with teacher-directed instruction as opposed to group work and class discussions. However, even in classrooms where educational interpreters were present or where cochlear implants and frequency modulation systems were used, deaf and hard-of-hearing adults report they often were still not fully included (Oliva & Lytle, 2014). Furthermore, the burden of navigating communication barriers in the classroom is often placed on the child. This may be especially true in schools with scarce resources and/or where awareness of issues faced by children who are deaf or hard-of-hearing is especially limited.

Contact theory, developed by Allport (1954), hypothesized that prejudice would be reduced and positive feelings would be enhanced among group members if they were together significant amounts of times and (a) had equal status, (b) were engaged in cooperative activities, (c) had common goals, and (d) were supported by social and institutional authorities. Using the parameters outlined by contact theory, deaf and hard-of-hearing students in general-education settings are, theoretically, exposed daily to cooperative learning and/or team activities with common goals (good grades, winning games) and these activities, generally speaking, are supported by school administrators and teachers. The first requirement of "equal status," however, may very well be problematic for students who are deaf or hard of hearing. Full access to conversations, and the information conveyed within, is necessary for equal status in classroom and other school environs. This access is limited, sometimes severely so, for deaf and hard-of-hearing students in general-education settings.

Recent applications of Allport's theory have demonstrated that simply bringing two cross-groups into contact with each can reduce prejudice, but that friendships are developed only with long-lasting contact and deep communication (Davies et al., 2011). Physical togetherness does not result in social connections if the cross-groups lack the language to communicate deeply (Keating & Mirus, 2003). Placing deaf and hard-of-hearing children in general-education classes may help hearing children learn to accept differences. Unless equal linguistic competence and access to informal conversation allows depth of friendship to develop, deaf and hard-of-hearing students may still feel lonely and isolated in general-education settings.

Dorminy (2013) interviewed 10 deaf and hard-of-hearing college students about their experiences in general-education classrooms. A major theme emerging from this study was the amount of effort and energy her participants described as necessary for navigating communication barriers in both learning and social environments each and every day. Into the effort/energy column went any kind of self-advocacy action such as asking a teacher to repeat information, asking that captions be turned on for movies, asking a friend for information, and requesting front-row seating or notes. Her participants also talked about the toll taken by the intense focus on lip-reading, listening, or watching the interpreter for hours at a time; and the copious amounts of reading and independent work done outside of class to make up for what they knew they were missing. Participants in the study by Oliva and Lytle (2014) talked about the same issues and included in their list the necessity of parents becoming involved in advocacy. In fact, they went so far as to say parents of deaf and hard-of-hearing children who were not willing or able to advocate for their child had no business putting them in a mainstream setting because it was just too hard for students to carry the advocacy burden alone. The task of actual learning became secondary to the enormous task of addressing barriers to learning.

The constant energy expended toward breaking down barriers was a central experience for Dorminy's (2013) participants, so much so that they developed a highly sensitive "energy expenditure radar" (p. 109) that helped them to do a kind of cost–benefit analysis for any actions they were considering in any given situation. For example, the cost of raising a hand in class to ask a question to clarify missing information was only beneficial if one had been following the lecture successfully up to that point. If there were significant chunks of information missing, the student could easily be worried about the appropriateness of her question or wonder where to start asking for clarification. Maybe the question would make it painfully obvious she had missed something already explained in detail or would point out clearly how totally lost she was. The student might very well determine there was little benefit to asking and instead decide to research the information independently later that evening. Thus, the cost of speaking up in a classroom setting often carries with it much more expense than benefit. Even if the student was to express the question successfully, her receptive communication would also need to be successful for the action of asking the question to be beneficial.

All this information about what deaf or hard-of-hearing learners face daily in school environments suggests their social capital reservoirs are not filling up in the ways they should. An individual's social capital typically begins to develop during the K–12 years, when opportunities for communication and resulting social connections are ever-present. However, clearly the barriers to friendships and social connections for most deaf and hard-of-hearing students in general-education settings are enormous. Although many hearing individuals maintain friendships with K–12 classmates throughout life, this is rare indeed for mainstreamed deaf and hard-of-hearing individuals. In the studies cited previously, there were exceedingly few stories of trust or cooperation between deaf and hard-of-hearing students and their hearing classmates. Many described, instead, feeling isolated and lonely, sometimes desperately so.

Research has shown that the flow of information between deaf and hearing schoolmates can be quite superficial. When connections are made, those connections are often unidirectional, from hearing teacher or classmate to deaf student. Little reciprocity—an important part of social capital—seems evident. As an illustration, Keating and Mirus (2003) observed interactions between deaf and hearing elementary students in their school setting for 5 months. They found significant differences in interaction patterns that left the deaf children observing more than interacting and participating in dyadic rather than multiparty conversations. In addition, they noted significantly less turn-taking by the deaf children (the deaf children had significantly fewer opportunities to say something or contribute) and turn-taking interactions were briefer in duration.

Ramsey (1997) eloquently described this lack of reciprocity. Based on her year-long observation of three second graders in their public school classrooms, she described how hearing classmates gave directives to their deaf and hard-of-hearing peers (for example, "turn to page 20" or "the teacher said ... "), but did not genuinely converse with them. Decades have passed since studies by Ramsey (1997) and Keating and Mirus (2003), and still it seems that the full participation desired for deaf and hard-of-hearing students in general-education settings is not happening. Ramsey (1997) concluded:

> For the purposes of learning and development, the interaction among deaf and hearing children in the mainstreaming classroom ... was highly constrained and not developmentally helpful ... few parents of hearing children would judge sufficient for their own children the personal contact and peer interaction that was available in the mainstream for deaf second graders at Aspen School [fictitious name]. (p. 74)

This limited kind of classroom interaction continues as students enter middle and high school (Oliva & Lytle, 2014). Significant daily effort is required to fit in and to develop friendships. Deaf and hard-of-hearing students often report they feel unknown by their hearing peers and have extremely limited friendships with them. In fact, in looking back on their K–12 school days, many deaf and hard-of-hearing adults called their classroom interpreter their best friend and advocate (Oliva & Lytle, 2014). Because of communication inaccessibility, they felt their interpreter was the one person who had a strong connection with them and truly knew them.

THEORIES RELATED TO SOCIAL CAPITAL AND IDENTITY

Theories from several disciplines outside of deaf education lend support to the fact that parents, educators, and policymakers need to be thinking about how and where deaf and hard-of-hearing school children will develop social capital. Kleiber (1999) studied the impact of leisure experiences on human development. He described "fourth environments" as places where people go to hang out and chat—away from home, school, and work. Conversations that take place in these environments are critical to the development of social support. Adults congregate in coffee shops, bars, or similar venues on some regular basis. In these fourth environments they "chillax" and talk about "stuff" and make sense of what is happening in their lives.

Adolescents crave such environments. Youth congregate in malls, on street corners, and in other designated venues. An important element of these environments is the absence of adults. School buses, hallways, cafeterias, and locker rooms are all fourth environments. Far too often the conversations taking place in these environments are totally inaccessible for deaf and hard-of-hearing students. In the 21st century, online communities offer an alternative. If students who are deaf or hard-of-hearing are able to participate equally (for example, they have pragmatic language skills), this could very well result in more inclusion. Several of the participants in the study by Oliva and Lytle (2014) relied heavily on their online friendships to get them through their day.

"Fourth environments" foster the development of social capital and thereby identity. Although identity development is based on numerous factors, one major influence is friendships and connections with those who are similar to us. Racial identity theory is built on this premise (Tatum, 1997). When black kids choose to sit together in the cafeteria (which is almost the exact title of one of Tatum's books [1997]), they are creating a fourth environment for themselves. There is a natural inclination to crave the company of others who we sense are like us, and it is in these friendships and connections that we are our most comfortable true selves and have the ability to stretch, compare ourselves with others, and, during the process, discover new parts of ourselves.

In another area of research, scholars developed identity theories for deaf and hard-of-hearing individuals. They used both racial identity theory with its focus on awareness of oppression, and developmental theory of identity, which encompasses an emerging self-acceptance of one's own uniqueness. Glickman's (1996) deaf cultural identity development theory places individuals on a continuum of four stages: hearing, marginal, immersion, and bicultural. His theory was intended to apply to all deaf and hard-of-hearing individuals, regardless of background. Melick (1998) developed a theory of identity focused exclusively on mainstreamed deaf and hard-of-hearing individuals from hearing families. She saw individuals moving developmentally through four stages: being an outsider, encountering/connecting, transitioning from outsider to insider, and self-definition.

Deaf identity theorists (Glickman, 1996; Leigh, 2009; Melick, 1998; Moschella, 1992) have consistently identified two elements that support movement toward positive self-esteem and a clear sense of identity. These elements—exposure to and embracing of a visual language (such as American Sign Language [ASL]), and affiliation and friendship with others who share key characteristics—are closely connected. It is the embracing of a visual language that creates opportunities to connect to others in the Deaf and hard-of-hearing community. Oral deaf and hard-of-hearing children and adults experience similar opportunities to connect with others like themselves through organizations such as the Alexander Graham Bell Association for the Deaf and Hard of Hearing. These opportunities and connections in turn move individuals from peripheral roles to fully participatory and inclusive roles in their own lives.

Friendships with other deaf and hard-of-hearing individuals are critical because they become a protective buffer against the rejection often found with hearing peers (Bat-Chava, 1993; Oliva & Lytle, 2014). Dorminy (2013) found that "becoming grounded in a community of others like themselves served as a key catalyst for shifting from an identity framework of denial, shame, and isolation to one of acceptance, pride, and belongingness" (p. 82). The sense of confidence and emerging identity supported by friendships with deaf and hard-of-hearing peers translates into better relationships with hearing peers as well (Dorminy, 2013; Musselman et al., 1996).

Deaf adults who are from other historically marginalized groups may have a different experience with friendships. For example, a deaf black woman in the study by Oliva and Lytle (2014) clearly valued her black hearing friends from her immediate neighborhood and worked hard to keep these friends in her life after she was placed in a mainstream program outside that neighborhood. However, it was not until she met deaf peers in the mainstream program that her self-esteem strengthened sufficiently for her to aim for college studies. Her black friends from the neighborhood had encouraged her to aim high, but she needed the encouragement that came from deaf peers to move forward. As she became increasingly a part of her deaf community, the friends she valued the most were deaf and hard-of-hearing people of color. Along with a few other respondents in the study by Oliva and Lytle (2014), she defined the community she needed as one that was both deaf and of color.

Clearly, more research needs to be done in this area, but there is this message: the development of full potential requires connections with others like oneself, in all the rich diversity that exists. This example also illustrates the importance of having an intersectional analysis of the development of social capital among deaf and hard-of-hearing students in K–12 settings. Intersectional analyses acknowledge that we occupy multiple social locations and have multiple social identities at the same time—for example, a person is not only "deaf," but also is a member of a racial/ethnic group, has a gender and a sexual orientation, and so on (see Crenshaw, 1993).

These studies illustrate a critical need for strategies to build both bridging and bonding social capital for K–12 students who are deaf or hard of hearing. Bridging social capital enables these students and their hearing peers to connect on meaningful levels so that reciprocity can be developed. Connecting deaf and hard-of-hearing students with each other builds bonding social capital for strong identity and awareness of common issues and remedies. A requirement for the development of both is the ability to engage easily in regular, frequent, and ongoing conversation with others.

LACK OF ACCESS TO INCIDENTAL LEARNING OPPORTUNITIES

So, how do we make it easy for deaf and hard-of-hearing students to engage with hearing peers in ways that at least approximate the rich language and social capital available to the latter? And before answering this question, how do we know the extent of missed information? With so many children using cochlear implants, are these children missing just as much as those from previous generations (such as the adults who have given their reports through the various aforementioned studies)? Experience in general-education settings—living with this ongoing, pervasive cacophony of inaccessible conversation—has spurred a number of deaf scholars and their hearing allies to delve more deeply into this phenomenon.

Hopper's (2011) study of incidental and informal learning in the public school environment is one of a handful of these new studies that uses a unique and creative design that emanates from her own experience of missing conversational content and other sources of social capital in general-education settings. Her work drew heavily from the work of Lave and Wenger (1991), who began their collaboration looking at human learning. They evolved terms such as "situated learning," "peripheral participation," and "mutual engagement" to describe the concept of "communities of practice," where individuals with a common goal can best take advantage of the knowledge and skills of each member. Although they focused mostly on communities of practice in the workplace, surely school environments contain many of the same or similar elements.

Following the work of Lave and Wenger, Rogoff (1994) argued that students engage in a "community of learners" when "learning is a process of transforming participation in shared socio-cultural endeavors" (p. 210). In other words, learning is not based on knowledge transmitted in only one direction; knowledge is free flowing from all directions. Participation results from learning that flows and accumulates as a result of various interactions. Deaf students in mainstreamed environments may feel free and safe while participating in group projects if they have full or at least considerable access to the relevant peer discussions. This access would exist if the deaf student has sufficient hearing, adequate language comprehension, and/or enough assistance from an FM system, some kind of real-time text transcription such as communication access real-time translation, or a sign language (or oral) interpreter. However, it is crucial to remember that actual in-classroom group work is often enhanced by outside-classroom planned gatherings and spontaneous interactions as well, and these might be less or not at all accessible to the deaf student.

A concrete example of a "community of learners" in the K–12 arena might be a project that a group of seventh graders is required to work on for some extended period of time, perhaps even an entire semester. Participants of such a group project might cross paths here and there on the school premises and blurt out a thought, or they might agree spontaneously to meet and then engage in rapid-fire conversation. If this happened in a hallway or locker room or cafeteria, it is considerably unlikely the deaf student would have access to these conversations. An additional point, practically universally overlooked, is that this means the hearing students in their community of learners is not able to include the deaf student's input, including his or her ideas and experiences.

Hopper (2011) also drew on Vygotsky's (1978) concept of scaffolding. Vygotsky argued that solitary exploration does not lead to learning; instead, learning results from stimuli exposed by surrounding interactions within the learner's environment. In addition, such stimuli are mediated by more experienced participants through language or communication. Upon accessing and learning from stimuli, a learner's fund of knowledge increases. The learner then reconstructs knowledge, values, beliefs, or stances. Within all of this, learners reexamine their connectedness to their community or world and knowledge is built on knowledge, enabling a progressively wider range of opportunities for participation.

Hopper (2011) argued scaffolding happens everywhere as students situate themselves in various contexts at school. However, if scaffolding opportunities are not accessible, deaf students' options for reconstructing knowledge and participation are hindered. Hopper (2001) tied the scaffolding phenomenon to incidental learning, which occurs when an individual becomes aware either consciously or subconsciously of some piece of information (such as a comment about an upcoming state test) and subsequently or simultaneously the individual (again, consciously or subconsciously) associates this information with prior knowledge. In Hopper's study, the lack of access to information that is part and parcel of incidental learning becomes crystal clear in a previously undemonstrated way.

Hopper's (2011) phenomenological case study included data from a survey, interviews, participant observations, and "freewriting" sessions. Her main participants were two eighth-graders, one deaf (identified as culturally deaf and from a deaf family) and one hearing, who were friends and spent time together regularly during the school day. These students were provided with electronic notebooks and were instructed to freewrite about what they heard, saw, or talked about during time spent on the school bus, walking through the hallways, and hanging out at their locker spaces and/or at the classroom entrance. They were given 2 minutes to freewrite—reflecting on the immediately previous 45-minutes of time spent on the school bus, going to their lockers, and walking to their classroom. This same freewriting procedure was repeated before the start of the students' first class after their lunch period. Hence, the students produced two 2-minute freewriting sessions per day. Hopper collected these daily freewriting entries twice a week for 4 weeks.

On analyzing and comparing these freewriting entries, Hopper (2011) found that the deaf student freewrote 59% of the time about what she saw and 40% about brief conversations in which she was involved. The majority of her entries were about people walking, running, standing, talking, and fiddling with things at their lockers. The entries about conversations indicated the deaf girl herself initiated them most of the time, and clothing was usually the topic. Hearing peers initiated only one-third of these brief conversations—for example, "New shirt?" "Yes." "Nice!" "Thanks!" Primarily, the hearing peers with whom the deaf student talked were those who could sign or fingerspell.

The hearing student's freewriting entries were almost entirely (97%) regarding things she heard (actually, overheard) from surrounding conversations. Although the instructions were to write about anything the student saw, heard, or talked about, this student wrote almost exclusively about what she heard. Among the topics about which she freewrote included sports, boys, the musical *Wicked* (currently showing), a nearby Six Flags amusement park, and state math tests. Essentially, these were all topics the hearing participant learned from conversations going on around her in informal school-related spaces—for example, the school bus, hallways, and so on. She was not actively involved in these conversations; she simply heard (or overheard) them.

After analyzing her data, Hopper (2011) discussed the freewriting sharing sessions with the deaf eighth grader and a deaf friend of hers who was mainstreamed in a different school. As they learned about the freewriting findings, they came to some realizations that found their way into Hopper's eventual theory development. One realization was that, although they had known all along they missed information daily, they did not realize the significant extent of information missed. In a moment of quite profound awakening, one of the students pointed to one of the hearing student's freewriting entries (representing 2 minutes of freewriting about a 45-minute time of informal banter) and declared, "That's more than I would have learned in one single day!"

Reading the freewriting entries of the hearing student made the deaf students profoundly aware of the inaccessibility of many daily conversations. They could access only what they could see or was told to them directly. All the conversations happening behind them, on the periphery or at a distance, were completely inaccessible. This led to their profound recognition of themselves as bystanders. Furthermore, they recognized this was not their choice, but rather a powerless position in which they were placed. They were "relegated" to this bystander status. With this awareness, the students expressed a desire for immediate access in informal spaces, such as hallways and the cafeteria. They perceived, and rightly so, that only ongoing immediate access would enable them to participate equally and thereby feel like equal members of their school community.

The sociocultural theories reviewed by Hopper (2011), as well as her unique study design, have given us a new lens through which to look at the lives of deaf and hard-of-hearing students as they navigate their way through public schools. Her adolescent participants' involvement as co-creators of knowledge and the awareness they obtained about their own lives (such as how much incidental learning they were missing day by day) are significant in and of themselves, because these factors are aligned with contemporary ideas about research with marginalized groups.

From her study, Hopper (2011) proposed a new theory that researchers and practitioners are encouraged to study further. *Access–participation theory* focuses on various levels of access to conversational interactions and how these levels influence participation by deaf and hard-of-hearing students in general-education settings. The theory suggests the more immediate or full access individuals have, the more choices they have for participation. If students are positioned, marginalized, or relegated at the periphery, their environment is not conducive to their social capital.

Hopper's (2011) proposed terminology "relegated periphery" and, in particular, the idea that the deaf students were "positioned as relegated bystanders" may provide a new "Aha!" moment for the many parents and school personnel who naturally have difficulty imagining what life is like for such children and youth. In other words, access to incidental learning opportunities has been taken for granted. The word *periphery* is a concept many people understand. The word *relegated*, on the other hand, critically depicts the powerlessness so many deaf and hard-of-hearing individuals have reported either when they were young or when they became adults and could articulate their experiences better. The terms *relegated* and *positioned* reveal that someone else or something else is doing the relegating or positioning. In plain terms, it is not the students' choice to be on the outside looking in. Deaf and hard-of-hearing students are being forced into this relegated behavior positioning, thus limiting their access and participation in school environments.

This evidence of deaf students' (lack of) incidental learning and active participation in K–12 spaces illuminates the sorely limited social capital acquisition alluded to by so many studies focused on adults who are deaf or hard of hearing. The design is one that should be replicated exactly or in variation all over the globe because it very clearly allows both parents and professionals to see explicitly the breadth and depth of what is missing day in and day out in the lives of mainstreamed deaf and hard-of-hearing students.

How can we use Hopper's (2011) findings and theory—as well as the numerous retrospective studies and first-person accounts deaf authors have provided to spur additional research into the experience of being a solitaire in the mainstream? Furthermore, how can we use her findings and theory to create remedies and activities to alleviate the results of day-to-day relegated bystander status among deaf and hard-of-hearing schoolchildren in general-education settings? Scholarly investigation into the work of cross-cultural allies provides some insight and ideas.

THE IMPORTANCE OF ALLIES

During the last half of the 20th century and into the 21st century, the concept of "allies" has been amply applied to activism on behalf of human liberation, where the term has been used to describe members of dominant groups who work with and on behalf of members of marginalized groups (Bishop, 2002). With this relatively recent conceptualization, allies are seen as individuals who are committed to eliminating inequality by acting in supportive and nondiscriminatory ways toward individuals who do not share their own key social identities.

Increasingly, psychological and sociological research on intergroup relations has enumerated the consistent qualities displayed by white people, heterosexual people, and nondisabled people who are allies, respectively, to people of color, LGBTQ people, and people with disabilities. This section reviews key theory and research on allies, focusing ultimately on research about hearing allies to deaf and hard-of-hearing individuals and the potential role of hearing peers, teachers, and educational interpreters as allies in K–12 classrooms.

To understand better the issues involved with hearing–deaf/hard-of-hearing alliances, it is helpful to look at work that has been done with other cross-group relationships. Although there are differences in some of the specific attitudes and actions that hearing allies can embrace, work in other domains has identified some general definitions and characteristics of allies that are useful for exploring the potential role of allies in building social capital for deaf and hard-of-hearing students.

In the domain of disability, Gill (2001) defined nondisabled allies as people who stand up against disability oppression, who appreciate "their disabled associates ... in their full glory and full ordinariness"—in short, who "get it" (p. 368). Critical race theorists have written extensively about white allies to people of color who speak out against and challenge racism (rather than "help" people of color) and are willing to engage in the difficult process of exploring their own identities and privileges related to being white (Tatum, 1997). Effective white allies deliberately cultivate friendships with people of color (Feagin & Vera, 2002), and they acknowledge their own racism. Furthermore, they understand that they cannot fully understand the experiences of people of color, but they make an effort nevertheless (Feagin & Vera, 2002).

Recent research has focused on identifying specific qualities exhibited by dominant-group allies. Much of this work has focused on straight allies to LGBTQ individuals (e.g., Brooks & Edwards, 2009; Fingerhut, 2011) and on white allies to people of color (e.g., Alimo, 2012; Case, 2012). Ostrove's work has focused in general on nondisabled allies to people with disabilities (e.g., Ostrove & Crawford, 2006) and more specifically on hearing allies to deaf and hard-of-hearing individuals (e.g., Ostrove et al., 2009a, b). All this work, within all the various cross-group relations, suggests those considered allies display a willingness to understand their own privileged identity, behave in a nondiscriminatory manner, and are proactive on behalf of the rights and successes of members of nondominant groups (see, for example, Reason et al. [2005]).

Some studies have asked people in targeted groups directly about the qualities they value in dominant-group allies. The themes are clear: people of color want to be listened to and respected by white people. They want white people to be knowledgeable about the histories and cultural practices of people of color. They also want privileged individuals to be willing to experiment with terminology and behavior, even at the risk of making a mistake. For example, people of color want white people to recognize they might use a word or phrase they thought was appropriate then later learn that someone is offended by it. And they want white people not to hesitate to interrupt or (in social media parlance) "call out," a discriminatory action, statement, or joke. People of color do not want white people to take over or make assumptions about the best way to do a project or make a decision (Kivel, 2006). As Freire (1970/2000) described in *Pedagogy of the Oppressed*, a theory applied widely to education practices including deaf education (see, for example, Fleischer [2008]), true solidarity across the "oppressor–oppressed" divide happens when those committed to liberation do not think of themselves as the "liberator of the oppressed" (p. 39), but instead are "fighting at their side to transform the objective reality which has made them these 'beings for another'" (p. 49).

Additional qualities mentioned explicitly in other studies of white allies include not treating people of color differently because of their race and taking action among their own groups by, for example, organizing white people to support the efforts of a group of students of color on campus (Brown & Ostrove, 2013). Women with physical disabilities in the study by Ostrove and Crawford (2006) wanted to be respected, accommodated, and seen as a person with multiple identities (not only as a "disabled person"). They did not want to be condescended to, pitied, or ignored.

Of note, much scholarly research and exposition on the topic of allies acknowledges the power imbalances within which alliances are built. Bishop (2002) suggested that oppressive societies have social structures "based on separation, hierarchy, and competition" (p. 25). Relations are typically characterized by domination and subordination (Baker-Miller, 2007), with members of dominant groups in positions of power and authority over members of marginalized groups. Taking these issues into account, then, key challenges for allies in general include acknowledging their dominant position vis-à-vis the group with whom they are allied, understanding the history of oppression that characterizes their own group's relations with members of the marginalized group, and supporting these members' access to power and leadership roles without simultaneously assuming control, being paternalistic, or doing things for them (Baker-Shenk, 1992).

The formation of alliances between deaf and hearing people also occurs in a context of hierarchy grounded in audism, or the systematic discrimination of individuals based on hearing ability (Bauman, 2004). Humphries (1975) defined audism as "the notion that one is superior based on one's ability to hear or behave in the manner of one who hears" (as cited in Bauman, 2004, p. 240). Deaf individuals report experiencing considerable discrimination based on the (misguided) notions that being able to hear is superior to not being able to, and that hearing (and speaking) conveys a basic humanness that is denied to people who do not hear (Bauman, 2004). Oliva and Lytle's (2014) focus group participants expressed being expected to "live up to the hearing standard" (p. 58) as one of their predominant challenges in hearing contexts. Thus, in addition to the key challenge for allies in general noted earlier, key challenges for hearing allies include recognizing their assumptions about deaf and hard-of-hearing individuals and paying careful attention to expectations about, and their role in, communication. The remainder of this section focuses specifically on deaf and hard-of-hearing individuals' perspectives on hearing allies.

In one research study, adult deaf women, some from deaf families and some from families in which they were the only deaf member, emphasized in focus group discussions that they expected allies to understand the importance of communication, show clear respect for deaf and hard-of-hearing individuals, and recognize the complicated nature of identity (Ostrove & Oliva, 2010). In the area of communication, participants in these groups focused on whether hearing individuals in their families, workplace, and neighborhoods were willing to modify their behavior to converse with them. The women expressed a desire that hearing individuals be willing to communicate in ways that make it possible for the deaf or hard-of-hearing individual to be fully involved. The women who preferred to use sign language wanted hearing family members and friends to learn and use sign language. In most cases, the participants expected their family and friends would make these adjustments to their own behavior, thus doing their share of the work of conversation. They considered this to be a critical representation of the hearing individual's acceptance of his or her own responsibility in the relationship.

Ostrove et al. (2009b) also analyzed the stories of deaf and hard-of-hearing adults reflecting on their experiences as solitaires during their K–12 school years. Their descriptions of positive experiences with hearing teachers and peers offer important insight into the qualities and potential roles of hearing allies in the K–12 public school environment. The best hearing teachers, in these participants' experiences, exhibited specific behaviors and attitudes: they took steps to ensure the student always understood what was happening, treated the student like any other student, and took an interest in deafness/hearing loss by asking questions and encouraging students to share their experiences related to being deaf. These best teachers were also encouraging with respect to academic and extracurricular activities (for example, they believed the student was intellectually capable, and encouraged the student to join the debate team), and were caring and sensitive.

Effective hearing peers also demonstrated very specific behaviors and attitudes; they sought ways to be helpful (such as served as a notetaker in class, helped the student understand what was happening in social situations) and treated the deaf student like other peers. These effective hearing peers were also protective in bullying or discriminatory situations, expressed a desire to understand what it meant to be deaf or hard of hearing, and in general were inclusive. They took time to get to know a deaf or hard-of-hearing peer and made it clear by their actions and/or words that their deaf or hard-of-hearing friend was a valuable and equal member of the friendship. The findings from this analysis suggest that hearing peers and teachers can be encouraged—even taught—to be accommodating, curious, inclusive, and caring toward deaf and hard-of-hearing students.

Sign language interpreters in K–12 settings can play critical roles in the lives of schoolchildren who are deaf or hard of hearing. Contemporary models describe the effective sign language interpreter as an ally, working to redress power imbalances between deaf and hearing people in the context of facilitating communication between members of these groups (e.g., Baker-Shenk, 1992; Humphrey & Alcorn, 2002). Baker-Shenk's (1992) ally model has been adopted as an important paradigm for interpreters, replacing the earlier "helper" and "machine/conduit" models of interpreting (Humphrey & Alcorn, 2002). Critically, Baker-Shenk's (1992) discussion hinged on the acknowledgment of a systemic power differential between deaf and hearing individuals, and an analysis of the power held by the (hearing) interpreter, and offers strategies for redressing this power imbalance in interpreting situations. Baker-Shenk (1992) suggested that, in their efforts to facilitate communication and adhere strictly to the accepted code of professional conduct, interpreters may maintain an unjust system—the power imbalance between deaf and hearing people—and disempower the deaf person even further.

One example of this support of power imbalance is well known to all who have knowledge of sign language interpreting. When an interpreter provides inadequate or low-quality voice interpretation for a deaf person without acknowledging to the hearing listeners that her skills are inadequate, it maintains a view of the deaf person as the one "owning" the inadequacy. In these cases, listeners often conclude the deaf person's command of language is responsible for the interpreter's halting or nonstandard utterances. Baker-Shenk (1992) exhorted interpreters to function instead as allies, "to use their power to help equalize the power relations between Deaf and hearing people" (p. 10). A perusal of articles and responses on the fairly new website Street Leverage (www.streetleverage.org) clearly indicates that working interpreters are paying attention to these exhortations and using this online public space to examine and rethink their roles, especially with respect to issues of power.

How does this apply to K–12 interpreting situations? Bowen-Bailey (2014) recently wrote about exactly this issue, describing a "new paradigm" for educational interpreting. This new paradigm acknowledges the (minimal) amount of authority (or power) a deaf child has in a given K–12 setting and stipulates the interpreter is ethically bound to make adjustments to provide the best educational experience possible for the deaf student.

In situations in which the student has low autonomy—for example, when their knowledge of English vocabulary is limited—interpreters may need to make more "liberal" decisions in which they provide more expansive interpretations to ensure *meaning* is conveyed. Zimmerman (2014) described the following situation: If a student knows a sign for a concept (such as mountain), but the interpreter never fingerspells the English word, the interpreter has offered an inadequate interpretation that does not enhance the autonomy of the student. Other examples concern students' social experiences in school. Interpreters can place themselves strategically but unobtrusively to be able to interpret peers' casual conversation (Metzger, 2014). Such decisions can have the effect of enhancing autonomy and empowering deaf students, who will be more informed, more engaged with the subject matter, and more connected to their peers or teachers.

Students who have more autonomy, who have developed strategies for engaging directly with their peers or who have high levels of knowledge going into a given educational situation, may benefit from more "conservative" interpreting decisions, in which the interpreter's presence is much more subtle and the interpreted information is a more "direct" (that is, English-based) reflection of what the teacher just said. Many educational interpreters are very aware of the often-compromised position they themselves are in with respect to the parameters and expectations of their role. They frequently recognize the challenges many deaf students face, and often they are the one adult in the school who best knows their particular students and can communicate directly with them. And thus often it is the interpreter who has the responsibility of "making things work." Yet, no one person or entity has "the answer" of to meet best the educational needs of deaf and hard-of-hearing students. As such, interpreters are slowly but surely coming to voice their potential as allies. They have increasingly discussed and debated about how the concept of ally in general can be deployed effectively to enhance the social and educational experience of deaf and hard-of-hearing students in general-education settings.

A recent issue of *VIEWS* (2014), a quarterly magazine published by the Registry of Interpreters for the Deaf in the United States, offered a good example of the ways in which K–12 interpreters and interpreter trainers are acknowledging issues of power in their work and underscoring the importance of being well trained and taking themselves and their role in deaf and hard-of-hearing students' lives very seriously. As noted earlier, recent discussions on the website Street Leverage (www.streetleverage.org) provide additional evidence of the ways in which interpreters—often in conversation with deaf individuals—are grappling with navigating their power in interpreting situations and recognizing the need to empower deaf and hard-of-hearing individuals further in interpreted contexts. This discourse is becoming increasingly more public, indicating a strong recognition of changes needed for deaf and hard-of-hearing individuals, including schoolchildren, to have the power that will allow them to move from periphery to centrality, and that will promote the building of social capital.

FROM PERIPHERY TO CENTRALITY: STRATEGIES FOR BUILDING BONDING SOCIAL CAPITAL

Anyone who cares about children who are deaf or hard of hearing should be thinking about where and how they can acquire ample social capital. Although there have been minimal empirical studies of this, evidence of its importance comes from several sources. First, qualitative studies and autobiographical work involving adults looking back on their school years "tell it like it was." Works cited earlier in this chapter tell us that deaf and hard-of-hearing adults wish they had opportunities to befriend others like themselves much earlier in their lives. They say their interactions with hearing peers were often of a superficial quality. Second, various human development and other theories tell us that all children need to be nurtured in environments that support optimal development.

Evidence of the importance of focusing on social capital comes from a third source as well. All over the world, summer, weekend, and after-school programs for deaf and hard-of-hearing youth have emerged; their goal is to build bonding social capital among today's deaf schoolchildren. That so many people have spent so much time, as volunteers, to develop these programs is in itself evidence of the cultural recognition that children who are deaf or hard of hearing have a critical need that general-education settings are not meeting. Oliva and Lytle (2014) draw this conclusion from Oliva's numerous onsite observations and interviews with both staff and campers at 15 different programs between 2005 and 2010. In essence, all the interviewees emphasized that attendance at these programs changes lives for children who have few if any contacts with other individuals, peer or adult, who are also deaf or hard-of-hearing.

These programs are so numerous that only a few of the more modern and innovative are mentioned here to highlight those that bring together students who are either marginalized within the community or are themselves members of marginalized groups. The film camp offered at Camp Mark Seven (a summer camp for deaf children) in 2014 resulted in an ASL performance of the song "Happy," which—as of this writing—has received more than one million YouTube views. Of the 24 campers involved, 17 were from general-education settings and, of these, 10 were solitaires. The video was named as one of "25 inspirational stories of 2014" by NBC News (2015). The director of Camp Mark Seven stated:

> I have so many examples of how the campers' lives are forever transformed from the "Happy" music video, and yet, this example stays with me—you see, many campers from last summer were the "only deaf" in their mainstream programs, and one camper called me in early September in *sheer delight* that the high school principal asked the camper for permission to screen the HAPPY music during their assembly on the first day of school!!!! :) (S. Lawrence, e-mail conversation, February 25, 2015)

Two other very new programs focus on special niches: bringing together both oral and signing deaf teens in outdoor programs, and bringing together ethnic minority deaf teens. In the first program, Kaitlyn Millen, a hearing individual who learned ASL in college and then spent 4 years working at the Clarke School in Northampton, Massachusetts, organized a trip to Peru in partnership with two different Peruvian school programs for deaf children. This trip, sponsored by Millen's employer (No Barriers, USA), took place in August 2015. Of note, oral students who signed up for this groundbreaking program eagerly learned Peruvian sign language in preparation for this trip. Thus, despite their lack of opportunity to learn ASL while in the United States, their exposure to communication and other diversity within deaf communities was enhanced in Peru.

Within the deaf community, the past 10 to 20 years have seen a growing presence of awareness of diversity and intersectionality among schoolchildren as well as adults. The National Black Deaf Advocates has been sponsoring a Youth Empowerment Summit since 1997. This program for black youngsters age 13 to 17 years has been held in conjunction with the National Black Deaf Advocates national conference. The National Council of Hispano Deaf and Hard of Hearing also sponsors a leadership retreat for high school juniors and seniors in conjunction with their biennial conference.

In addition to the relatively longer programs (1–3 weeks) that can be offered over the summertime, deaf individuals and their hearing allies have developed both weekend and after-school programs that take place during the regular school year. These programs are promoted on social media—many have Facebook pages—and generally focus on middle and high school students within a given state. Texas,

Wisconsin, and Maine are three states that have pioneered programs, and the developers/managers of them have carefully designed the activities to enhance various areas of both academics and social capital. Youngsters meet each other in these programs and are then able to stay in touch via webcams, social media, and face-to-face meetings when transportation allows.

Day camps spread across the summer are also offered in certain localities. Of note is Camp Summer Sign in Nashville, Tennessee. The sponsors of this program, which has been in operation since 1995, have developed an innovative approach to teaching about teen risk behaviors by engaging participants in the development of a film. The campers conceive the story, write the script, assign acting parts (including bringing in hearing members of the nearby community as needed), plan/build the sets, film, edit, and then debut on YouTube. During the 2014 season, they had 72 campers, of whom 35 were hearing siblings of 51 deaf campers. Of these deaf and hard-of-hearing campers, 47 attend mainstream schools (Corey & Lekowicz, 2015). Parents, teachers, audiologists, interpreters—anyone who has a child or teenager who is deaf or hard of hearing—should know about these programs and plan actively for the child to attend as many as possible during their K–12 years, especially the middle and high school years. Many of the existing programs have developed their curricula to meet the needs of children who spend their school days in general-education classrooms and in neighborhoods where there are few, if any, peers who are also deaf or hard-of-hearing. And when a concerned adult determines there are not enough programs proximate enough for their particular charge, it behooves them to develop a new program, be it for summer, weekends, or after school.

Bonding social capital is so important. It changes lives. The first time a deaf person meets and truly connects with another deaf person is often an "Aha!" moment that jolts them with a sense of possibilities where they can—often for the first time—use their energy to be themselves, rather than scanning their environment vigilantly for potential communication problems or opportunities. Attendance at summer and weekend programs can and should be written into individualized education programs so that funds are made available to children from all socioeconomic backgrounds.

Bringing together families, and including families of all backgrounds, is also important. In creating opportunities for deaf and hard-of-hearing children and youth to be together, additional attention must be focused on deaf youth and their families from marginalized groups such as black, Asian, Latino, and other ethnic minority families. The best way to do that is to be sure the organizers of the events are as diverse as the membership.

FROM PERIPHERY TO CENTRALITY: STRATEGIES FOR BUILDING BRIDGING SOCIAL CAPITAL

Although being aware of, and making arrangements for, a deaf or hard-of hearing child's need for bonding social capital, certainly there is a need for bridging social capital as well. Because bridging social capital is built between others different from ourselves, it often presents more challenges. When communication barriers exist, the challenges become even greater. To ensure bridging capital is enhanced, parents, teachers, and advocates need to be looking at students' involvement with their hearing peers in general-education settings. Given related scholarly work that suggests that bridging social capital may not evolve on its own between hearing and deaf schoolchildren, parents, educators, and allies are encouraged to think outside the proverbial box. What would that mean in practice? How can parents and teachers "fix" the situation demonstrated so starkly by Hopper's (2011) study? How can deaf and hard-of-hearing students develop effective hearing allies?

The website of the Listening and Spoken Language Center of the Alexander Graham Bell Association includes an article "How Students can A.D.A.P.T in Life." In part, it suggests the following:

> Students with hearing loss who listen and use spoken language must employ creative strategies at an early age in order to be successful, especially in the area of social interaction with peers. These tactics can include speech reading to enhance listening skills, asking questions from those next to them and uttering the well-known "What?" response when engaged in conversation. (Altman & Rothwell-Vivian, 2010)

These would obviously be the minimal requirements for a deaf child's success in a spoken language setting such as a public school. The article goes on to mention self-advocacy, determination, attitude, and a few other related behaviors or standpoints. Those behaviors and standpoints will help any student, but they place the burden of success predominantly on the shoulders of the deaf children, who are often least able to assert themselves. It is important to consider the responsibility of schools and school systems—and especially to focus on the responsibility of adults in the school system—to become more aware of the systemic oppression that exists for many deaf and hard-of-hearing schoolchildren and to address this issue directly. In short, adults in the school system must become allies.

Oliva and Lytle (2014) suggested a major paradigm shift in that concerned persons need to look at deaf children not from a deficit framework, but as a part of the fabric of rich multiculturalism within the school. When deaf and hard-of-hearing students are seen as part of the broad diversity of the school as a whole, they have an increased chance of being valued; adults will be more likely to seek or invent activities that support bridging social capital. It is also more likely that viewing deaf and hard-of-hearing students through a diversity lens would illuminate more clearly their need for connections with others like themselves. So often school personnel are focused solely on the idea that deaf and hard-of-hearing students need to learn how to fit into the so-called "inclusive" environment of the school. The multicultural lens will support their need to be part of a community of others like themselves as well as their need to be accepted by their own local school community.

One very concrete way to support this diversity lens is through artwork—and, more specifically, the genre of Deaf Culture Art, or De'VIA Art.

> De'VIA represents Deaf artists and perceptions based on their deaf experiences. It uses formal art elements with the intention of expressing innate cultural or physical Deaf experience. These experiences may include Deaf metaphors, Deaf perspectives, and Deaf insight in relationship with the environment (both the natural world and Deaf cultural environment), spiritual and everyday life. (Miller et al., 1989)

One can view this work, which focuses on the common experiences of persons who are deaf or hard of hearing, on the Internet. In February 2015, a 28-day challenge was issued and 15 to 20 artists posted work daily. This art, some quite raw, conveys many of the common experiences the artists had as children, demonstrating powerfully that "a picture is worth a thousand words." Providing assignments in which all students create "art to change the world" and then share with classmates the meaning in the art would enable hearing classmates to gain an understanding of their hard-of-hearing or deaf classmates as facing challenges and having concerns "just as we all do."

Encouragement and support for direct communication is a major theme in changing the school environment for a deaf or hard-of-hearing child. This includes encouraging teachers and peers to learn to communicate directly with deaf or hard-of-hearing students. Along with this, teachers and peers should be expected to develop meaningful relationships with deaf students that do not include the classroom interpreter (Oliva & Lytle, 2014) and that go beyond the kind of "caretaker talk" that Ramsey (1997) identified. Even in schools or programs where the emphasis is on spoken language in formal classroom activity, sign language should be introduced as a tool that can further connections in informal settings. This means that students in a cooking class can learn signs for "fork," "stir," "boil," and similar vocabulary. Coaches and teammates should work together to learn basic sign vocabulary for their sport—"free throw," "homerun" "intercept," and so on. Not only does this enable quicker and easier communication, but also it fosters a greater acceptance of the diversity that exists with regard to hearing and speaking.

The establishment of ASL classes and clubs (Oliva & Lytle, 2014) and individualized education program planning that includes and empowers (Mitchell et al., 2009; Oliva & Lytle, 2014), and greater flexibility with resource room regulations and requirements have all been suggested. With regard to the latter, deaf adults have reported that the resource room was frequently a "waste of time"; they suggested these spaces could be used in more productive and creative ways. For example, maybe this is where a deaf or hard-of-hearing student could be guided in the development of learning modules to educate peers and adults about deaf culture and sign languages. Modules could be developed that focus on the achievements of certain deaf and hard-of-hearing adults in a variety of careers, key activities of the deaf community (local, national, and international), the breadth and depth of literature and art by deaf individuals, visual learning and language, as well as the obvious "how to communicate with a deaf person."

Increased training to school counselors would also be of great help, because many do not have information about programs and resources from which deaf students could benefit (Oliva & Lytle, 2014). Oliva and Lytle (2014) and Wilkens and Hehir (2008) strongly recommended more system-wide accountability for assessment data and increased training for both teachers of the deaf and classroom interpreters.

Educators, policymakers, and parents need to consider carefully how the fourth environments within schools can be made more accessible to students who are deaf or hard of hearing, because this is key to the development of their social capital. It is the fourth environments that are most closed off to incidental learning—school buses, hallways, cafeterias, locker rooms, and other spaces where students congregate. Hopper (2011) made some specific recommendations that would be applicable to these environments, emphasizing that transforming these environments to be accessible for all students, including deaf and hard-of-hearing students, is necessary if schools want to be truly inclusive. Her participants suggested innovative uses of electronic devices as "text translators" that could be placed in such environments, where voice recognition software could pick up conversation. Another suggestion from her study is for schools to collaborate with interpreter preparation programs to provide internships where interpreting students would "follow" a hard-of-hearing or deaf student and make notes of conversations passing around to share with the student. As an extension of this, a creative approach might be to make this part of English or journalism classes in which hearing peers would have the job of recording conversations taking place in fourth environments.

As part of a focus group experience, Oliva and Lytle (2014) asked their informants to brainstorm the "ideal system" for deaf education. One strong recommendation emanating from this was the idea of a "new profession"—an expert to keep tabs on all the deaf and hard-of-hearing students within some defined geographic area. Although systems may have special education directors, audiologists, teachers of the deaf, and other individuals who attempt—to varying degrees—to fill this role, existing training programs do not prepare them to *oversee* the range of issues faced by the range of children who are deaf or hard of hearing. This may be the most crucial recommendation because it is focused on remedying systematic problems that have resulted in the current status of education for deaf and hard-of-hearing children. Such a professional would not only monitor the whole student, with some reasonable student caseload, but plan training and programs, as needed, focused on reducing isolation and increasing connections for these students, ultimately creating an environment that provides the enriching opportunities for social capital development, both bridging and bonding.

From the work of Ostrove and others focused on cross-cultural alliances, especially alliances from privileged to marginalized individuals or groups, parents and teachers can take steps to ensure the deaf or hard-of-hearing student is always "in the loop" in the classroom. Teachers can model for peers, treating the student like any other student and showing an interest in the student including, but also going beyond, deafness. Teachers can also model for peers ways to be helpful to each other, taking care to model reciprocal relationships, going out of their way to teach the idea that everyone has something to offer. Teachers can model behavior that is accommodating, curious, inclusive, and caring.

With regard specifically to the emerging role of educational sign language interpreters as allies, clearly, research and professional deliberation need to take place in this area as well as in the entire realm of social capital for deaf and hard-of-hearing schoolchildren. One might ask if interpreters are best suited to perform this advocacy role. Is asking an interpreter to have such multiple roles in the best interests of diverse children? Or, would it be better if the proposed "expert" suggested by Oliva and Lytle's (2014) focus groups oversaw the involvement of interpreters, auditory–verbal therapists, counselors, and so on? Obviously, implementation of this latter recommendation would take time (and motivation). Meanwhile, as a stop-gap measure, someone already in the school (possibly a highly qualified interpreter, teacher of the deaf, a motivated parent, or deaf adult) who knows clearly about the needs of children who are deaf or hard of hearing, and particularly about local events and resources that would be important vehicles for developing the child's social capital, should be identified. Individuals such as these have knowledge and expertise that is often unrecognized, underused, and unappreciated within the school system. Instead, their knowledge should be shared with school personnel and, perhaps more important, with the child and family.

Ultimately, the answer to the question of who should be overseeing the educational experiences of schoolchildren who are deaf or hard-of-hearing should come down to this: what will result in daily educational experiences wherein these diverse children and youth are engaged and included—no longer merely peripheral participants in daily school life? The much-needed reforms should result in educational oversight that includes attention to their social capital as well as their language development and academic skills.

RESEARCH DIRECTIONS

The social isolation of deaf and hard-of-hearing students in general-education settings has been studied directly (Hopper, 2011; Keating & Mirus, 2003; Ramsey, 1997) and reported through retrospective studies (Oliva & Lytle, 2014). This critical element has received only a small portion of all research efforts expended with this population. Interested researchers could help increase our knowledge about informal and incidental learning, avenues for increasing social capital with other deaf and hard-of-hearing students, and strategies for improving the overall experience in general-education classrooms.

With regard to informal and incidental learning, Hopper's (2011) study could be replicated with various grade levels and/or students with various backgrounds, including geographic location (urban vs. rural) and family language factors. Exploring school personnel's perspectives of the deaf students attending their schools, particularly with regard to their participation in informal interactions with hearing peers, could yield interesting findings.

Another area where research would be helpful is in regard to the short- and long-term impact of participation in various nonschool activities, such as summer and weekend programs (or elements thereof) on identity development, self-esteem, and other factors known to affect educational success and/or social–emotional well-being. There are many existing programs, and access to them is not prohibitive; investigators can examine associations between general participation and specific activities and various measures of school success.

Interventions designed to address communicative challenges within general-education settings need to be implemented and evaluated. Giving teachers and hearing classmates basic sign language and visual communication skills, allowing all signing children to eat together in the cafeteria, using voice recognition software to provide visual representation of outside classroom conversation have all been suggested. Action research could provide insight for choosing interventions that are most likely to work with particular students and/or in particular settings.

Finally, we need to know more about the characteristics and behaviors that deaf and hard-of-hearing students find empowering in their hearing peers, teachers, sign language interpreters, note-takers, and other school personnel. Based on knowledge of these elements, schools can develop programs leading to strong, effective, and mutually respectful relations between deaf and hard-of-hearing students and hearing students.

REFERENCES

Alimo, C. J. (2012). From dialogue to action: The impact of cross-race intergroup dialogue on the development of white college students as racial allies. *Equity & Excellence in Education, 45,* 36–59.

Allport, G. W. (1954). *The nature of prejudice.* Reading, MA: Addison Wesley.

Altman, J., & Rothwell-Vivian, K. (September 2010). How students can A.D.A.P.T in life. *Volta Voices.* http://www.listeningandspokenlanguage.org/Document.aspx?id=1262#sthash.

Baker Miller, J. (2007). Domination and subordination. In P. Rothenberg (Ed.), *Race, class, and gender in the United States* (7th ed., pp. 108–115). New York, NY: Worth Publishers.

Baker-Shenk, C. (1992). The interpreter: Machine, advocate, or ally? In J. Plant-Moeller (Ed.), *Expanding horizons: Proceedings of the 12th National Convention of the Registry of Interpreters for the Deaf* (pp. 120–140). Silver Spring, MD: RID Publications.

Bat-Chava, Y. (1993). Antecedents of self-esteem in deaf people: A meta-analytic review. *Rehabilitation Psychology, 38,* 221–234.

Bauman, H. L. (2004). Audism: Exploring the metaphysics of oppression. *Journal of Deaf Studies and Deaf Education, 9,* 239–246.

Bishop, A. (2002). *Becoming an ally: Breaking the cycle of oppression in people* (2nd ed.). London: Zed Books.

Bowen-Bailey, D. (2014). New paradigms for the interpreted classroom. *RID VIEWS, 31*(2), 18–21.

Brooks, A. K., & Edwards, K. (2009). Allies in the workplace: Including LGBT in HRD. *Advances in Developing Human Resources, 11*(1), 136–149.

Brown, K. T., & Ostrove, J. M. (2013). What does it mean to be an ally?: The perception of allies from the perspective of people of color. *Journal of Applied Social Psychology, 43,* 2211–2222.

Case, K. A. (2012). Discovering the privilege of whiteness: White women's reflections on anti-racist identity and ally behavior. *Journal of Social Issues, 68*(1), 78–96.

Corey, B. and Lekowicz, L. (2015). A summer camp with a bonus: True-to-life film making experiences. *The Endeavor,* Winter 2015.

Crenshaw, K. (1993). Mapping the margins: Intersectionality, identity politics, and violence against women of color. *Stanford Law Review, 43,* 1241–1299.

Davies, K., Tropp, L. R., Aron, A., Pettigrew, T. F., & Wright, S. C. (2011). Cross-group friendships and intergroup attitudes: A meta-analytic review. *Personality & Social Psychology Review, 15,* 332–351.

Dorminy, J. L. 2013. The experiences of non-signing deaf and hard-of-hearing students and their academic and social integration into a primarily signing deaf university environment. Order no. 3590754. Available from ProQuest Dissertations & Theses Full Text; ProQuest Dissertations & Theses Global. (1432725117). http://search.proquest.com/docview/1432725117?accountid=27346.

Drolsbaugh, M. (2013). *Madness in the mainstream.* Spring House, PA: Handwave Publications.

Feagin, J., & Vera, H. (2002). Confronting one's own racism. In P. S. Rothenberg (Ed.), *White privilege: Essential readings on the other side of racism* (3rd ed.,pp. 153–157). New York, NY: Worth.

Fingerhut, A.W. (2011). Straight allies: What predicts heterosexuals' alliance with the LGBT community? *Journal of Applied Social Psychology, 41*(9), 2230–2248.

Fleischer, L. (2008). Critical pedagogy and ASL videobooks. In H.-D. L. Bauman (Ed.). *Open your eyes: Deaf studies talking* (pp. 158–166). Minneapolis, MN: University of Minnesota Press.

Freire, P. (1970/2000). In Myra Bergman Ramos (Ed., Trans.), *Pedagogy of the oppressed.* 30th anniv. New York, NY: Continuum Press.

Gill, C. J. (2001). Divided understandings: The social experience of disability. In G. L. Albrecht, K. D. Seelman, & M. Bury (Eds.). *Handbook of disability studies* (pp. 351–372). Thousand Oaks, CA: Sage.

Glickman, N. (1996). The development of culturally deaf identities. In N. Glickman and M. Harvey (Eds.), *Culturally affirmative psychotherapy with deaf persons* (pp. 115–153). Mahwah, NJ: Lawrence Erlbaum Associates.

Hopper, M. (2011). Positioned as bystanders: Deaf students' experiences and perceptions of informal learning phenomena. PhD dissertation, University of Rochester.

Humphrey, J. H., & Alcorn, B. J. (2001). *So you want to be an interpreter? An introduction to sign language interpreting* (3rd ed.). Seattle, WA: H&H Publishing.

Keating, E. & Mirus, G. (2003). Examining interactions across language modalities: Deaf children and hearing peers at school. *Anthropology & Education Quarterly, 34*(2), 115–135.

Kivel, P. (2006). Guidelines for being strong white allies. Retrieved November 18, 2008, from http://www.paulkivel.com/articles/guidelinesforbeingstrongwhiteallies.pdf.

Kleiber, D. (1999). *Leisure experience and human development: A dialectical interpretation.* New York, NY: Basic Books.

Kluwin, T., Moores, D., & Gaustad, M. (Eds.) (1992). *Towards effective public school programs for deaf students: Context, process, and outcomes.* New York, NY: Teachers College Press.

Lane, H., Hoffmeister, R., & Bahan, B. (1996). *Journey into the Deaf-World.* San Diego, CA: Dawn Sign Press.

Lave, J., & Wenger, E. (1991). *Situated learning: Legitimate peripheral participation.* New York, NY: Cambridge University Press.

Leigh, I. W. (2009). *A lens on deaf identities.* New York, NY: Oxford University Press.

Melick, A. M. (1998). Deaf identity development: A qualitative inquiry. PhD dissertation, Pennsylvania State University.

Metzger, M. (2014). Educational interpreting: Much more than a language event. *RID VIEWS, 31*(2), 36–38.

Miller et al. (1989). What is deaf art? http://www.deafart.org/Deaf_Art_/deaf_art_.html.

Mitchell, V. J., Moening, J. H., & Panter, B. R. (2009). Student-led IEP meetings: Developing student leaders. *Journal of the American Deafness and Rehabilitation Association (JADARA), Conference Issue*, 230–240.

Moschella, J. G. (1992). The experience of growing up deaf or hard-of-hearing: Implications of sign language versus oral rearing on identity development and emotional well-being. PhD dissertation, Antioch University.

Musselman, C., Mootilah, A., and MacKay, S. (1996). The social adjustment of deaf adolescents in segregated, partially integrated, and mainstreamed settings. *Journal of Deaf Studies and Deaf Education, 1*, 52–63.

NBC News (February 10, 2015). *25 Inspirational stories of 2014.* http://www.nbcnews.com/pop-culture/lifestyle/25-most-inspirational-stories-year-n274941.

Oliva, G. A. (2004). *Alone in the mainstream: A deaf woman remembers public school.* Washington, DC: Gallaudet University Press.

Oliva, G. A., & Lytle, L. R. (2014). *Turning the tide: Making life better for deaf and hard-of-hearing schoolchildren.* Washington, DC: Gallaudet University Press.

Ostrove, J. M., Cole, E. R., & Oliva, G. A. (2009). Toward a feminist liberation psychology of alliances. *Feminism & Psychology, 19*, 381–386.

Ostrove, J. M., & Crawford, D. (2006). "One lady was so busy staring at me she walked into a wall:" Interability relations from the perspective of women with disabilities. *Disability Studies Quarterly, 26*(3). Retrieved from http://www.dsq-sds.org/article/view/717/894

Ostrove, J. M., & Oliva, G. A. (2010). Identifying allies: Explorations of deaf–hearing relationships. In S. Burch & A. Kafer (Eds.), *Deaf and disability studies: Interdisciplinary perspectives* (pp. 105–119). Washington, DC: Gallaudet University Press.

Ostrove, J. M., Oliva, G., & Katowitz, A. (2009b). Reflections on the K–12 years in public schools: Relations with hearing teachers and peers from the perspective of deaf and hard-of-hearing adults. *Disability Studies Quarterly, 29*(3). Retrieved from http://www.dsq-sds.org/article/view/931/1107

Putnam, R. D. (2000). *Bowling alone: The collapse and revival of American community.* New York, NY: Simon & Schuster.

Ramsey, C. L. (1997). *Deaf children in public schools: Placement, context, and consequences.* Washington, DC: Gallaudet University Press.

Reason, R. D., Millar, E. A. R., & Scales, T. C. (2005). Toward a model of racial justice ally development. *Journal of College Student Development, 46*(5), 530–546.

Rogoff, B. (1994). Developing understandings of the idea of community of learners. *Mind, Culture, and Activity: An International Journal, 1*(4), 1–11.

Stewart, D., & Ellis, M. (2005). Sports and the deaf child. *American Annals of the Deaf, 150*, 59–66.

Stinson, M., & Antia, S. (1999). Considerations in educating deaf and hard-of-hearing students in inclusive settings. *Journal of Deaf Studies and Deaf Education, 4*(3), 163–175.

Tatum, B. D. (1997). *"Why are all the black kids sitting together in the cafeteria?" And other conversations about race.* New York, NY: Basic Books.

VIEWS. (2014). *31*(2) [entire issue].

Vygotsky, L. (1978). In M. Cole, V. John-Steiner, S. Scriner, & E. Souberman (Eds.), *Mind in society: The development of higher psychological processes*. Cambridge, MA: Harvard University Press.

Wilkens, C. P., & Hehir, T. P. (2008). Deaf education and bridging social capital: A theoretical approach. *American Annals of the Deaf, 153*(3), 275–284.

Zimmerman, K. (2014). Educational interpreting: Plan B or perfect fit? *RID VIEWS, 31*(2), 30–31.

13

The Inclusion of Deaf and Hard-of-Hearing Students in Mainstream Classrooms: Classroom Participation and Its Relationship to Communication, Academic, and Social Performance

Naama Tsach and Tova Most

FROM SEGREGATION TO INCLUSION

World trends show a transition of deaf and hard-of-hearing (DHH) students from segregated special schools to mainstream education. As a result, many DHH students currently attend regular education settings. In the United States, for example, the percentage of DHH students who attend mainstream education is currently more than 80%, and the percentage of students who attend special schools for DHH students has decreased by half during the past 25 years (Gallaudet Research Institute, 2011; Karchmer & Mitchell, 2003; Power & Hyde, 2002).There are different kinds of mainstreaming for DHH students, including regular education, resource rooms, and self-contained classrooms. DHH students who attend self-contained classrooms stay with special education teachers for most of their classes. However, students who attend regular education and resource rooms have to cope with the same instruction as their hearing classmates. Some of these students receive special accommodations, such as a few classes per week with special education teachers (Karchmer & Mitchell, 2003). In United States, 85% of the students who attend regular schools and 75% of the students in resource rooms received speech-based instruction (Karchmer & Mitchell, 2003). In Israel, about 80% of DHH students attend regular schools (National Council for the Child, Israel, 2013), most of whom receive a few classes per week of specialized educational services. Because they are not provided with sign language interpreters and they have to communicate in school using spoken language, they are required to have certain spoken language skills that enable them to cope with the spoken instructions and communication challenges.

Various factors contribute to the transition of DHH students from segregated special schools to mainstream education settings. First, technological developments have improved auditory accessibility (Anderson & Goldstein, 2004). Second, there has been a decline in the age of detection of hearing loss and earlier intervention (Spivak et al., 2009; see also Chapter 2). Third, values of individualism and diversity in education contribute to the integration of children with special needs rather than isolation in segregated educational settings. Last, parents of DHH students, who in most cases have normal hearing, prefer to integrate their children into mainstream education (Gallaudet Research Institute, 2011).

FACTORS THAT CONTRIBUTE TO INCLUSION

Studies that evaluate the inclusion of DHH students refer to various factors that affect their performance. The main factors affecting those who use spoken language are presented here. However, it is important to recognize there is not one single factor that affects these mainstream students. Instead, it is a combination of all factors and the interactions among them.

Student Factors That Contribute to Inclusion

Auditory Ability

Various studies have indicated that students with severe to profound hearing loss have greater chances of experiencing difficulties in acquiring spoken language and academic skills when compared with students with less severe hearing loss (Wake et al., 2004). However, poorer academic achievement of mainstream DHH students compared with hearing students was also found among students with mild or unilateral hearing loss (McKay et al., 2008; Most, 2004). In addition to the severity of the hearing loss, the students' auditory ability is also influenced by the age of the onset of the hearing loss and the duration of the hearing loss. These factors have a major impact on the inclusion through their effects on students' spoken language development (Damen, et al., 2006; Power & Hyde, 2002).

Auditory Rehabilitation

Inclusion is also affected by factors related to auditory rehabilitation, such as age of the detection of the hearing loss, age when auditory rehabilitation began, type of hearing device, consistency of use of the hearing device, and use of assistive devices (Damen et al., 2006; Most, 2004, 2006; Powers, 2003; Powers et al., 1999; Wake et al., 2004). Cochlear implants, for example, improve access to auditory communication and therefore contribute to the inclusion of students with severe to profound hearing loss. Various studies have indicated that among students with the same severity of hearing loss, students with cochlear implants have an advantage over students with hearing aids in inclusion rates and academic skills (Damen et al., 2006; Vermeulen et al., 2007; see also Chapter 18). Francis et al. (1999) reported that the longer the students used the implant, the less they required special educational assistance and the better they were integrated at school. Another device that was found to have a positive impact on DHH student inclusion is the personal frequency modulation (FM(system. The FM system consists of a transmitter microphone used by the teacher and a receiver used by the student, connected to the student's hearing aid or cochlear implant (Anderson & Goldstein, 2004; Powers, 2003).

Language Skills

As a result of auditory deprivation, many DHH children have deficits in their spoken language skills, showing semantic difficulties in receptive and expressive spoken vocabulary (Fegan & Pisoni, 2010; Wake et al., 2004) as well as in the areas of phonology, morphology, and syntax. These difficulties are expressed in word repetition and grammatical judgments, as well as in production of nominal adjectives, irregular plurals, prepositions, passive structure, finite verbs, and relative clauses (Delage & Tuller, 2007; Friedmann & Sztrezman, 2006; Norbury et al., 2001). DHH students may also have difficulties in the pragmatic aspects of language. Toe and Paatsch (2010; see also Chapter 9) reported that DHH students make more requests for clarification compared with hearing students. Other pragmatic difficulties reflected in these children's spoken interactions relate to taking part in group discussions, and resolving misunderstandings and communication breakdowns (Eriks-Brophy et al., 2006; Jeanes et al., 2000; Stinson & Liu, 1999).

Difficulties in spoken language affect DHH students' ability to cope with the communication, social, and academic requirements in mainstream education. Studies have found correlations between the spoken language skills of mainstream DHH students and their achievements in reading and writing (Geers, 2003; Vermeulen et al., 2007) as well as in math (Kelly & Gaustad, 2007). In addition, correlations were found between these students' spoken language ability and their self-concept, learning motivation, and peer relationships (Bat Chava & Deignan, 2001; Fellinger et al., 2009; Silvestre et al., 2007; Stinson & Whitmire, 2000).

Speech Intelligibility

Speech intelligibility plays a central role in the quality of communication between DHH students and their teachers and hearing peers. Examination of the relationship between the speech intelligibility and the social–emotional status of mainstream DHH students 12 to 14 years old revealed a significant correlation between speech intelligibility and feelings of loneliness (Most, 2007). Stinson and Whitmire (2000) reported that better speech intelligibility increased the social interactions of DHH adolescents with their hearing classmates, and improved their motivation and sense of control.

Learning Disabilities

Having any disability in addition to hearing loss may have a negative effect on learning as well as on the inclusion in mainstream education. DHH students who have learning disabilities have complex educational needs requiring multidisciplinary educational teams that usually are not available in general education schools (Soukup & Feinstein, 2007). McCain and Antia (2005) compared DHH students with and without learning disabilities who were enrolled in the same coenrolled classroom. According to their study, students who had learning disabilities in addition to the hearing loss found the communication with their hearing classmates more challenging. They also experienced more frustration and demonstrated more negative behaviors in school compared with DHH students without learning disabilities.

Educational Setting Factors That Contribute to Inclusion

Acoustical Conditions in the Classroom

Most of the instructions and communication in regular classrooms are based on speech and hearing (Crandell & Smaldino, 2000). However, many classrooms are not adjusted acoustically for studying. Knecht et al. (2002), for example, measured noise levels and reverberation times in 32 classrooms in the United States and only one classroom met the American National Standards Institute's (ANSI) acoustical standards (noise level did not exceed 35 dB in an unoccupied classroom and reverberation time did not exceed 0.6 second). DHH students, especially those with sensorineural hearing loss, experience difficulties in speech perception that worsen in noisy environments. Therefore, classroom acoustic conditions characterized by noise generated from inside and outside the classroom by reverberation and by the distance of the student from the teacher and other classmates cause extreme challenges for DHH students (Crandell & Smaldino, 2000; Eriks-Brophy et al., 2006; Mather & Clark, 2012). The use of assistive hearing devices, such as FM systems, can help DHH students to understand the teacher in a noisy classroom. However, many DHH students are not equipped with FM systems and, in some cases, the teachers do not use the systems properly (Anderson & Goldstein, 2004).

The Classroom Teacher

Mainstream DHH students depend largely on the willingness of teachers to make various adjustments to meet their educational needs. Eriks-Brophy et al. (2006) and Stinson et al. (1996) reported that teachers were perceived as the main factor contributing to inclusion success. Itinerant teachers, parents, and DHH students emphasized the following as critical for inclusion success: the style and teaching methods the teachers chose, the teachers' understanding of the students' speech perception disabilities and special communication needs in class, and the teachers' ability to cooperate with other teachers and therapists involved in rehabilitation (Eriks-Brophy et al., 2006; Luckner & Muir, 2001; Mather & Clark, 2012; Reed et al., 2008; Stinson & Antia, 1999).

MEASURES OF SUCCESSFUL INCLUSION

Thus far, we have considered factors that have an effect on the success of the inclusion of DHH students in regular classrooms. This section presents common measures to evaluate inclusion. There is no consensus on the definition of "success" regarding the inclusion of DHH students (Eriks-Brophy et al., 2006; Foster et al., 1999; Powers, 2002; Silvestre et al., 2007; Stinson & Liu, 1999). According to the literature, as well as to conversations with teachers and parents of DHH children, it is common to assess the quality of inclusion by academic achievements as well as by social and emotional aspects.

Academic Inclusion

Various studies have evaluated academic performance of mainstream DHH students and pointed out two main findings. First, many mainstream DHH students need academic support to keep pace with the average academic level of the class. Power and Hyde (2002), for example, reported that, among DHH students, 27% were described by teachers as students who are dependent on intensive individual learning support to function academically. Only 31% of the DHH students were described as having the ability to cope with academic requirements without individual support. Second, many mainstream DHH students do not reach their classes' academic standards. Teacher reports revealed that only 69% of mainstream DHH students functioned at a good academic level and qualified academically according to regular classroom standards (Power & Hyde, 2002). Comparisons of national test results in language, math, and science of 16-year-old DHH students and hearing students revealed significant differences between the two groups. The differences were found to be to the detriment of the DHH students in terms of the percentage of students who passed the exams and of the percentage of students who achieved higher scores (Powers, 2003).

Studies that have evaluated the reading, writing, and math achievements of mainstream DHH students in comparison with hearing students, have demonstrated several differences. In the area of reading, studies have found a large distribution in DHH students' reading comprehension results (Karchmer & Mitchell, 2003). Overall, lower reading comprehension results have been reported for hearing-aid and cochlear implant users compared with hearing students (Antia et al., 2005; Vermeulen et al., 2007; Wake et al., 2004).

Difficulties of DHH students compared with their hearing peers also have been demonstrated in their writing performance (see Chapter 10). Antia et al. (2005) assessed stories written by mainstream third-grade to 12th-grade DHH students. Results showed that 51% of the students performed below average relative to hearing students, whereas students with moderate to profound hearing loss achieved lower results in relation to students with less severe hearing losses. In addition, the gap between DHH students and hearing students increased with age, suggesting that writing difficulties become more severe as academic requirements increase (Antia et al., 2005).

The academic difficulties of DHH students are also reflected in their performance in mathematics. Mainstream DHH students face various challenges in mathematics because of its use of linguistic knowledge (Kelly & Gaustad, 2007). Kelly et al. (2003) interviewed itinerant teachers of mainstream DHH students in grade 6 to grade 12. The teachers noted the students lacked spoken language skills, limiting the ability of the instructors to teach them advanced mathematical concepts. Special difficulties were reported in solving word problems. Ninety-two percent of the teachers reported they taught their students at the class level, but they focused on solving math problems rather than solving word problems. McCain and Antia (2005) monitored 10 mainstream DHH students every year for three years in a coenrolled classroom and found lower math achievement compared with their hearing classmates.

Social Inclusion

Various researchers have argued that DHH students appear to be at risk for developing social–emotional difficulties (see Chapter 12). These difficulties arise from the restricted accessibility to auditory information, social interaction, and academic content (Antia, 2007; Bat-Chava & Deighnan, 2001; Eriks-Brophy et al., 2006; Preisler et al., 2005; Reed et al., 2008). The hearing loss may also be accompanied by neurological problems, which can have a negative influence on the mental–emotional development of DHH students (Knoors & Marschark, 2013).

Kent (2003) compared the results of a self-reported health behavior questionnaire of mainstream DHH students and hearing students age 11, 13, and 15 years. He reported that DHH students experienced more feelings of loneliness compared with hearing students. In addition, among mainstream DHH students, those who defined themselves as "hard of hearing " or "deaf" felt lonelier and experienced more bullying than those who did not define themselves in that way. Feelings of loneliness and adjustment problems were also found by Most (2007) in both mainstream DHH students and in those who attended special classes for DHH students. Based on these findings, it is not surprising that many mainstream DHH students report they do not have meaningful social relationships with their classmates (Stinson & Whitmire, 2000). The absence of meaningful social relationships, evident by lack of preference for a classmate or playmate, becomes prominent with age (Tvingstedt, 1995).

Punch and Hyde (2011) collected reports from parents, itinerant teachers, and mainstream cochlear implant users regarding the students' behavior in different situations during the school day. The researchers found a correlation between hearing loss and social behaviors of isolation and avoidance. DHH students tended to stay away from or to avoid interactions with hearing classmates in situations including multitalker conversations or multiplayer games, as well as in noisy environments. However, further analysis revealed the reason for these behaviors was the students' feelings that, in noisy or group situations, they might lose important auditory information and would not be able to respond appropriately. These findings demonstrate the complexities of social challenges faced by mainstream DHH students and explain the common misperceptions of teachers and hearing classmates regarding these students' social behaviors.

Thus far, we have described inclusion results with reference to the academic and social aspects. This description, however, provides only a limited perspective, focusing on the results but ignoring the process. A comprehensive description of inclusion is incomplete without referring to the everyday learning process itself. How do DHH students face everyday challenges during class? What are their difficulties and which strategies do they use to participate and to be involved in class? Stinson and Antia (1999) claimed the evaluation of school performance of mainstream DHH students should relate to two main components: academic achievement and classroom participation. It should also be noted that retrospective reports of DHH adults on their school experience, as well as self-reports of mainstream DHH students, indicate that class participation plays a key role in their perception of their inclusion experience (Antia et al., 2007; Stinson et al., 1996).

CLASSROOM PARTICIPATION

Classroom participation is an important part of students' learning process. The classroom discourse provides an opportunity for students to speak and to be heard. It exposes them to a variety of points of view and allows social and cognitive development by encouraging critical thinking, self-awareness, social involvement, and taking a stand (Dallimore et al., 2004). Classroom participation requires students to focus on the teachers' instructions, explanations, and questions. However, the process of listening in the classroom is not easy or natural for many students, regardless of their hearing ability. Listening in class requires students to deal with different psychological and physiological distractions such as fatigue, lack of interest, difficulties in attention, or sensory impairments (Lau et al., 2008; Peterson, 2012). Other factors such as language impairment, difficulties in memory, difficulty in interpreting nonverbal cues, poor self-confidence, and social difficulties may also worsen students' classroom participation. The negative impact of these factors on class participation might become more prominent when students are exposed to new learning material, especially in the presence of a noisy classroom, rapid speech, or foreign dialect of the teacher (Bosacki et al., 2014; Swain et al., 2004).

The existence of hearing loss adds significant difficulties to the inherent challenges of classroom participation. Because classroom learning is based on auditory–verbal communication, the restricted language skills and the difficulties in perception and production of spoken language limit the classroom participation of many DHH students. This is especially true for those who do not have the assistance of sign language interpreters and use spoken language in class.

Spoken language deficits might limit DHH students' ability to cope with academic requirements. Language difficulties further reduce these students' abilities to deal with misunderstandings and to take part in group activities during class (Damen et al., 2006; Stinson & Liu, 1996). The level of speech intelligibility of DHH students plays a central role in the quality of communication between them and their teachers and classmates, and might prevent many DHH students from speaking in class (Most, 2007; Stinson & Whitmire, 2000).

The auditory speech perception skills of DHH students who depend on spoken language affect their ability to participate in class. Because learning in a regular classroom is based mainly on listening, DHH students face significant challenges in perceiving their teachers' oral instructions and understanding the students who participate in class. Many DHH students, especially those with sensorineural hearing loss, experience difficulties in speech perception that worsen in noisy and reverberant environments typical in many classrooms (Crandell & Smaldino, 2000; Eriks-Brophy et al., 2006; Powers, 2002). In addition, the physical distance of the students from the teacher and classmates makes communication during class even more challenging. (Antia, 2007; Crandell & Smaldino, 2000; Luckner & Muir, 2001; Mather & Clark, 2012; Preisler et al., 2005, Stinson & Liu, 1999; Tvingstedt, 1995).

As a result of the negative impact of the classroom acoustic conditions on the spoken communication abilities of DHH students, they need the support of visual cues of speech-reading. However, in most classrooms, eye contact between all the speakers in class is not possible because of common seating arrangements in rows or in groups. Such seating arrangements prevent direct eye contact between the students. In addition, classroom interactions are characterized by quick exchanges of speakers, and sometimes more than one person speaks at the same time. This kind of interaction challenges DHH students who have to integrate visual and auditory information from multiple sources, and have to decide what information to give up at any given time. This process results in a loss of information and places a heavy load on working memory (Mather & Clark, 2012; Stinson & Liu, 1999; Tvingstedt, 1995). The situation is worse when classmates speak too softly or too fast, or when they comment briefly, or are unwilling to repeat themselves (Antia, 2007; Foster et al., 1999; Preisler et al., 2005; Stinson & Antia, 1999; Tvingstedt, 1995).

Some teachers' behaviors can make participating in class even more difficult for DHH students. These added difficulties may occur when the teacher is unorganized in the presentation of class materials, speaks too fast or too softly, or does not use visually cued instruction. Teacher behaviors such as moving constantly, not repeating the words of other students, refusing to use an FM system, and not maintaining eye contact with the students may also harm the classroom participation of DHH students (Hyde et al., 2009; Luckner & Muir, 2001; Preisler et al., 2005; Reed et al., 2008; Stinson & Antia, 1999; Tvingstedt, 1995).

Social–emotional issues arising from hearing loss might also worsen the students' situation in class. Insecurity, shyness, and negative attitudes toward hearing people may be expressed in a reluctance to communicate with hearing classmates, in passive behavior, and in denial of classroom participation (Stinson & Liu, 1996). Previous research results, based on teachers' and students' reports, have indicated that mainstream DHH students may refrain from new activity during class before verifying the actions of hearing students. They rarely raise their hand and, if they do, it is only after other students do so. Their willingness to answer the teacher's questions occurs on very selective occasions (Antia et al., 2007; Foster et al., 1999; Tvingstedt, 1995). Many mainstream DHH students feel dependent on their classmates' help to understand the teacher during class (Luckner & Muir, 2001; Preisler et al., 2005). Difficulties in classroom participation have been reported among various groups of DHH students, including students with mild or unilateral hearing loss (McKay et al., 2008) and cochlear implant users with severe to profound hearing loss (Damen et al., 2006). Older students, in college, have reported similar difficulties (Hyde et al., 2009).

Reed et al. (2008) found the classroom participation of DHH students to be related to various areas of school performance. Participation in class allows DHH students to cope better with academic requirements, and many of them reported that classroom participation was a major factor in their academic success. In addition, a sense of involvement in class has been shown to be associated with feelings of better social inclusion (Antia et al., 2007; Foster et al., 1999; Preisler et al., 2005; Stinson & Liu, 1999). Antia et al. (2011) found that participation in the classroom was one of the two best predictors of social functioning of mainstream DHH students. A retrospective study by Stinson et al. (1996) based on interviews of DHH adults who were mainstream students during their school years revealed that, of the various factors contributing to their school inclusion experience, classroom participation left the strongest impression in their memories.

Despite the fact that classroom participation is a factor that impacts other aspects of school experience and has a unique contribution to the sense of inclusion of DHH students, there are only a few research studies that have focused on classroom participation. Most of these studies based their findings on reports of parents and teachers, and students' self-reports (Damen et al., 2006; Foster et al., 1999; Hatamizadeh et al., 2008; McCain & Antia, 2005; Stinson et al., 1996, Stinson & Liu, 1999). A few studies have based their findings on limited classroom observations and reported qualitative descriptions of students' performance in class (Stinson & Liu, 1999; Tvingstedt, 1995). Considering that most DHH students currently attend regular education settings and that classroom participation has a major impact on their inclusion, further research on classroom participation of mainstream DHH students is required. The remainder of the chapter describes research designed to explore further the classroom participation profile of mainstream DHH students.

CLASSROOM PARTICIPATION OF MAINSTREAM DHH STUDENTS

Seventy students (20 boys and 50 girls), fourth to sixth graders, participated in a study of classroom participation. There were 35 students with moderate to profound hearing loss who attended 34 different regular classrooms in 32 different general education elementary schools located in various regions in Israel, and 35 normally hearing classmates. None of the students were suspected of having or been diagnosed with learning disabilities.

All DHH students used sensory aids. Nineteen students used conventional hearing aids and one used a bone-anchored hearing aid. Fifteen students used cochlear implants, five of whom had bilateral implants. None of the students were supported by a sign language interpreter and all of them communicated through spoken language at school.

In this study, direct assessment of classroom participation was conducted through the use of observations of students during class. The observations enabled quantitative assessment of students' behaviors in typical classroom situations, such as when the teacher asks questions or gives instructions, classmates are speaking, and when students participate without the teacher's prompt. Class observation was accompanied by the collection of information that included the students' feelings during class and their communication skills, academic achievements, and social performance. As detailed here, the information was obtained through the use of tests and questionnaires completed by the researcher, the teachers, and the students themselves. The performance of DHH students was compared with the performance of their hearing classmates. The study also sought to analyze the relationship between classroom participation of DHH students and the physical conditions of the classroom, their communication skills, academic achievements, and social performance.

How Do Mainstream DHH Students Participate in Class Compared with Hearing Students?

To evaluate and quantify the students' behavior during class, an observation tool was developed on the basis of interviews with teachers, DHH students, and adults with hearing loss who were in mainstream classes during their school years. The goals of the interviews were to set up common situations that occur during class and to define the behaviors reflecting classroom participation, especially those behaviors that are particularly challenging for DHH students. Thus, the observation tool focused on the students' behaviors in four different situations.

The first situation included the teacher asking questions. The number of questions asked by the teacher was documented. Each question was followed by a documentation of the students' responses. There were five possible student responses: answers the question correctly, answers the question incorrectly, raises a hand to answer the question but does not receive permission to speak, makes eye contact with the teacher, or ignores the question (does not make any eye contact).

The second situation included the teacher giving instructions. The number of times the teacher gave instructions in class was documented. Each teacher's instruction was followed by a documentation of the students' responses. There were three possible responses: the student follows the instructions independently, the student follows the instructions with the help of the teacher or classmate, or the student doesn't follow the instructions.

The third situation included classmate speaking. The number of times that classmates spoke was documented as well as one of three possible student responses: makes eye contact with the student who spoke, responds verbally to the student who spoke, or ignores the student (does not make eye contact).

The fourth and last situation included students participating without prompts from the teacher. There were four types of responses: raises a new topic, asks a question, asks for help, or raises a hand but does not get permission to speak.

The findings of the observations indicated that DHH students were more likely than hearing students to follow the instructions with help from both the teacher and classmates. No differences between the two groups were found in their responses to teachers' questions. However, the DHH students made more eye contact with the students participating in class compared with the hearing students. No differences between the two groups were found in their classroom participation without prompts from the teacher.

Difficulties in following the teachers' instructions were reported in previous studies based on students' and teachers' reports. Preisler et al. (2005) interviewed students who claimed to have difficulties in understanding teachers' instructions, mainly because of the teachers' rapid and disorganized speech. Similar findings were reported by Luckner and Muir (2001) based on interviews with parents and teachers of academic and socially successful mainstream DHH students, as well as on interviews with the students themselves.

The findings showed that DHH students were more likely to follow the instructions with help, yet there were no differences between the two groups in their responses to teachers' questions. These findings suggest that classroom observation can discern the difficulties that DHH students experience in following the teacher's instructions, however, classroom observation cannot reflect completely the difficulties they might have in understanding the teacher's questions. This can be explained by the fact that the students' ability to answer the teacher in class is affected by various factors beyond hearing ability, including knowledge of the curriculum, verbal expression abilities, as well as social and emotional factors (Bosacki et al., 2014).

The students' responses to their classmates who spoke in class and the number of times they were speaking during class without prompts from the teacher were also evaluated. The results indicated that DHH students made more eye contact with the students participating in the class compared with hearing students. Unlike hearing students, who most of the time do not need to make eye contact with the different speakers in class, many DHH students need the support of visual information during spoken language interactions. For DHH people, eye contact serves as a necessary condition for communication and has a unique pragmatic role (Skelt, 2013). However, of the 35 DHH students who participated in the study, only one student was located in a seat that allowed her to make eye contact with most of her classmates. This was possible as a result of a U-shape seating arrangement in her classroom. All the other participants were seated in columns, rows, or groups. In addition, in most cases the DHH students were sitting at the front of the class, close to the teacher, and therefore visual access to their classmates' face was limited. These findings support the recommendation by Mather and Clark (2012) that seating arrangements in the classroom should enable mainstream DHH students to have a 360-degree visual access to the faces of their classmates to be able to participate in the class.

The last part of the classroom observation focused on students' participating without prompts from the teacher. It should be noted that, overall, behaviors of participating in class without the teachers' prompts were rarely seen in the current study. The results indicated no differences between the DHH students and the hearing students in participating in class without the teachers' prompts. Reports on observations taken in classrooms without DHH students (e.g., Shepherd, 2010), however, can contribute to our understanding of the learning environment that DHH students face when in a mainstream classroom. Interestingly, the reports revealed that teachers generally ignore students' hand-raising when not in response to a direct question or instruction from them. Shepherd (2010) reported that more than 70% of the time when students raised their hand without a teacher's prompt, they were ignored by the teacher. In addition, when teachers accepted the unsolicited students' hand-raising, they asked the students to shorten their questions and requests. These findings may indicate that the learning environments in many classrooms discourage classroom participation. A learning environment that discourages students from expressing themselves is problematic for students, regardless of their hearing status. However, the impact of such a learning environment on DHH students is particularly negative because it prevents direct communication with the teacher, including asking questions to make sure they understand the learning material (Tvingstedt, 1995). Therefore, it is important that teachers get the required assistance to implement teaching methods that encourage classroom participation in general, and encourage the participation of mainstream DHH students in particular.

How Do Mainstream DHH Students Feel during Class Compared with Hearing Classmates?

In addition to the classroom observations, each student reported on his or her subjective experience in class using the Classroom Participation Questionnaire (CPQ) (Antia et al., 2007). The questionnaire relates to the students' understanding of the teacher and the other students, as well as to their positive and negative affect during class.

DHH students rated their own abilities to understand the teacher and classmates as less than that of the hearing students. They also had less positive affects during class and more negative affect compared with their hearing peers. These findings support previous studies that assessed elementary school to college-level DHH students (Antia et al., 2005, 2007; Foster et al., 1999; Hyde et al., 2009; Luckner & Muir, 2001; McCain & Antia, 2005; Preisler et al., 2005; Reed et al., 2008). Significant differences between DHH students and hearing students regarding their self-perceived ability to understand the teacher and their classmates were also reported by Hatamizadeh et al. (2008). These researchers compared elementary school students with mild to moderate hearing loss and hearing students. They found that only 55% of the DHH students reported they understood the teacher, and only 50% reported they understood their classmates. Thus, professionals should be aware of the fact that these difficulties are not unique to students with more severe hearing loss and should take into account that students with a wide range of hearing loss experience difficulties understanding their teacher and classmates during class.

With regard to students' feelings during class, the findings that DHH students had less positive affect during class and more negative affect compared with hearing students support the previous findings of Richardson et al. (2010), who reported more negative affect among college DHH students who attended mainstream programs (with hearing students) compared with DHH students who attended separate programs (without hearing students) at the same institution. It is interesting to note that McCain and Antia (2005) did not find significant differences in positive and negative affect between DHH students who attended a coenrolled classroom and their hearing classmates. It is possible the students in that study felt better in class than the students of the current study because they were integrated as a group and were supported continuously by a teacher and a sign language interpreter.

To understand more fully the source of the negative feelings during class, future studies should examine the relationships between the feelings of mainstream DHH students during class and different factors such as classroom atmosphere, student–teacher relationships, self-esteem, and social status. Understanding the source of these difficulties may contribute to these students' mental well-being, improve their motivation to learn, and, indirectly, maximize their academic performance (Antia et al., 2007).

Are There Differences between Mainstream DHH Students and Hearing Students in Their Communication, Social Functioning, and Academic Performance?

In addition to the observed classroom participation and to the students' feelings during class, the study examined the communication, social functioning, and academic performance of the DHH students compared with their hearing classmates. Communication performance included a hearing through the use of the child's audiogram, assessment of speech perception of sentences in the presence of noise, assessment of speech intelligibility using the Speech Intelligibility Rating scale (McDaniel & Cox, 1992), and assessment of language through the use of specific tests that evaluated the semantic, morphological, and syntactic aspects of language.

Academic achievement was assessed using grades in two core subjects—mathematics and language—as in previous studies (Powers et al., 1999). The scores were determined by the average of the grades of the last two tests reported by teachers. The social performance of the students was assessed through teachers' report using the School Social Behavioral Scale Questionnaire (SSBS [Merrel, 2002]). The questionnaire relates to two areas: social behaviors (including peer relationships, self-control, and academic behavior) and antisocial behaviors (including bullying and hostility, aggressiveness, and discipline problems).

With regard to communication performance (speech perception in noise, speech intelligibility, and language performance), the results revealed there was a significant difference between DHH students and hearing students in their speech perception performance in background noise. Not surprisingly, DHH students performed worse than hearing students (Crandell & Smaldino, 2000). Teachers should be aware of these difficulties, take care to adapt and improve environmental conditions in the classroom, use auditory assistive devices, and offer the appropriate help.

No significant differences were found between the two groups in their speech intelligibility or their semantic, morphological, and syntactic skills. It should be noted that, in the current study, there were 20 participants with moderate to severe hearing loss who used their hearing aids regularly. In addition to the hearing-aid users, there were 15 participants who used cochlear implants from an early age (11 of the 15 underwent cochlear implantation before the age of two years; the other four, before the age of five). Thus, all these students who used implants had a relatively long experience with them. These two factors, early implantation and duration of implant use, are significant factors that contribute to spoken language development (Francis et al., 1999; Nicholas & Geers, 2007). All the DHH participants received individual educational support at school. It is possible that factors such as early detection of hearing loss, early use of hearing aids and/or cochlear implants, and early educational intervention (which characterized the students enrolled in this study) had significant positive contributions to their spoken language performance (Damen et al., 2006; Most, 2006; Powers, 2003; Wake et al., 2004). The current findings support previous research by Norbury et al. (2001), which indicated no differences in vocabulary, grammatical structures, and morphological expressive skills between hearing students and students with mild to moderate hearing loss age 5 to 10 years.

Contrary to these findings, Friedmann and Sztrezman (2006) evaluated the syntactic skills of students with moderate to profound hearing loss using the same evaluation tool used in the current study. They found significant inferiority in their relative clause production skills compared with hearing students. The difference between these findings and the current study's findings may be explained by the fact that almost all the participants evaluated by Friedman and Sztrezman (2006) had prelingual hearing loss (12 of 14) whereas in the current study only about two-thirds of the participants (22 of 35) had prelingual hearing loss. Many previous studies have indicated that a later occurrence of hearing loss has a major positive impact on developing age-appropriate spoken language performance (Damen et al., 2006; Power & Hyde, 2002).

The current study's measures of academic performance were the grades in mathematics and language (Hebrew). Many parents and educators perceive grades as the main indicator of academic success. The results revealed no differences in the grades of the DHH students and the hearing students in both areas. These findings did not support many previous studies that reported the inferiority of the academic achievements of mainstream DHH students compared with hearing students (Antia & Reed, 2005; Kelly et al., 2003; McCain & Antia, 2005; Nicholas & Geers, 2007; Power, 2002; Punch & Hyde, 2011; Tvingstedt, 1995). A partial explanation for this inconsistency may be that, unlike the current study, in most of these studies no distinction was made between students with or without additional disabilities. Inclusion of students with additional disabilities in the sample may decrease the results of the DHH students as a group. The lack of consistency may also be a result of environmental and cultural differences between the countries in which the data were collected. These differences may be reflected in different assessment methods in the teachers' evaluations.

It should be noted that although the use of grades as a measure of academic achievement is common in educational systems, it has various disadvantages. First, the grades reflect specific knowledge in a certain area and do not provide all the information that represents students' academic abilities. In addition, because grades can be improved through tutoring, the comparison between mainstream DHH students and hearing students can be problematic. Although most mainstream DHH students receive individual assistance provided by itinerant teachers, hearing students usually do not benefit from this kind of service. Hence, grade comparisons may be biased toward the group of DHH students. Another disadvantage of using grades as an academic measure is that grades may be affected by the teacher. It should be noted, however, that the statistical analysis in the current study took into account this limitation and evaluated the contribution of class affiliation to the students' grades by using a hierarchical, multilevel statistical model that included explanatory variables at two levels: the student level and the level of class affiliation (Twisk, 2006). Evaluation of grades of DHH students and hearing students found class affiliation to be insignificant.

The social performance of the students was assessed through the use of the SSBS as completed by the teacher. The results revealed no differences between DHH students and hearing students in terms of antisocial behaviors, including bullying and hostility, aggressiveness, and discipline problems. This finding was expected, mainly because the sample did not include students with additional difficulties. However, in terms of social behaviors, differences were found between the two groups to the detriment of DHH students in their self-control as well as in their interpersonal relationships with their hearing classmates.

Many previous studies have evaluated different aspects of social skills and used different assessment tools administered by different evaluators (parents, teachers, and students with and without hearing loss). In addition many previous studies have evaluated different groups of DHH students that differ by various factors such as severity of the hearing loss and educational placement. Some of the studies did not compare the performance of DHH students with the performance of hearing students. The large variance between studies in all these aspects is reflected in the large variation in findings. On the one hand, there is evidence that DHH students experience social difficulties in comparison with students with normal hearing (Damen et al., 2006; Fellinger et al., 2009; Hatamizadeh et al., 2008; Punch & Hyde, 2011; Wauters & Knoors, 2008). On the other hand, there is evidence that such differences do not exist (Antia et al., 2011; Noll, 2007).

Based on reports from parents, teachers, and mainstream students with cochlear implants, Punch and Hyde (2011) found that DHH students were less involved in group activities compared with hearing students. Wauters and Knoors (2008) reported that mainstream DHH students were rated lower by their classmates regarding their willingness to help friends and their ability to cooperate with others compared with hearing students. Studies have indicated more adjustment problems in DHH students compared with hearing students (Eriks-Brophy et al., 2006: Most, 2007).

In contrast to these findings, Noll (2007) reported that teachers did not perceive mainstream DHH students as having a lack of discipline or problematic social skills. In addition, the teachers did not report significant problems in adjustment of students who graduated from oral–deaf programs during the past two years. Antia et al. (2011), who used the Social Skills Rating Scale questionnaire filled out by the teachers, also found no differences between mainstream DHH students and hearing students. Interestingly, Antia et al. (2011) pointed out that teachers' evaluation of social performance may not be sensitive enough to reflect difficulties that are not expressed in the students' outward behavior. Teachers' evaluations may also have limited reliability as a result of misinterpretation of student behaviors, especially because teachers in mainstream education are often unaware of the effects of hearing loss on the communication and social abilities of these students (Punch et al., 2011). Hence, teacher reports of normal social functioning do not necessarily contradict the possibility that DHH students experience social difficulties (Antia et al., 2011).

These findings demonstrate the challenge in evaluating social behaviors of mainstream DHH students. To evaluate their social functioning more completely, it is recommended we use tools designated specifically or adjusted for these students, so they reflect their social rather than their communication skills. When using a nonspecific tool for mainstream DHH students, it is important to monitor the items that represent complex acoustic and communication conditions. The SSBS that was used in the current study evaluated the students' social behaviors as well as their antisocial behaviors and revealed differences between the two groups in certain social skills) self-control and interpersonal relationships). These findings suggest this kind of differentiation can contribute to the understanding of the specific social difficulties experienced by mainstream DHH students.

Did Classroom Variables Affect Student Classroom Participation and Their Feelings during Class?

The students included in this study were mainstream pupils in 34 different classes. Therefore, the two factors of classroom acoustic conditions and the number of students per classroom were examined to access their contributions to student performance. Classroom acoustic conditions were assessed through an observation tool that included seven items, with each item scored from 0 to 2. The tool is based on ANSI (2010) recommendations, which determine whether classroom acoustical learning conditions are affected by the follow main components: reverberation, mechanical noise, noise from internal and external sources, and the volume of the teacher's voice.

Regardless of hearing status, a larger number of students in the classroom reduced the students' ability to understand the students who speak during class and increased their eye contact with the teacher. These findings support previous results reported by Blatchford et al. (2005), who evaluated the classroom behavior of hearing students. They found that in a classroom with at least 31 students, the students retain more eye contact with the teacher compared with smaller classes of 25 students or less. The noise and distractions that are inevitable results of a large number of students per class cause hearing students to seek visual cues of speech-reading to understand the teacher.

The results of the self-report Classroom Participation Questionnaire indicated that, regardless of hearing status, better acoustics provided a better sense of understanding of the teacher and the students, as well as more positive affects during class. These findings supported previous research by Klatte et al. (2010), who found the acoustic conditions influence the degree of understanding and feelings of students with normal hearing in class. They demonstrated a significant effect of reverberation time on word understanding and on students' sense of discomfort. Although students, both with and without hearing loss, found it difficult to comprehend in a noisy classroom, it is important to note that DHH students require better acoustics. It is known that understanding speech in the presence of background noise or competitive speech is harder for people with hearing loss compared with people with normal hearing (Best et al., 2010). Thus, the education staff should consider acoustic aspects as an issue of major impact on the learning and behavior of the students. In addition, classroom amplification systems should be used. Furthermore, classrooms of mainstream DHH students should be accommodated specifically to meet their special auditory needs.

Is There a Relationship between Mainstream DHH Students' Observed Classroom Participation and Their Communication, Academic, and Social Performance?

Two measures of classroom participation correlated significantly with other assessment measures: following the teachers' instructions and making eye contact with students. Note that these two classroom participation measures were also found to differ between DHH students and their hearing classmates.

The students' ability to follow the teachers' instructions correlated significantly with semantic performance, speech perception in noise, and social behavior. The need for semantic knowledge to follow teachers' instructions was supported by Haynes et al. (2006). They described the consequences of poor linguistic ability, such as children with specific language impairment, on their class listening skills, which was reflected in their comprehension of teacher instructions.

The correlation between the ability to follow teachers' instructions and speech perception of sentences in background noise emphasizes the need to assess speech perception in noise as an indicator of students' ability to understand the teacher during class. This finding supports previous studies that demonstrated that noisy environments affect speech understanding of DHH students negatively (Crandell & Smaldino, 2000; Eriks-Brophy et al., 2006; Mather & Clark, 2012; Powers, 2002) as well as show a positive impact of improving the signal-to-noise ratio by using FM systems (Davies et al., 2001). Thus, to facilitate mainstream DHH students' classroom understanding of teacher instructions, it is necessary to improve acoustic conditions in the classroom as well as to use assistive hearing devices.

A significant relationship was found between student ability to follow teacher instructions and their social behavior. This finding supports previous findings by Antia et al. (2011), which indicated that classroom participation is related to positive social relationships inside and outside the classroom. Students who participated in the classroom were perceived positively by the teacher and other students. They also found that the variable that predicted social performance most strongly was classroom participation.

Regarding the students making eye contact with the students who were speaking during class, findings indicate that students with more severe hearing loss made less eye contact with their classmates. However, it was expected that students with more severe hearing loss would seek more visual cues, and therefore would increase their eye contact with students participating in class. It is possible that this finding results from the fact that all students with profound hearing loss participating in the current study used cochlear implants. In other words, it is possible that our findings reflect the effectiveness of cochlear implants, which allow students to rely less on visual cues and more on auditory cues. On the other hand, it is also possible that this finding reflects the situation in which students with more severe hearing loss who, in general, have greater difficulties in speech perception, might not invest resources in seeking visual cues and may actually give up on the opportunity to understand their classmates during class. To understand this finding more fully, future studies should examine the effect of hearing loss severity regardless of the type of assistive hearing device.

SUMMARY AND EDUCATIONAL IMPLICATIONS

As a result of technological advances and changes in educational values, most DHH students are currently enrolled in mainstream educational settings. This trend provides schools, teachers, and students with significant educational challenges. Most studies to date have focused on the academic and social challenges of these students, whereas their classroom participation has hardly been investigated. The study described in this chapter focused on classroom participation of DHH students who attend regular classrooms with minimal education support (a few classes per week with specialized educational services), and base their communication at school on their spoken language skills. The use of a class observation tool, focusing on the behaviors of the students in common class situations, allowed a glimpse into the ongoing learning process of DHH students and provided unique insight regarding the daily challenges they face in class. Results indicated that DHH students made more eye contact with their classmates who speak during class, and they had more difficulty in following teacher instruction in comparison with hearing students. In addition to the observation results, DHH students reported greater difficulty understanding the teacher and the students, and had more negative and less positive affect during class. In addition, teacher ratings of social behaviors revealed differences between the two groups to the detriment of DHH students.

The findings also revealed that, regardless of hearing status, a large number of students per classroom causes students to make more eye contact with the teacher. In addition, poor acoustic conditions reduced students' understanding of the teacher and classmates, and reduced their positive feelings during class, regardless of their hearing status. These findings support the need to reduce the number of students per class and to improve acoustic conditions in the classrooms. This is especially important when integrating a DHH student, who needs the most accessible learning environment possible.

Contrary to the differences found between the two groups, reflecting the difficulties experienced by mainstream DHH students, no differences were found between the two groups in their language performance, speech intelligibility, and grades. Today, the support that most mainstream DHH students receive focuses successfully on improving academic achievement. However, classroom participation gets minimal or no attention at all. Many mainstream DHH students reported a gap between their self-learning ability and their ability to follow the ongoing discourse in class (Stinson et al., 1996). This gap can be expressed in high grades based on independent learning or on the assistance of the itinerant teacher, regardless of the level of involvement during class. Therefore, relying exclusively on grades as a measure of academic inclusion may present a false impression of high academic performance and may obscure the existence of problems and difficulties. Thus, the participation of DHH students in class should be evaluated as a separate measure that has its own importance, and the academic support given to mainstream DHH students should include specific attention to their classroom participation difficulties. Improving students' classroom participation and their feelings during class should be done by supporting the students and instructing their teachers. The students should be taught how to use strategies that enable them to communicate in a variety of situations during class. Teachers should be instructed by the itinerant teachers of the DHH students to recognize the difficulties of mainstream DHH students, to use assistive devices, and to use teaching methods that enhance student learning and communication in class, thereby improving their feelings.

The current findings highlight the fact that even mainstream DHH students who perform similar to their hearing classmates in terms of language, speech intelligibility, and grades are expected to experience significant difficulties in social functioning and classroom participation. High-functioning mainstream DHH students may mislead teachers and parents who perceive them as "normal," without recognizing their unique needs and challenges. Many mainstream DHH students have to deal with unrealistic parent and teacher expectations to "be like everyone else," thus denying legitimacy to express difficulties or to seek and receive proper assistance. This situation causes many difficulties to remain unaddressed. When DHH students do not receive professional support, it may perpetuate their difficulties and increase their frustration. The behaviors and feelings, social inferiority, and general difficulties that DHH students experience at school should not be ignored. The findings demonstrate the need for a wider educational point of view regarding the inclusion of DHH students. Comprehensive evaluations of DHH students, which includes classroom participation, will allow for better understanding of the daily challenges and difficulties they face at school. This knowledge will create a platform for more efficient rehabilitation programs that will lead to more successful inclusions of DHH students.

REFERENCES

Anderson, K. L., & Goldstein, H. (2004). Speech perception benefits of FM and infrared devices to children with hearing aids in a typical classroom. *Language, Speech, and Hearing Services in Schools, 35*(2), 169–184.

Antia, S. (2007). Can deaf and hard of hearing students be successful in general education classrooms? The teachers college record. http://www.tcrecord.org ID Number: 13461.

Antia, S. D., Jones, P., Luckner, J., Kreimeyer, K. H., & Reed, S. (2011). Social outcomes of students who are deaf and hard of hearing in general education classrooms. *Exceptional Children, 77*(4), 489–504.

Antia, S. D., Reed, S., & Kreimeyer, K. H. (2005). Written language of deaf and hard-of-hearing students in public schools. *Journal of Deaf Studies and Deaf Education, 10*(3), 244–255.

Antia S. D., Sabers, D. L., & Stinson, M. S. (2007). Validity and reliability of the classroom-participation questionnaire with deaf and hard of hearing students in public schools. *Journal of Deaf Studies and Deaf Education, 12*(2), 158–171.

ANSI (American National Standards Institute, Inc.) & ASA (Acoustical Society of America). (2010). *American National Standard acoustical performance criteria, design requirements and guidelines for schools: Part one: Permanent schools.* Acoustical Society of America (ASA), Melville, NY, S12. 60–2010.

Bat-Chava, Y., & Deignan, E. (2001). Peer relationships of children with cochlear implants. *The Journal of Deaf Studies and Deaf Education, 6*(3), 186–199.

Best, V., Gallun, F. G., Mason, C. R., Kidd, J., & Shinn-Cunningham, B. G. (2010). The impact of noise and hearing loss on the processing of simultaneous sentences. *Ear & Hearing, 31*(2), 213–220.

Blatchford, P., Bassett, P., & Brown, P. (2005). Teachers and pupils behavior in large and small classes: A systematic observation study of pupils aged 10–11 years. *Journal of Education Psychology, 97*(3), 454–467.

Bosacki, S., Rose-Krasnor, L., & Coplan, R. S. (2014). Children's talking and listening within classroom: Teacher's insights. *Early Child Development and Care, 184*(2), 247–265.

Crandell, C. C., & Smaldino, J. J. (2000). Classroom acoustics for children with normal hearing and with hearing impairment. *Language, Speech, and Hearing Services in Schools, 31*(4), 362–370.

Dallimore, E. J., Hertenstein, J. H., & Platt, M. B. (2004). Classroom participation and discussion effectiveness: Student-generated strategies. *Communication Education, 53*(1), 103–115.

Damen, G. W., van den Oever-Goltstein, M. H., Langereis, M. C., Chute, P. M., & Mylanus, E. A. (2006). Classroom performance of children with cochlear implants in mainstream education. *The Annals of Otology, Rhinology, and Laryngology, 115*(7), 542–552.

Davies, M. G., Yellon, L., & Purdy, S. C. (2001). Speech: In noise perception of children using cochlear implants and FM systems. *Australian and New Zealand Journal of Audiology, 23*, 52–62.

Delage, H., & Tuller, L. (2007). Language development and mild to moderate hearing loss: Does language normalize with age? *Journal of Speech, Language, and Hearing Research, 50*, 1300–1313.

Eriks-Brophy, A., Durieux-Smith, A., Olds, J., Fitzpatrick, E., Duquette, C., & Whittingham, J. (2006). Facilitators and barriers to the inclusion of orally educated children and youth with hearing loss in schools: Promoting partnerships to support inclusion. *The Volta Review, 106*(1), 53–88.

Fegan, M. K., & Pisoni, D. B. (2010). Hearing experience and receptive vocabulary development in deaf children with cochlear implant. *International Journal of Deaf Studies and Deaf Education, 15*(2), 149–161.

Fellinger, J., Holzinger, D., Beitel, C., Laucht, M., & Goldberg, C. (2009). The impact of language skills on mental health in teenagers with hearing impairments. *Acta Psychiatrica Scandinavica, 120*(2), 153–159.

Foster, S., Long, G., & Snell, K. (1999). Empirical paper: Inclusive instruction and learning for deaf students in postsecondary education. *Journal of Deaf Studies and Deaf Education, 4*(3), 225–235.

Francis, H. W., Koch, M. E., Wyatt, J. R., & Niparko, J. K. (1999). Trends in educational placement and cost–benefit considerations in children with cochlear implants. *Archives of Otolaryngology-Head & Neck Surgery, 125*(5), 499–505.

Friedmann, N., & Sztrezman, R. (2006). Syntactic movement in orally trained children with hearing impairment. *Journal of Deaf Studies and Deaf Education, 11*(1), 56–76.

Gallaudet Research Institute (2011). *Regional and national summary report of data from the 2009–2010 annual survey of deaf and hard of hearing children and youth.* Washington, DC: Gallaudet University.

Geers, A. E. (2003). Predictors of reading skill development in children with early cochlear implantation. *Ear and Hearing, 24*(1), 59S–68S.

Hatamizadeh N., Ghasemi, M., Saeedi, A., & Kazemnejad, A. (2008). Perceived competence and school adjustment of hearing impaired children in mainstream primary school setting. *Child: Care Health and Development, 34*(6), 789–794.

Haynes, W. O., Moran, M. J., & Pindzola, R. H. (2006). School-age and adolescent language disorders. In W. O. Haynes, M. J. Moran, & R. H. Pindzola (Eds.), *Communication disorders in classroom: An introduction for professionals in school settings* (pp. 173–188). Boston, MA: Jones and Bartlett Publishers.

Hyde, M., Punch, R., Power, D., Hartley, J., Neale, J., & Brennan, L. (2009). The experiences of deaf and hard of hearing students at a Queensland University: 1985–2005. *Higher Education Research & Development, 28*(1), 85–98.

Jeanes, R., Niehearing, T., & Rickards, F. (2000). The pragmatic skills of profoundly deaf children. *Journal of Deaf Studies and Deaf Education, 5*(3), 237–247.

Karchmer, M. A., & Mitchell, R. E. (2003). Demographic and achievement characteristics of deaf and hard-of-hearing students. In M. Marschark & P. E. Spencer (Eds.), *Oxford handbook of deaf studies, language, and education* (pp. 21–37). New York, NY: Oxford University Press.

Kelly, R. R., & Gaustad, M. G. (2007). Deaf college students' mathematical skills relative to morphological knowledge, reading level, and language proficiency. *Journal of Deaf Studies & Deaf Education, 12*(1), 25–37.

Kelly, R. R., Lang, H. G., & Pagliaro, C. M. (2003). Mathematics word problem solving for deaf students: A survey of practices in grades 6–12. *Journal of Deaf Studies and Deaf Education, 8*(2), 104–119.

Kent, B. A. (2003). Identity issues for hard-of-hearing adolescents aged 11, 13, and 15 in mainstream setting. *The Journal of Deaf Studies and Deaf Education, 8*(3), 315–324.

Klatte, M., Lachmann, T., & Meis, M. (2010). Effects of noise and reverberation on speech perception and listening comprehension of children and adults in a classroom-like setting. *Speech Perception and Understanding, 12*(49), 270–282.

Knecht, H. A., Nelson, P. B., Whitelaw, G. M., & Feth, L. L. (2002). Background noise level & reverberation times in unoccupied classrooms: Predictions and measurements. *American Journal of Audiology, 11*, 65–71.

Knoors, H., & Marschark, M. (2013). Learning and social and emotional development. In H. Knoors & M. Marschark (Eds.), *Teaching deaf learners: Psychological and developmental foundations* (pp. 132–158). New , NY: Oxford University Press.

Lau, S., Liem, A. D., & Nie, Y. (2008). Task-and self-related pathways to deep learning: The mediating role of achievement goals, classroom attentiveness, and group participation. *British Journal of Educational Psychology, 78*(4), 639–662.

Luckner, J. L., & Muir, S. (2001). Successful students who are deaf in general education settings. *American Annals of the Deaf, 146*(5), 435–445.

Mather, S. M., & Clark, M. D. (2012). An issue of learning: The effect of visual split attention in classes for deaf and hard of hearing students. *Odyssey: New Directions in Deaf Education, 13*, 20–24.

McCain, K. G., & Antia, S. D. (2005). Academic and social status of hearing, deaf, and hard of hearing students participating in a co-enrolled classroom. *Communication Disorders Quarterly, 27*(1), 20–32.

McDaniel, D. M., & Cox, R. M. (1992). Evaluation of the Speech Intelligibility Rating (SIR) test for hearing aid comparisons. *Journal of Speech, Language and Hearing Research, 35*(3), 686–693.

McKay, S., Gravel, J. S., & Tharpe, A. M. (2008). Amplification considerations for children with minimal or mild bilateral hearing loss and unilateral hearing loss. *Trends in Amplification, 12*(1), 43–54.

Merrel, K. W. (2002). *School social behavior scales* (2nd ed.). Eugene, OR: Assessment-Intervention Resources.

Most, T. (2004). The effects of degree and type of hearing loss on children's performance in class. *Deafness and Education International, 6*(3), 154–166.

Most, T. (2006). Assessment of school functioning among Israeli Arab children with hearing loss in the primary grades. *American Annals of the Deaf, 151*(3), 327–335.

Most, T. (2007). Speech intelligibility, loneliness, and sense of coherence among deaf and hard-of-hearing children in individual inclusion and group inclusion. *The Journal of Deaf Studies and Deaf Education, 12*(2), 495–503.

National Council for the Child, Israel. (2013). *Children with special needs*. Jerusalem, Israel (Hebrew): The national Council for the Child Publications.

Nicholas, J. G., & Geers, A. E. (2007). Will they catch up? The role of age at cochlear implantation in the spoken language development of children with severe to profound hearing loss. *Journal of Speech, Language, and Hearing Research, 50*(4), 1048–1062.

Noll, D. L. (2007). Activities for social skills development in deaf children preparing to enter the mainstream. Master's thesis, Washington University, School of Medicine.

Norbury, C. F., Bishop, D. V. M., & Briscoe, J. (2001). Production of English finite verb morphology: A comparison of SLI and mild-moderate hearing impairment. *Journal of Speech, Language and Hearing Research, 44*, 165–178.

Peterson, S. A. (2012). The labor of listening. *The International Journal of Listening, 26*, 87–90.

Power, D., & Hyde, M. (2002). The characteristics and extent of participation of deaf and hard-of-hearing students in regular classes in Australian schools. *Journal of Deaf Studies and Deaf Education, 7*(4), 302–311.

Powers, S. (2002). From concepts to practice in deaf education: A United Kingdom perspective on inclusion. *Journal of Deaf Studies and Deaf Education, 7*(3), 230–243.

Powers, S. (2003). Influences of student and family factors on academic outcomes of mainstream secondary school deaf students. *Journal of Deaf Studies and Deaf Education, 8*(1), 57–78.

Powers, S., Gregory, S., & Thoutenhoofd, E. D. (1999). The educational achievements of deaf children: A literature review executive summary. *Deafness & Education International, (9)*, 1–9.

Preisler, G., Tvingstedt, A., & Ahlstrom, M. (2005). Interviews with deaf children about their experiences using cochlear implants. *American Annals of the Deaf, 150*(3), 260–267.

Punch, R., & Hyde, M. (2011). Social participation of children and adolescents with cochlear implants: A qualitative analysis of parent, teacher and child interviews. *Journal of Deaf Studies and Deaf Education, 16*(4), 474–493.

Reed, S., Antia, S. D., & Kreimeyer, K. H. (2008). Academic status of deaf and hard-of-hearing students in public schools: Student, home, and service facilitators and detractors. *The Journal of Deaf Studies and Deaf Education, 13*(4), 485–502.

Richardson, J. T. E., Marschark, M., Sarchet, T., & Sapere, P.(2010). Deaf and hard-of-hearing student's experiences in mainstream and postsecondary education. *International Journal of Deaf Studies and Deaf Education, 15*(4), 358–382.

Shepherd, M. A. (2010). A discourse analysis of teacher–student classroom interactions. PhD dissertation. http://www.proquest.com/en-US/products/dissertations/individuals.shtml.

Silvestre, N., Ramspott, A., & Pareto, I. D. (2007). Conversational skills in a semi-structured interview and self-concept in deaf students. *Journal of Deaf Studies and Deaf Education, 12*(1), 38–54.

Skelt, L. (2013). Recipient gaze and the resolution of overlapping talk in hearing impaired interaction. *Journal of Interactional Research in Communication Disorders, 4*(1), 71–94.

Soukup, M., & Feinstein, S. (2007). Identification, assessment, and intervention strategies for deaf and hard of hearing students with learning disabilities. *American Annals of the Deaf, 152*(1), 56–62.

Spivak, L., Sokol, H., Auerbach, C., & Gershkovich, S. (2009). Newborn hearing screening follow-up: Factors affecting hearing aid fitting by 6 months of age. *American Journal of Audiology, 18*(1), 24–33.

Stinson, M., & Antia, S. (1999). Considerations in educating deaf and hard-of-hearing students in inclusive settings. *Journal of Deaf Studies and Deaf Education, 4*(3), 163–175.

Stinson, M., & Liu, Y. (1999). Empirical paper: Participation of deaf and hard-of-hearing students in classes with hearing students. *Journal of Deaf Studies and Deaf Education, 4*(3), 191–202.

Stinson, M., Liu, Y., Saur, R., & Long, G. (1996). Deaf college students' perceptions of communication in mainstream classes. *Journal of Deaf Studies and Deaf Education, 1*(1), 40–51.

Stinson, M. S., & Whitmire, K. A. (2000). Adolescents who are deaf or hard of hearing: A communication perspective on educational placement. *Topics in Language Disorders, 20*(2), 58–72.

Swain, K. D., Mary, F., & Harrington, J. M. (2004). Teaching listening strategies in the inclusive classroom. *Intervention in School and Clinic, 40*(1), 48–54.

Toe, D. M., & Paatsch, L. E. (2010). The communication skills used by deaf children and their hearing peers in a question-and-answer game context. *Journal of Deaf Studies and Deaf Education, 15*(3), 228–241.

Tvingstedt, A. L. (1995). Classroom interaction and the social situation of hard-of-hearing pupils in regular classes. Paper presented at the 18th International Congress on Education of the Deaf. Tel-Aviv, Israel.

Twisk, J. W. R. (2006). *Applied multilevel analysis: A practical guide for medical researchers.* Cambridge, UK: Cambridge University Press.

Vermeulen, A. M., van Bon, W., Schreuder, R., Knoors, H., & Snik, A. (2007). Reading comprehension of deaf children with cochlear implants. *Journal of Deaf Studies and Deaf Education, 12*(3), 283–302.

Wake, M., Hughes, E. K., Poulakis, Z., Collins, C., & Rickards, F. W. (2004). Outcomes of children with mild-profound congenital hearing loss at 7 to 8 years: A population study. *Ear and Hearing, 25*(1), 1–8.

Wauters, L. N., & Knoors, H. (2008). Social integration of deaf children in inclusive settings. *Journal of Deaf Studies and Deaf Education, 13*(1), 21–36.

14

Mental Health Problems of Deaf Children and Adolescents: An Overview

Tiejo van Gent and Ines Sleeboom-van Raaij

In principle, deaf children and adolescents will experience comparable mental health difficulties as their hearing peers. However, additional physical problems, cognitive and communicative shortcomings, and the presence of other sources of social distress can complicate diagnosis and treatment considerably (Van Gent, 2012). Most deaf children and adolescents do not have a lifetime mental health disorder (e.g., Fellinger et al., 2009b; Van Gent et al., 2007), although many may experience psychological difficulties or even distress at some moments in their life, as do their hearing peers. Because this chapter describes mental health functioning of deaf children and adolescents from a psychiatric perspective, the primary focus is to address the origin of mental health difficulties and mental disorders, their causes, course, symptoms, and treatment options.

EPIDEMIOLOGY OF DEAFNESS AND MENTAL HEALTH PROBLEMS

A child may be called deaf when he or she has little or no functional hearing in the better ear and depends primarily on visual communication when without a hearing aid or other device. From an audiological–medical perspective, this description of deafness corresponds to bilateral severe to profound hearing loss as defined by mean thresholds (in decibels) of hearing, which may vary across reports and international standards (e.g., Van Gent, 2012).

The number of children who are deaf is lowest in high-income countries (for example, around 0.85 per thousand live births in the United Kingdom [Fortnum et al., 2001]) and is higher in low-income countries (World Health Organization, 2010). Deafness does not decrease over time, but the relative distribution of causes does (Fortnum et al., 2001).

The causes of deafness vary from nonsyndromic simple genetic deafness, not associated with other signs or symptoms; syndromic deafness, occurring as part of a syndrome together with other medical conditions, organ involvement, or specific physical features; acquired deafness, such as through intrauterine or postnatal infections, perinatal problems, ototoxic medication; tumor or trauma; and unknown causes. Although simple genetic deafness has remained the most prevalent kind throughout the years, syndromic genetic deafness and deafness caused by perinatal factors have increased as a result of improved diagnostics and therapeutic possibilities, whereas deafness caused by prenatal and postnatal infections have decreased (Fortnum et al., 2002), at least in countries with advanced healthcare facilities. Technological advances in diagnosis will further reduce the number of cases of unknown etiology.

Epidemiological studies have shown that populations of children who are deaf or hard of hearing show higher mean rates of emotional and behavioral difficulties than normative or comparison groups of hearing peers (Stevenson et al., 2015; Van Gent et al., 2007). In studies using comparable versions of the same rating scale, the Achenbach System of Empirically Based Assessment (Achenbach & Rescorla, 1999), two to two and a half times increased rates of difficulties have been reported in school populations of deaf children with roughly normal levels of intelligence (Van Gent, 2012). To date, studies on the prevalence of general mental health disorder—based on a diagnosis by a multimethod assessment including a diagnostic interview with the deaf child to assess general psychopathology—are few. In the only study including a diagnostic interview with all participants (a representative sample of school-age deaf adolescents in the Netherlands; n = 70; age range, 12–21 years; severe to profound hearing loss; average intelligence), the prevalence of general mental health disorders was 46% (Van Gent et al., 2007). Independent of the degree of hearing loss or the etiology of the deafness, half the subjects were shown to have a mild mental health disorder, with the other half having a more severe mental health disorder as indicated by a greater social impact or handicap (Van Gent, 2012). Comparably high disorder rates were found in a study in the United Kingdom that used diagnostic interviews with a select number of the participating deaf and hard-of-hearing children (Hindley et al., 1994) and in a study in Austria that used diagnostic interviews with parents of deaf and hard-of-hearing children (Fellinger et al., 2009b).

ETIOLOGY AND PATHOGENESIS RELATED TO MENTAL HEALTH PROBLEMS

Genetic Factors

Inherited deafness without other physical symptoms or disability accounts for the majority of genetically determined cases, with syndromic deafness accounting for the minority. There is a considerable number of syndromes in which distinctive physical conditions are associated with deafness. Syndromes that interfere with prenatal central nervous system development may show developmental delay, learning disability, or features of autism spectrum disorder (ASD). Syndromes with other organ system involvement may be associated with other, sometimes serious and recurring physical health problems. Syndromes in which there are facial dysmorphisms or other features involving physical appearance may lead to social difficulties, including bullying, and emotional problems including anxiety and depression.

Neurobiological Factors

A considerable number of deaf children have a history of neurological disorder (16% [Freeman et al., 1975]), and children with a neurological disorder, such as neurological motor disorder (36%) or epilepsy (6%), are overrepresented among deaf and hard-of-hearing children and adolescents with serious mental health problems (Van Gent et al., 2012b). The chance of central nervous system disorder is greatest when deafness is generated by a syndrome or an acquired cause.

Central nervous system involvement resulting from the underlying cause of deafness, concomitant neurodevelopmental delay or disabilities, or other distinctive physically handicapping conditions all add to the risk of mental health problems as well as to the complexity of the clinical picture. For instance, children with congenital deafness from an intrauterine rubella infection who are referred for psychiatric assessment belong to the subgroup of referred patients with the most serious mental health needs, especially when they come along with additional complex health needs resulting from physical comorbidity. They may present with severe problems in impulse control, including self-harm and aggression, relatively often related to ASD (Van Gent et al., 2012b), which in itself may hinder social understanding and coping with physical distress. Not unexpectedly, the chance of serious problems in impulse control in rubella patients is associated with the presence of brain damage (Chess & Fernandez, 1980).

Another example indicating complex mental health needs related to specific etiologies of deafness is congenital cytomegalovirus (CMV) infection through intrauterine maternal transmission. It is the leading cause of bilateral nongenetic congenital hearing loss, with a reported rate of 23% among children with a profound permanent hearing loss (Korver et al., 2009). The hearing loss caused by congenital CMV infection may show variability in onset, severity, and fluctuations over time. It may be missed at early neonatal hearing screening and may only be recognized at a later age because the onset of hearing loss frequently occurs later, and may be progressive in nature, even years after birth. Because of its often unpredictable course, it may be especially difficult for parents and other caregivers to find early accommodating communication strategies and interaction with a child with fluctuating and progressive hearing loss of late onset.

That physical comorbidity in general is an important risk factor of emotional dysregulation and mental health problems in children and young people (Friedman & Chase-Landsdale, 2002) may be supported by the finding that a history of physical disorder appeared to be the only one of a large number of demographic and medical variables to be associated with the presence of emotional disorder among deaf adolescents in the study by Van Gent et al. (2007).

Last, long-term risks of specific, acquired causes of deafness have been demonstrated in adults, too. In prenatal rubella, CMV, and toxoplasmosis, a greater frequency of nonaffective psychosis was observed in adult psychiatry with this population (Blomström et al., 2015; Brown et al., 2001).

Environmental Influences

Deaf children may be found to be at an increased risk of mental health problems when faced with a variety of heterogeneous developmental challenges related to the nature, degree, and age of onset, diagnosis of deafness and subsequent additional long-term complications—such as blindness, learning problems, physical illness or hospitalization—as well as adverse social circumstances. A serious limitation in one sensory function can be particularly challenging for the development of a child if the remaining sensory functions cannot be used optimally (e.g., see Hindley & Van Gent, 2002; Van Gent, 2012). Most deaf and hearing children have enough resources to cope and adapt successfully to limited amounts of environmental stress without serious consequences to their mental health. However, deaf children and adolescents may be exposed to a range of additional environmental risk factors that may be regarded as stressors that induce more or less chronic adverse circumstances. Examples include persistent communication problems, social misunderstandings, social deprivation, loneliness, rejection and discrimination, traumatic life events (bullying, victimization, exposure to violence), familial distress and parental discord, or socioeconomic risk related to low parental educational level or immigrant status (Hindley & Van Gent, 2002; Van Gent, 2012). For instance, limited hearing or suffering from physically handicapping conditions may elicit recurrent negative thinking of serious personal shortcomings in deaf children, especially in deaf children with low self-esteem (Van Gent et al., 2011).

The accumulation of risk—that is, of many such factors being present at the same time—in particular contributes to an increase in vulnerability to mental health problems (Friedman & Chase-Lansdale, 2002). The effect of adversities on social and cognitive functioning depends on how they interact with individually varying inherent predispositions, comprising gender, genetics, physical health, and temperament, to influence intrapersonal processes. The main processes that are elementary to healthy emotional, social, and cognitive functioning are the formation of secure attachment relationships, the regulation of emotions, and cognitive processes such as internal representations of the world, belief systems, and cognitive appraisals, in addition to physiological systems and their responses (Friedman & Chase-Lansdale, 2002).

DEVELOPMENTAL ASPECTS

The way deafness influences the development of a child depends on the interplay of many factors. Interactions among deafness-related and intra- and interpersonal factors eventually results in very heterogeneous, highly individualized competencies and outcome in all developmental domains, including formal and informal learning and academic achievement (see Chapter 18). To a large extent, vulnerability to mental health problems of a deaf child is determined by the consequences of being deaf in a world adjusted primarily to the needs of hearing people (e.g., Hindley & Van Gent, 2002; Van Gent, 2012). The quality of social interaction between deaf children and the environment is, to a great degree, determined by the way parents, other caregivers, siblings, teachers, and other significant people in the direct environment respond and adapt to the visual/spatial, linguistic/communicative, and emotional needs of the child.

Here we discuss significant aspects of interactive and social–emotional processes related to the social–emotional development of deaf children in greater detail. Discussions of the effect of cognitive and language/communication development can be found in several other chapters in this volume.

Attachment

Parental involvement, availability, and emotional security are among the key features of the interaction between parents and their child underlying safe attachment relationships, adequate emotion regulation, and, later, adequate social and cognitive functioning (e.g., Calderon & Greenberg, 2011; see also Chapter 5). They are also powerful predictors of language development (e.g., Yoshinaga-Itano, 2003).

Most deaf children (approximately 95%) are born into hearing families, and most of their parents will not have had prior contact with deafness and deaf people. Many may experience an emotional crisis (Calderon & Greenberg, 2011) or feelings of shock on discovering and realizing their child is deaf (e.g., Freeman et al., 1975). Anxiety, guilt, and depressive reactions can vary strongly among these parents (Marschark, 2007). Those reactions may complicate important aspects of the interaction between a parent and the child, such as sharing attention, meaning, involvement, and reciprocity. A very premature birth, hospitalization, and physical deformities can create additional risks.

Ideally, parents and siblings come to terms with the deaf child being different, not disabled (Young, 1999). In general, the quality of the early interaction between parents and their deaf child is promoted by the extent to which parents succeed in establishing visual communication patterns by the early use of visual–tactile communication strategies (Loots & Devisé, 2003; Loots et al., 2005), even if, ultimately, the child uses spoken language. Visual and communicative attunement provide advantages in the development of a deaf child. Research with 18- to 24-month-old deaf infants and their mothers suggests that visual–tactile communicative fine-tuning and signing promotes the development of symbolic intersubjectivity, implying a mutual exchange and sharing of linguistic and symbolic meaning between deaf or hearing parents and their deaf child (Loots et al., 2005). The interaction between deaf children and hearing parents who selectively preferred spoken communication tended to stagnate in the transition from more basic to symbolic intersubjectivity (Loots & Devisé, 2003).

Deaf parents may have an advantage over hearing parents in this respect. Deaf parents may demonstrate greater sensitivity to the visual initiatives to interact (Smith-Gray & Koester, 1995) and may perceive bodily signals of their deaf infant as attempts to communicate and so reciprocate, setting up early communicative interactions. For instance, deaf parents are probably more likely than hearing parents to recognize and respond to babbling with the hands, a rhythmic syllabically organized linguistic activity in their deaf infant (Baker et al., 2006; Pettito & Marentette, 1991). Deaf parents may rely on a greater variety of communicative methods (Harris, 2001), using both visual and tactile signals to attract visual attention, and they may be more consistent in signing in their child's visual signing space, and more apt to wait to obtain the child's visual attention before signing than hearing parents (Loots & Devisé, 2003). Deaf children who are subject to more restricted communication patterns with hearing parents and teachers are at risk of developing a delay in language development (Hauser & Marschark, 2008); they will have fewer opportunities to identify and differentiate meaning and to become familiar with the use of abstract concepts (Marschark, 1993). They will experience less environmental and social diversity (Marschark, 2007), less incidental learning (Calderon & Greenberg, 2011), and less exposure to a variety of cause–effect relationships reflecting differences in problem solving, and may show a tendency to focus on individual item processing rather than on sequential processing and relations among them (Marschark, 2003, 2007).

Current programs for neonatal hearing screening and early intervention contributed strongly to the early detection of deafness and meeting the needs of the child and his family; to the provision of information, emotional, and social support to all parents; as well as the promotion of effective communication between parents and their deaf child (see Chapter 2). Moreover, the introduction of cochlear implants (CIs), an advanced electronic device delivering hearing sensations by stimulating electrically the auditory nerve inside the inner ear, has led to more young deaf children, especially in industrialized countries, being able to hear better under favorable conditions and to use spoken language. However, sign language remains important in the future, not only for children and adults who have not received implants but also as an aid to learning spoken language in situations in which a CI is less useful as an effective form of communication before and after implantation (Knoors & Marschark, 2012), and when meeting deaf friends who sign (De Raeve, 2014).

Social–Emotional Development

Parents of deaf children may experience many obstacles in parenting as a result of communication problems, such as problems in understanding and limited options to socialize with their child (Calderon & Greenberg, 2011) in all phases of development. Limited communication between parents and their deaf child may seriously affect the quality of interaction between them, with negative consequences to the developing ability of a child to articulate experiences; to recognizes, identify, and share emotions; to solve social dilemmas; and to develop a positive self-image later in life (Calderon & Greenberg, 2011). In contrast, good sign language proficiency of the parents, regardless of their hearing status, is associated with greater levels of self-esteem in their deaf children (Bat-Chava, 1993; Desselle, 1994), whereas support for signing early in life as well as good-quality social communication between parents and deaf adolescents as perceived by both is related to greater levels of global self-worth in deaf adolescents (Van Gent et al., 2012a).

Lags in language development may also affect the development of play, at least in part because of limited access to interaction with parents (Marschark, 2007) and other caregivers. However, deaf children with sufficient access to suitable language and without a delay in language development may engage in age-appropriate play behavior and interactions similar to those in hearing peers (Musyoka, 2015; Spencer & Deyo, 1993).

Rieffe (2012) reported less effective emotion regulation strategies in deaf children (mean age, 11 years) compared with those of hearing, age- and gender-matched peers. The deaf children showed fewer problem- and emotion-focused coping strategies and made almost no use of avoidance to diminish the negative impact of the situation, in contrast to their hearing peers. Less emotion awareness and fewer emotion regulation skills may contribute to a greater vulnerability to negative mental health outcomes (Rieffe, 2012). Long-lasting communicative problems, misunderstandings, shortcomings, and social isolation may be particularly troublesome during adolescence (Van Gent et al., 2011, 2012a). During this developmental period, belonging to a social network as well as having intimate relationships with both parents and peers are especially important for the development of a sense of self-esteem and identity (Calderon & Greenberg, 2011). But, the challenge to become a more or less successful member of a broader social context than before might be hindered for deaf adolescents because of either restricted opportunities of getting access to outside activities, in the case of schools for the deaf (Musselman et al., 1996), or considerable communicative differences with less familiar and predominantly hearing others in new sociocultural environments (Van Gent et al., 2012a). Consequently, this is when deaf adolescents become particularly at risk of feeling socially isolated, especially in a hearing environment, in regular schools, and in the surrounding neighborhood (Calderon & Greenberg, 2011).

Research by Van Gent et al. (2012a) with a representative sample of deaf adolescents of average intelligence in the Netherlands revealed no difference in the mean level of global self-esteem between them and a hearing comparison group with a comparable educational level. However, deaf adolescents reported, on average, a lower level of self-perceived competence in peer-related social domains, particularly in the domain of social acceptance. The lowest level of social acceptance was found in the subgroup of adolescents who also reported the lowest level of close friendships in addition to a normal level of global self-esteem compared with the other subgroups, either with low self-perceptions in all self-concept domains or with increased competences in both the social and the global domain. Interestingly, membership of the first competence cluster (low social acceptance and few close friendships but normal self-esteem) was associated significantly more often with attending regular school and the highest mean level of sociocognitive maturity. Moreover, adolescents from this subgroup appeared to exhibit the highest risk of emotional mental health problems relative to the adolescents from the other two clusters (Van Gent, 2012). These results may be in line with findings in other studies showing that feeling isolated from the majority of hearing peers adds to the risk of emotional problems for deaf children (Farrugia & Austin, 1980; Van Gurp, 2001). Such findings support the view that communicative barriers in a hearing world especially affect social well-being and self-concept in social interactions (Calderon & Greenberg, 2011; Schlesinger & Meadow, 1972).

DIFFERENTIAL DIAGNOSTIC ASPECTS OF MENTAL HEALTH PROBLEMS

Clinical Picture

A large clinical sample of children and adolescents (n = 389) who were referred to the national in- and outpatient mental health service for the deaf and hard-of-hearing in the Netherlands for a study period of 15 years appeared to differ significantly from a large clinical comparison group of new hearing referrals to a specialist mental health service (n = 3339) in a number of areas (Van Gent et al., 2012b). This referred sample may be regarded as representative for the total population of deaf and hard-of-hearing children and adolescents with serious mental health problems in the Netherlands.

First, the average age of referral among the deaf and hard-of-hearing to the mental health center was 1 to 3 years older, depending on the presence or absence of complicating circumstances such as lower intelligence or other complexities. A number of factors may play a role in explaining the delay in seeking help for deaf or hard-of-hearing children with serious mental health problems. Most obviously, linguistic communication problems between the predominantly hearing environment and the deaf or hard-of-hearing child with mental health problems may impede sharing and recognition of such problems. For deaf children, especially those with limited language skills, it may be difficult to recognize, name, share, and nuance emotions, thoughts, and experience in general. This is particularly likely with parents, siblings, teachers, and professionals with whom communicative tuning is limited and, therefore, exploring problems might be difficult for them. Parents, teachers, and professionals also may have different frames of reference and perceptions of a child and his or her problem behavior, and the same child may show variations in problem behavior according to varying settings and persons (Fombonne, 2002). This may explain limited agreement between informants on who has a significant problem and who does not in epidemiological research (Fombonne, 2002), which has been observed in research with deaf populations as well (Van Gent et al., 2007). In addition, the coexistence of deafness or hearing loss and mental health problems may lead caregivers and others to assume prematurely that deafness or hearing loss explains all— the phenomenon of diagnostic shadowing (Kitson & Thacker, 2000). Especially in very complex cases such as ASD among patients with IQ and other, mostly physical, comorbidity and communication problems, it may be difficult to differentiate developmental delays resulting from physical inferences or cognitive disability in a child with limited communication skills from a developmental disorder characterized by restricted or abnormal social involvement and often-occurring atypical sensory responses (Rogers & Ozonoff, 2005). Last, another factor may be the limited availability of specialized mental health services that contribute to the undesirable prolongation of help seeking.

Second, a preponderance of ASD was observed in the target population compared with the comparison group in the study by Van Gent et al. (2012b). This may be explained by the increased frequency of ASD among deaf and hard-of-hearing children resulting from brain dysfunction or damage as underlying cause of both deafness or hearing loss and ASD (Jure et al., 1991). This is in line with the finding that 43% of the relatively large subgroup (21%) of deaf and hard-of-hearing patients with very complex physical health problems, either related to congenital rubella, or visual disorders, neurological motor disorder or epilepsy resulting from other causes, was diagnosed with ASD.

Third, a variety of chronic contextual stressors and putative risk factors were found to be present more frequently in the population in the study by Van Gent et al. (2012b) than in the comparison group. Deaf and hard-of-hearing referrals more often lived in single-parent families (38% vs. 29%), suggesting a higher rate of parental divorce, had parents with a lower educational backgrounds (44% vs. 31%), or had parents of with a nonwhite or Mediterranean background (35% vs. 8%). Such a finding may illustrate the occurrence of higher levels of environmental adversity in the referred target population, supporting the view that accumulation of health-related and chronic social and socioeconomic risk factors render children more vulnerable to mental health problems, as has been argued before. Alternatively, better educational and mental health care facilities in an industrialized country may attract families from abroad to present their children with special needs to available services. In addition, the educational level of deaf or hard-of-hearing parents differed significantly from hearing parents of the referred children. This is consistent with the finding of lower educational (Antia et al., 2009) and employment (Winn, 2007) outcome among deaf school leavers and adults, both of which are recognized as two cumulative risk factors. Last, the documented or presumed existence of sexual abuse in 7% to 11% of the referred target population illustrates the risk of abuse in children with disabilities in general (Sullivan et al., 2000), warranting specific attention during assessments because many cases may be missed.

Specific Disorders That Raise Specific Complexities

Autism Spectrum Disorder

The rate of ASD is increased in deaf and hard-of-hearing children (5.3%) compared with the general population (Jure et al., 1991), and approximately 3.5% of children with ASD are deaf or hard of hearing (Rosenhall et al., 1999). Brain damage as a result of interference with normal prenatal development of the central nervous system has been related etiologically to deafness as well as ASD. Examples include intrauterine viral infections such as rubella (Jure et al., 1991), CMV (Yashamita et al., 2003), and CHARGE association—a congenital disorder originally characterized by the combination of *c*oloboma, *h*eart abnormalities, *a*tresia of the choanae, *r*etardation of growth and development, defects of the *g*enitalia, and anomalies of the *e*ar, associated with hearing loss (Johansson et al., 2006).

The age of diagnosis of ASD is often later in deaf children than hearing children (Jure et al., 1991) because of differential diagnostic issues (Van Gent et al., 2012b), in part reflecting diagnostic shadowing (Hindley & Van Gent, 2002). Although the symptoms of ASD are the same in deaf and hearing children, differences in language skills and communication patterns between hearing and deaf children may complicate the clinical picture and the recognition of features typical of ASD. For instance, poor language skills resulting from a delay in language development in a nonautistic deaf child must be differentiated from an impaired ability to use language effectively in social contexts among deaf children with ASD. Sign language has grammatical constructs such as the use of repetition to emphasize a point, it omits the pronoun "I" in directional verbs that point in a different direction or order, and there are differences in the use of time and localization compared with many spoken languages. As well as a delay in spoken language, such constructs must not be confused with language use, which is often seen in children with autism: pronominal reversal, neologisms, direct and postponed echolalia, and formal language use. When assessing signing children psychiatrically for ASD and comorbid disorders, subtle deviations in hand forms, movements, or abnormal localizations pointing at analogies of neologisms or language defects can be missed easily.

Difficulties in social interaction and reciprocity, impaired imaginative play, or restricted interests may help to indicate children with ASD. Research involving hearing children suggests that co-occurrence of ASD and specific language impairment is not associated with increased severity of ASD symptoms, but rather with greater impairment in receptive language and functional communication (Loucas et al., 2008). In children with ASD, difficulties in making eye contact and avoiding looking at faces can hinder learning and use of sign language. However, in line with clinical impressions (e.g., Hindley, 2000), research in the United Kingdom has demonstrated deaf signing children with ASD to have relatively unimpaired face recognition skills for communication purposes (Denmark, 2011). Deaf children with ASD in the study by Denmark (2011) performed comparably with deaf children without ASD in making functional eye contact with a purely linguistic function, but they showed greater impairments in recognition and production of affective facial expressions. These findings suggest that linguistic face processing is far less confusing than processing emotional expression in purely social eye contact in signing deaf children with ASD (Denmark, 2011). When coming to a diagnosis of ASD, the quality and quantity of eye contact must be interpreted in this context. Another regularly occurring diagnostic dilemma may be differentiation between interactive, communicative, and behavioral symptoms resulting from an *inability* to give meaning to social stimuli in respect of ASD as opposed to *not knowing how* to give meaning to social–communicative deficiencies as a result of serious social deprivation and understimulation (O'Connor et al., 2000), a cognitive handicap (Vig & Jedrysek, 1999), or blindness (Jan et al., 1977).

The diagnosis of ASD may be especially complicated in deaf children who also have serious vision problems in combination with intellectual disability. In a study of deaf–blind children with severe intellectual disability, children with autism differed from nonautistic children with respect to the quality of social interaction, initiative, and use of communicative signals and functions in particular, but less so in respect to the quality of play, exploration, problem solving, and the existence of stereotypes (Hoevenaars-Van den Boom et al., 2009). Currently, observational tools with promising psychometric properties, such as the Observation of Autism in People with Sensory and Intellectual Disabilities, are being developed to help clinicians differentiate the origin of typical and atypical problem behavior and to diagnose ASD in deaf–blind individuals with additional intellectual disabilities as a prerequisite to intervention planning (de Vaan et al., 2015).

Attention Deficit Hyperactivity Disorder and Disruptive Behavioral Disorder

With regard to the broad category of behavioral disorders including disruptive behavior and attention deficit hyperactivity disorder (ADHD), Van Gent et al. (2012b) found more disorders in deaf or hard-of-hearing children with hearing parents (35%; n = 362) than in children with deaf or hard-of-hearing parents (30%; n = 27) or hearing children with hearing parents (29%; n = 3339), although the difference did not reach significance. Remarkably, the rate of behavioral disorder in the deaf and hard-of-hearing population of referrals declined over the years, suggesting that the most urgent demand for assessment and treatment of serious problem behavior had been dealt with during the first phase of the existence of a new specialized mental health service for deaf and hard-of-hearing children and adolescents. Alternatively, more focus toward the specific communicative needs of deaf children during the past few decades has probably contributed considerably to the gradual reduction in numbers of referrals of deaf children and adolescents to mental health centers for attention deficit disorders and behavioral disorders (Sinkkonen, 1994) in recent decades (Van Gent et al., 2012b).

In a recent meta-analysis of studies on the prevalence of emotional and behavioral problems using the Strengths and Difficulties Questionnaire (Goodman, 1997), no indication of an increased risk for deaf or hard-of-hearing children to exhibit ADHD-type symptoms was found (Stevenson et al., 2015). From a differential-diagnostic viewpoint, disruptive behavior, impulsivity, hyperactivity, and other symptoms such as attention deficit may have various backgrounds. First, these types of behavior may be associated with brain pathology that is found more frequently with some types of deafness (Kelly et al., 1993), particularly acquired or syndromic deafness. In a longitudinal study of children affected by congenital rubella (Chess & Fernandez, 1980; Chess et al., 1971), early impulsiveness in children with hearing loss alone disappeared as the children acquired language and self-control skills. In contrast, impulsiveness persisted in deaf children with neurological signs of brain damage resulting from congenital rubella. ADHD-like symptoms and behavioral problems may also indicate communicative and social deprivation that, in itself, is not specific to deafness. Second, oppositional behavior, distractibility, and overactivity can be an expression of underlying feelings of impotence, anxiety, sadness, or frustration with communication difficulties (Hindley & Kroll, 1998); a distracting visual environment; or poor language and visual attention matching in the classroom (Dye et al., 2008; Kelly et al., 1993). Deaf individuals are likely to be distracted by visual information in their peripheral vision, and, with respect to attentional allocation, there may be a conflict between the demands of the environment and the default allocation of resources (Dye et al., 2008). Alternatively, or at the same time, behavioral and attention problems may reflect problems with learning, undetected cognitive problems, problems with executive functioning (Hintermair, 2013), or problems with language, both directly or indirectly via an effect on sustained attention (Barker et al., 2009).

Attention problems also have been associated with absence seizures or petit mal epilepsy (very brief attacks of impaired consciousness, sometimes accompanied by muscle spasms, often followed by confusion and unawareness of the attack), as well as the side effects of drugs (Kelly et al., 1993). Last, exaggerated self-appraisal of social acceptance has been associated with behavioral mental health problems, both in deaf and in hearing adolescents (Van Gent et al., 2011). Hypothetically, this could reflect the impact of a younger mental age and lower social–cognitive maturity in a number of deaf adolescents, as has been found in hearing peers (Harter, 2006; Van Gent et al., 2012a). Such differential diagnostic considerations can be weighted only with the aid of diagnostic interviews and other assessment tools that are aimed adequately at the communicative abilities of the child/adolescent or his or her parents.

Affective Disorder

Most prevalence studies in deaf children and adolescents have found increased rates of emotional difficulties or disorders in deaf children and young people compared with the general population (Stevenson et al., 2015; Van Gent et al., 2007). Emotional mental health problems were even found more often than behavioral problems in representative samples of schoolchildren with moderate to profound hearing loss (Fellinger et al., 2009b) and deaf adolescents (Van Gent et al., 2007).

A range of underlying factors has been related to emotional problems: communicative interactional, parental, and intrapersonal. The risk of an emotional disorder increases in adolescents who are rejected (Van Gent et al., 2011), teased, isolated or maltreated (Fellinger, et al., 2009b), or victimized (Kouwenberg et al., 2012) by family members or peers. Both depressive disorder and teasing have been associated with the child's ability to make himself understood as perceived by the parents (Fellinger et al., 2009b). The finding that the chance of emotional problems is more pronounced when deaf children have lower language skills in the dominant language mode of the majority of pupils at school (Fellinger et al., 2009a) supports the view that intra- and interpersonal factors act in concert to predict emotional mental health outcome. With regard to parental factors, low parental sensitivity and expectations of their deaf or hard-of-hearing child have been associated with more victimization (Kouwenberg, 2013). In general, the perception of high-quality parent–child communication as perceived by both has been related positively to global self-esteem in deaf adolescents, which in itself may protect from emotional mental health problems (Van Gent et al., 2012a). With regard to intrapersonal factors, emotional mental health problems have been related to various characteristics of the child. Examples include a low sense of social acceptance in deaf adolescents who report average levels of global self-esteem and a relatively high level of social–cognitive maturity (Van Gent, 2012); low global self-esteem in deaf adolescents with functional residual hearing, past or present neurological disorder, or an acquired or syndromic cause of deafness (Van Gent et al., 2011); low levels of emotion awareness and theory of mind (Kouwenberg et al., 2011); and lower language skills regardless of language modality or degree of hearing loss (Dammeyer, 2009).

Although the rate of emotional problems is increased in deaf children and adolescents, emotional and other disorders may be underdiagnosed (Van Gent et al., 2007). This might be the case especially with deaf children with mental health problems exhibiting only limited disturbing behavior. The factors that may contribute to problems in recognizing and diagnosing emotional and other psychological problems in deaf children have been mentioned earlier.

Special attention must be paid to possible factors underlying emotional disorders in children who become deaf at a later age, although this will be a minority of cases. Gradually or suddenly becoming deaf at an age when basic or more advanced levels of spoken language have been acquired has far-reaching consequences for the experience of a child. It can cause a great shock for the child as well as the parents, a great loss, and a social handicap, the significance of which may only gradually become clear. Loss of control, helplessness, loneliness, and low self-esteem (Herbst, 2000) can result and can increase the chances of developing emotional disorders.

Depression, anxiety disorders, and acceptation problems may also occur in deaf children who are confronted with an often-unexpected progressive loss of sight. A child who is born deaf and who, throughout the course of his or her development loses vision progressively (as with Usher's syndrome), will almost certainly experience serious distress. This may be a result of tensions in the family during an intensive period of genetic assessments of family members, the uncertain prognosis of loss of sight (from night blindness to tunnel vision to complete loss), or still other factors underlying the necessity for the child and his or her family to modify expectations of the future. For example, loss of sight may strongly interfere with a child's needs to expand his or her world socially during puberty, and this may give rise to serious emotional and social problems. Such complex cases in particular illustrate the importance of adopting a family approach to assessment and intervention.

As described earlier, professionals must be aware that behavioral problems can be an early or late expression of emotional mental health problems. One must also recognize that somatic conditions such as the Jervell-Lange-Nielsen syndrome can present with anxiety and/or mood disorders as an early symptom. This syndrome is also called the *long QT syndrome*, after a prolongation of the interval between the Q wave and the T wave in the electrical cycle of the heart, which is the time to recharge between heartbeats. This symptom may trigger increased and irregular heartbeats (arrhythmia), especially during exertion or anxiety, which when left untreated may lead to fainting or even sudden death through acute heart failure. About 0.75% of deaf children for whom the cause of deafness is unknown has Jervell-Lange-Nielsen syndrome (Ocal et al., 1997). A child with this undiagnosed and untreated syndrome can present with anxiety and feelings of despair and insufficiency, together with avoidance of circumstances that elicit the irregular heartbeats, such as bodily exertion of otherwise distressing conditions, with avoidance being a coping mechanism to avoid misunderstood but potentially life-threatening situations. Diagnostic confusion can occur when this avoidance behavior is interpreted prematurely as a symptom of conversion or phobia, or even affectation or posing, and treated as such. Early recognition of this syndrome is essential because the potentially life-threatening heart rhythm disorders can be treated easily with beta-blockers. Before starting psychopharmacological treatment it is important to exclude this syndrome because certain psychopharmacological drugs can prolong the QT interval.

Psychotic Disorders

Psychotic disorders are no more frequent in deaf than in hearing adolescents. However, accurate assessments of thought disorder and abnormal experiences can be difficult to obtain (Kitson & Thacker,

2000). For instance, deaf children and adolescents are often referred to specialized mental health services because of presumed paranoid ideation and uncertainty. In many cases, the perception of being looked at, being discussed or pointed at by hearing people when signing with others or trying to make contact with others than signing deaf people must be distinguished from real paranoid delusions in a deaf person. In general, good sign language proficiency—or the assistance of a professional sign language interpreter as a necessary alternative—is essential to explore psychological states of signing deaf children and adolescents to differentiate between not unusual grammatical constructs in sign language and associative thinking and other thought disorders indicating psychosis. Because the syntax of sign language is very different from that of spoken language, disorders of thinking can be easily misattributed (Evans & Elliott, 1987; Jenkins & Chess, 1996). Nevertheless, phenomena such as clang associations and flight of ideas have been clearly identified in deaf adults with psychotic disorders (Kitson & Thacker, 2000).

Visual or somatic hallucinations are observed more often in deaf patients with schizophrenia (in about 50% of cases) than in hearing patients (in about 15% [visual] or 5% [somatic] of cases) (Cutting, 1985). Contrary to expectations, auditory hallucinations do occur in deaf patients with schizophrenia (Du Feu & McKenna, 1999). It is highly likely that only deaf patients with some functional residual hearing and memory of hearing speech can experience hallucinations comparable with those of hearing patients with aural hallucinations (Atkinson et al., 2007). Perceptual characteristics of voice hallucinations may closely reflect the variety of experiences of real-life communication, language, and sound among deaf individuals (Atkinson et al., 2007). In deaf patients with no auditory memory, this is more a matter of vibrations or visual hallucinations in which signing or mouth images are seen. Occasionally "hearing voices" can be interpreted as a desire to hear. Establishing a diagnosis in deaf adolescents can take time because early symptoms are difficult to recognize. Associated restlessness and agitation can easily be confused with ADHD, and negative symptoms can be mistaken for depression.

MENTAL HEALTH EXAMINATION

Diagnostic Process

In the absence of a gold standard for the diagnostic process of mental health problems in children and young people, a multimethod and multi-informant approach—that is, bringing together data from meaningful informants and weighing the relative contribution of their specific information by trained mental health professionals using multiple methods of assessment—seems the process of choice (Goodman et al., 1996). Its value has also been demonstrated in research with deaf young people (Van Gent et al., 2007). Diagnosing mental health problems, including judging the presence or absence of psychopathology, based on the selective use of screening instruments or single informants must be avoided, especially when working with deaf children and young people. As noted earlier, the clinical picture may be relatively complicated through communication issues, multiple risk factors, and physical complexities. Ideally, in the case of deaf children and young people, a multidisciplinary team of mental health professionals (psychiatrist, psychologist, and family counselor) and others, including a pediatrician, cooperate to create a diagnostic process involving open and (semi-) structured interviews, standardized questionnaires, observations, tests, and examinations (Hindley &Van Gent, 2002; Van Gent, 2012, 2015). All mental health professionals working with deaf children and their families need to have sufficient knowledge in many domains, including the medical and audiological aspects of deafness and hearing loss; the influence of deafness and other background variables on development (such as parental hearing status and social–cultural preferences, educational placement, and additional physical health problems); cultural aspects of deafness including differences in identification and cultural style within the heterogeneous population of deaf people; and consequences of acculturation preferences. In addition, good communication skills in various modalities are required.

Psychiatric Assessment

As described elsewhere (Hindley & Van Gent, 2002), adaptations have to be made to promote the social interaction with deaf and hard-of-hearing children and their families. When interviewing a deaf child who relies on visual communication, the room needs to be uncluttered and well lit, but without backlight for deaf individuals, such as a window behind the interviewer. Likewise, walls painted a too-bright white may reflect light too much. Speech-reading requires a clear view of the lips, and facial obstacles (such as bushy beards and objects in the visual space between interviewer and interviewee) can cause problems. No more than 25% of spoken language is seen through lip patterns alone (Conrad, 1979), and deaf people have to make educated guesses when speech-reading (Beck & De Jong, 1990). A strong foreign accent can make that even more difficult (Hindley & Van Gent, 2002).

One of the primary goals for clinicians should be to minimize the impact of language barriers during the assessment and treatment process (Mathos & Broussard, 2005). When clinicians have limited signing skills, their efforts to engage signing deaf children can blunt their capacity to detect affective signals, thereby missing pertinent cues for emotional (Hindley et al., 1993) and other disorders. Even more experienced clinicians may misjudge a deaf child's linguistic capacities in either signed or spoken language, particularly during the first interview (for instance, when dealing with children with CIs). In these cases, it is preferable to engage a professional sign language or oral interpreter, primarily with experience in children's mental health (Hindley & Van Gent, 2002). Aspects of communication, content of the interview, procedure, and cooperation with the interviewer must be discussed with the interpreter, both before and after the interview (Hindley & Van Gent, 2002). Most important, the interpreter will have eye contact with the child and may pick up subtle emotional cues (Turner et al., 2000) that may help the clinician to assess the nature of any problems.

A diagnostic family interview is essential in dealing with deaf children and their families, as well as with hearing children in families with deaf parents or deaf siblings, perhaps even more so than with all-hearing families. As a rule, vital information on the experience of all members, family interactions, involvement, and intimacy, and on the impact of communication within the family can thus be obtained.

In a study into the effect of communication on the quality of the psychiatric interview with deaf children, it was shown that many signed, verbal, and nonverbal clues expressing emotional experience, ideas, and imagination are missed resulting from limited expertise and communication skills with deaf children and their families on the part of the hearing psychiatrist or other mental health professional (Hindley et al., 1993). As a consequence, professionals may be insufficiently able to place themselves in the inner world of the deaf child (Hindley et al., 1993). In many such cases, the attention of interviewer and interviewee is focused primarily on how rather than what is being discussed during interview. As a rough guideline, a professional who does not possess sufficient skills in the preferred form of communication of a deaf child should always ask the assistance of a qualified interpreter. It might be even better to call in a qualified interpreter in all those circumstances that it is reasonable to expect that the interviewer's proficiency in the preferred communication modality of the child will not equal the skills of the deaf child (Jenkins & Chess, 1996).

Substantial deafness-related themes within the psychiatric examination include, among others, the experience and perception of being deaf, the perception of the quality of social interactions and communication with others (and ideas on how others perceive him- or herself), social–cultural preferences and identification, self-perceptions in different domains, the development in these areas, identification with others, quality of life in general, and physical well-being. In general, it is essential for the mental health professional to realize that many deaf people do not see themselves as handicapped or as having "lost something," but rather as healthy individuals with their own language, culture, identity, and style.

Psychiatric evaluation may be more challenging when deafness is combined with an intellectual disability. For deaf individuals with a profound disability, it may be necessary to consider other communicative strategies, including the use of caregivers as interpreters of communication, and careful observations of behavior in different contexts (Carvill, 2001) that may have to be spread out over a longer period of time.

The assessment of children and young people with a combined hearing and vision loss may be especially complicated. One should always be quite sure that a visual disorder can be ruled out in children and adolescents with a hearing loss. One should take particular care not to miss sensory impairments when a complex, multicausal neuropsychiatric syndrome is combined with serious communicative problems. More frequently than in the examination or treatment of a child who is deaf only, the clinician will encounter a need for more assistive resources, which may be hard to distinguish from abnormal psychological dependency (Van Gent, 2012, 2015). More than 60% of deaf–blind people have been found to have IQs less than 50 in a nationwide survey in the United States (Klein Jensema, 1980), indicating that serious intellectual disability often complicates the clinical picture with deaf–blind children and adolescents even more.

Psychological Assessment and Testing

Psychological information based on test scores of cognitive, linguistic, neuropsychological, academic, and other aspects of functioning, including personality assessment, is one of the keystones of the multiaxial and multi-informant psychiatric assessment process as a whole. Caution should be exercised when conducting psychological assessments of deaf children because most of the psychological tests have been validated exclusively in hearing children and adolescents. Restrictions in applying psychological tests to deaf people are found in both presenting and understanding test instructions. Many of the tests require a high degree of verbal proficiency, reading skills, and comprehension, and do not sufficiently take into account specific aspects of the linguistic and cultural background of deaf children and adolescents. Deaf people may interpret the texts differently from what is intended, particularly when figurative and abstract language is used. It is a well-known pitfall to assess the intelligence of deaf children and young people based on the combined use of verbal and performance scales of intelligence tests, measuring a full-scale IQ. Often, professionals from regular mental health services refer deaf children with suspected deficits in cognitive functioning based on a full-scale IQ to specialized mental health services for deaf children and young people. However, verbal scales may reduce the IQ falsely. They are better used as literacy measures for reading and writing achievement rather than as an index for intelligence in deaf subjects. That said, even performance-based intelligence tests may be too verbal, especially for deaf people with limited receptive language abilities (Blennerhassett, 2000).

Tests standardized or developed specifically for use with deaf people are still few in number, and many frequently used tests also demand relatively high levels of intellectual and communicative abilities. Several studies (Blennerhassett, 2000; Maller & Braden, 2011) provide thorough accounts of the psychological assessment of deaf children. In a pilot study of the applicability of existing personality tests for deaf children, Spronk (1994) made a number of recommendations for the adaptation of existing personality tests for use with deaf children. Examples of these are (a) testing using signing when necessary, (b) avoiding items that related insufficiently to the world of deaf people or are confusing, and (c) inserting themes relating to the perception of deafness and contact with the hearing world.

In everyday practice, psychological assessments of deaf children and young people take about twice as long as those of their hearing peers. This is, in part, because of the child's communication needs and, in part, because examiners need more time to be certain of the validity of their findings (Boer & Van Gent, 1996).

Physical Examination in Relationship to the Mental Health Examination

More than 50% of all children referred to the national mental health service for deaf and hard-of-hearing children and adolescents in the Netherlands have one or more additional physical disorders compared with 8% of referred hearing control subjects (Boer & Van Gent, 1996). Considering the degree to which this group is representative for the deaf population of children and adolescents with significant mental health problems nationwide throughout the years, a pediatric assessment, including a general physical and exploratory neurological examination, can be regarded as one of the keystones of the psychiatric assessment of deaf and severely hard-of-hearing children. Symptoms that are often missed include motor coordination problems, vertigo, vision problems in semidarkness, and tinnitus (sensation of noise within the ear or head without an external cause) or even hyperacusis (oversensitivity to sound).

INTERVENTION

Specialized Services Versus Generic

Probably the earliest psychiatric study of deaf individuals was performed in Norway by Hansen (as cited by Vernon and Daigle-King [1999]), who reported in 1929 that deaf adults were overrepresented in psychiatric hospitals and that the average duration of stay was significantly longer than that of hearing patients. More systematic clinical and scientific interest in mental health problems in deaf people began around 1950. In 1955, the first specialist mental health clinic for deaf adults opened in the United States, and in 1972, Schlesinger and Meadow opened the first ambulatory treatment service for deaf children in the United States (Vernon, 1980). Although these initial mental health services for deaf adults (Rainer & Altschuler, 1966) and children (Schlesinger & Meadow, 1972; Vernon, 1980) were being established in North America, similar interest was developing in northern Europe (Van Gent, 2012). Although mental health services for deaf children and adolescents are better developed in western European countries and the United States than elsewhere, facilities are still few and many of them deliver basic services only. As exemplified by the special-interest group for deaf children and families of the European Society for Mental Health and Deafness, this foundation of international networks of professionals promotes an exchange of information, resources, and experience among practitioners, thus creating an international platform for cooperation and support in this low-incidence, highly specialized area of care (Van Gent, 2015).

The fundamental characteristic of specialized mental health services for deaf children and their families involves adaptation to heterogeneous needs of deaf clients, including various degrees of visual–spatial experience of the world and heterogeneous communication needs (Hindley & Van Gent, 2002). Most services emphasize the importance of the sociocultural model of deafness, consultation with both the deaf community and parents of children with a hearing loss, as well as a mixed team of deaf and hearing professionals in which all are expected to achieve high levels of sign language proficiency (Hindley & Van Gent, 2002). In addition, qualified interpreters (in sign language, sign-supported spoken language, or in hand-on-hand signing in cases of deaf–blindness) should be available to assist when language skills of staff members are not sufficient.

Following a thorough assessment of the children, the same range of outpatient and inpatient treatments should be provided as for hearing children and their families. Because of their scarcity, specialized services are often provided by consultants to local clinics or ambulatory services (Hindley & Van Gent, 2002). The distance to specialized mental health services is often great. To promote accessibility of services, both assessment and treatment have to be organized as near as possible to the child's home or school. School-based mental health programs aiming at early detection and treatment of psychological problems and comprehensive collaborative working between educational, care, and mental health care services have now been developed in the Netherlands, the United Kingdom, and Austria. Where specialist services are unavailable, clinicians should seek additional resources (such as sign language interpreters) and be prepared to use nonverbal means of communication.

Psychotherapy and Other Psychological Interventions

The deaf mental health care services have learned from experience that all forms of psychotherapy must be available for deaf children and their parents. Therapists must match their communication with that of the child. This means psychotherapists must be able to sign fluently with signing deaf children and young people, but also be able to use other forms of communication. As an alternative, a signing interpreter may be brought in as member of the therapy team, but this may complicate interaction, especially within the individual therapeutic process. Interpreters in family and group therapy may be very useful but, again, an increase in the complexity of transference relationships (Hoyt et al., 1981) has to be dealt with. Evans and Elliott (1987) described specific pitfalls in both the psychotherapy of deaf and hard-of-hearing children and the value of deaf therapists.

Psychopharmacological Treatment: Effects, Side Effects, and Psychoeducation

Psychopharmacological treatment of deaf and hard-of-hearing children with mental health disorders is a complex process in which general, ontogenic, and deafness-related factors play an important role. Pharmacotherapy as part of a broader treatment plan needs a careful approach in which these factors are taken into account.

General and Ontogenic Factors in Psychopharmacological Treatment in Children

Lack of psychopharmacological research with children makes it necessary for clinicians to prescribe medication to children "off label." They often have to use their best judgment based on adult literature and the clinical experience of themselves and others accumulated over the years. It is important to recognize that developmental changes during childhood affect profoundly the responses to medication; the absorption, metabolism, distribution, and excretion of the medication; and produce a need for age-dependent adjustments in doses (Correll, 2008; Kearns et al., 2003).

Deafness-Related Factors

In contact with their general practitioner and mental health professionals, deaf children and young people often experience a linguistic and cultural barrier (Pereira & De Carvalho Fortes, 2010; Steinberg et al., 1998). They may have difficulties in expressing their feelings and thoughts, which can hinder the report of symptoms of their psychological problems, as well as effects and side effects of medication prescribed. On the other hand, limited language in the preferred modality of the child, inexperience in working with deaf children, and restricted time may hinder (a) prescribing the medication adequately, (b) providing psychoeducation, and (c) exploring and monitoring effects and side effects of the medication during psychopharmacological treatment of the child.

Not always is the cause of the deafness known to the child and/or the parents. Various causes of deafness, however, come with comorbidities such as vision disturbances, cardiovascular abnormalities, renal abnormalities, tinnitus and vertigo, thyroid function disorder, and epilepsy. Side effects of psychopharmacological medication can aggravate the symptoms of these comorbidities with possibly dangerous consequences (Sleeboom-van Raaij, 1997). For example, several psychopharmacological drugs can have an epileptogenic effect and may increase the risk of epileptic seizures (Ruffmann et al., 2006). Influence of drugs on the electrical activity of the heart can cause severe cardiovascular dysfunction. Because physical comorbidities, especially neurological disorder, occur more often in deaf children than hearing children, and because some forms of medication carry side effects that occur more frequently as a result of brain damage, the therapeutic window may be changed and smaller in deaf children, especially deaf children with a cognitive disability (Advokat et al., 2000).

Several side effects can also affect the everyday life of deaf and hard-of-hearing children. Movement disorders such as dystonia, tremor, muscle rigidity, and muscle weakness can affect the signing of the child (Advokat et al., 2000; Nobutomo & Inada, 2012). Vision disturbances such as blurred vision can hinder visual communication, and retina damage and glaucoma are other harmful, potential side effects of some medications (Richa & Yazbek, 2010). A decline in communication skills reduces the opportunities of taking part in life within the family, school, and society, and hinders the development of the child (Sleeboom-van Raaij, 2015). Increased perspiration—that is, profuse sweating on the face and scalp, which is a frequent side effect of antidepressants—can cause damage in the CI or hearing aid by short circuit or oxidation. Excessive perspiration also can make it impossible to wear a hearing aid during physical exercise. The sound the hearing aid produces can become inaudible or distorted by the sweat (Marcy & Britton, 2005; Sleeboom-van Raaij, 2010).

In relation to these general ontogenic and deafness-related factors in psychopharmacological treatment, physical examination by a pediatrician can be of great value in excluding physical causes of the psychiatric disorder, in treating concomitant somatic disorders, and in preventing physical problems during psychopharmacological treatment (Correll, 2008; Sleeboom-van Raaij, 2015). For the pediatrician and child and adolescent psychiatrist, it is essential to have information about the medical history, the current medical treatment, vital signs, cardiovascular and respiratory functioning, allergies, weight, length, body mass index (BMI), results of laboratory tests, electroencephalograms, and electrocardiograms. Based on all these factors, it is evident that the psychopharmacological approach should be tailored to the individual child (Landsberger & Diaz, 2010, Sleeboom-van Raaij et al., 2008). In addition to the medication itself, possible side effects should determine the choice of the drugs (Sleeboom-van Raaij et al., 2008).

Psychoeducation During Psychopharmacological Treatment

Psychoeducation implies provision of information and education to a person with severe and enduring mental health problems about the diagnosis, treatment, appropriate resources, prognosis, and common coping strategies (Pekkala & Merinder, 2002). Psychoeducation is important to improve loyalty to treatment and therapy (Bäuml et al., 2006; Pekkala & Merinder, 2002). Regardless of the way psychoeducation is provided—in individual sessions, group therapy, or family therapy—all can have a positive effect on the outcome of treatment and relapse (Rummel-Kluge et al., 2013). For deaf and hard-of-hearing children, psychoeducation should be adapted to their specific needs in communication and language (Du Feu & Fergusson, 2003; Landsberger & Diaz, 2010; Sleeboom-van Raaij et al., 2008). The information should be about the usefulness and necessity of medication, effects and side effects, treatment of side effects, results of discontinuation of the medication, interactions with other medication, and regimen of daily living, such as food, alcohol, exercise, outside activities, school, or work. Psychoeducation is an intervention that should be offered to the deaf and hard-of-hearing child or adolescent as well as to the parents, siblings, caretakers, and school personnel (American Academy of Child and Adolescent Psychiatry, 2007). Note-taking by a staff member during the psychoeducation session can help the child to concentrate on the conversation and repeat the content of the session together with the parent, caretaker, or staff member. Communication and cultural barriers can be overcome by the mental health service by providing treatment with deaf staff members together with adequately trained medical professionals.

CHILDREN WITH COCHLEAR IMPLANTS

CIs can bypass the ear and stimulate the neurobiological and neurocognitive substrates for speech and spoken language perception and promote cognitive development (Kral & O'Donoghue, 2010). They have a positive effect on auditory perception, speech perception and production, and spoken language development in a deaf child. Early age of implantation, longer duration of implant, bilateral implantation, and postimplantation spoken communication are beneficial. Effects of cochlear implantation may also vary among children and adolescents. In general, the beneficial effects of CIs are most marked in the least adverse communicative circumstances (such as low background noise, dyadic interactions, and being supported to join and maintain interaction in groups [Martin et al., 2010; Punch & Hyde, 2011]).

There is a growing body of research on the long-term effects of cochlear implantation on psychosocial development. In a longitudinal study in Sweden (Tvingstedt & Preisler, 2006), for example, children with CIs reported a positive appreciation of their implant, but they and their parents shared the awareness that they are still deaf. Overall, studies indicate that language ability, regardless of modality, is an important predictor of psychosocial well-being in children with CIs (Dammeyer, 2009). Children with CIs showed a faster improvement in social skills following the development of communication skills over time than children with conventional hearing aids (Bat-Chava et al., 2004). Whether this reflects an improvement in the forming of a mental perspective, as has been suggested by Bat Chava et al. (2004) and others (e.g., Remmel & Peters, 2009), remains a subject for further research. Although delayed development of theory of mind was reported for both deaf children with CI and with conventional hearing aids compared with hearing children, longitudinal research suggests that those who missed early conversational inputs continue to improve their understanding of theory of mind at advanced ages (e.g., Wellman et al., 2011).

Research into the effect of CIs on executive functioning—the regulation and control over cognitive processes based on working memory, mental flexibility, and self-control—is still inconclusive. Figueras et al. (2008) found no differences in executive functioning between deaf children with and without CIs despite the finding of a positive association between language ability and executive functioning (Hintermair, 2013). Children with CIs showed difficulties in executive functioning domains, too, especially in the domains of working memory inhibition and behavior regulation (Beer et al., 2011).

To date, findings from studies into the effect of cochlear implantation on self-concept in children need further exploration. Despite the suggestion of a positive effect of a longer duration of implant use on global self-esteem and cognitive competence in young children (Martin et al., 2010), no differential effect on all self-concept domains was found with regard to the presence or absence of a CI in deaf adolescents (Leigh et al., 2009) nor with regard to the type of hearing device (CI or hearing aid [Theunissen, 2013]). More discrepant findings have been reported with regard to presumed effects of cochlear implantation on the occurrence of psychosocial difficulties. Some researchers have found a positive effect of implantation on behavioral outcome (Edwards et al., 2006; Theunissen, 2013), whereas others have not (e.g., Dammeyer, 2009; Fellinger et al., 2009b; Leigh et al., 2009). One quality-of-life study of profoundly deaf children (n = 44; mean age, 10.7 years) suggested barely any difference between profoundly deaf children with or without CIs, except regarding satisfaction with school, which was less for pupils with CIs (Fellinger et al., 2008). In a study of deaf children (n = 157; mean age, 14.1 years) both unaided participants and participants with CIs scored higher on quality of life as measured by the Youth Quality of Life Instrument—Deaf and Hard-of-Hearing than those using hearing aids, regardless of the type of school (Meyer et al., 2013). With regard to mental health disorder, no effect of CIs on psychiatric diagnosis was observed in a population-based study with children and adolescents (age, 6–16 years), using diagnostic parental interviews and parental and teachers' questionnaires (Fellinger et al., 2009b). In another population-based study, Theunissen et al. (2015) found lower levels of anxiety and other both internalizing and externalizing problems in children with CIs than in children with hearing aids. Based on these research findings, the authors speculated that it is not the type of hearing device but rather the intensity of the rehabilitation program that explains the difference in findings between children with and without CIs.

Differences in study design, measures, participants, and composition of samples hamper comparisons across studies of children with CIs. Research findings should be interpreted with caution, in as much as failure to control for some variables (such as gender, age of onset of deafness, co-occurring disabilities, socioeconomic status) may lead to an overestimation of the effectiveness of CIs (Stacey et al., 2006). Failure to control for other variables, such as average hearing level and age (Stacey et al., 2006) or shorter use of CIs (Figueras et al., 2008) may lead to an underestimation. As described earlier, a multimethod approach in which multiple informants, diagnostic interviews, and expert judgments are combined seems the best choice when examining the presence or absence of mental health problems in deaf children with and without CIs. For instance, studies relying on parents or teachers as unique sources of information may tend to overrate adjustment of children with CIs, and risk missing significantly different views from self-reports of the children, for example, in the domain of quality of life regarding school (Fellinger et al., 2008). Thus, more research on psychological development and the prevalence of mental health problems in well-described homogeneous samples of children with and without a CIs is much needed.

From a perspective based on a combination of current cultural values and empirical findings, a bilingual approach to the education of most deaf children is still advocated (Petitto & Holowka, 2002; Preisler, 2007). However, at least in industrialized countries, a growing number of children who have received a CI early on have opportunities to learn a spoken language, and spoken language will become a first language for many of them (Knoors & Marschark, 2012). At the same time, sign language will likely remain important not only for other children and adults, but also for younger children with CIs and their parents, for whom it can serve as both an adjunct to spoken language and an effective bridge before and after implantation. Research variations notwithstanding, CIs have definitively changed the face of deafness (Marschark, 2007).

In current day-to-day clinical practice, a deaf child with a CI will not be completely hearing, but will be moderately or severely hard-of-hearing when the CI is turned on. A number of children will still be dependent on sign language or will prefer sign language to communicate in varying circumstances, which may change after a period of time. Occasionally, in mental health services, children are seen who experience sounds that are new to them as painful and disturbing, which sometimes may become overwhelming. Acceptance and ambivalence regarding their deafness or their device may play a role. In rare cases, the extra auditory stimuli may (temporarily) exceed the integrative capacity of a child, which may lead to deterioration in general function and even borderline psychotic decompensation. In the case of a suspicion of ASD in a child before implantation , it is important to assess to what extent the impact of a CI, the operation, and the rehabilitation program (including speech therapy and educational guidance) will interfere with the capacity to process information and to integrate social meaning before a positive indication for a CI is made. Problems with the child's stimulus regulation can thus be identified and treated early.

CONCLUSIONS

In principle, deaf children will experience mental health difficulties comparable with their hearing peers. However, the rate of mental health difficulties is increased in deaf and severely hard-of-hearing children and adolescents compared with the general population, according to most studies. Deafness may have significant consequences for the development of the child. At least from a psychiatric perspective, every child with psychological problems or a disorder is unique and should be treated as such. Early recognition, screening, assessment, and intervention are essential to support parents and children adequately, and to prevent communicative and social deprivation. Children and adolescents with mental health problems who are deaf or hard of hearing may have very diverse needs related to their deafness or hearing loss, as well as additional special needs regarding their visual, cognitive, and linguistic strengths and weaknesses, and their general health. They and their families benefit from multidisciplinary and highly specialized mental health services that warrant combined expertise in these domains as well as effective communication (Fellinger et al., 2012; Van Gent, 2012). Although basic mental health care for deaf and deaf–blind children and young people has been developed in a number of countries for many decades, mental health services for these children and young people are still underrepresented. Notwithstanding the benefits of programs for neonatal hearing screening, early intervention, and other technical advances, the need to meet the special, often complex, heterogeneous needs of these children, adolescents, and their families—to bundle knowledge, clinical expertise, research, and organizational power—is as urgent as it was some 50 years ago (Schlesinger & Meadow, 1972; Van Gent, 2012, 2015).

REFERENCES

American Academy of Child and Adolescent Psychiatry. (2007). Practice parameters for the assessment and treatment of children and adolescents with depressive disorders. *Journal of the American Academy of Child and Adolescent Psychiatry, 46,* 1503–1526.

Achenbach, T. M., & Rescorla, L. A. (1999). *Mental health Practitioners' guide for the Achenbach System of Empirically Based Assessment (ASEBA).* Burlington, VT: University of Vermont Department of Psychiatry.

Advokat, C. D., Mayville, E. A., & Matson, J. L. (2000). Side effects profiles of atypical antipsychotics, typical antipsychotics, or no psychotropic medications in persons with mental retardation. *Research in Developmental Disabilities, 21,* 75–84.

Antia, S. D., Jones, P. B., Reed, S., & Kreimeyer, K. H. (2009). Academic status and progress of deaf and hard-of-hearing students in general education classrooms. *Journal of Deaf Studies and Deaf Education, 14,* 293–311.

Atkinson, J. R., Gleeson, K., Cromwell, J., & O'Rourke, S. (2007). Exploring the perceptual characteristics of voice hallucinations in deaf people. *Cognitive Neuropsychiatry, 12*(4), 339–361.

Baker, S. A., Michnick Golinkoff, R., & Petitto, L. A. (2006). New insights into old puzzles from infants' categorical discrimination of soundless phonetic units. *Language Learning and Development, 2,* 147–162.

Barker, D. H., Quittner, A. L., Fink, N. E., Eisenberg, L. S., Tobey, E. A., Niparko, J. K., & CDaCI investigative team (2009). Predicting behavior problems in deaf and hearing children: The influences of language, attention, and parent–child communication. *Development and Psychopathology, 21,* 373–392.

Bat-Chava, Y. (1993). Antecedents of self-esteem in deaf people: A meta-analytical review. *Rehabilitation Psychology, 38,* 221–234.

Bat-Chava, Y., Martin, D., & Kosciw, J. G. (2004). Longitudinal improvements in communication and socialization of deaf children with cochlear implants and hearing aids: Evidence from parental reports. *Journal of Child Psychology and Psychiatry, 46,* 1287–1296.

Bäuml, J., Froböse, T., Kraemer, S., Rentrop, M., & Pitschel-Walz, G. (2006). Psychoeducation: A basic psychotherapeutic intervention for patients with schizophrenia and their families. *Schizophrenia Bulletin, 32*(Suppl. 1), 1–9.

Beck, G., & de Jong, E. (1990). *Opgroeien in een horende wereld* [Growing up in a hearing world]. Twello: Van Tricht.

Beer, J., Kronenberg, W. G., & Pisoni, D. P. (2011). Executive functioning in everyday life: Implications for young cochlear implant users. *Cochlear Implants International, 12*(Suppl. 1), S89–S91.

Blennerhassett, L. (2000). Psychological assessments. In P. Hindley & N. Kitson (Eds.), *Mental health and deafness* (pp. 185–205). London: Whurr Publishers.

Boer, F., & Van Gent, T. (1996). *Evaluatie 1993 1994 1995 Afdeling voor doven en ernstig slechthorenden de Vlier. Intern evaluatierapport Academisch Centrum Kinder- en Jeugdpsychiatrie Curium.* [Evaluation 1993 1994 1995 Department for deaf and severely hard-of-hearing children and adolescents de Vlier: Internal evaluation report Academic Center Child and Adolescent Psychiatry Curium]. Oegstgeest: Curium.

Blomström, Å., Gardner, R. M., Dalman, C., Yolken, R. H., & Karlsson, H. (2015). Influence of maternal infections on neonatal acute phase proteins and their interaction in the development of non-affective psychosis. *Translational Psychiatry, 5*, e502.

Brown, A. S., Cohen, P., Harkavy-Friedman, J., Babulas, V., Malaspina, D., Gorman, J. M., et al. (2001). Prenatal rubella, premorbid abnormalities, and adult schizophrenia. *Biological Psychiatry, 49*, 473–486.

Brown, R., R. P. Hobson, A. Lee, & J. Stevenson. (1997). Are there "autistic" features in congenitally blind children? *Journal of Child Psychology and Psychiatry, 38*, 693–703.

Calderon, R., & Greenberg, M. T. (2011). Social and emotional development of deaf children: Family, school, and program effects. In M. Marschark & P. E. Spencer (Eds.), *The Oxford handbook of deaf studies, language, and education* (2nd ed., Vol. 1, pp. 188–199). New York, NY: Oxford University Press.

Carvill, S. (2001). Sensory impairments, intellectual disability and psychiatry. *Journal of Intellectual Disability Research, 45*, 467–483.

Chess, S., & Fernandez, P. (1980). Do deaf children have a typical personality? *Journal of the American Academy of Child Psychiatry, 19*, 654–664.

Chess, S., Korn, S. J., & Fernandez, P. B. (1971). *Psychiatric disorders of children with congenital rubella.* New York, NY: Brunner & Mazel.

Conrad, R. (1979). *The deaf school child.* London: Harper & Row.

Correll, C. U. (2008). Antipsychotic use in children and adolescents: minimizing adverse effects to maximize outcomes. *Journal American Academy Child and Adolescent Psychiatry, 47*, 9–20.

Cutting, J. (1985). *The psychology of schizophrenia.* London: Churchill Livingstone.

Dammeyer, J. (2009). Psychosocial development in a Danish population of children with cochlear implants and deaf and hard-of-hearing children. *Journal of Deaf Studies and Deaf Education, 15*, 50–58.

Denmark, T. (2011). Do deaf children with autism spectrum disorder show deficits in the comprehension and production of emotional and linguistic facial expressions in British Sign Language? PhD dissertation, University College, London.

De Raeve, L. (2014). Paediatric cochlear implantation: Outcomes and current trends in education and rehabilitation. PhD dissertation, Radboud University Nijmegen.

Desselle, D. D. (1994). Self-esteem, family climate, and communication patterns in relation to deafness. *American Annals of the Deaf, 139*, 322–328.

de Vaan, G., Vervloed, M., Peters-Scheffer, N. C., Van Gent, T., Knoors, H., & Verhoeven, L. (2015). Behavioural assessment of autism spectrum disorders in people with multiple disabilities. *Journal of Intellectual Disability Research.*

Du Feu, M., & Fergusson, K. (2003). Sensory impairment and mental health. *Advances in Psychiatric Treatment, 9,* 95–103.

Du Feu, M., & Mckenna, P. J. (1999). Prelingually profoundly deaf schizophrenic patients who hear voices: A phenomenological analysis. *Acta Psychiatrica Scandinavica, 99,* 453–459.

Dye, M. W. G., Hauser, P. C., & Bavelier, D. (2008). Visual attention in deaf children and adults. In M. Marschark & P. C. Hauser (Eds.), *Deaf cognition. Foundations and outcomes* (pp. 250–263). New York, NY: Oxford University Press.

Edwards, L., Kahn, S., Broxholme, C., & Langdon, D. (2006). Exploration of the cognitive and behavioural consequences of paediatric cochlear implantation. *Cochlear Implants International, 7,* 61–76.

Evans, J. W., & Elliott, H. (1987). The mental status examination. In H. Elliott, L. Glass, & J. W. Evans (Eds.), *Mental health assessment of deaf clients: A practical manual* (pp. 83–92). San Diego, CA: Little, Brown.

Farrugia, D., & Austin, G. F. (1980). A study of social-emotional adjustment patterns of hearing-impaired students in different educational settings. *American Annals of the Deaf, 125,* 535–541.

Fellinger, J., Holzinger, D., Beitel, C., Laucht, M., & Goldberg, D. P. (2009a). The impact of language skills on mental health in teenagers with hearing impairments. *Acta Psychiatrica Scandinavia, 120*(2), 153–159.

Fellinger, J., Holzinger, D., & Pollard, R. (2012). Mental health of deaf people. *Lancet, 379,* 1037–1044.

Fellinger, J., Holzinger, D., Sattel, H., & Laucht, M. (2008). Mental health and quality of life in deaf pupils. *European Child and Adolescent Psychiatry, 17,* 414–423.

Fellinger, J., Holzinger, D., Sattel, H., Laucht, M., & Goldberg, D. (2009). Correlates of mental health disorders among children with hearing impairments. *Developmental Medicine & Child Neurology, 51,* 635–641.

Figueras, B., Edwards, L., & Langdon, D. (2008). Executive function and language in deaf children. *Journal of Deaf Studies and Deaf Education, 13,* 362–377.

Fombonne, E. (2002). Case identification in an epidemiological context. In M. Rutter & E. Taylor (Eds.), *Child and adolescent psychiatry* (4th ed., pp. 52–69). London: Blackwell.

Fortnum, H. M., Marshall, D. H., & Summerfield, A. Q. (2002). Epidemiology of the United Kingdom population of hearing-impaired children including characteristics of those with and without cochlear implants: Audiology, etiology, co-morbidity, and affluence. *International Journal of Audiology, 41,* 170–179.

Fortnum, H. M., Quentin Summerfield, A., Marshall, D. H., Davis, A. C., & Bamford, J. M. (2001). Prevalence of permanent childhood hearing impairment in the United Kingdom and implications for neonatal hearing screening: questionnaire based ascertainment study. *British Medical Journal, 153,* 437–443.

Freeman, R. D., Malkin, S. F., & Hastings, J. O. (1975). Psychological problems of deaf children and their families: A comparative study. *American Annals of the Deaf, 120,* 275–304.

Friedman, R. J., & Chase-Lansdale, P. L. (2002). Chronic adversities. In M. Rutter & E. Taylor (Eds.), *Child and adolescent psychiatry* (4th ed., pp. 261–276). Oxford: Blackwell Publishing.

Goodman, R. (1997). The Strengths and Difficulties Questionnaire: A research note. *Journal of Child Psychology and Psychiatry, 38*, 581–586.

Goodman, R., Yude, C., Richards, H., & Taylor, E. (1996). Rating child psychiatric caseness from detailed case histories. *Journal of Child Psychology and Psychiatry, 37*, 369–379.

Harris, M. (2001). It's all a matter of timing: sign visibility and sign reference in deaf and hearing mothers of 18-month-old children. *Journal of Deaf Studies and Deaf Education, 6*, 177–185.

Harter, S. (2006). Self-processes and developmental psychopathology. In D. Cicchietti & D. J. Cohen (Eds.), *Developmental Psychopathology* (pp. 370–418). Hoboken, NJ: Wiley.

Hauser, P. C., & Marschark, M. (2008). What we know and what we don't know about cognition and deaf learners. In M. Marschark & P. C. Hauser (Eds.), *Deaf cognition: Foundations and outcomes* (pp. 439–457). Oxford: Oxford University Press.

Herbst, K. G. (2000). Acquired deafness. In P. Hindley & N. Kitson (Eds.), *Mental health and deafness* (pp. 253–281). London: Whurr Publishers.

Hindley, P. (2000). Child and adolescent psychiatry. In P. Hindley & N Kitson (Eds.), *Mental health and deafness* (pp. 42–74). London: Whurr Publishers.

Hindley, P. A., & van Gent, T. (2002). Psychiatric aspects of specific sensory impairments. In M. Rutter & E. Taylor (Eds.), *Child and adolescent psychiatry: Modern approaches* (4th ed., pp. 842–858). Oxford: Blackwell Science.

Hindley, P. A., Hill, P. D., & Bond, D. (1993). Interviewing deaf children, the interviewer effect: A research note. *Journal of Child Psychology and Psychiatry, 34*, 1461–1467.

Hindley, P. A., Hill, P. D., McGuigan, S., & Kitson, N. (1994). Psychiatric disorder in deaf and hearing impaired children and young people: a prevalence study. *Journal of Child Psychology and Psychiatry, 35*, 917–934.

Hindley, P. A. & Kroll, L. (1998) Theoretical and epidemiological aspects of attention deficit and overactivity in deaf children. *Journal of Deaf Studies and Deaf Education, 3*, 64–72.

Hintermair, M. (2013). Executive functions and behavioral problems in deaf and hard-of-hearing students at general and special schools. *Journal of Deaf Studies and Deaf Education, 18*, 344–359.

Hoevenaars-van den Boom, M. A. A., Anthonissen, A. C. F. M., Knoors, H., & Vervloed, M. P. J. (2009). Differentiating characteristics of deafblindness and autism in people with congenital deafblindness and profound intellectual disability. *Journal of Intellectual Disability Research, 53*, 548–558.

Hoyt, M. F., Siegelman, E. Y., & Schlesinger, H. S. (1981). Special issues regarding psychotherapy with the deaf. *American Journal of Psychiatry,138*, 807–811.

Jan, J. E., Freeman, R. D., & Scott, E. P. (1977). *Visual impairment in children and adolescents*. New York, NY: Grune and Stratton.

Jenkins, I. R., & Chess, S. (1996). Psychiatric evaluation of perceptually impaired children: hearing and visual impairments. In M. Lewis (Ed.), *Child and adolescent psychiatry; a comprehensive textbook* (pp. 526–534). Baltimore, MD: Williams & Wilkins.

Johansson, M. R., Råstam, M., Billstedt, E., Danielson, S., Strömland, K., Miller, M., & Gillberg, C. (2006). Autism spectrum disorders and underlying brain pathology in CHARGE association. *Developmental Medicine & Child Neurology, 48,* 40–50.

Jure, R., Rapin, I., & Tuchman, R. F. (1991). Hearing impaired autistic children. *Developmental Medicine and Child Neurology, 33,* 1062–1072.

Kearns, G. L., Abdel-Rahman, S. M., Alander, S. W., Blowey, D. L., Leeder, J. S., & Kauffman, R. E. (2003). Developmental pharmacology: drug disposition, action, and therapy in infants and children. *New England Journal of Medicine, 349,* 1157–1167.

Kelly, D., Forney, J., Parker-Fischer, S., & Jones, M. (1993). The challenge of attention deficit disorder in children who are deaf or hard of hearing. *American Annals of the Deaf, 138,* 343–348.

Kitson, N., & Thacker, A. (2000). Adult psychiatry. In P. Hindley & N. Kitson (Eds.), *Mental health and deafness* (pp.75–98). London: Whurr Publishers.

Klein Jensema, C. (1980). A profile of deaf–blind children with various types of educational facilities. *American Annals of the Deaf, 125,* 896–900.

Knoors, H., & Marschark, M. (2012). Language planning for the 21st century: revisiting bilingual language policy for deaf children. *Journal of Deaf Studies and Deaf Education, 17,* 291–305.

Korver, A. M. H., de Vries, J. J., Konings, S., de Jong, J. W., Dekker, F. W., Vossen, A. C., Frijns, J. H., Oudesluys-Murphy, A. M., & DECIBEL Collaborative Study Group (2009). DECIBEL study: Congenital cytomegalovirus infection in young children with permanent bilateral hearing impairment. *The Netherland Journal of Clinical Virology, 36*(Suppl. 4), S27–S31.

Kouwenberg, M. (2013). Social–emotional factors underlying internalizing problems & peer relations in deaf and hard of hearing youth. PhD dissertation, Leiden University.

Kouwenberg, M., Rieffe, C., & Theunissen, S. C. P. M. (2011). Intrapersonal and interpersonal factors related to self-reported symptoms of depression in DHH youth. *International Journal of Mental Health and Deafness, 1,* 46–57.

Kouwenberg, M., Rieffe, C., Theunissen, S. C. P. M., & de Rooij, M. (2012). Peer victimization experienced by children and adolescents who are deaf or hard of hearing. *PLoS One, 7,* e52174.

Kral A., &. O'Donoghue, G. M. (2010). Profound deafness in childhood. *New England Journal of Medicine, 363,* 1438–1450.

Landsberger, S., & Diaz, D. R. (2010) Inpatient psychiatric treatment of deaf adults: Demographic and diagnostic comparisons with hearing inpatients of psychiatric services. *Psychiatric Services, 61,* 196–199.

Leigh, I. W., Maxwell-McCaw, D., Bat-Chava, Y., & Christiansen, J. B. (2009). Correlates of psychosocial adjustment in deaf adolescents with and without cochlear implants: A preliminary investigation. *Journal of Deaf Studies and Deaf Education, 14,* 244–259.

Loots, G., & Devisé, I. (2003). The use of visual-tactile communication strategies by deaf and hearing fathers and mothers of deaf infants. *Journal of Deaf Studies and Deaf Education, 8,* 31–42.

Loots, G., Devisé, I., & Jacquet, W. (2005). The impact of visual communication on the intersubjective development of early parent-child interaction with 18- to 24- month old deaf toddlers. *Journal of Deaf Studies and Deaf Education, 10,* 357–375.

Loucas, T., Charman, T., Pickles, A., Simonoff, E., Meldrum, & Baird, G. (2008). Autistic symptomatology and language ability in autism spectrum disorder and specific language impairment. *Journal of Child Psychology and Psychiatry, 49*, 1184–1192.

Maller, S. J., & Braden, J. T. (2011). Intellectual assessment of deaf people: A critical review. In M. Marschark & P. E. Spencer (Eds.), *The Oxford handbook of deaf studies, language and education* (Vol. 2, pp. 473–485). New York, NY: Oxford University Press.

Marcy, T. R., & Britton, M. L. (2005). Antidepressant-induced sweating. *Annals of Pharmacotherapy, 39*, 748–752.

Marschark, M. (1993). *Psychological development of deaf children*. New York, NY: Oxford University Press.

Marschark, M. (2003). Cognitive functioning in deaf adults and children. In M. Marschark & P. E. Spencer (Eds.), *The Oxford handbook of deaf studies, language, and education* (pp. 464–477). New York, NY: Oxford University Press.

Marschark, M. (2007). *Raising and educating a deaf child* (2nd ed.). New York, NY: Oxford University Press.

Martin, D., Bat-Chava, Y., Lalwani, A., & Waltzman, S. B. (2010). Peer relationships of deaf children with cochlear implants: Predictors of peer entry and peer interaction success. *Journal of Deaf Studies and Deaf Education, 16*, 108–120.

Mathos, K. K., & Broussard, E. R. (2005). Outlining the concerns of children who have hearing loss and their families. *Journal of the American Academy of Child and Adolescent Psychiatry, 44*, 96–100.

Meyer, A., Sie, K., Skalicky, A., Edwards, T. C, Schick, B., Niparko, J., & Patrick, D. L. (2013). Quality of life in youth with severe to profound sensorineural hearing loss. *JAMA Otolaryngology-Head & Neck Surgery, 139*, 294–300.

Musselman, C., Mootilal, A., & MacKay, S. (1996). The socials adjustment of deaf adolescents in segregated, partially integrated, and mainstreamed settings. *Journal of Deaf Studies and Deaf Education, 1*, 52–63.

Musyoka, M. (2015). Understanding indoor play in deaf children: An analysis of play behaviors. *Psychology, 6*, 10–19.

Nicolas, J. G., & Geers, A. E. (2003). Personal, social, and family adjustment in school-aged children with a cochlear implant. *Ear & Hearing, 24*, 69S–81S.

Nobutomo, Y., & Inada, T. (2012). Dystonia secondary to use of antipsychotic agents. In R. Rosales (Ed.), *Dystonia: The many facets* (pp.55–64). Croatia: In Tech Europe.

Ocal, B., Imamoglu, A., Atalay, S., & Ercan Tutar, H. (1997). Prevalence of idiopathic long QT syndrome in children with congenital deafness. *Pediatric Cardiology, 18*, 401–405.

O'Connor, T. G., Rutter, M., Beckett, C., Keaveney, L., & Kreppner, J. M., and the English and Romanian Adoptees Study Team (2000). The effects of global severe privation on cognitive competence: extension and longitudinal follow-up. *Child Development, 71*, 376–390.

Pekkala, E., & Merinder, L. (2002). Psychoeducation for schizophrenia. Review. *Cochrane Data Base Systematic Reviews, CD002831*, 1–41.

Pereira, P. C. A., & De Carvalho Fortes, P. A. (2010). Communication and information barriers to health assistance for deaf patients. *American Annals of the Deaf, 155*, 31–37.

Petitto, L. A., & Holowka, S. (2002). Evaluating attributions of delay and confusion in young bilinguals: Special insights from infants acquiring a signed and spoken language. *Sign Language Studies, 3,* 4–33.

Pettito, L. A., & Marentette, P. F. (1991). Babbling in the manual mode: Evidence for the ontogeny of language. *Science, 251,* 1493–1496.

Preisler, G. (2007). Will learning from the past give us insight for the future concerning the psychosocial development of deaf children with cochlear implants? Plenary presentation at the Seventh European Congress on Mental Health and Deafness, "Joining Forces." Haarlem, The Netherlands.

Punch, R., & Hyde, M. (2011). Social participation of children and adolescents with cochlear implants: A qualitative analysis of parent, teacher, an child interviews. *Journal of Deaf Studies and Deaf Education, 16,* 474–493.

Rainer, J. D., & Altschuler, K. Z. (1966). *Comprehensive mental health services for the deaf.* New York, NY: New York State Psychiatric Institute, Department of Medical Genetics.

Remmel, E., & Peters, K. (2009). Theory of mind and language in children with cochlear implants. *Journal of Deaf Studies and Deaf Education, 14,* 218–236.

Richa, S., & Yazbek, J. C. (2010). Ocular adverse effects of common psychotropic agents: A review. *Central Nervous System Drugs, 24,* 501–526.

Rieffe, C. (2012). Awareness and regulation of emotions in deaf children. *British Journal of Developmental Psychology, 30,* 477–492.

Rogers, S. J., & Ozonoff, S. (2005). Annotation: What do we know about sensory dysfunction in autism? A critical review of the empirical evidence. *Journal of Child Psychology and Psychiatry, 46,* 1255–1268.

Rosenhall, U., Nordin, V., Sandstrom, M., Ahlsen, G., & Gillberg, C. (1999). Autism and hearing loss. *Journal of Autism and Developmental Disorders, 29,* 349–357.

Ruffmann, C., Bogliun, G., & Beghi, E. (2006). Epileptogenic drugs: A systematic review. *Expert Review Neurotherapeutics, 6,* 575–689.

Rummel-Kluge, C., Kluge, M., & Kissling, W. (2013). Frequency and relevance of psychoeducation in psychiatric diagnoses: Results of two surveys five years apart in German-speaking European countries. *BMC Psychiatry, 13,* 170.

Schlesinger, H. S., & Meadow, K. P. (1972). *Sound and sign: Childhood deafness and mental health.* London: University of California Press.

Sinkkonen, J. (1994). Hearing impairment, communication and personality development. Unpublished PhD dissertation, University of Helsinki.

Sleeboom-van Raaij, C. J. (1997). Psychopharmacological treatment and deafness: hazards and highlights. Paper presented at the Fourth International Congress of the European Society for Mental Health and Deafness. Manchester, UK.

Sleeboom-van Raaij, C. J. (2010). Overmatige transpiratie bij antidepressiva. [Hyperhydrosis and antidepressants]. *Psyfar, 3,* 38–41.

Sleeboom-van Raaij, C. J. (2015). Important issues in the psychopharmacological treatment of deaf and hard of hearing people with mental health disorders: Theory and practice. In Benito Estrada Aranda & Ines Sleeboom-van Raaij (Eds.), *Mental health services for deaf people: Treatment advances, opportunities, and challenges* (pp. 15–39). Washington, DC: Gallaudet University Press.

Sleeboom-van Raaij, C. J., Bogers, J. P. A. M., Knoppert-Van Der Klein, E. A. M. (2008). Psychofarmaca bij de psychiatrische behandeling van doven en slechthorenden. [Psychopharmacological treatment of deaf and hard-of-hearing patients]. *Psyfar, 4,* 40–43.

Smith-Gray, S., & Koester, L. S. (1995). Defining and observing social signals in deaf and hearing infants. *American Annals of the Deaf, 140,* 422–427.

Spencer, P., & Deyo, D. (1993). Cognitive and social aspects of deaf children's play. In M. Marschark & M. Clark (Eds.), *Psychological perspectives on deafness* (pp. 65–91). Hillsdale, NJ: Lawrence Erlbaum Associates.

Spronk-Van Hal, C. M. (1994). Research into psychological instruments for deaf children and adolescents: A pilot study. Paper presented at the E.S.M.H.D. Third International Congress. Paris, France. December 14–16.

Stacey, P. C., Fortnum, H. M., Barton, G. R., & Summerfield, A. Q. (2006). Hearing-impaired children in the United Kingdom, I: Auditory performance, communication skills, educational achievements, quality of life, and cochlear implantation. *Ear & Hearing, 27,* 161–186.

Steinberg, A. G.; Sullivan, V. J.; & Loew, R. C. (1998). Cultural and linguistic barriers to mental health service access: The deaf consumer's perspective. *American Journal of Psychiatry, 155,* 982–984.

Stevenson, J., Kreppner, J., Pimperton, H., Worsfold, & Kennedy, C. (2015). Emotional and behavioural difficulties in children and adolescents with hearing impairment: a systemic review and meta-analysis. *European Child and Adolescent Psychiatry, 24,* 477–496.

Sullivan, P., Brookhouser, P., & Scanlan, M. (2000). Maltreatment of deaf and hard of hearing children. In P. Hindley & N. Kitson (Eds.), *Mental health and deafness* (pp. 149–184). London: Whurr Publishers.

Theunissen, S. C. P. M. (2013). Psychopathology in hearing impaired children. PhD dissertation, Leiden University.

Theunissen, S. C. P. M., Rieffe, C., Soede, W., Briaire, J. J., Ketelaar, L., Kouwenberg, M., & Frijns, J. H. M. (2015). Symptoms of psychopathology in hearing impaired children. *Ear & Hearing, 36,* e190–e198.

Turner, J., Klein, H., & Kitson, N. (2000). Interpreters in mental health settings. In P. Hindley & N. Kitson (Eds.), *Mental health and deafness* (pp. 297–310). London: Whurr Publishers.

Tvingstedt, A. L., & Preisler, G. (2006). *A psychosocial follow-up study of children with cochlear implants in different school settings.* EDUCARE. Malmö: Holmbergs.

Van Gent, T. (2012). Mental health problems in deaf and hard of hearing children and adolescents: Findings on prevalence, pathogenesis and clinical complexities, and implications for prevention, diagnosis and intervention. PhD dissertation, Leiden University.

Van Gent, T. (2015). Mental health problems in deaf children and adolescents. Part II: Aspects of psychopathology. In B. D. Estrada Aranda & C. J. Sleeboom-van Raaij (Eds.), *Mental health services for deaf people: Treatment advances, Opportunities, and Challenges* (pp. 167–191). Washington, DC: Gallaudet University Press.

Van Gent, T., Goedhart, A. W., Hindley, P. A., & Treffers, Ph. D. A. (2007). Prevalence and correlates of psychopathology in a sample of deaf adolescents. *Journal of Child Psychology and Psychiatry, 48,* 950–958.

Van Gent, T., Goedhart, A. W., Knoors, H., Westenberg, P. M., & Treffers, Ph. D. A. (2012). Self-concept and ego development in deaf adolescents: Associations with social context and deafness-related variables, and a comparison with hearing adolescents. *Journal of Deaf Studies and Deaf Education, 17,* 333–351.

Van Gent, T., Goedhart, A. W., & Treffers, Ph. D. A. (2011). Self-concept and psychopathology in deaf adolescents: preliminary support for moderating effects of deafness-related characteristics and peer problems. *Journal of Child Psychology and Psychiatry, 52*, 720–728.

Van Gent, T., Goedhart, A. W., & Treffers, Ph. D. A. (2012). Characteristics of children and adolescents in the Dutch national in- and outpatient mental health service for deaf and hard of hearing youth over a period of 15 years. *Research in Developmental Disabilities, 33*, 1333–1342.

Van Gurp, S. (2001). Self-concept of secondary school students in different educational settings. *Journal of Deaf Studies and Deaf Education, 6*, 55–69.

Vernon, M. (1980). Perspectives on deafness and mental health. *Journal of Rehabilitation of the Deaf, 13*, 8–14.

Vernon, M., & Daigle-King, B. (1999). Historical overview of inpatient care of mental patients who are deaf. *American Annals of the Deaf, 144*, 51–61.

Vig, S., & Jedrysek, E. (1999). Autistic features in young children with significant cognitive impairment: autism or mental retardation? *Journal of Autism and Developmental Disorders, 29*, 235–248.

Wellman, H. M., Fang, F., & Peterson, C. C. (2011). Sequential progressions in a theory-of-mind scale: Longitudinal perspectives. *Child Development, 82*, 780–792.

Winn, S. (2007). Employment outcome for people in Australia who are congenitally deaf: Has anything changed? *American Annals of the Deaf, 152*, 382–390.

World Health Organization. (2011). *International statistical classification of diseases and related health problems* (10th rev., ICD-10). Geneva: World Health Organization.

Yashamita, Y., Fujimoto, C., Nakajima, E., Isagai, T., & Matsuishi, T. (2003). Possible association between congenital cytomegalovirus infection and autistic disorder. *Journal of Autism and Developmental Disorders, 33*, 455–459.

Yoshinaga-Itano, C. (2003). From screening to early identification and intervention: discovering predictors to successful outcomes for children with significant hearing loss. *Journal of Deaf Studies and Deaf Education, 8*, 11–30.

Young, A. M. (1999). Hearing parents adjustment to a deaf child: The impact of a cultural linguistic model of deafness. *Journal of Social Work Practice, 13*, 157–172.

15

A Comprehensive Reading Intervention: Positive Postsecondary Outcomes and a Promising Practice for Students Who Are Deaf or Hard of Hearing

Greta Palmberg and Kendra Rask

This chapter examines the development and implementation of a comprehensive reading intervention and its corresponding effects on college enrollment and postsecondary outcomes for young deaf and hard-of-hearing (DHH) adults age 18 to 21 years. For three years this approach has led to increases in reading and college-ready student skills, and has played a vital role in opening postsecondary education paths for a diverse group of students.

THE NEED FOR A READING INTERVENTION

In spring 2012, a critical issue had emerged for some of the DHH students in the Vocational Education, Community Training, and Occupational Relations (VECTOR) transition program in Minnesota—an issue pivotal enough to have the power to limit their futures. A core group of students had postsecondary goals, but did not have the reading skills that would allow them to begin postsecondary enrollment. In fact, they were not eligible to take developmental reading coursework that would allow them to move into college-level reading. Because instruction to lift them out of those levels did not exist in the program, the DHH staff held several brainstorming sessions. The question of whether significant gains could even be made at this age required frank discussion. Was it advisable or realistic to attempt to make several grade levels of reading growth, when even one grade level of growth in a year had not happened in years? The team decided it was worth creating a powerful, research-based reading innovation and developing these proven strategies into a course framework. The stakes were too high not to give it a chance.

Twenty-six students had enrolled in the College Reading Readiness Program during the past three years. Twenty students successfully completed a minimum of three academic quarters. The reading data reflect the learning of these 20 students, who began the program with reading skills at approximately the third- to fifth-grade levels. The diversity of these learners and their postsecondary aspirations presented a unique opportunity and challenge. Most students had just one or two years to make the reading growth needed to take a postsecondary path. After completing the College Reading Readiness course, students averaged a yearly increase of 3.8 grade levels, and 80% of students increased their reading levels on the college placement test to the developmental levels. By spring 2016, 70% of the students will be enrolled in developmental or college coursework at the postsecondary level. This chapter outlines what was required from a systemic and educational standpoint to deliver the goal of helping students make educationally significant reading growth in a short time.

VECTOR Transition Program

VECTOR is a nationally recognized transition program offered by Intermediate District 287, for 18- to 21-year-olds who have a variety of disabilities in the state of Minnesota. Transition programming focuses on services for young adults with disabilities as they progress from an educational setting (K–12) to living and working as independently as possible in the community. From its inception, the program has believed strongly in student self-determination and the guided development of self-advocacy skills and personal responsibility. VECTOR uses an advisor/advisee process model that assists students in developing meaningful plans to empower them to accomplish their career or life goals. Students have access to a broad transition curriculum that includes academic and student skill development, independent living classes, vocational skills training, and employment opportunities. Recent statistics show that 90% of VECTOR's DHH students were enrolled in postsecondary education or successfully employed at the time of graduation.

Diverse Students

Students who are DHH form a highly diverse population. Students come to school with a range of hearing losses from mild to profound, along with different preferred modes of communication (sign, speech, or both). Students have variations in language knowledge of English and American Sign Language (ASL), (U.S. Government Accountability Office, 2011) and bring a wide range of academic skills in reading, writing, and mathematics. These academic skills vary more widely than those of their hearing counterparts. Last, students come from a variety of educational settings (residential, mainstream, and so on) and varying levels of special education support (U.S. Government Accountability Office, 2011). Students referred to transition programming represent a unique subpopulation of students identified as having additional public education needs in the areas of education and training, employment, and independent living.

VECTOR has been customizing transition services for students who are deaf or hard of hearing since 1987. About one-third of the student population is made up of students who are deaf, hard of hearing, and deaf–blind. The students in the reading program come from traditionally underserved groups, including immigrants and refugees (60%), low socioeconomic backgrounds (85%), diverse racial and cultural groups, rural locations, those who have a parent at home who does not use sign language or speaks a language other than English, and those who are lower achieving academically. Secondary or co-occurring disabilities are present in 65% of the DHH reading population, including mental health diagnoses, language processing difficulties, learning disabilities, and physical disabilities. Their hearing losses vary widely and include students who identify as Deaf and use ASL to students who are deaf and do not sign, hard-of-hearing students who sign, and hard-of-hearing pupils who do not sign. Some students use hearing aids or cochlear implants, whereas other students prefer personal FM systems in the classroom setting. For students who rely on sign language, there is also a diversity of sign language skill and proficiency. Of the 20 students described in this chapter, 60% are hard of hearing and 40% are deaf. For communication needs, 35% of the students use ASL primarily, 40% of the students use sign-supported English, and 25% of the students use spoken English only.

Community and Technical College Placements

A lower reading ability is a barrier to accessing higher education (Cuculick & Kelly, 2003). Placement testing scores on the Accuplacer, an integrated system of computer-adaptive assessments designed to evaluate student skills in reading, writing, and mathematics, verified this conclusion (The College Board, 2016). An existing VECTOR program component of established collaboration with a local technical and community college became part of the solution to addressing our students' reading difficulties.

Reading: A Postsecondary Obstacle

Reading is a key postsecondary skill. It is a prerequisite for many courses, programs, and degrees. At the postsecondary level, many students who are DHH struggle with reading. These students can sometimes lack the reading skills to enter even the developmental (postsecondary preparation) coursework. When a text is more complex than a student's instructional level, frustration sets in and it becomes difficult for learning to occur. The result of this mismatch is that students cannot read enough of the text to learn the course content adequately. This has implications for a student's entire educational experience and is often a factor for never completing a postsecondary degree or program. Research indicates that about 35% of deaf students across all U.S. postsecondary institutions graduate from two-year programs compared with about 40% of their hearing peers. In four-year postsecondary programs, around 30% of deaf students graduate compared with about 70% of their hearing peers (Marschark et al., 2002).

Placement Testing: A Barrier to Postsecondary Enrollment

The Accuplacer is a postadmission course placement exam used by most technical and community colleges in Minnesota. The Accuplacer tests current skills in reading, sentence skills, and math. The scores are used as a counseling tool and to determine placement. The reading portion of the Accuplacer indicates a student's independent ability to comprehend college-level reading materials. To earn a degree and function in a skilled profession, students need these reading skills in place. At Hennepin Technical College (HTC), scores indicate either college-ready, developmental, or adult basic education (ABE)/community education levels (Table 15.1). In reading, a score of 78 points or more is considered college ready. A score of 38 to 77 points is developmental. Students need to take and pass developmental reading classes before moving into higher level courses required for their degree or program. A score of 37 or less is the ABE or community education level. The significance of the ABE reading level is that students cannot take reading coursework at that school until they build their reading skills in places outside of college, such as ABE or community education programs. Students with scores in this range cannot take developmental coursework at the college or courses in their major because most of the coursework has college-ready reading requirements. ABE scores (37 points or less) close the door to postsecondary

Table 15.1 Accuplacer Reading Chart: Reading Course Placement

Accuplacer Score, pt	College Placement
0–37	Adult basic education
38–55	Developmental (ENGL0901 *Reading Techniques*)
56–77	Developmental (ENGL0921 *Applied Reading Techniques*)
78+	College-ready reading

Source: Hennepin Technical College, Brooklyn Park, Minnesota.

plans. A large percentage of students who are DHH in VECTOR scored in the ABE range.

Postsecondary Collaboration

A key element of the VECTOR transition program, and an essential component to the reading program design, is the collaborative relationship between the transition program and two local colleges: Hennepin Technical College (HTC) and North Hennepin Community College (NHCC). These partnerships exist to provide the supports needed to be successful in the college environment. At HTC, VECTOR's postsecondary liaison teacher has a classroom on campus and works closely with students to prepare for the college setting, and then supports students who enter the postsecondary setting as a transition student. Ultimately, students are being prepared for independent college enrollment and/or completion of occupational certificates, diplomas, or associate's in applied science or associate's in science degrees.

Academic counseling typically includes helping students select an appropriate course of study or develop a clearer understanding of their career plan and the skills needed to meet their goals. Advising is aimed at helping students gain access to postsecondary education: how to apply to college, how to select appropriate coursework, how to navigate the college culture, how to maintain satisfactory progress and work toward a career goal, and how to pay for college and access systems and supports independently. Students are taught how to identify needed accommodations and make those requests in accordance with the Americans with Disabilities Act. The disability services directors of both colleges have noted that students from VECTOR are better prepared to handle the rigors of college because of the enhanced supports and emphasis on self-advocacy training. These relationships are critical to building students' knowledge of the postsecondary system, creating personalized postsecondary plans, and adding to the intrinsic motivation to improve reading.

PROGRAM DESIGN: THE FOUR PRINCIPLES

The first task for the VECTOR Transition Program was to design a powerful reading intervention that would accelerate academic reading skills. Research indicates that adolescence is not too late to provide reading intervention, and older students who participate in interventions can benefit (Scammacca et al., 2007). But what about young adults who are DHH? Could a reading intervention be designed for these students, who need to double or triple their reading rates in a year? Special education research is not so favorable. Special education placements tend to stabilize reading growth of students with reading disabilities rather than accelerate it. Students who enter special education with reading levels that are two or more years less than those of their peers can be expected to maintain that disparity, or fall further behind (Denton et al., 2003). To design an intensive reading intervention, VECTOR focused on four critical principles: academic reading skills, metacognition skills, college-ready student skills, and high expectations.

Academic Reading Skills

To help students access and succeed in postsecondary education, the reading course needed to equip students for the demands of reading college textbooks, classroom resources, and written materials they would encounter in their career fields. The goal of the course was to improve the reading comprehension of academic, nonfiction texts. Students would need to develop reading strategies to focus their thinking and construct meaning from these texts. Struggling readers can improve their reading comprehension when taught comprehension strategies. Studies indicate that comprehension practices that engage students in thinking about text, learning from text, and discussing what they know are likely to be associated with improved comprehension outcomes for students with reading difficulties and disabilities (Edmonds et al., 2009). The research also shows that remedial students who "were explicitly taught strategic reading" outperformed remedial students who were not. In addition, students were found to transfer these skills to more reading-intensive courses (Caverly et al., 2004).

There were eight primary reading skills and strategies integrated into the reading course: the Four-Step Reading Process (preview, read actively, highlight/annotate, review), vocabulary skills (context clues and word parts), topic, main idea (stated and implied), supporting details (major and minor), drawing conclusions, patterns of organization, and critical thinking skills (fact vs. opinion, author's tone, author's bias, intended audience). Each skill was introduced by the teacher and practiced with multiple texts by the students until mastery. As students acquired each reading skill, these skills were scaffolded onto the previous reading strategies and used to build reading comprehension. Together, these reading skills became the language of the classroom. Metacognition discussions were also infused into this language. To illustrate this classroom culture, observe the following dialog between the teacher and students after completing a reading selection about alternative energy:

> TEACHER: If you were taking notes on this reading selection, how would you organize the notes?
> STUDENT 1: The topic is about different energy alternatives.
> TEACHER: That might be the title of your notes, but it doesn't help us with organization. Let's look at the pattern of organization of the reading.

STUDENT 2: It has some cause and effect when it describes the problems of nonrenewable fuel sources.
TEACHER: Yes, that's right. The first half of the reading gives the negative effects of these fuel sources.
STUDENT 1: I think it is simple listing because it lists and describes different alternative energies like nuclear power, wind power, solar power, and geothermal energy. It also defines each type of energy.
TEACHER: So the two patterns of organization found in this passage are cause and effect, and listing with definitions. How can you use these patterns to organize your notes? Work in your small groups to create notes for this reading selection. Remember that the topic, main idea, and major supporting details should show up in your notes. The visual structure of the notes should match your patterns of organization.

Metacognition Skills

Beyond reading skills, students need to learn metacognition skills and effective study skills. Teaching effective study skills, as well as metacognitive skills, may provide the necessary boost for more deaf students to persist and succeed in college (Albertini et al., 2011). In simple terms, metacognition refers to "thinking about thinking." Using metacognition skills is a reflective process and helps students apply reading strategies in different contexts to increase their learning potential. Several ways instructors can encourage ABE learners to become more strategic thinkers is to help them focus on the ways they process information through self-questioning and discussing their thought processes with other learners (TEAL Center, 2012). These were two strategies incorporated into the reading course. Self-regulated learning, an aspect of metacognition, is another strategy used to create independent and strong readers (Maitland, 2000). These metacognition skills enabled students to become active and engaged in their reading—students who would ultimately become more independent in their learning.

College-Ready Student Skills

Although reading skills were a major focus of the instruction, college-ready student skills were of equal importance. In fact, both were happening simultaneously. The course design simulated the college environment to prepare students more effectively for its rigors. Early in the program it became apparent that our students lacked the college-ready student skills needed to participate in the college environment.

During our first year, on the first day of class, the teacher displayed a paragraph on the SMART Board and asked students to read it. To her amazement, all eyes turned instantly to the interpreter. The students were waiting for the interpreter to sign the paragraph or someone to read the paragraph to them. This was the pivotal moment when we realized our students had become passive learners. We knew that active learning would be one of the first college-level expectations we would model and teach. After so many years of frustration, students had stopped trying; not understanding was their norm.

VECTOR staff cultivated a classroom in which students felt comfortable asking questions and taking an active role in their learning. Staff also, increasingly and incrementally, raised the level of the material and classroom expectations. A variety of student skills were woven into the reading curriculum: how to organize a notebook, how to take notes from the textbook, how to create a planner to keep track of assignments, and how to apply time management techniques to complete work on time and to expectations. Other student skills included test-taking strategies, self-management strategies, and teamwork skills. Teamwork skills required a great deal of modeling and shaping. These collaborative skills took almost a full semester before surface answer responses evolved into introspective discussions. For example, in the autumn, students would discuss a reading activity by responding in this fashion: "I got B for number one. What did you get?" In the second semester, student discussions during teamwork activities reflected more collaboration and critical thinking skills:

> "I think number one is B because that sentence is what the paragraph is mostly about, so it's the main idea."
>
> "I thought B was a supporting detail because only one part of the paragraph discussed this idea. I thought the main idea was C because it contains the topic and tells what the passage is mostly about. Let's read it one more time to make sure."

Writing skills, although not the focus of this course, were developed in the context of reading. Students improved their ability to summarize and paraphrase in their writing. They learned how to write short-answer and essay questions on chapter tests and practiced several outlining formats in note taking. The teaching and modeling of these study strategies took time away from reading, but these critical skills are necessary for students wanting to succeed in the postsecondary environment.

Several classroom expectations helped create the structure of the collegelike environment. The first expectation was attendance and punctuality. Successful college students are in class. Students were expected to have at least 85% attendance each quarter. Students were expected to demonstrate positive adult behaviors. The syllabus contained a calendar of assignments and test dates for each chapter. Students were responsible for any work missed outside of class. Classroom grading tracked both assignments completed during class time and assignments completed outside the school day. This strategy enabled the teacher to evaluate a student's time management and assignment completion skills. Due dates were enforced; late assignments were either not accepted or resulted in lower grades. To pass the class each quarter, students were required to have an overall grade of 70% or better. By modeling these college-level expectations, students were able to develop these student skills before entering the postsecondary environment, where the stakes are higher.

High Expectations

Last, students and staff would need to establish and maintain high expectations for student participation and learning. The expectations that teachers and staff set for their students are foundational in terms of how they then interact. Bosso (2014) argued that these high expectations correlate directly to academic outcomes. Students would also need to develop these high expectations in the form of self-efficacy—a person's belief about his or her ability to accomplish a task. Students with a strong sense of efficacy are more likely to challenge themselves with difficult tasks and be motivated intrinsically (Lang, 2002). These four principles: academic reading skills, metacognition skills, effective study skills, and high expectations became the framework for the College Reading Readiness course and, as a result, students achieved unprecedented growth in academic reading and became empowered and responsible for their own learning.

SYSTEMIC CHANGE

As the College Reading Readiness course began to develop, the DHH staff realized to make educationally significant outcomes in reading would require systemic change beyond our program's reach. This systemic change is best discussed using Dean L. Fixsen's work on implementation research (Blase et al., 2015; Fixsen et al., 2005). Systemic change, a change that occurs in all aspects and levels of the educational process, is needed to produce educational significant outcomes. The implementation research suggests three factors are needed to make educationally significant outcomes. The factors include effective innovations (research-based practices or programs), effective implementation (staff with the knowledge, skill, and ability to provide the innovation to students), and enabling contexts (the changes the district/school/community agencies need to make to support the work effectively). All these factors need to be present at significant levels for significant outcomes to occur (De Klerk et al., 2015). In many situations when new interventions are implemented, schools do not change the existing system, but change the effective innovations to fit the system. What is needed is to change the existing system to support the effectiveness of the innovation.

After identifying research-based reading interventions and selecting qualified staff, the biggest obstacle for VECTOR was changing the existing system. This meant doubling the class period, obtaining district funding for technology and curriculum, changing from a four-day-a-week to a five-day-a-week course, mandating a year-long commitment to the course (the transition courses run nine weeks), and having the approval from the technical college to be able to retest students using the Accuplacer for summative reading data. The reading program was designed for our DHH students. However, after the student reading results were shared at the end of the first year, VECTOR staff wanted to include hearing students as well. The DHH staff felt strongly that because of the unique literacy needs of this DHH population, we continue to have a separate class for these students. Today, VECTOR offers two sections of the reading class: one course for hearing students who have a variety of disabilities and one for students who are DHH. Each year, VECTOR staff must ensure all levels of the educational system are kept informed of and remain supportive to the needs of this significant reading intervention.

METHODOLOGY: CONSTRUCTING THE LEARNING AND DELIVERY

To build a researched-based intensive reading intervention, teaching staff gave careful consideration to designing the classroom environment in which reading growth could take place. Staff wrestled with the following questions: How much time should be devoted to reading to make substantial gains? What type of reading text and technology are needed to engage the older, diverse learner? How will reading growth be measured during the school year? And last, how should the learning environment be structured to create a classroom culture that prepares a student for postsecondary education?

Instructional Minutes

A dramatic increase in time spent on reading was required for students to make unprecedented growth and to develop college-ready student skills. The greater the catch-up growth needed in reading, the more intensive the intervention. There are three ways to increase the intensity of the reading intervention: decrease the class size, increase the time for learning, or both (Kamil et al., 2008). The VECTOR program already had the luxury of small class sizes as a result of the low-incidence population; class sizes were between 9 students and 12 students each year. The real problem became scheduling intervention periods so dramatic that increases in reading growth would actually occur. VECTOR staff committed to doubling the class period. Instead of 50 minutes a day for four days a week, the College Reading Readiness class would run

100 minutes a day for five days a week. In addition, the class would not follow the typical quarter schedule of the transition program; it would be a year in length. This was a significant systemic change. It was also a significant commitment by students, using two of the six class periods per day for reading instruction. As a result, it would affect participation in other transition programming and activities, such as work experience and independent living skills classes, during the school day.

Blended Classroom/Hybrid Teaching

A hybrid teaching model was used in constructing the learning for the College Reading Readiness course. A hybrid model, also known as a *blended classroom*, is instruction that uses a balance of face-to-face and online environments. In the U.S. Department of Education, Office of Planning, Evaluation, and Policy Development (2010) evaluation of online learning studies, research findings suggest that blends of online and face-to-face instruction had stronger learning outcomes than face-to-face alone. These types of classrooms use the learning opportunities afforded by technology. The physical classroom design maintains the teacher's ability to provide direct instruction and plan reading activities delivered in a variety of instructional groupings—small collaborative groups, teacher-led whole group, and independent practice (see Chapter 8).

In the College Reading Readiness course, explicit instruction was used for the introduction of reading skills and strategies. Explicit instruction occurs when the teacher models and teaches skills and concepts clearly. Studies have shown, especially for low-achieving students, explicit instruction in reading also makes a difference in student outcomes (Denton et al., 2003).

Another instruction model used in this blended-learning course was interactive learning. The teacher designed these activities so students would have the opportunity to process key learning objectives and practice reading skills in group settings. Students worked on promoting their own ideas and learning from each other as they completed assignments in partners, teams, or small groups. Through these interactive activities, students learned to work in a team and took accountability for their own learning. Effective teamwork behaviors were modeled and shaped during the year. By the end of the course, students were more successful in working within time limits, recognizing the strengths each member brought to the team, and completing an activity in a collegial relationship. A major portion of the online component of the class was tied to the curriculum used in the course: MyReadingLab by Pearson/Longman/Prentice Hall. This online curriculum combined reading diagnostics, practice exercises and activities, tests, and teaching videos. Study materials, such as notes, PowerPoint presentations, and graphic organizers were also made available to students online.

Instructors are able to individualize the reading activities for students and encourage their progress. Through this online part of the course, students could ask the teacher questions about assignments outside of class. The teacher could also give feedback on work completed online. Every week students worked individually on reading comprehension exercises and diagnostic tests through the MyReadingLab online curriculum.

Measuring Reading Growth

When selecting a data collection model to measure the reading growth of students in our transition program, it was important the assessment be in line with our college partners (HTC and NHCC) to ensure student readiness for enrollment. For this reason, we chose the Accuplacer (On-Target Testing) for our summative assessment, which is the colleges' placement test. Using the Accuplacer also helped the students understand the content and cutoff scores of these postsecondary institutions. Students learned quickly the meaning and consequences of ABE and developmental scores. They also had a greater understanding of their current reading skills in relation to "college-ready" reading.

Lexile scores, a widely adopted reading measure by MetaMetrics, were used as a formative assessment to monitor growth in reading development and measure progress toward college reading readiness. The Lexile Framework provides teachers with a tool for determining a student's reading ability relative to the difficulty of the text (Blackburn, 2000) and is measured by an assessment. It should be noted that the Lexile Framework is not a reading program or a method of teaching literacy. Lexile measures were taken eight times a quarter and reading growth was recorded at the end of each quarter. Students could monitor this growth through the online MyReadingLab curriculum.

The Lexile measurement was also used as a preassessment to determine students' instructional level through the Initial Lexile Locator Test. A Lexile score of 600L or greater was encouraged before entering the reading program. This score was needed to match the lowest reading difficulty of the course textbook, which was designed for grades 6 through 9. Most of our DHH students had initial Lexiles in the range of 545L to 715L. Table 15.2 shows text difficulty measured by grade levels using the Lexile Framework and based on research from the Common Core State Standards Initiative (Nelson et al., 2012). Our students' initial Lexile scores are comparable with text difficulty at the elementary levels. Typical text measures of high school material begin at 960L. This was not enough growth, however, for reading at the postsecondary level. Current research shows the typical postsecondary reading materials have text complexity measures ranging from 1200L to 1380L; the median text complexity measure is 1300L (Stenner et al., 2012).

Table 15.2 Text Difficulty Based on Grade Levels: Common Scale for Band-Level

Text Difficulty Ranges

Grade	Lexile Band
K–1	N/A
2 and 3	420L–820L
4 and 5	740L–1010L
6–8	925L–1185L
9–10	1050L–1335L
11–college/career	1185L–1385L

K, kindergarten; N/A, not applicable.

During the first year, the reading instructor hypothesized that students would need to increase their Lexile to at least the 1000L level by the end of the year to test into the developmental college reading courses. Students strived for this number and the class celebrated individual reading growth each quarter. At the end of the first year, most students who reached this Lexile range tested into the developmental levels. The high correlation between the Accuplacer and Lexile scores was also recognized by the developmental reading instructors at HTC (Larson, 2014). Their developmental reading courses are eight weeks each, so students can finish the developmental reading requirements in one semester. HTC data show that students in the first developmental course, Reading Techniques, have initial Lexiles around 800L to 900L. Students in the second developmental course, Applied Reading Techniques, typically start between 900L and 1000L. Although the course moves much faster than VECTOR's College Reading Readiness course, students who test into these developmental levels have the student skills and Lexile levels to pass these courses successfully and move on to their course of study.

Authentic Academic Reading Material

Choosing a reading text and curriculum for this diverse student population was challenging. Despite exhaustive searches, staff were unable to find reading materials used successfully with DHH students that had an emphasis on postsecondary readiness, so community and technical colleges were contacted to see what was working for English-language learners in their developmental reading courses. English-language learners are generally defined as students who were not born in the United States or whose native language is a language other than English and who lack sufficient mastery of English to meet state standards and excel in an English-language classroom. This information set the course and tone for the rest of the course development process. Several other considerations were used when selecting a reading text. First, it was imperative that students be exposed to the type of texts that they will encounter in college-level coursework. The developmental level students' success in college depends on their "ability to engage in strategic reading of extensive academic or informational text" (Caverly et al., 2004, p. 25). Next, the text should align with transition philosophy and be relevant and engaging to the students. Last, the text should also meet the literacy needs of our DHH students.

After much research, the text we chose was *Reading for Life* (Fennessy & Dorling, 2011), a college developmental text for students at a sixth- to ninth-grade reading level. *Reading for Life* was selected because it paired reading skill instruction with career exploration. Each chapter contained stories and vocabulary around different careers, and this matched our transition program's focus. We also chose a second book, *Breaking Through College Reading* (Smith & Morris, 2013), which had a secondary focus on teaching college student skills. These books allowed staff to create a two-year reading curriculum for students who needed more than one year of reading instruction. Both of these reading texts had chapters devoted to our essential reading skills: vocabulary, main idea, supporting details, patterns of organization, drawing conclusions, and critical thinking skills, which was the core of the reading instruction. These texts were paired with Pearson's MyReadingLab, which was being used successfully with developmental readers at community and technical colleges across the United States.

MyReadingLab is an online program created specifically for the developmental reader at the college level that delivers instruction beginning at the fourth-grade level (Pearson Education, 2016). The program uses the Lexile system to measure text difficulty and to analyze students' reading levels as the levels change over time. As students read academic passages and take diagnostic tests, their scores are adjusted incrementally based not only on their scores for specific test, but also on their history in the Lexile system. MyReadingLab provides authentic practice with "real-world" texts that challenge and hold the students' interest. It combines diagnostics, practice exercises, and tests to help improve student reading skills and reading level. MyReadingLab also allows students to monitor their Lexile progress and chart their reading growth. Instructors are able to track student data, manage their students' reading comprehension, and evaluate student Lexile growth.

Building Vocabulary and Background Knowledge

To help meet the special literacy considerations for our DHH learners, special emphasis was placed on developing language skills through increasing vocabulary and background knowledge. Research evidence is clear that the stronger the reading and language skills deaf students acquire during their K–12 experiences, the stronger the foundation for success in both college and careers (Cuculick & Kelly, 2003; see also Chapter 17). As a result of the English language deficits of our students, vocabulary instruction was expanded from the general vocabulary activities in the textbook. In addition, extended background knowledge was taught before each story and career content. Although time-consuming, adding additional background knowledge paid off in dividends throughout each chapter. It not only increased comprehension, but also equipped students with the knowledge they needed to discuss story concepts using critical thinking skills.

Vocabulary development not only focused on definitions, but also on learning multiple meanings of words in context. Students needed to understand that *server* is not only a waitress at a restaurant, but it has a completely different definition in the context of computer careers. For each chapter, students were responsible to learn 15 to 20 new words presented in the two stories. In addition, students were encouraged to look up any word they did not know in the MyReadingLab Lexile passages. Students shared with each other their favorite dictionary and grammar sites on the Web, as well as apps on their phones and other electronic devices. Apps and websites for making flash cards, studying, and playing vocabulary games were also shared. While completing reading assignments, students were encouraged to use technology to look up independently people, places, and events to add to their background knowledge. This vocabulary and language enrichment became as important as the studying students were completing outside of class for each reading skill chapter test.

The instructional team, including interpreter, teacher, and educational assistant, discussed how they would promote vocabulary growth when working with students. If the teacher talked about a college *course*, we made sure not only to sign the word (which in Minnesota is the same for *class* and *group*), but also to fingerspell and display the word in printed form. Advanced vocabulary skills were enhanced when specific words were fingerspelled and displayed visually on a whiteboard. When answering comprehension questions, students were encouraged and rewarded for using chapter vocabulary as well as vocabulary introduced in previous chapters. Slowly, vocabulary growth was demonstrated. Student questions progressed from identifying unfamiliar words, "What is this word?" to defining words using context clues, "Does this mean ___?" Expecting students to take accountability for increasing vocabulary, not for a grade, but for their own future success in college and future careers, was cultivated throughout the school year.

REVIEW OF THE READING DATA

Results of the three-year College Reading Readiness program have confirmed our diverse students who are DHH and older (age, 18–21 years) can still make educationally significant reading growth. Using student Lexile scores to measure reading growth, Figure 15.1 shows that each year the classroom average Lexile growth was at least 300 points. Annually, students made an average grade-level increase of 3.8 years. Individual student Lexile growth and Accuplacer testing results are presented in Table 15.3. Results of the final student Lexiles indicate that 70% of students reached or exceeded the Lexile levels comparable with developmental students in HTC's second developmental course, where students typically start between 900L and 1000L (Larson, 2014). A high bar was set for students to reach the 1000L level, and 65% of our students had final Lexiles scores near or above the 1000L level. To reach this goal, individual student Lexile growth ranged from 278 to 756 points of growth from their initial Lexile scores. These students also had a higher probability of testing from the ABE levels to the developmental college reading level.

These Accuplacer results played a vital role in opening postsecondary education paths for a diverse group of students. Overall, 80% of our students increased their reading levels on the college placement test to the developmental levels. As mentioned, by spring 2016, 70% of the students will be enrolled in developmental or college coursework at the postsecondary level. There are 14 students who have now graduated from the VECTOR Transition Program and who have completed the College

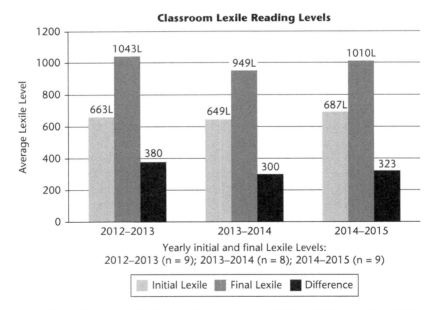

Figure 15.1 Classroom Lexile reading levels for 2012 to 2013 (n = 9), 2013 to 2014 (n = 8) and 2014 to 2015 (n = 9).

Table 15.3 Student Reading Data (2012–2015)

Students	Quarters Enrolled	Initial Accuplacer	Final Accuplacer	Initial Lexile	Final Lexile	Lexile Growth	College Enrollment
Student A	4	29 ABE	65 DEV 2	715L	1028L	313	DEV/College
Student B	6	40 DEV	36 ABE	580L	1045L	465	DEV/College
Student C	4	33 ABE	38 DEV	615L	994L	379	
Student D	4	51 DEV	72 DEV 2	785L	1159L	374	DEV/College
Student E	4	29 ABE	56 DEV	820L	1098L	278	
Student F	4	36 ABE	40 DEV	650L	1121L	471	
Student G	4	31 ABE	29 ABE	505L	878L	373	
Student H	8	27 ABE	38 DEV	650L	1221L	571	DEV/College
Student I	4	32 ABE	41 DEV	650L	1095L	445	DEV/College
Student J	10	30 ABE	43 DEV	530L	1286L	756	DEV
Student K	8	38 DEV	39 DEV	650L	1379L	729	DEV
Student L	8	35 ABE	49 DEV	650L	886L	236	
Student M	8	42 DEV	65 DEV 2	715L	1089L	379	DEV
Student N	5	48 DEV	50 DEV	580L	795L	215	DEV
Student O	5	44 DEV	52 DEV	683L	1121L	438	DEV
Student P	8	27 ABE	32 ABE	545L	779L	234	
Student Q	4	—	44 DEV	580L	976L	396	DEV/College
Student R	4	28 ABE	39 DEV	580L	926L	346	
Student T	4	—	45 DEV	615L	868L	253	
Student U	4	—	46 DEV	685L	728L	43	

ABE, adult basic education (not college ready); College, college-level coursework; DEV, developmental college coursework.

Reading Readiness course. Nine of these students are currently enrolled in college coursework at local technical and community colleges.

What cannot be truly measured is the increase in student skills. However, passing developmental college coursework or regular college coursework is an indication that these students have the independent student skills needed to succeed at the postsecondary level. Throughout the course of five semesters, from spring 2013 to spring 2015, these students completed 54 credits in developmental courses, earning an overall grade point average of 3.5 out of 4.0, and completed 38 credits in college-level coursework, earning an overall grade point average of 3.2 out of 4.0.

STUDENT CASE STUDIES

The following case studies (students' names have been changed) represent a sampling of the personal stories behind the reading data. We had hoped that the College Reading Readiness course would result in reading gains; what the students' achieved was so much more. It changed their futures.

The Case of Debra

Debra was born in Liberia, Africa, and moved to Minnesota when she was 11 years old. During childhood, she lost her hearing and became deaf. When she arrived in America, she knew some British Sign Language, but soon began learning ASL at school. Her family uses spoken English and Liberian, and none of her family members sign. After graduating from high school, she started in the VECTOR program and is currently in her second year. English is a third language for Debra and, as a result of her delayed English skills, her reading growth has not been easy journey. Debra benefited from learning the reading skill strategies that helped unlock the English language, such as recognizing patterns of organization, telling the difference between major and minor details, and using context clues to help discover word meaning. Vocabulary development and expanding background knowledge also helped increase reading comprehension. Most important, Debra developed metacognition strategies that allowed her to think about a reading passage and decide which reading strategies to apply to create meaning.

Debra completed two years in the College Reading Readiness program. Her initial Lexile was 650L; her last measured Lexile was 1379L—a growth of 729 Lexile points. She tested into developmental reading courses at HTC and began her first postsecondary experience in fall 2015. Debra worked actively with staff on the steps to enrollment, and her postsecondary plan is to pursue a diploma in child development, which matches her current skills and abilities. Her goal is to serve others internationally, much like the assistance she and her family received. She wants to teach children in developing countries to read and write, and to help others like herself.

The Case of Katya

An immigrant from Russia, Katya's hearing loss was not identified for many years and she was unaware she suffered from hearing loss. In her home country, she was considered to have an intellectual disability. In Russia, she recalls watching the seasons change out the window while other students were busy listening and learning in the classroom. When she arrived in Minnesota, she was identified to be hard of hearing and was fitted with hearing aids. Katya uses spoken English and a personal frequency modulation (FM) system in the classroom.

Katya's high school staff recognized she was unprepared for postsecondary education, although this was a hope for Katya and her family. Her reading skill growth took time and patience. She also needed to develop the ability to work and learn independently, because she had become highly dependent on one-on-one support to access and complete any academic work during her middle school and high school years. While at VECTOR, Katya developed her independent student skills in following directions, managing her time, working effectively in a group, and taking notes from a textbook. She increased her skills from full dependence on school staff to college-ready student skills by her last semester.

Katya completed 2.5 years in the College Reading Readiness class. Her initial Lexile was 530L and her last measured Lexile was 1286L—a growth of 756 Lexile points. After twice testing into the ABE level in reading, with scores of 30 points and 34 points on the Accuplacer, she tested this spring into developmental reading with a score of 43 points. Katya understood her Lexile scores and the needed Accuplacer scores for college enrollment. So when she saw her score, she was fully cognizant of what she had achieved.

Katya completed developmental writing coursework successfully during the spring 2015 semester at HTC and is graduating from VECTOR in spring 2015. She plans to continue at HTC independently. Katya registered for developmental reading coursework for fall 2015 and then plans to be able to move on to her chosen course of study.

The Case of Mark

One of the original students for whom this program was developed, Mark is a young deaf man whose primary mode of communication is ASL. When entering transition education after high school, he did not envision attending college. Mark became interested in the culinary arts when he obtained an entry-level position in a restaurant. He continued exploring this career while taking secondary vocational culinary arts classes, in which he excelled. Mark had a strong desire to enroll in culinary arts at the technical college; however, he was unable to register because of the reading prerequisite. Mark completed two years of the College Reading Readiness course. His initial Lexile was 650L and his last measured Lexile was 1221L—a growth of 571 Lexile points. After twice testing into the ABE level in reading on the Accuplacer, Mark tested into developmental reading courses. He is now able to start working on his college goal of becoming a chef.

His journey in VECTOR provided him with the time to become an active, engaged, goal-oriented learner. As his skills began to improve, he started purchasing books about cooking and e-mailing chefs who are deaf to learn more about the industry. He has an acute awareness of the growth he has made, and feels successful and unafraid to move forward. In his last semester in VECTOR, he completed full-time culinary arts training for a 16-credit Occupational Certificate at HTC. He has since adjusted his goal and plans to acquire a culinary arts diploma or associate's in applied science degree. He began this coursework as an independent college student in fall 2015. Mark's future career goal is to open his own restaurant someday.

The Case of Kaim

Another of the original students who presented with ABE reading scores, Kaim was born in America, and his parents came from Thailand and speak Hmong. He is hard of hearing and communicates using ASL, English, and Hmong.

Kaim completed one year of the College Reading Readiness course because he only had a year of eligibility left in K–12 education. His initial Lexile score was 650L and his last measured Lexile was 1095L—a growth of 445 Lexile points. Kaim wanted to pursue a career in computers. Early that year, he tested into ABE reading, which closed the door to further postsecondary education. A few weeks before graduating from VECTOR, Kaim increased his Accuplacer score by nine points and tested into developmental reading courses at HTC. Kaim found that being able to read and understand his work has helped him continue in his college coursework. After graduating VECTOR, Kaim continued on to HTC and completed all his developmental coursework. Today he is an independent college student nearing completion of his desktop support specialist degree.

The Case of Amina

Amina was born in Kenya, East Africa, and came to the United States during the late 1990s. She is hard of hearing and uses ASL and English. Amina completed one year of the College Reading Readiness course. Her initial Lexile score was 715L, and her last measured Lexile was 1028L—a growth of 313 Lexile points. Before attending the College Reading Readiness course, Amina wanted a career as a certified nursing assistant, and she was successful in the hands-on portion of the course, even passing the state skills test. However, she was still unprepared to meet the reading and literacy requirements of her career. She could not pass the certified nursing assistant written exam, also required for certification. Amina wanted to develop the reading skills that would allow her to pursue a health career. Her initial Accuplacer reading score of 29 points was ABE level. At the end of the year, she scored into developmental reading with a score of 65 points. This growth of 36 points not only elevated Amina to the developmental level, but also allowed her to skip the first developmental reading classes altogether.

Amina adjusted her goals when her reading scores improved, and she is pursuing a career in radiologic technology at a technical college. Reflecting on her experiences in VECTOR, Amina feels accomplished and confident moving forward in college. No longer nervous, Amina notes that choosing a career path is hard for anyone and that, as a person who is deaf, she works on her goals like anyone else. Amina hopes to take her medical training and work overseas to help people in other countries.

FINAL REFLECTIONS

Twenty-six DHH students have participated in this program during the past three years and 20 succeeded in completing at least three-quarters of the program. Beyond students' hearing loss, these diverse students, ages 18 to 21, also faced other challenges and obstacles, which affected their ability to learn. Some of these issues included mental health, homelessness, pregnancy, chemical health, and unstable family circumstances. In addition, some students had more severe learning difficulties that prevented achieving the reading level and student skills required for college enrollment. Despite these struggles, students did increase their current reading levels and had more information about themselves to be able to self-advocate for transition plans that met their skills and abilities.

During the past two years of implementation, College Reading Readiness was successful for not only students with a hearing loss, but also for hearing students as well. The hearing students were special education students with transition needs. Some of these disabilities included learning disabilities, autism, mental health issues, and physical disabilities. The classroom mean beginning Lexile score in the hearing section was 941L; the DHH classroom initial Lexile mean score was 639L. This difference of 300 points may account for greater Accuplacer achievements for the hearing students. There were 19 hearing students who completed the course during the two years it has been offered. Sixteen of these students took the Accuplacer testing at the end of the year and 50% increased scores either to the first or second developmental college reading course. In addition, 44% of the students increased from developmental to college-ready reading scores. In the case of the hearing students, the benefit of the College Reading Readiness course was that it not only increased student skills, but also it afforded students the opportunity to enter into postsecondary education at the highest level of developmental education or become college ready with no developmental requirements needed.

Intensive reading instruction or intervention programs are rarely found at the secondary level. This is quite significant because many struggling readers in older grades (6–12) are not provided effective instruction in reading comprehension (Edmonds et al., 2009). Further exploration is needed to determine what would happen if middle school and high school students who are DHH were able to take part in an intensive reading program to prepare for postsecondary education.

By integrating evidence-based practices in reading, a research to practice model was created. The students in this reading program did not follow the traditional postsecondary path from high school to a four-year college or university. Rather, a unique postsecondary path was created that allowed students to gain the reading and student skills needed for enrollment in the local community and technical college system.

ACKNOWLEDGMENTS

Preparation of this chapter was made possible by the financial support of the Minnesota Department of Education. The reading course intervention described in the chapter would not have been possible without the additional support and assistance from the dedicated and amazing VECTOR staff (Dori Beach, Kayla Beccue, Kathy Manlapas, Donna Moe, and Tina Sunda) and the courageous students who committed to continue working on their reading skills despite many years of struggles and failure.

REFERENCES

Albertini, J. A., Kelly, R. R., & Matchett, M. K. (2011). Personal factors that influence deaf college students' academic success. *Journal of Deaf Studies and Deaf Education, 17*(1), 85–101.

Blackburn, B. R. (2000). Best practices for using Lexiles? *Popular Measurement, 3*(1), 22–24.

Blase, K. A., Fixsen, D. L., Sims, B. J., & Ward, C. S. (2015). *Implementation science: Changing hearts, minds, behavior, and systems to improve educational outcomes.* Oakland, CA: Wing Institute.

Bosso, E. (2014). Letters from the vice president. *Odyssey, 15,* 3.

Caverly, D. C., Nicholson, S. A., & Radcliffe, R. (2004). The effectiveness of strategic reading instruction for college developmental readers. *Journal of College Reading and Learning, 35*(1), 25–49.

The College Board (2016). About ACCUPACER.https://accuplacer.college-board.org/professionals

Cuculick, J. A., & Kelly, R. R. (2003). Relating deaf students' reading and language scores at college entry to their degree completion rates. *American Annals of the Deaf, 148*(4), 279–286.

De Klerk, A., Fortgens, C., & Van der Eijk, A. (2015). Curriculum design in Dutch deaf education. In H. Knoors & M. Marschark (Eds.), *Educating deaf learners: Creating a global evidence base* (pp. 573–593). New York: Oxford University Press.

Denton, C., Vaughn, S., & Fletcher, J. (2003). Bringing research-based practice in reading intervention to scale. *Learning Disabilities Research & Practice, 18*(3), 201–211.

Edmonds, M. S., Vaughn, S., Wexler, J., Reutebuch, C., Cable, A., Tackett, K. K., & Schnakenberg, J. W. (2009). A synthesis of reading interventions and effects on reading comprehension outcomes for older struggling readers. *Review of Educational Research, 79*(1), 262–300.

Fennessy, C., & Dorling, K. (2011). *Reading for life.* Upper Saddle River, NJ: Longman/Pearson Education.

Fixsen, D. L., Naoom, S. F., Blase, K. A., Friedman, R. M., & Wallace, F. (2005). *Implementation research: A synthesis of the literature*. FMHI publication no. 231. Tampa, FL: University of South Florida, Louis de la Parte Florida Mental Health Institute, National Implementation Research Network.

Kamil, M. L., Borman, G. D., Dole, J., Kral, C. C., Salinger, T., & Torgesen, J. (2008). *Improving adolescent literacy: Effective classroom and intervention practices: A practice guide*. NCEE no. 2008-4027. Washington, DC: National Center for Education Evaluation and Regional Assistance, Institute of Education Sciences, U.S. Department of Education. http://ies.ed.gov/ncee/wwc

Lang, H. G. (2002). Higher education for deaf students: Research priorities in the new millennium. *Journal of Deaf Studies and Deaf Education, 7,* 267–280.

Marschark, M., Lang, H., & Albertini, J. (2002). *Educating deaf students: From research to practice.* New York: Oxford University Press.

Maitland, L. E. (2000). Self-regulation and metacognition in the reading lab. *Journal of Developmental Education, 24*(2), 26–36.

Nelson, J., Perfetti, C., Liben, D., & Liben, M. (February 2012). *Measures of text difficulty: Testing their predictive value for grade levels and student performance.* Technical Report to the Gates Foundation. Washington, DC: Council of Chief State School Officers.

Pearson Education (2016). Learn About MyReadingLab. http://www.pearson-mylabandmastering.com/northamerica/myreadinglab/educators/features/index.html

Scammacca, N., Roberts, G., Vaughn, S., Edmonds, M., Wexler, J., Reutebuch, C. K., & Torgesen, J. K. (2007). *Interventions for adolescent struggling readers: A meta-analysis with implications for practice.* Portsmouth, NH: RMC Research Corporation, Center on Instruction.

Stenner, J., Sanford-Moore, E., Ph.D., & Williamson, G. (2012). The Lexile® Framework for Reading Quantifies the Reading Ability Needed for "College & Career Readiness". *MetaMetrics Research Brief.* https://lexile.com/research/152/.

Smith, B., & Morris, L. (2013). *Breaking Through College Reading.* Upper Saddle River, NJ: Pearson.

U.S. Department of Education, Office of Planning, Evaluation, and Policy Development (2010). *Evaluation of evidence-based practices in online learning: A meta-analysis and review of online learning studies* Washington, DC: U.S. Department of Education.

U.S. Government Accountability Office (May 2011). *Report to congressional requesters: Deaf and hard of hearing children: Federal support for developing language and literacy.* Washington, DC: GAO Publications.

U.S. Department of Education, Office of Vocational and Adult Education (2011). *Just Write! Guide.* Washington, DC: Author.

16

Critical Factors Toward the Inclusion of Deaf and Hard-of-Hearing Students in Higher Education

Merv Hyde, Magda Nikolaraizi, Denise Powell, and Michael Stinson

In most developed and many developing nations, the compulsory years of schooling mandated within national education systems are open to deaf and hard-of-hearing (DHH) students. Most of these students are included in mainstream education with appropriate accommodations of communication, curriculum choice, pedagogy, and assessment, and some degree of individualized support in recognition of their rights to learn, engage, and succeed in publicly funded education. Although most nations have recognized and ratified the conditions of the UN Convention on the Rights of People with a Disability (2006) for equitable engagement in education at all levels, inclusive outcomes within the compulsory years of schooling are not well reflected within postsecondary education, particularly in higher education. Many challenges remain in the higher education sector internationally. As one student in Greece concluded:

> The interpreter helps and I also get some notes from my co-students and my teachers and I also do tutorials in maths. I go together with the interpreter to teacher's office for individual tutorials. I do not go [to] his lecture because I do not understand anything.

This represents an ongoing challenge for the tenets of inclusive education, if the capacities and career development of diverse deaf students are to be recognized and realized. This chapter examines a number of education systems that have addressed this challenge within their social, economic, and national frameworks; and outlines a number of characteristics of higher education programs that may promote the academic, social, and vocational inclusion of DHH students.

Attaining a degree and graduating from a higher education institution can produce significant socioeconomic benefits throughout an individual's life span, including enhanced employment potential, broader career options, greater career mobility, and increased earnings (Boutin, 2008; Schley et al., 2011; see also Chapter 17). However, research indicates that although more DHH students are able to experience some of the benefits of inclusion in higher education, such as enhanced access and some degree of participation, many are not able to complete their study programs. Several factors can contribute to this restricted outcome, including the students' academic preparedness and other personal characteristics, as well as external factors related to the communication and learning environments available and the support services provided by the higher education systems (Boutin, 2008; Hyde et al., 2009; Marschark et al., 2005, 2008; Polich, 2001; Powell et al., 2013).

DHH students, compared with their hearing peers, often enter higher education with reduced educational and academic attainments and knowledge of the spoken and written language used in the institution (Marschark & Wauters, 2008). In addition, the diverse personal characteristics of DHH students themselves, such as their levels of motivation and interest in higher education, levels of anxiety, study habits and strategies, self-advocacy skills, and identity issues, can play a critical role in their success in higher education (Albertini et al., 2011).

In addition to students' personal characteristics, a range of external factors extends beyond inclusive opportunities for access and participation into the more complex domains of accommodated communication and learning environments, and associated support systems, services, and technologies. These factors can influence significantly the extent of their academic and social engagement and course achievement in higher education, and, ultimately, program completion. If all the principles of inclusive education are to be applied in higher education, the outcome measures of engagement and program completion need to be prioritized.

University teachers with high levels of subject knowledge, effective communication skills (Lang et al., 1994), knowledge of diverse learning styles, and a learner-centered approach are more likely to respond to the needs of DHH students, and to promote deeper approaches to learning and more successful study outcomes (Marschark et al., 2008; Richardson et al., 2010). DHH students, however, often report dissatisfaction with their higher education teachers, who may not be aware of the students' communication and learning needs, who make poor accommodations of these needs, or assume they do not play a role in the students' access to learning because interpreters or note-takers have such a role (Foster et al., 1999; Hyde et al., 2009; Powell et al., 2013; Stinson et al., 1996).

Available and effective support services for DHH individuals are of major importance to students' communication access, learning, and academic performance. Sign language interpreting and a real-time display of captions are common support services that postsecondary programs use to enhance the academic access of DHH students (Marschark et al., 2005; Stinson et al., 2014).

Interpreting is of major importance for students who have a good knowledge of a native sign language. Unfortunately, there is frequently a shortage of qualified interpreters, and many deaf students remain unsatisfied with the level of interpreting services (Hyde et al., 2009) and may not receive adequate access to the content of lectures through interpreting (Marschark et al., 2005; Napier & Barker, 2004; Powell et al., 2013) even in situations when interpreters are experienced and consider the communication needs of their students who might also be highly proficient in a sign language (Marschark et al., 2005). University-level interpreters require both: knowledge of the subjects taught (conceptually and lexically) as well as a highly developed interpreting capacity.

The communication and learning support services for students who are hard of hearing and who, under accommodated communication conditions, may understand and learn through the use of a spoken language, can also be quite different from those of deaf students using a sign language interpreter. Their particular needs are reported to be neglected or assumed to be minimal (Hyde et al., 2009). They may be neglected for two reasons. First, the teacher may assume that, because students have a cochlear implant or other effective speech amplification, they do not need any specific services or teaching and learning accommodations. Second, it is often assumed that the services provided for deaf students also address the needs of hard-of-hearing students. This has been shown not to be the case (Hyde et al., 2009). Students who have effective spoken language reception with suitable communication and learning accommodations may use some of the same services as deaf students (such as note-taking, captioning, small-group tutoring), but they may use these services with different emphases, reflecting the diversity of their individual backgrounds, competencies, and abilities. In addition to their engagement academically, their patterns of identify formation and social engagement may vary from those of deaf students.

The cases that follow serve to illustrate the variety and diversity of ways in which DHH students may find an inclusive higher education through effective transition, support for learning, social and academic engagement, and program achievement; and how the education systems of the countries involved have responded, and continue to respond, to their rights and needs. The cases presented range from enduring, highly structured, and individualized systems of support at the National Technical Institute for the Deaf (NTID) in the United States, to more recent developments in Greece and New Zealand. Each case is instructive for how it shows the inclusive processes at work and the different contexts of the national education systems involved.

A CASE IN AUSTRALIA

In Australia, few universities have specialist support programs for DHH; more commonly, the 39 universities' generic disability support offices provide services and hire interpreters and tutors as needed. Griffith University, which has an enrollment of more than 32,000 students across five campuses in Southeast Queensland, is one of the few with a specialist program. Griffith has a long history of enrollment of deaf students; the Deaf Student Support Program (DSSP) began in 1985 and continues as part of the University's student support network.

Power and Hyde, then directors of the Centre for Deaf Studies and Research, undertook a retrospective examination of the experiences of DHH students across a 20-year period at Griffith, and subsequently the graduates' experiences in work and further study. The objectives were to identify those support services and academic and social experiences that were of greatest benefit to supporting the students' graduation and the extent to which their university experiences helped the DHH graduates move successfully into the workplace.

The participants consisted of 72 former and current students of Griffith University. The majority (70%) were recent graduates and current students, having attended the university from 2000 to 2005. In addition, 25% had attended between 1991 and 1999, and 13% had attended from 1985 to 1990. The 262 students who had identified their hearing loss when they enrolled at Griffith University in the 20-year period were surveyed to ascertain the nature of their career and workplace experiences since graduation.

The survey had questions about respondents' primary means of communication (such as spoken English, Australian Sign Language, signed English), cultural/linguistic affiliations (hearing, deaf, bicultural), type of school setting in both primary and high school, degree of hearing loss, time in life when hearing loss occurred, and use of hearing aids or cochlear implants. Other questions asked about communication tools used, and DSSP generic and external support services accessed at the university. Open-ended questions asked about major challenges, highlights, and recommendations from their time at the university.

Thirty-one percent of the participants reported their hearing losses as being in the mild/moderate range, 36% in the moderate/severe range, and 33% indicated they had a profound hearing loss. The majority of respondents (68%) reported that spoken English was their primary means of communication in everyday life, and 32% reported that Australian Sign Language was their primary means of communication. Similarly, the majority (60%) identified primarily with a hearing community, whereas 14% identified with a deaf community and 26% reported a bicultural/bilingual (deaf/hearing) identity.

University records showed that of the 262 students who had initially identified as being deaf or hard-of-hearing on enrollment at the university, 41% had completed the degree in which they enrolled. A further 13% were currently enrolled, but with deferred studies. Sixteen percent of students had withdrawn from their studies for personal reasons, and only 2% had been excluded for poor academic performance.

Less than half of the 262 students who identified themselves as being deaf or hard-of-hearing on enrollment at the university during the 20-year period had accessed the DSSP support services. Overall, the program completion rate for the group was 70%. For students who had accessed DSSP services, the completion rate was 76%, and for students who had not used DSSP services, the completion rate was 65%.

Participants strongly indicated that the major reason for their choice of the university was the availability of their desired study program (76%). In addition, 21% reported that their awareness of Griffith University's support services for DHH people was a key reason for their choice.

Twenty-seven of the participants reported having studied teacher education programs at diploma, bachelor's, or master's levels, and it appeared that most of these individuals were working in the field of deaf education. Twenty other programs of study were reported by the remaining respondents, including law, science, arts, social sciences, visual arts, human services, health sciences, communication, multimedia, information technology, and hotel management.

Of the supports offered by the DSSP, the most commonly used was peer note-taking (65%), with a further 19% using laptop computer note-taking. Interpreters were used by 36% of the students and 35% reported having used technological and communication aids, listed as hearing aids, frequency modulation (FM) aids, induction loops, TTYs, Web services, e-mail, and short message service messaging. Other supports such as recording of tutorials, captioned videos, peer support groups, and specialist tutorial assistance were also reported.

The quantitative data on students' use of communication services was elaborated by qualitative data from written responses to questions, one asking about most useful communication tools and the other asking about major challenges experienced with studying at the university. A large number of respondents nominated manual/peer note-taking as the communication support they found most useful. Respondents also mentioned interpreting as a support service they especially appreciated. Typical responses included, "Interpreters are a huge plus—allows for real-time interaction in lectures and tutorials. Note-taking allowed me to watch interpreter. This allowed maximum understanding."

However, several responses pointed out the uneven quality and availability of interpreting and note-taking. In relation to ongoing challenges, the majority of responses came from students who relied on their residual hearing rather than sign language interpreters in classes. These responses described their difficulties in lectures and tutorials. Mentioned frequently were lecturers with "foreign" accents, lecturers speaking indistinctly or not using a microphone, lecturers speaking while walking around the room or writing on the whiteboard, and lecturers not repeating audience responses or questions. In addition, problems associated with poor acoustics and background noise were reported.

Several respondents commented that the social aspects of university life constituted an area of particular difficulty and challenge. Feelings of social isolation were intertwined with academic life and frequently resulted from difficulties in group work situations, as this response illustrates: "The greatest challenge was mixing with peers— other students—trying not to remain isolated; this was always the challenge. You learn a lot from others and the sharing. Assignments in teams were hard." Others reflected on their experience more positively:

> [Because of] the support provided to me [FM, note-taking, interpreting and social–emotional support], I didn't spend so much time trying to catch up on what I missed and so had spare time to actually relax and not be so tired. For once, I actually felt like I was intelligent rather than not very bright and having to study so much harder to understand what others understood with ease.

In terms of graduate outcomes, 77% of respondents were working and 29% were current postgraduate students or out of the workforce as a result of family responsibilities. Their fields of work were closely aligned with their original fields of study and included teaching, government departments, private sector, and self-employment. Seventy-nine percent reported their first job, and 58% reported their current job, was related to their field of university study.

A range of difficulties in the work place was reported, mostly in situations when spoken communication was required, performance evaluations, supervision of others, workplace noise, and lack of necessary accommodations. Deaf workers reported more difficulties than those with effective spoken communication. Others reported that some people at work responded to them as if they were "rude or stupid" or "abrupt and loud" because of the effect of their hearing loss on their spoken communication (see Chapter 17).

Clearly there is much to be done by the university in preparing for transition to the vocational sector in terms of perceived direct and indirect discrimination. It was noted that a greater proportion (than the general Australian population) of these graduates were working in self-employed situations because to their perceived difficulties in communication and noisy environments.

It is interesting to note that more than of the students who reported their hearing losses at enrollment did not use the services of the DSSP. It may be that some of these individuals did not consider they needed help, especially if they had received little assistance at school. The students who used the DSSP showed a slightly higher rate of program completion and lower levels of withdrawal and deferral from their study programs, suggesting a benefit to students who availed themselves of the support services.

Although it is difficult to compare exactly the Griffith DHH students with national and other Griffith University groups, the overall rate of completion of 70% for this group of students during the past 20 years is comparable with the retention and completion rates for other students in undergraduate studies—that is, about 75% year-to-year retention and 70% program completion. In other words, the support services were a sound "investment."

The wide range of fields of study, from education to law, health to hotel management, suggested that these DHH people were not allowing their hearing losses to circumscribe their career aspirations and choices at this stage. It was reported by those in the workplace that their experiences at Griffith were critical for their sustained employment.

Analysis of workplace experiences identified a strong pattern of sustained employment within fields of study. There was, however, a narrower range of workplaces than those apparent within the general Australian population, and lower rates of in-work promotion. A number of attitudinal, environmental, and communication barriers remain within many Australian workplaces. It was also notable that few of the DHH workers sought workplace accommodations, suggesting that part of their university programs could well focus on self-advocacy strategies and study-to-work transition.

Overall, there was strong and effective engagement displayed academically, socially, and vocationally by the DHH students enrolled at this university. Since this study was conducted almost 10 years ago (Hyde et al., 2009) and the reported success of the DSSP at Griffith, most other universities in Australia have developed a range of support services for DHH students.

A CASE IN GREECE

Most research regarding the academic inclusion of DHH students in higher education has taken place in institutions with specialized support services and has indicated that DHH learners have mixed experiences regarding their academic participation. However, there is diversity in the nature and range of support services across different countries. In Greece, for example, national legislation and policy do not mandate designated support services for DHH students in higher education. Therefore, few higher education institutions provide support services, and rely primarily on volunteer participation, because institutions have limited or no budget provision for these services.

Considering the growing number of DHH students seeking or gaining access to Greek higher education institutions and the poor support services available, a study was conducted to examine the perspectives and experiences of these DHH individuals regarding their academic inclusion in higher education across Greece. Participants were 19 DHH students from 10 higher educational institutions from four cities in Greece. Of these institutions, two universities had accessibility centers for DHH students. The students' views were elicited with a semistructured interview developed from a review of the literature regarding the access of DHH students to higher education (Foster et al., 1999; Hyde et al., 2009; Lang, 2002; Stinson et al., 1996). Data were analyzed qualitatively and the identification of broad themes was guided by the research questions, and "middle-order" categories and subcategories (Dey, 1993) emerged from the students' comments.

The findings presented in this section concern the DHH participants' experiences in relation to the type and level of support they received toward their academic inclusion. This was not an intervention study, but part of an ongoing study that explores the views and perspectives of the DHH students. Based on the qualitative data analysis four broad themes are presented in this section—namely, the types of support, the role of the teachers, the role of interpreters, and the role of peers in the academic inclusion of DHH students in higher education in Greece.

To gain access to the lectures and enhance their inclusion, DHH students used diverse sources of support, including notes from their teachers and other students, tutoring, and Greek Sign Language (GSL) interpreting during classes. Rather than relying on any single type of support, most used a combination to attempt to obtain their best outcome:

> The interpreter helps, I also get some notes from my co-students and my teachers and I also do tutorials in maths. I go together with the interpreter to the teacher's office for individual tutorials rather than going to his lecture because I do not understand anything there. There is an interpreter 3 days per week, Tuesday, Thursday and Friday. Also, I met a deaf student at the second year who gives me her notes that she has from the first year. Also, there is another student from my class who will help me if I ask her to.

The participants commented on the important role of teachers who applied techniques that responded to their communication needs and enhanced their access during the lectures:

> There was a teacher who asked me to sit at the front and she also tried to keep visual contact with me and did not move. Some teachers

speak more carefully than others, especially the ones who also had deaf students in the past. Some teachers come close to me and ask me questions to check whether I understand, they repeat to me some things, they may ask my co-students to give me notes.

Also, the students referred to teachers' support after their lectures:

> If I do not understand something, I go to the teacher and ask her. I never ask something during the lecture because there are many students, it is very noisy and the teacher will not understand me. Some teachers dedicate more time to me than to my co-students. For example they explain to me in detail how to do an assignment.

Candidate interpreters played a key role in communication for the 13 students who knew GSL. Candidate interpreters enhanced the academic access of the students during and after lectures; some students received individual tutoring with their teachers, during which their interpreters were always present.

> I do not care that the teacher walks all the time and does not watch me because I have my interpreter. If my interpreter cannot come I do not go to the lectures. I go together with the interpreter to the teacher's office for individual tutorials rather than going to his lecture because I do not understand anything there.

However, a few students underlined some of the difficulties that occurred because interpreters were not specialized in specific fields:

> The interpreters help but they cannot interpret correctly if they have not the specific knowledge. When the content of the lectures have very specialized vocabulary it is very difficult for the interpreters. There is no way to translate maths, computer language and such things. Therefore, some interpreters may quit and at the end I have no interpreter.

All the DHH students interviewed reported that other students supported them, either by taking notes or providing individual tutorials after the lectures. Some students were appointed by the university as peer tutors, where accessibility centers provided such services.

> There is a student who is my peer tutor and helps me a lot to do the assignments, to study during the exams. There are two students who are learning GSL and they help me. Also, my peer tutor helps me during the lectures. When I do not understand something she might explain it to me. She helps me during the lectures and also we met after the lectures to discuss issues that I do not understand.

Based on the findings of the study to date, the DHH students' academic inclusion was highly dependent on teachers, peer tutors, and candidate interpreters who were reported as being supportive in diverse and complementary ways. The students also commented on the positive role of teachers who, in agreement with previous studies (Lang et al., 1993, 1994; Marschark et al., 2002, 2005; Marschark & Wauters, 2008; Powell et al., 2013), tried to adjust their teaching to the communication and learning needs of DHH students during lectures. The teachers who supported the DHH participants after the lectures by providing individual tutoring, were most valued. One participant, for example, preferred to attend only these tutorials, instead of attending lectures. As stressed in previous studies, tutoring is a valuable service for supporting the academic access of DHH students (Lang, 2002; Lang et al., 2004; Orlando et al., 1997; Stinson, 1987). However, in Greece, there are no official positions for such tutors in universities and no associated tutor training. For participants in this study, any extra tutoring offered by the lecturers or by student peers helped to clarify issues during or after the lectures. Peer tutors can play a dynamic role in the inclusion of DHH students in higher education, but the effectiveness of peer tutoring in supporting students' access and learning is associated with their training and course knowledge (Colvin, 2007; Hyde et al., 2009; Nikolaraizi et al., 2013; Osguthorpe, 1976).

Last, the role of candidate interpreters was reported to be critical to participants' academic access and engagement during lectures as well as during individual tutoring with teachers. However, the DHH participants emphasized that interpreting was not effective when the lectures used specialized vocabulary—for example, mathematics terminology. The need for highly qualified and experienced sign language interpreters with specific subject knowledge of the lecture material has been stressed in previous studies (Marschark et al., 2005; Napier & Barker, 2004). This is a challenge in many countries, but in Greece it remains a major barrier for effective academic engagement. The interpreters identified in this study were candidate GSL interpreters who were doing their practicum at university, as part of their training, during which they were not allowed to be paid. In Greece, it is not mandatory to employ GSL interpreters in higher education institutions or other levels of education, and the government does not finance such positions. As a result of the lack of funding and agreed position descriptions, there are only about 80 qualified GSL interpreters in the entire country. These interpreters have other jobs and may only work as university GSL interpreters on a part-time basis. Therefore, even if there was funding for qualified GSL interpreters, it would remain difficult to find experienced GSL interpreters in higher education who also have the subject knowledge necessary to interpret fully and accurately.

In conclusion, this Greek study found that significant goodwill and commitment were apparent among university staff, peer students, and DHH students themselves. In the absence of professional-level appointments and associated funding, the DHH participants reported in this study valued the support of their teachers, volunteer peer-tutors, and candidate interpreters who enabled them to gain some academic access, participate in their studies, and engage with academic challenges. Although the role of volunteering is important, DHH students in higher education have the right in an inclusive education model to professional support services to enhance their access, increase their participation in classes, and ensure their academic and social outcomes are successfully so they may become proficient vocationally and professionally.

At this stage, there is a need for the development of a legal and policy framework that requires universities to develop support centers and provide specific support services for DHH students, such as interpreting and tutoring, as well as technological support (such as real-time captioning), which was not mentioned by students in this study. Furthermore, if there was such a legal framework, universities in which DHH students are enrolled would be better positioned to seek funding from government sources as well sponsorships or grants from sources within the private sector or through European or other international organizations.

A CASE IN NEW ZEALAND

In New Zealand, DHH students are now entering higher education in larger numbers than ever before. A study by Powell (2011) examined the learning and social participation experiences of DHH students in New Zealand higher education settings. The majority of DHH students in New Zealand attend postsecondary institutions where there are few other DHH students, with most institutions reporting fewer than 10 deaf and 20 hard-of-hearing students. Furthermore, specialist support services for the few DHH students enrolled in any particular institution are frequently not provided. Instead, each institution's generic disability support offices attempt to assess DHH students' needs and provide a range of resources.

A key feature of the study by Powell (2011) was an examination of the transition process from the compulsory and inclusive years of secondary schooling to higher education. Transitioning from secondary school to higher education is particularly difficult for students with disabilities, with many students leaving high school without the self-advocacy skills they need to learn to survive in tertiary education (Eckes & Ochoa, 2005; Fiedler & Danneker, 2007; Madaus, 2005). Several studies have emphasized the need for transition programs aimed specifically at DHH students because of the unique needs these students have before starting their postsecondary studies (Bonds, 2003; Garay, 2003; Kolvitz & Wilcox, 2002; Punch et al., 2005).

Punch and Hyde (2005), in an Australian study, shed light on students' social self-concepts and the way in which these interacted with their career aspirations and thoughts about occupational futures. These authors suggested that a loss of confidence in social interactions may have transferred to the students' career decision making. In addition, Stinson and Walter (1997) suggested that strong career decision-making skills were likely to reduce the rate of noncompletion of university degrees among this population. Consistent with this suggestion, Punch et al. (2006) found that DHH young people circumscribed their career options prematurely based on their beliefs about what occupations they would be able to undertake, thus affecting their future study options in higher education.

The New Zealand research had a national focus and included 64 students studying at 13 postsecondary institutions. The gender split in the study was male (36%) and female (64%). Using a mixed-methods design, quantitative and qualitative methods were applied in a manner that allowed the broader features of participants' experiences to be identified and examined in a written survey, and individual perspectives to be reflected through their responses to open-ended questions and interviews (Morse & Richards, 2002).

The survey was informed by studies undertaken at Rochester Institute of Technology, which includes the NTID (Foster et al., 1999), and an Australian study (Hyde et al., 2009) that examined students' access to academic information and the students' sense of belonging and engagement in the postsecondary environment. Fixed-choice questions gathered demographic data, including age, gender, current educational qualifications, preferred method(s) of communication, and primary cultural/linguistic affiliation. Open-ended questions asked participants to describe highlights and barriers they encountered during the postsecondary setting as well as any recommendations they may have to give DHH students thinking about postsecondary study.

Eight of the 64 participants were selected for interviews, using maximum variation sampling, which selects cases from the widest possible range across the sample "to ensure strength and richness to the data, their applicability, and their interpretation" (Cohen et al., 2007, p. 115). Furthermore, using this form of sampling enabled the diversity within this DHH student population to be captured. During semistructured interviews, these participants were asked about their perception of their academic, social, and emotional readiness for postsecondary education.

One aspect of successful and meaningful transition from secondary school to higher education is an understanding or knowledge about different careers and preparation for study. Many participants reported receiving little or no advice about building a degree that would be beneficial to a career path, or knowing what to expect or how to access appropriate support. In hindsight, one student said:

> I definitely wasn't prepared at all. I didn't know what was going to happen. I had just left school so I hadn't really found my path I don't think and I was just carrying on doing something that I enjoyed. It wasn't a really good year for me.

Students reported that before undertaking higher education they felt academically prepared, but found that reality was somewhat different. Many students knew what teachers expected of them in high school and knew how to be successful academically. Comments such as, "I needed to work much harder to get the same results" or "Studying independently—there was no one I could look to for a while," were typical of many responses, and illustrated some of the differences that exist for all students between secondary school and higher education, not just those who are DHH.

The qualitative findings indicated that the ability of students to advocate on their own behalf and knowledge of how to access and use services were critical factors in improving their tertiary education experience.

> Ummm, well at school things were a wee bit different. There was a disability support person so she did everything. Whereas, at university I had to organize everything.

There was also a feeling among participants that if they did not ask for services, they would not be offered.

> I mean a friend of mine was saying "oh there's no interpreters" and I was saying "why don't you talk to the office?" They knew it was the office's job to do it but you have to be assertive to get them on to doing it. A lot of deaf people sort of just stand back. They don't want to make a fuss.

Of those students who had declared their hearing status on enrollment, 15% did not make use of the disability coordinator, or services of the disability support office, and these findings are consistent with earlier studies (e.g., Hyde et al., 2009; Luckner, 2002). Reasons identified for this nonuse included some students admitting they had not fully understood what their specific needs were or did not always have the necessary knowledge, skills, or confidence to advocate their own needs in this new environment.

> I had a new FM after school. . . . but I didn't want to walk up at the front of the lecture and put it in front of the lecturer. I realized later that that was because I thought uni was the same as school, but it wasn't. Therefore, the obstacles were greater than I had imagined so. . . .

I found asking for help and the support I needed difficult as I felt I should have known these things before starting.

This study's findings suggest that assisting prospective higher education students to source appropriate information about study programs and support services available, when they are making decisions about future study options, could increase their chances of successful transition and their initial forays into higher education.

The study also found there was a lack of knowledge about newer technology, such as speech-to-text or real-time captioning, in that there was minimal reported use of technology such as electronic note-taking (21%), speech-to-text translation, and video conferencing (13%) by participants. Often, exposure to such potentially advantageous technology did not occur when the students were at high school and, furthermore, it appeared from some interviewees' reactions to probes about other forms of technology they often were not informed about what assistive technology options might be available to them and did not know to ask for them, as this profoundly deaf oral student's response illustrates: "Wow! No, I have never heard of those. I have never been offered anything like that. That sounds really good!"

The findings that the disability support offices did not offer use of such technology routinely is disappointing, given that various technologies have the ability to provide environments that are more accessible for those who are DHH. As Lang (2002) emphasized, there is a necessity for postsecondary programs to stay abreast of new technologies and be innovative in incorporating technology into the curriculum to achieve students' greater inclusion and engagement.

Participants described a variety of solutions they had implemented, including self-advocacy and self-reliance, ensuring they knew the supports to which they were entitled, and what was available to them in terms of human resources and technological aids. Participants viewed educating other students and staff about deafness, and having the perseverance to see things through to completion, as important.

> My parents always told me I could do anything I wanted; they encouraged me to try things, and this is what I did. This helped to build a sense of esteem and confidence that helped me to push past barriers that I, and others, inadvertently put in the way.

Students further identified the need to disclose their hearing status to staff and students to gain understanding and appropriate assistance, and to make participation academically and socially a better experience. Underlying this was the need for strong self-advocacy skills and self-belief, because these are a key part of empowerment for these students.

In terms of academic readiness and transition to postsecondary study, many students found the progression from secondary school to postsecondary study challenging, and initial concerns about study skills, time management, exams, and achieving good marks were commonplace. These findings reflected those of earlier researchers (Eckes & Ochoa, 2005; Fiedler & Danneker, 2007; Madaus, 2005) who reported that many participants left school without the self-advocacy skills they needed to negotiate higher education systems. Similar to Gardynik's (2008) findings on parental support for postsecondary students with learning disabilities, the findings in the current study revealed instances of parental support in advocating within the higher education system. At a time in their lives when young people generally are developing greater independence from parents, it would be preferable if DHH students were better equipped before finishing high school to advocate on their own behalf.

In line with earlier studies (Danermark et al., 2001; Punch et al., 2005; Schroedel, 1991, 1992), students interviewed in the current study described their difficulties making career choices, their limited knowledge of occupations, and their perceptions of barriers related to their hearing loss. In New Zealand, the area of transition from secondary school to further education, training, or employment for DHH students is addressed in a decidedly ad hoc fashion and largely falls to the teacher of the deaf (ToD) and/or advisor on deaf children who work with the students in compulsory school settings (Logan, 1995). Hyde and Power (2004) studied itinerant ToDs in Australia, and McKee and Smith (2004) surveyed itinerant teachers in New Zealand. Both studies reported that itinerant teachers had very little time to collaborate with other professionals, including career advisors and guidance counselors. Therefore, DHH students may not be getting the best advice, or support, in terms of planning their future options. Given that career-planning skills can reduce the high rate of noncompletion of higher education courses by DHH students (Stinson & Walter, 1997), this lack of guidance and support is potentially significant for this group of students.

The survey data showed that most students in this study (60%) had not received regular ToD support during their secondary schooling. One could surmise that a lack of ToD support during their secondary schooling influenced these students' feelings of independence and perceptions about the assistance they would require accessing the postsecondary learning environment. Certainly, some students spoke about their unpreparedness for study and not understanding the accommodations that were potentially available to them. The findings thus identified that failure to access such supports meant some students had negative results and experiences when commencing postsecondary education. The findings reinforce the need for transition programs specifically aimed at DHH students and their teachers as a result of the unique needs they have in postsecondary studies (Bonds, 2003; Garay, 2003; Kolvitz & Wilcox, 2002; Punch et al., 2004, 2005). Students who accessed support services when they commenced postsecondary study had to make the switch from being passive recipients of support in high school to active consumers of support services at this level. As in Sameshima's (1999) findings, many students in this study had little or no training in how to use supports such as note-takers or interpreters and, consequently, had to learn quickly how to work effectively with such support staff.

It is imperative that future students arrive at higher education understanding the differences between high school and postsecondary education, and with the necessary skills to negotiate the higher education environment. The years immediately before leaving school may be the optimum time in which to educate students so they are well prepared with knowledge and skills, thus enabling them to make the best use of the resources that can be provided at the postsecondary level. In conclusion, the study findings related to transition indicated that strong self-advocacy skills, an understanding of their own learning styles and needs, and being familiar with the range of resources available, including new technology, were critically influential to New Zealand DHH students' learning and participation experiences when they commenced postsecondary study. Being able to self-identify support needs confidently and knowledgeably was a valuable skill and often one that students had not been required to implement at secondary school.

Although this study was undertaken in 2010/2011, it is the only one to date that has examined the transition process for DHH students in New Zealand, and the issues identified are still relevant today (pers. comm., 2014). The way support services are provided to this diverse population has not changed since the study, and the use and knowledge of various technological supports have not altered. There is still no specific transition planning for DHH students available nationally.

DHH students need assistance to develop these skills before entering higher education and, therefore, decisions should be made about whose role it is to ensure these students do not "fall through the cracks." An increased awareness within compulsory education of DHH students' academic and social needs before transitioning to higher education must be at the forefront of any move toward inclusive education at the postsecondary level, where both deaf and hearing students are equal participants.

A CASE IN THE UNITED STATES

The NTID is a college of Rochester Institute of Technology (RIT), established in 1965 to provide DHH students with technical and professional education programs, complemented by a strong liberal arts and sciences curriculum, to prepare them to live and work in the mainstream of a rapidly changing global community. The case presented here examines an important communication technology developed at NTID, the C-Print real-time captioning service that is used to facilitate communication access of DHH students at RIT and at other institutions of higher education.

Increasingly, DHH students attend college with hearing peers in mainstream settings. Of the 25,000 DHH students in postsecondary education in the United States, more than 23,000 are enrolled in programs with primarily hearing students (Gallaudet Research Institute, 2007; McGinnis & Stefanich, 2007; Newman, 2006; Richardson et al., 2010). Despite their motivation to attend postsecondary education programs, graduation rates for DHH students are low. Nationally, 25% to 30% of these students receive either a 2- or 4-year degree (Cawthon et al., 2014). When DHH students participate in classes with hearing students, they often have difficulty understanding the speaker and other participants. Access services help DHH individuals understand the participants who speak.

One reason that providing appropriate access services is difficult is that DHH students have diverse communication needs. Some DHH students use sign language. Other students rely on speech-reading and a hearing aid or cochlear implant and know little sign language. Another challenge is the setting: DHH students' communication access needs may be different for a history class and a business meeting. Real-time captioning, also called *speech-to-text*, is one way to provide communication access for DHH students. Other options for communication access are sign language interpreting and note-taking.

With real-time captioning, a service provider (called a *captionist*), who is often in the classroom or other setting with the DHH individual produces text as it is being spoken by a presenter (such as a teacher) and displays it on a device so the DHH student can understand what is happening in the class, meeting, and so on. For the past 25 years, a group of researchers and developers at NTID has been developing the C-Print real-time captioning system (Stinson et al., 2008, 2014). The C-Print captioning technology is used to produce a text display of spoken information for students who are DHH (or other individuals who may have difficulty understanding speech). Usually, C-Print is the only accommodation the student receives if there is only one DHH student in the class. If there is more than one DHH student, there are often other accommodations, such as an interpreter.

One of the latest and ongoing developments of the C-Print group has been to enable viewing of a display of C-Print captions on mobile devices such as tablets. The work described here has involved field trials in college-level science, technology, engineering, and mathematics (STEM) classes where DHH students use C-Print for communication access. This work currently is examining effects of using C-Print

Mobile on students' self-reported communication and motivation in STEM laboratory courses.

The new C-Print Mobile app allows users to view captioning in a variety of settings—for example, in traditional classrooms, labs, and meetings. Users can also use the Mobile app to view captioning in remote settings, such as a classroom field trip. C-Print Mobile was developed in part to incorporate advances in technology, such as wide use of iPads other tablet devices and smartphones, and to enable C-Print to meet DHH communication access needs effectively in situations when it has not been possible to provide effective services with standard laptops. For example, in laboratory settings, lab tables often have considerable paraphernalia, and a laptop for viewing captions takes up a good deal of table space.

In situations such as a laboratory setting, one way of delivery of captions, such as use of C-Print Mobile on a relative small, mobile device, may be more effective than another form of delivery, such as on a standard laptop, for facilitating student comprehension of information. Use of the smaller, more portable device may contribute to comprehension because student users can place the device more easily on a cluttered lab table where they can easily shift visual attention between the captions and laboratory work than they can with a standard laptop that needs to be placed in a less desirable location. Furthermore, quality of communication in such settings such as laboratories may be relevant to STEM interest and motivation for DHH students because these students' views of their communication experiences are likely to be closely associated with their actual commitment to a STEM major and career. If these students do not feel they understand well what is happening in a class, including the laboratory section, then they are unlikely to feel they are in control of outcomes associated with performance in that situation and they are unlikely to be engaged in learning—that is, they will show little motivation (Stinson & Whitmire, 2000). Students with little motivation may not persist in their STEM major because they do not make the necessary commitment and put forth the necessary effort.

The purpose of the research described here was to examine effects of students' use of C-Print Mobile in laboratory sections of STEM courses. The dimensions of interest were student-rated quality of communication and participation in the laboratory section of the course, motivation for the laboratory section of the course, and students' confidence and interest in their STEM major. In addition, the study included qualitative interviews with students to obtain additional perceptions regarding communication and STEM interests, and to identify student perceptions regarding use of C-Print Mobile that may relate to communication and interests.

The 67 student participants were enrolled in diverse STEM laboratory courses in which all, or almost all, the other students in the course had normal hearing. More females than males participated. They were 17 to 25 years of age, except for two who were 26 to 35 years of age. All the participants were enrolled in a STEM major or interested in entering a STEM major. They were enrolled in either an upper division laboratory course or a course that is attended primarily by students who will enter a STEM major (e.g., organic chemistry) and for which C-Print services are available at a university in the northeastern United States (55 participants) or in a university in the Southeast or the Midwest, or in a community college in the Midwest (12 participants). Most of the participants were at the northeastern university because it has a large population of DHH students in classes with hearing students, of whom a relatively large proportion are enrolled in STEM majors, and because it has a large C-Print service that serves many students. All study participants had requested C-Print services for the laboratory course for communication access. Typically students who request the service are familiar with it and have used it previously.

To provide C-Print services to the study participants, a trained transcriptionist used computerized abbreviations primarily based on phonetic rules (C-Print uses a standard QWERTY keyboard) and condensing strategies to produce the text display of spoken information. At almost the same time, the spoken information was displayed on a computer or mobile device. The content was saved and distributed as a transcript afterward. The C-Print captionist is trained to include all information being said in producing the text display. C-Print Mobile is the app that students used to view C-Print real-time captions on mobile devices. It is a free download from the Apple iTunes and Google Play stores.

To assess student participants' perceptions of their experience with viewing C-Print captions with a laptop (comparison group) or mobile device, each student responded to an online survey that included questions about student demographics, communication preferences, and experiences in a prior laboratory course. The survey also asked about experiences in the current course, such as communication ease, confidence to complete the course, and motivation to remain in STEM given the access service (C-Print Mobile or traditional C-Print on a standard laptop). These questions included one that asked students to rate how much of the lab instructor's comments they thought they understood on a scale of seven response alternatives that ranged from 0 (0%–20% understanding) to 6 (90%–100% understanding). A second question asked students to rate the extent to which using C-Print Mobile helped them feel confident they could succeed in their laboratory class. A third question asked them to rate the extent to which using C-Print Mobile would help them complete their major. Students rated these two questions on a 5-point scale that went from "strongly disagree" to "strongly agree." The survey also included the following open-ended question: If you have other things to tell us about using C-Print on a cell phone, please do so here. Responses to the question were analyzed qualitatively (Bogdan & Biklen, 2007).

The study used an experimental design in which courses were assigned randomly to a C-Print Mobile device group (n = 36; 31 from the northeastern university and 5 from the midwestern or southeastern institutions) or to a comparison (standard laptop) group (n = 31; 26 from a northeastern university and 5 from the Midwest or Southeast). There was a wide range of different laboratory courses for the comparison group and also for the mobile group. The project conducted multiple trials in a number of these courses, which ranged from biology to engineering. Project staff working with student disability services offices at the four participating campuses identified laboratory courses in which students had requested C-Print support services for the course. The identification took place about 3 weeks after the start of the marking period, so that schedules would be stabilized. Students were contacted and invited to participate. When students agreed to participate, they were randomized *by course* to either a mobile trial or a comparison group. Students completed a survey near the conclusion of the academic term.

For the trials that involved C-Print Mobile, regular C-Print captionists who worked at one of the four participating campuses delivered the captions. Captionists used their regular laptop computers and the campus wireless network to transmit the real-time captioning to students' mobile devices. Students viewed the display on the mobile devices. A member of the research team accompanied the captionist to the classroom and was responsible for connecting each mobile device to the C-Print display. Throughout the laboratory class, the research team member monitored the mobile devices, reconnecting them (if necessary), and maintained a log, documenting any technical issues that arose during class. For students in the C-Print Mobile group, each student participant in the class was assigned a specific mobile device that was distributed at the beginning of each laboratory session and collected at the end of the session. Mobile devices used included the Apple iPad2, Apple iPad Mini, and various Android devices such as the Samsung Galaxy Tab. Screen quality, screen size (4.3 inches as the minimum acceptable size), and the mobile device operating system were criteria used to select the devices.

Students in the comparison group viewed the C-Print display on a standard laptop. To determine the effects of C-Print Mobile on students' perceptions of communication and interest in a STEM career, mean ratings of understanding of the laboratory instructor for the C-Print Mobile and for the comparison group were compared. In addition, the mean ratings of confidence in succeeding in their laboratory course and in completing their major were compared for the two groups. With respect to understanding the instructor, students in the C-Print Mobile group perceived the instructor as easier to understand than students in the comparison group. The mean rating for students in the C-Print Mobile group was 5.27 (standard deviation [SD] = 0.85) and that for the comparison group was 4.39 (SD = 1.33). These mean ratings are equivalent to rated percentages of understanding of 83% for the C-Print Mobile group and 74% for the comparison group. A between-group *t*-test indicated the difference was statistically significant. For the question on confidence in completing their (STEM) major, use of C-Print Mobile, in contrast to using C-Print on a laptop, seemed to increase students' confidence that they could succeed in their major. Students in the C-Print Mobile group agreed more strongly with the statement that having C-Print would help them succeed in their major (mean = 4.19, SD = 0.78, n = 36) than students in the comparison group (mean = 3.96, SD = 0.71, n = 31); however, the difference was not statistically significant. Students in the C-Print Mobile group also agreed more strongly with the statement they were likely to succeed in class (mean = 4.05, SD = 0.75, n = 36) than those in the comparison group (mean = 3.96, SD = 0.71, n = 31), a difference that also was not statistically significant.

In addition, students were given the opportunity to comment about the C-Print service they received. Students who received the C-Print Mobile trials made some specific comments about the devices they used. These comments were associated with three themes: size, portability, and readability. Sample quotes from participants in the Mobile trials arranged according to theme include the following:

- *Size*: "The size of the mobile device was really convenient. I was able to have more space with the mobile device and computer I was using for class" (Advanced Computational Techniques). "It wasn't so bulky on the lab bench; I was allowed a lot more room to do my work" (Molecular Biology).
- *Portability*: "It was portable and could be moved with me" (General Biology). "It was definitely much more portable, and easier; was not heavy to carry like the laptop" (Molecular Biology). "I was able to carry it around the lab with me, to hold it in my hand while the instructor is talking, and was able to scroll up and down to see what was previously said" (Molecular Biology).
- *Readability*: "It was easy to read, especially white on black makes it easier. The print was big enough for me to sit back and read" (Molecular Biology).

The DHH students in STEM laboratory classes responded more positively to C-Print caption displays on a mobile device than on a standard laptop. This finding supports the proposition that when captioning technology has features that may make it a better accommodation in a specific educational setting, this improvement increases students' comprehension of communications. The accommodation issue here is that standard laptops are awkward to use in laboratories because they take up too much table space and are not sufficiently mobile. Results suggested that students while may be more confident they will be successful when they use a mobile device; however, differences between mean ratings for the two groups were not statistically significant in this current study.

Students' comments on the open-ended question suggest reasons why students with C-Print Mobile gave higher ratings of comprehension for the course. Students stated that the small size, greater portability, and easily read display of the mobile device benefited them in laboratory settings. Students' comprehension ratings may have been associated with these perceptions.

CONCLUSIONS AND LOOKING AHEAD

The cases presented here reflect the national, social, economic, and technological contexts in which each is embedded at this point in time. There are, however, a number of common themes evident among the needs expressed by students, the support services provided, the university staff involved, and the outcomes achieved.

First, it is clear that all four nations, having ratified the UN Convention on the Rights of People with Disability (2006), are attempting to open access to their higher education systems to DHH learners. There is some diversity to be observed perhaps, in the extent to which there is current implementation of all the principles of inclusive education. The transitions observed from access, to participation, to forms of active engagement and, last, to equitable outcomes show variation across the cases. Factors that may constrain or afford implementation of these principles are frequently viewed in economic terms, such as available budget funding, or in legal terms, such as in human rights or antidiscrimination legislation. In these cases, we see that the role of individuals and of institutional initiatives can be important. Some universities can lead the way, and staff within those institutions can establish effective practices despite political, economic, or social constraints. To sustain and systematize these initiatives across the higher education systems is, of course, a major challenge over time.

In addition to common themes, there is evidence among the experiences of the DHH students in the cases described in this chapter, a diversity of needs and interests. Such diversity is to be expected, given the range of national and cultural contexts in which these students live, their individual spoken language and sign language communication proficiencies, their levels of academic preparedness, their self-advocacy skills, the range of technologies available to them, the education systems in which they learn, as well as the normal range of human potential and identity. Responding to the diversity of their needs as individuals remains as great a challenge as institutional and systemic responses to the common trends identified in studies such as the ones described earlier.

Sign Language Interpreters

There is a need expressed to provide skilled sign language interpreters for those students who use sign language who also have knowledge of the fields of study involved. Being a skilled interpreter, but without such knowledge, can create a major limitation to student learning. Also evident is a continuing problem with workforce issues related to finding enough interpreters with such skills and knowledge, and the potential for these key staff to find adequately remunerated careers in their field. Schick et al. (2006) pointed out the need for more skilled interpreters and stressed that interpreters with weak signing skills might modify or distort the conceptual components of instruction, thus impeding DHH students' access to learning. Additional factors, which might also affect the level and outcome of interpreting on DHH students' learning, apart from the important role of interpreters' skills, include the challenges DHH students face in monitoring and evaluating their own comprehension through an interpreted lecture and the instructors' capacities to respond to the learning needs of DHH students, considering the interpreted lectures are largely structured by hearing teachers who usually teach hearing students and therefore have little knowledge and experience in accommodating the learning needs of DHH students (Marschark et al., 2004, 2005, 2008). Interpreting where it is used needs to be provided in combination with other communication and learning support systems to respond to student diversity and also to provide DHH students with multiple sources of information and learning opportunities.

The Use of Technology

An interesting parallel to the shortage of skilled interpreters is seen in the RIT/NTID case, using C-Print where many students are able to access, through relatively inexpensive hand-held devices, accurate, comprehensive real-time classroom discourse through print and to retain this record for further study. This recent extension of the use of C-Print technology at RIT has the capacity to assist all DHH students, regardless of whether they are users of a sign language. Some constraints still exist in the use of such technology, such as availability and cost of trained captionists (whose salary is similar to or less than that of an interpreter) and the literacy levels of the DHH users, but technologies such as C-Print and interactive learning technologies developed within the context of open and distance learning and social media have the capacity to enhance DHH students' access to coursework and increase their independence in higher education learning and social environments. Within the framework of inclusive education, the use of modern technologies, now available more generically and economically, would seem to be a priority. Indeed, although as university staff or administrators we may often lament the lack of funds for such technological applications, many DHH students are solving some issues of social and academic engagement themselves, using Facebook, FaceTime, messaging, Glide, Skype, cloud-share systems (such as Google Docs), and other communication technologies. Deaf people have been shown for many years as being among the earliest adopters of such technologies in their lives (Breivik, 2013). Many universities now use such social media as their default communication software in open and distance learning and teaching environments.

In addition, multinational organizations developing such technologies and their applications may well be open to supporting the learning of DHH students in relation to the corporate social responsibility obligations they need to honor within the various nations and states in which they legally operate. There are many examples of significant funding being made available under corporate social responsibility requirements in developing and developed nations, and this pattern of support could well include DHH students in postsecondary education.

Last, there is considerable scope for universities to work together to create and share online and related resources with countries and across borders in geographic regions. This is not to suggest that technology is the complete answer to the communication and learning needs of DHH students. Although such technologies can increase choice and independence, the role of people and goodwill are paramount in teaching, tutoring, counseling, planning, and evaluating if inclusive education outcomes are to be achieved.

Inclusive Education: Cost or Investment?

As noted earlier, one of the major concerns expressed about achieving greater inclusion of DHH students in higher education is the perceived costs associated with necessary support services and differentiated pedagogies. In many ways this concern reflects a view of education as community cost, rather than an investment in future capacity and economic benefit for all. In this context, the NTID and RIT have, for many years, been able to demonstrate strong national economic benefits in supporting DHH students in higher education. Their long-term tracking studies show the costs of university support services and accommodations of teaching and learning result in economic and vocational benefits nationally and for the individuals involved (Schley et al., 2011). These benefits are well evidenced in increased employment rates, increased earnings and increased tax contributions, and decreased dependency on federal income support programs.

Economic and vocational benefits were also shown in the Australian case presented in this chapter. This case is an example of a particular university taking the initiative to lead nationally and support DHH students with a range of support services and staff development strategies. Such initiative is also seen in the Greek universities' case, where they have established accessibility centers within universities to further inclusive education of DHH students. The Australian university case showed that DHH students graduated from a diversity of fields of study and achieved program completion rates that were equal to or greater than the rates for hearing students nationally. This study also showed high rates of sustained employment in a field of study for up to two decades. Although the human rights of DHH students are justified and served through inclusive higher education systems, collation of economic benefit and outcome data by institutions is important for demonstrating the broader social, academic, and vocational benefits of investment in such systems.

DHH Student Use of Support Services and Transition Implications

Many of the students enrolled at the Australian university did not seek the support services on offer, seemingly because they had not experienced these services during their secondary schooling. This was a conclusion also reached by Powell (2011) in her New Zealand study. Although strong student approval levels were evident for tutorial services, interpreters, note-taking services, and the universities' standard learning support resources, many students remained reticent about asking for support. Therefore, it would appear that either the students did not have the knowledge or the self-advocacy skills required to access or request specific supports to study successfully. The lack of self-advocacy skills among some DHH students might be attributed to the fact that some students with disabilities are brought up and educated in a protective home and school environment where parents or teachers make choices and advocate for them. As a result, when they move to higher education they might expect that support services will be provided to them in a similar way to high school and they might not have skills to self-advocate and ask for support services (Barnard-Brak et al., 2010; Hadley, 2006; Powell et al., 2013). However, support services have a value in furthering the objectives and outcomes of inclusive higher education, and if students do not self-advocate obtaining support services, they may feel excluded, fail, and quit their studies.

Considering the critical role of self-advocacy in the academic inclusion of DHH students, there is a need for primary and secondary school education to offer DHH students opportunities to develop and exercise self-advocacy skills to facilitate the transition from secondary to higher education (Lartz et al., 2008; Luckner 2012). In addition, empowering students so they feel confident about their career options, technology, and their ability to use support services successfully, such as notetakers and interpreters, plays a significant role (Bullard & Luckner, 2013). This learning needs to occur well before any transition to higher education takes place, ideally throughout their compulsory education as appropriate for age and stage.

Hard-of-Hearing Students

Another trend observed in the Australian, U.S., and New Zealand cases regards the support needs for students who are functionally hard of hearing. These students, many now with cochlear implants and other technology-based communication systems, are at times neglected because support provision may focus on interpreting, tutoring, and other services with deaf students in mind. Although no clear dichotomy should be suggested among the diverse range of needs of DHH learners, it is apparent there may be different emphases in their communication and learning needs and, ultimately, individual choices. Systems such as C-Print and other communication technologies are equally applicable for DHH students. Arising from the Australian, New Zealand, and Greek cases, however, is a view that recognition of the potential for technologies to support DHH students is not always filtering down to institutional levels and students themselves. This area needs urgent attention because these technologies have the capacity to alter the learning and lives of DHH students in higher education.

A significant feature of the Greek study is the level of volunteering among staff, teachers, and, more important, DHH students themselves. Such commitment is the foundation on which relevant and effective services are established and diversified. It was also evident in the New Zealand study that the parents and families of the DHH students often accepted roles as advocates and support agents. This is an area that requires greater recognition. These studies also highlight ongoing challenges for many students' participation in class discussion and small-group work, noisy backgrounds in some instruction settings, the quality of interpreting services, and the need for greater institutional policy and budget recognition of the potential of DHH students as learners.

Staff Development

Identified with each of the university cases are approaches that have been used within the universities for staff development. University staff were generally shown to be responsive to having DHH students in their classes, willing to spend extra time assisting them and interested in supporting their inclusion. Structured staff development programs could cover a range of topics, such as the principles of inclusive education, differentiated pedagogies for achieving inclusive education, accommodations of assessment and learning to respond to DHH students' learning styles and competencies, and the use of communication systems and technologies directed toward greater emphasis on visual learning processes. Such staff development should also emphasize the diversity of communication and learning needs among DHH students and avoid a one-size-fits-all orientation toward the provision of greater access and participation in higher education by DHH students.

Another important conclusion that can be drawn from the university cases presented is that DHH students require national responses to their learning needs in higher education. Although one university or a small number of universities may lead the way, as in the U.S., Greek, New Zealand, or Australian cases, all universities have the responsibility to follow and respond with access for DHH students, and academic and communication support toward their graduation and employment.

If the basic principles of inclusive education do not cease at the end of compulsory schooling, DHH students need equitable access to higher education so that their potential and rights may be realized in this sector of learning. However, creating access and participation for DHH students to higher education is only part of inclusive education, and these early steps are not ends in themselves. Authentic evaluation of inclusive higher education for DHH students rests in the quality of the engagement they experience, their sense of belonging in universities and colleges, and, ultimately, the graduate trajectories they create as individuals.

ACKNOWLEDGMENTS

This research was supported in part by grants from the National Science Foundation (awards HRD-072659 and HRD-0726591). C-Print is a registered trademark that belongs to the Rochester Institute of Technology.

REFERENCES

Albertini, J. A., Kelly, R. R., & Matchett, M. K. (2011). Personal factors that influence deaf college students' academic success. *Journal of Deaf Studies and Deaf Education, 17*, 85–101.

Barnard-Brak, L., Lechtenberger, D., & Lan, W. (2010). Accommodation strategies of college students with disabilities. *The Qualitative Report, 15*, 411–429.

Bogdan, R. C., & Biklen, S. K. (2007). *Qualitative research for education* (5th ed.). Boston, MA: Allyn & Bacon.

Bonds, B. G. (2003). School-to-work experiences: Curriculum as a bridge. *American Annals of the Deaf, 148*, 38–48.

Boutin, D. (2008). Persistence in postsecondary environments of students with hearing impairments. *Journal of Rehabilitation, 74*, 25–31.

Breivik, J.-K. (2013). *Deaf identities in the making: Local lives, transnational connections*. Washington, DC: Gallaudet University Press.

Bullard, C., & Luckner, J. L. (2013). *The itinerant teacher's handbook* (2nd ed.). Hillsboro, OR: Butte Publications.

Cawthon, S. W., Schoffstall, S. J., & Garberoglio, C. L. (2014). How ready are postsecondary institutions for students who are d/Deaf or hard-of-hearing? *Education Policy Analysis Archives, 22* [entire volume].

Cohen, L., Manion, L., & Morrison, K. (2007). *Research methods in education* (6th ed.). New York, NY: Routledge.

Colvin, J. W. (2007). Peer tutoring and social dynamics in higher education. *Mentoring & Tutoring, 15*, 165–181.

Danermark, B., Antonson, S., & Lundstrom, I. (2001). Social inclusion and career development - transition from upper secondary school to work or post-secondary education among hard of hearing students. *Scandinavian Audiology, 30*, 120–128.

Dey, I. (1993). *Qualitative data analysis. A user-friendly guide for social scientists*. London; New York, NY: Routledge.

Eckes, S. E., & Ochoa, T. A. (2005). Students with disabilities: Transitioning from high school to higher education. *American Secondary Education, 33*, 6–20.

Fiedler, C. R., & Danneker, J. E. (2007). Self-advocacy instruction: Bridging the research-to-practice gap. *Focus on Exceptional Children, 39*, 1–20.

Foster, S., Long, G., & Snell, K. (1999). Inclusive instruction and learning for deaf students in postsecondary education. *Journal of Deaf Studies and Deaf Education, 4*, 225–235.

Gallaudet Research Institute (2007). *Regional and national summary report of data from the 2006–2007 annual survey of deaf and hard of hearing children and youth*. Washington, DC: GRI Gallaudet University.

Garay, S. V. (2003). Listening to the voices of deaf students: Essential transition issues. *Teaching Exceptional Children, 35*, 44–48.

Gardynik, U. (2008). Defying the odds: Academic resilience of students with learning disabilities. Unpublished doctoral dissertation, University of Alberta, Edmonton, Canada. [abstract]. Retrieved from http://proquest.umi.com/pqdlink?did=1671872341&Fmt=7&clientI d=79356&RQT=309&VName=PQD. Accessed January 26, 2016.

Hadley, W. M. (2006). L.D. students' access to higher education: Self-advocacy and support. *Journal of Developmental Education, 30*, 10–16.

Hyde, M. B., & Power, D. J. (2004). Inclusion of deaf students: An examination of definitions of inclusion in relation to findings of a recent Australian study of deaf students in regular classes. *Deafness and Education International, 6*, 82–99.

Hyde, M., Punch, R., Power, D., Hartley, J., Neale, J., & Brennan, L. (2009). The experiences of deaf and hard of hearing students at a Queensland University: 1985–2005. *Higher Education Research and Development, 28*, 85–98.

Kolvitz, M., & Wilcox, H. D. (2002). Gates to adventure: Transition to post-secondary training for deaf and hard-of-hearing students [electronic version]. Paper presented at the Tenth Biennial Conference on Postsecondary Education for Persons who are Deaf or Hard of Hearing. Knoxville, TN.

Lang, H. G. (2002). Higher education for deaf students: Research priorities in the new millennium. *Journal of Deaf Studies and Deaf Education, 7*, 267–280.

Lang, H., Biser, E., Mousley, K., Orlando, R., & Porter, P. (2004). Tutoring deaf students in higher education: A comparison of baccalaureate and sub-baccalaureate student perceptions. *Journal of Deaf Studies and Deaf Education, 9*, 189–201.

Lang, H. G., Dowaliby, F. J., & Anderson H. P. (1994). Critical teaching incidents: Recollections of deaf college students. *American Annals of the Deaf, 139*, 119–127.

Lang, H. G., McKee, B. G., & Conner, K. (1993). Characteristics of effective teachers: A descriptive study of the perceptions of faculty and deaf college students. *American Annals of the Deaf, 138*, 252–259.

Lartz, M. N., Stoner, J. B., & Stout, L. (2008). Perspectives of assistive technology from Deaf students at a hearing university. *Assistive Technology Outcomes and Benefits, 5*, 72–91.

Logan, S. (1995). *Deaf and hearing impaired students: Access to postsecondary education.* Auckland, New Zealand: National Foundation for the Deaf.

Luckner, J. L. (2002). *Facilitating the transition of students who are deaf or hard of hearing.* Austin, TX: Pro-Ed.

Luckner, J. L. (2012). Transition education for adolescents who are deaf or hard of hearing. In M. L. Wehmeyer & K. W. Webb (Eds.), *Handbook of transition for youth with disabilities* (pp. 417–438). New York, NY: Routledge, Taylor & Francis Group.

Madaus, J. W. (2005). Navigating the college transition maze: A guide for students with learning disabilities. *Teaching Exceptional Children, 37*, 32–37.

Marschark, M., Lang, H. G., & Albertini, J. A. (2002). *Educating deaf students: From research to practice.* Oxford: Oxford University Press.

Marschark, M., Sapere, P., Convertino, C. M., & Pelz, J. (2008). Learning via direct and mediated instruction by deaf students. *Journal of Deaf Studies and Deaf Education, 13*, 446–461.

Marschark, M., Sapere, P., Convertino, C., & Seewagen, R. (2005). Access to postsecondary education through sign language interpreting. *Journal of Deaf Studies and Deaf Education, 10*, 38–50.

Marschark, M., Sapere, P., Convertino, C., Seewagen, R., & Maltzen, H. (2004). Comprehension of sign language interpreting: Deciphering a complex task situation. *Sign Language Studies, 4*, 345–368.

Marschark, M., & Wauters, L. (2008). Language comprehension and learning by deaf children. In M. Marschark & P. C. Hauser (Eds.), *Deaf cognition: Foundations and outcomes* (pp. 309–350). New York, NY: Oxford University Press.

McGinnis, J. R., & Stefanich, G. P. (2007). Special needs and talents in science learning. In S. K. Abell & N. G. Lederman (Eds.), *Handbook of research on science education* (pp. 287–318). Mahwah, NJ: Lawrence Erlbaum Associates.

McKee, R. L., & Smith, E. (2004). *Itinerant teacher of the deaf survey: Deaf learners in the mainstream.* Wellington, New Zealand: Victoria University.

Morse, J., & Richards, L. (2002). *README FIRST for a user's guide to qualitative methods.* Thousand Oaks, CA: Sage.

Napier, J., & Barker, R. (2004). Accessing university education: Perceptions, preferences, and expectations for interpreting by deaf students. *Journal of Deaf Studies and Deaf Education, 9*, 228–238.

Newman, L. (2006). Facts from NLTS2. NCSER 2006–3001. Washington, DC: Institute of Education Sciences. Retrieved from http://www.nlts2.org. Accessed January 26, 2016.

Nikolaraizi, M., Karagianni, K., & Filippatou, D. (2013). The role of peer tutoring for students with and without disabilities in higher education. In *Proceedings of the fifth Annual International Conference on Education and New Learning Technologies* (pp. 6328–6334). Barcelona, Spain.

Orlando, R., Gramly, M. E., & Hoke, J. (1997). *Tutoring deaf and hard-of-hearing students*. A report of the National Task Force on quality of services in the postsecondary education of deaf and hard of hearing students. Rochester, NY: Northeast Technical Assistance Center, Rochester Institute of Technology.

Osguthorpe, R. (1976). The hearing peer as a provider of educational support to deaf college students. Paper presented at the annual meeting of the American Educational Research Association, April 19–23. San Francisco, CA.

Polich, L. G. (2001). Education of the deaf in Nicaragua. *Journal of Deaf Studies and Deaf Education*, 6, 315–326.

Powell, D. (2011). Floating in the mainstream: New Zealand deaf students learning and social participation experiences in tertiary education. PhD dissertation, Griffith University. Retrieved from https://www120.secure.griffith.edu.au/rch/file/50908dc2-8eda-37b0-aeb7-913daa656a3a/1/Powell_2011_02Thesis.pdf. Accessed January 26, 2016.

Powell, D., Hyde, M., & Punch, R. (2013). Inclusion in postsecondary institutions with small number of deaf and hard-of-hearing students: Highlights and challenges. *Journal of Deaf Studies and Deaf Education*, 19, 126–140.

Punch, R., Creed, P. A., & Hyde, M. B. (2005). Predicting career development in hard of hearing adolescents in Australia. *Journal of Deaf Studies and Deaf Education*, 10, 146–160.

Punch, R., Creed, P. A., & Hyde, M. B. (2006). Career barriers perceived by hard of hearing adolescents: Implications for practice from a mixed methods study. *Journal of Deaf Studies and Deaf Education*, 11, 224–237.

Punch, R., & Hyde, M. B. (2005). The social participation and career decision-making of hard of hearing adolescents in regular classes. *Deafness and Education International*, 7, 121–137.

Punch, R., Hyde, M., & Creed, P. A. (2004). Issues in the school-to-work transition of hard of hearing adolescents. *American Annals of the Deaf*, 149, 28–38.

Richardson, J. T. E., Marschark, M., Sarchet, T., & Sapere, P. (2010). Deaf and hard-of-hearing students' experiences in mainstream and separate postsecondary education. *Journal of Deaf Studies and Deaf Education*, 15, 358–382.

Sameshima, S. (1999). Deaf students in mainstream universities and polytechnics: Deaf student perspectives. Unpublished master's thesis, Victoria University.

Schick, B., Williams, K., & Kupermintz, H. (2006). Look who's being left behind: Educational interpreters and access to education for deaf and hard-of-hearing students. *Journal of Deaf Studies and Deaf Education*, 11, 3–20.

Schley, S., Walter, G. G., Weathers, R. R., Hemmeter, J., Hennessey, J. C., & Burkhauser, R. V. (2011). Effect of postsecondary education on the economic status of persons who are Deaf or hard of hearing. *Journal of Deaf Studies and Deaf Education*, 16, 524–536.

Schroedel, J. G. (1991). Improving the career decisions of deaf seniors in residential and day high schools. *American Annals of the Deaf*, 136, 330–338.

Schroedel, J. G. (1992). Helping adolescents and young adults who are deaf make career decisions. *The Volta Review*, 94, 37–46.

Stinson, M. (1987). Perceptions of tutoring services by mainstreamed hearing-impaired college students. *Journal of Postsecondary Education and Disability, 5,* 18–26

Stinson, M., Elliot, L., & Easton, D. (2014). Deaf/hard of hearing and other postsecondary learners' retention of STEM content with tablet computer based notes. *Journal of Deaf Studies and Deaf Education, 19,* 251–269.

Stinson, M. S., Elliot, L. B., & Francis, P. (2008) The C-Print system: Using captions to support classroom communication access and learning by deaf and hard of hearing students. In C. Schlenker-Schulte & A. Weber (Eds.), *Barrieren überwinden—Teilhabe ist möglich! Villingen-Schwenningen* (pp.102–122). Villingen-Schwenningen, Germany: Neckar-Verlag.

Stinson, M., Liu, Y., Saur, R., & Long, G. (1996). Deaf college students' perceptions of communication in mainstream classes. *Journal of Deaf Studies and Deaf Education, 1,* 40–51.

Stinson, M. S., & Walter, G. (1997). Improving retention rate for deaf and hard of hearing students: What the research tells us. *Journal of the American Deafness and Rehabilitation Association, 30,* 14–23.

Stinson, M. S., & Whitmire, K. A. (2000). Adolescents who are Deaf or hard-of-hearing: A communication perspective on educational placement. *Topics in Language Disorders, 20,* 58–72.

Convention on the Rights of People with Disability. United Nations (2006). Retrieved from http://www.un.org/disabilities/default.asp?id=150. Accessed January 26, 2016.

17

21st-Century Deaf Workers: Going Beyond "Just Employed" to Career Growth and Entrepreneurship

Ronald R. Kelly, Andrew B. Quagliata,
Richard DeMartino, and Victor Perotti

Increased educational attainment comes with higher expectations for greater work opportunities, sustained employment, and improved compensation, along with potential for promotion and career advancement. During the mid-20th century, following World War II, only about 400 deaf and hard-of-hearing (DHH) men and women were estimated to attend college annually in the United States, with graduation rates never exceeding more than 50 to 60 per year (Moores, 1987). Today, in contrast, of the 2.93 million DHH people between the ages of 25 years and 59 years identified in the 2010 United States census data, approximately 16% (n = 474,047) reported they had a bachelor's degree or higher (U.S. Census Bureau, 2010). The selected age range of 25 to 59 years for DHH corresponds approximately to the prime working age group in the U.S. labor market of 25- to 54-year-olds (Toossi, 2012).

As more DHH people earned university and college degrees during the past 50 years, researchers examined the effects of educational attainment on their professional life and career growth. Welsh and Walter (1988) studied the workforce mobility of three DHH groups with (a) no college degree, (b) 2-year associate degrees, and (c) bachelor degrees. To assess vertical mobility, they used the Duncan Socioeconomic Index to measure gains of DHH individuals within each of the three groups over 15 to 20 years of employment experience. Their results showed a stunning lack of vertical mobility for both DHH high school graduates and bachelor degree recipients compared with DHH 2-year college graduates with associate degrees who made modest gains. Although DHH individuals with bachelor degrees had the highest Duncan Socioeconomic Index scores, their gains over time were negligible. Welsh and Walter (1988) speculated that this lack of vertical mobility might have resulted from factors such as difficulty in receiving incidental information, thus making it harder to stay current professionally at higher occupational levels. Another possible explanation offered was that DHH bachelor graduates were hired into professional roles where the next step on the career ladder was management. Welsh and Walter (1988) observed: "Relatively few DHH college graduates move into management ... perhaps because management positions place excessive demands on communication skills that are limited by deafness itself" (p. 19).

Luft (2000) identified communication as one of the primary barriers to career advancement of DHH people. The perception that interactive or spoken communication is a barrier to promotion and management also is held by working DHH adults (Wells, 2008) and DHH high school students (Punch et al., 2006; Weisel & Cinamon, 2005). Furthermore, Foster (1992) found that hearing managers evaluating the communication skills of DHH employees perceived communication as a barrier to their promotion. As for written communication, it is not only a barrier to career growth but also employment opportunities (Hartmann, 2010). The findings of Boutin and Wilson (2009) and Boutin (2010) showed that significantly more hard-of-hearing people obtain competitive positions compared with deaf people, presumably as a result of the expectation of hiring managers that competitive jobs require more interactive (written) communication with coworkers, managers, and customers or clients.

Welsh (1993) identified six dimensions of career mobility (personal choice to work or not, change jobs, change type of employer, exercise control over how much is earned, pursue more responsibility, and seek jobs with higher socioeconomic status) and showed that DHH people as a group are less mobile in every dimension compared with their hearing peers. For those DHH individuals in the United States who had career mobility equal to their hearing peers, three important conditions accounted for the difference relative to those less mobile: English ability, education level, and career options.

If DHH people desire career options and a growth trajectory, they need to be intentional and goal driven starting early during their career. Research shows that early job status is related to career growth (Rosenbaum, 1984). Furthermore, Lewis and Allee (1992) found that for people with disabilities working for the U.S. government, promotions were more likely for those with additional education, but as age and length of service in the same relative position increased, the probability for promotion decreased, regardless of education.

In Australia, Winn (2007) found lower employment outcomes for congenitally deaf adults even with increased access to higher education and legislation that prohibits discrimination. Deaf males were disproportionately employed as tradespeople, whereas both deaf females and males were underrepresented in "professional" positions. Furthermore, the unemployment rate for deaf males in the state of South Australia was 37.5% and for females was 33.3% compared with the state unemployment rate of 10.6%. Winn (2007) concluded that congenitally deaf adults continued to be marginalized in Australia, with deaf women being even further marginalized in employment and income compared with men. Eighty-six percent of the respondents in Winn's (2007) study believed deafness limited their employment opportunities, whereas 76% reported it also limited promotion. Similarly, Willoughby (2011) examined Australian census data and found DHH sign language users persisted at lower employment and income levels, although census data showed they approached parity with the general population on several measures of educational attainment.

More recently Kelly et al. (2015) confirmed the persistent difficulty that DHH university graduates have in achieving promotions and career advancement. Their survey of 1196 DHH and 940 hearing alumni who graduated from the same large technical university between 1970 to 2012 revealed that the DHH alumni in the working age range of 22 to 59 years showed significantly less movement into management positions.

As shown in Table 17.1, DHH alumni with 2-year college associate-level degrees had the lowest percentage of promotions into management compared with DHH and hearing graduates with 4-year bachelor degrees. Furthermore, although DHH and hearing bachelor graduates looked similar in terms of their job roles during their 20s, from age 30 years onward, their hearing peers moved increasingly into management positions. For the DHH and hearing alumni with comparable 4-year bachelor degrees, the hearing graduates had a significantly greater probability of being promoted throughout their careers: 3.2 times more likely to become a middle manager, 5.7 times more likely to become a senior manager, and 7.3 times more likely to be an owner/entrepreneur.

In the United States, federal statistical agencies use a Standard Occupational Classification system defined by the U.S. Bureau of Labor Statistics to classify workers into occupational categories (U.S. Department of Labor, 2015). The Standard Occupational Classification codes examined for the 2.93 million DHH people in the age range of 25 to 59 years in the 2010 U.S. Census showed that less than 1% (0.88%) of

Table 17.1 Percent of DHH and Hearing College Graduates by Job Title Regardless of Age

Group	Nonmanagement	Mid Management	Senior Management	Owner/ Entrepreneur
DHH 2-year associate degree	86.2	8.1	0	2.0
DHH 4-year bachelor degree	76.3	15.2	1.6	1.6
Hearing 4-year bachelor degree	50.7	33.3	7.4	8.2

DHH, deaf and hard of hearing.

them held positions categorized as chief executives or general/operational managers, whereas 5.20% of them held positions that could be categorized as mid-level management. This percentage appears to compare somewhat favorably to the 132.64 million hearing people (nondisabled) in the same age range of 25 to 59 years that show 1.4% categorized as chief executives, or general/operational managers, and 8.0% categorized as mid-level management. However, to put this in perspective, DHH people are part of the total labor force (2.93 + 132.64 = 135.57 million), and in this larger context, only two-hundredths of 1% (0.02%) of DHH people are categorized as chief executives or general operational managers compared with 1.39% of hearing people, and only one-tenth of 1% (0.11%) of DHH people held mid-level management positions compared with 7.7% of hearing people.

In the United States, everyone, including DHH college graduates, will face a labor force that continues to grow more slowly (Toossi, 2002). Furthermore, everyone will be competing for employment opportunities that involve more sophisticated skills and technological knowledge that require greater levels of English literacy and numeracy (Allen, 1994). Now and in the future, DHH individuals will be competing for jobs in a world of rapid technological change that increasingly involves digital business, online marketing, and entrepreneurship. In addition to the importance of communication, what other factors will influence DHH people's ability to participate and thrive in work environments and the ever-changing labor market?

A continuing reality for DHH people is that they will be competing for employment opportunities in primarily hearing work environments as a result of the low incidence of significant hearing loss in the total population. In the United States, there are approximately one million functionally deaf people, representing only 0.38% of the population, and approximately eight million hard-of-hearing, equaling 3.7% of the population (Mitchell, 2006). Furthermore, DHH people between the ages of 25 years and 59 years make up only about 1.6% of the labor force in the United States (U.S. Census Bureau, 2010). To be recognized and achieve promotions to advance their careers, DHH individuals will have to understand and attend to the same factors that contribute to career success for all people, regardless of hearing status.

EDUCATION, EMPLOYMENT, AND JOB/CAREER SATISFACTION OF DHH PEOPLE IN THE UNITED STATES

> The population of DHH children is more diverse than the population of hearing children ... there are DHH children who succeed with spoken language ... with sign language, and ... with both....
>
> MARSCHARK ET AL. (2014, p. 470)

During the past 50 years there have been significant increases in the number of DHH students pursuing education beyond high school to acquire advanced skills certification, as well as graduating with a range of 2-year and 4-year degrees. In addition to spoken and sign language diversity, there appears to be greater diversity among DHH students' use of cochlear implants, academic readiness, and ethnicity entering postsecondary programs since the early 1980s, when enrollments nearly doubled as a result of the rubella epidemic in the United States, known as the "rubella bulge" that occurred between 1963 and 1965 (Karmel, 1982). This increased diversity results from changes in educational policy and technology during the past three decades. For example, in the 2014 entering class at the National Technical Institute for the Deaf at Rochester Institute of Technology (NTID/RIT) nearly one-third (32.5%) used cochlear implants, up from 24.4% in 2012 (National Technical Institute for the Deaf, 2014). Also, the 2014 entering class consisted of 34% minority students—triple the number of entering DHH minority students in 1995. In terms of academic diversity, during the 2014 academic year, 27.1% of the DHH students at RIT were in bachelor's programs with another 22.1% in 2-year associate programs leading to bachelor's programs. The baccalaureate graduation rates for DHH students in other RIT colleges is 61% and 41% for 2-year NTID associate degrees, which compares favorably to the average graduation rates of public higher education with traditional admission standards at 4-year institutions (59%) and 2-year institutions (31%). Although there continues to be diversity in the academic readiness of DHH students entering postsecondary programs, more DHH students are increasingly finding success at the bachelor's level and beyond.

In addition to the current annual average enrollments of 1500+ DHH students at Gallaudet University and 1300+ DHH students at NTID/RIT, postsecondary educational opportunities exist throughout the United States for DHH students at numerous universities, colleges, and community college programs. Other countries have also established college and university programs for DHH students, such as Griffith University in Australia established in 1985 and Tsukuba College of Technology in Japan established in 1987.

Compared with the estimate that only about 400 DHH students in the mid 20th century attended college annually in the United States (Moores, 1987), by the early 1990s, approximately 20,000 DHH students were enrolled in colleges and universities (Lewis et al., 1994). By 2011, the estimated number of DHH students enrolled in all postsecondary education programs in the United States increased to approximately 31,000 (Aud et al., 2011). However, enrollment numbers do not translate to successful program completion and graduation rates as a result, primarily, of the diversity in qualifications of DHH students, many of whom enter college underprepared.

Educational levels for the majority of DHH people remain problematic in relation to the total population of the United States. Figures for the general population from the Census Bureau's annual Current

Population Survey show that 30.4% of people older than 25 years of age in the United States held at least a bachelor's degree and 10.9% held a graduate degree (U.S. Census Bureau, 2011). In contrast, 10.7% of DHH people ages 25 to 59 years in the 2010 U.S. Census data had a bachelor's degree and 5.5% had earned a graduate degree. As summarized by Schley et al. (2011), national demographics continue to point to inequities in education, employment, and earnings for DHH individuals. Table 17.2 provides further details on the educational attainment of DHH people ages 25 to 59 years in the United States.

Beyond differences in graduation rates, research suggests that many DHH college students may not graduate with the same knowledge levels as hearing students. On average, DHH students go into and leave college classrooms with less content and world knowledge compared with hearing students (Marschark et al., 2008; Richardson et al., 2010). Although it is generally assumed that sign language interpreters provide equal access to classroom instruction, DHH college students acquire less information on average from interpreted college-level classes compared with their hearing peers (Marschark et al., 2005).

In terms of employment, of the 2.93 million DHH people between the ages 25 to 59 years in the 2010 U.S. Census, 53.35% were employed, 6.57% were unemployed, and the remaining 40.08% were not in the labor force. Regarding the impact of educational attainment on employment for DHH people ages 25 to 59 years, the average employment rate was highest (93.52%) for those with college degrees, next

Table 17.2 Highest Educational Level and Related Employment Rates of DHH Individuals (Age, 25–59 Years) in the 2010 U.S. Census (n = 2,931,883)

Highest Educational Level	Frequency	Percent	Percent Employed	Percent Unemployed
No high school diploma, 12th grade or less	552,722	18.85	84.39	15.35
GED or alternative credential	186,282	6.35	83.68	16.32
Regular high school diploma	770,132	26.27	88.87	11.13
Some college, no degree	700,763	23.90	88.01	11.99
College 2-year associates degree	247,937	8.46	91.34	8.66
College 4-year baccalaureate degree	313,924	10.71	92.62	7.38
Master's degree	115,810	3.95	96.61	3.39
Professional degree beyond baccalaureate	25,712	0.88	94.91	5.09
Doctoral degree	18,601	0.63	92.13	7.87
Total	2,931,883	100.00		

GED, general educational development.

highest (88.44%) for those with a high school diploma or some college but no degree, and lowest (84.65%) for DHH with no high school degree. Table 17.2 provides further details on the employment status of DHH people per educational level attained for those still active in the labor force.

Regarding the data reported in Table 17.2, Burkhauser et al. (2014) have cautioned that information on working-age people with disabilities retrieved from the American Community Survey may provide underestimates of the population if one uses only a work-limitation question or the six-question sequence alone to query the data. Both must be used in combination to obtain an accurate estimate of the population.

With regard to career attainments and related quality-of-life satisfaction, Schroedel and Geyer (2000) conducted a 15-year longitudinal study of DHH college graduates during 1985, 1989, 1994, and 1999, reporting results only for respondents who participated in every survey to assess changes over a 15-year period. Although initially 490 DHH individuals participated in 1985, 51% attrition reduced the participants to 240 who completed all subsequent surveys. Of the respondents included in the report, 53% were female, 93% were white, and, by 1999, 28% had completed a vocational degree; 24%, a 2-year associates degree; 32%, a bachelor's degree; 15%, a master's degree; and 1%, a doctorate. Despite the fact that a persistent 15% of these 240 respondents continued to work in less than challenging jobs 15 years into their careers, their responses suggested that "a majority ... were relatively successful in their careers, ... making sustained progress in their career attainments, and ... satisfied with their quality of life" (Schroedel & Geyer, 2000, p. 313). However, only 64% were satisfied with their income. Results also indicated that 85% of the 240 respondents persisted in the labor force, were employed in a wide range of occupations, were self-sufficient economically, and had worked for the same employer for a long time. These findings confirmed that economic benefits resulted from postsecondary training consistent with other research (Schley et al., 2011; Walter et al., 2002; Welsh & MacLeod-Gallinger, 1992), but also showed that men made more consistent gains in income than females.

Geyer and Schroedel (1998) examined DHH college graduates' job satisfaction and, not surprisingly, showed those with lower levels of satisfaction were more likely to experience periods of unemployment longer, have lower level jobs on the Socioeconomic Index scores, and perceive on-the-job limitations. Low salaries and less satisfaction with one's job were significantly related to job search behavior. Kelly et al. (2015) showed that DHH college graduates are generally less satisfied with both their current positions and their careers compared with their hearing alumni peers with comparable college degrees. However, when job status levels are factored into the analysis (no management role, middle manager, and senior manager), satisfaction was equivalent for DHH and hearing individuals at each level. Specifically, satisfaction was statistically equivalent for DHH and hearing comparisons within nonmanagement positions, middle management roles, and senior management roles. Furthermore, regardless of hearing status, senior managers were significantly more satisfied than middle managers with both their job and career. In turn, middle managers were significantly more satisfied with their job and career compared with individuals in nonmanagement positions. The findings of Kelly et al. (2015) show that promotions into mid-level and senior management positions increase one's satisfaction with career and current job for both DHH and hearing people.

Factors That Influence Educational Attainment and Employment

In the United States, two critical areas associated with attending college and subsequent graduation are English language skills and mathematical ability. For DHH students, Garberoglio et al. (2014) showed that English literacy is a significant predictor for attending postsecondary education. They examined a sample of more than 1000 DHH students from the National Longitudinal Transition Study-2, during which students were administered the Woodcock-Johnson III Tests of Achievement between the ages of 13 years and 16 years. Using the passage comprehension score on the Woodcock-Johnson III as the predictor variable in a logistic regression model, they calculated that the odds of attending postsecondary education were 2.75 times greater for DHH individuals who scored one standard deviation higher on the literacy measure. Cuculick and Kelly (2003) examined graduation outcomes of DHH students for a 10-year period from one large technical university and found that higher reading and language skills were critically important to graduating with 4-year bachelor degrees and 2-year associate degrees. Furthermore there is evidence that DHH college students' English language reading abilities are associated significantly with their performance in college mathematics courses (Kelly & Gaustad, 2007). Rose and Betts (2001) showed that mathematics was linked to both college graduation and subsequent employment earnings for people in general, whereas quantitative literacy has been shown to impact employability directly (Rivera-Batiz, 1992).

The evidence to date on DHH students in the United States acquiring sufficient English language and literacy skills, as well as mathematical skills, for success in the workplace is not encouraging. Qi and Mitchell (2012) examined five cohorts of DHH students' performance on the Stanford Achievement Test representing approximately three decades from 1974 to 2003. For reading comprehension, they found that DHH students' "performance levels are slightly higher for each age cohort from age 8 through 17, but median performance never exceeds the fourth-grade equivalent for any cohort" (Qi & Mitchell, 2012, p. 5). For mathematical problem solving, the median performance for 17-year-old DHH students approached the equivalent of sixth grade, and for mathematical procedures, their median performance varied between sixth grade and a 7.5-grade equivalent. Other research has also shown gaps in achievement performance. Shaver et al. (2011) examined data from the National Longitudinal Transition Study-2 and found that gaps exist for DHH secondary school students on academic achievement with the general secondary school population for reading, mathematics, science, and social studies as measured by the Woodcock-Johnson III.

Both reading comprehension and mathematical problem solving continue to challenge DHH students when they attend college. Morphographic analysis of printed English, for example, is a word identification tool used by advanced readers, and, more important, is used to improve their word comprehension and reading literacy. Research has shown that DHH college students appear to have approximately the same morphological knowledge and word segmentation skills as hearing middle school students (Gaustad et al., 2002), whereas further examination shows clear nuanced differences in the morphological skills favoring hearing middle school readers over DHH college students when matched for reading levels (Gaustad & Kelly, 2004). Specifically, Gaustad and Kelly (2004) found that hearing middle school readers were more accurate with the meaning of derivational morphemes and roots of words, as well as the segmentation of words containing multiple types of morphemes.

For mathematical word problem solving, which involves both reading comprehension and mathematical problem solving skills, Blatto-Vallee et al. (2007) found that the performance of DHH college students in baccalaureate programs was also generally equivalent to hearing middle school students. For college-bound DHH students who took the American College Test (ACT), Kelly (2008) reported that

> five entering freshman cohorts from 2002–2006 had average ACT composite scores at least one standard deviation below the general population of students ([National Technical Institute for the Deaf], 2006). For these deaf students, only 20%, on average, met or exceeded the ACT College Readiness Benchmarks (ACT, 2005) for English and Reading, while 10% and 15%, on average, met or exceeded the benchmarks for science reasoning and mathematics, respectively. (p. 227–228)

Albertini et al. (2011) found both reading and mathematical skills of DHH students at entry to college contributed significantly and positively to their initial quarter grade performance average. Their results also reveal that the majority of DHH students entering college show less confidence in their verbal, mathematical, and science skills compared with typical hearing students entering college. As noted previously, mathematical skills have been linked to college success for all students in general (Rose & Betts, 2001), whereas English literacy has been shown to be a predictor for DHH students to enter college (Garberoglio et al., 2014), and reading comprehension and language skills are associated significantly with DHH students' college success culminating in graduation (Cuculick & Kelly, 2003).

Welsh (1993) emphasized that DHH individuals must set the highest possible standards for themselves in terms of a college degree and avoid preset limits on their educational attainment stating, "Career mobility is not beyond the grasp of deaf people ... goals must be set high; there must be no mind set [sic] that deafness is in any way limiting; and that mind set [sic] must be dispelled in others" (Welsh, 1993, p. 338). More recently, Weisel and Cinamon (2005) examined the attitudes of DHH and hearing Israeli high school students and found that both groups evaluated occupations involving intensive communication levels less suitable for DHH people compared with positions requiring less interaction and communication. Also, both DHH and hearing participants expressed some biased stereotypic evaluations regarding DHH women's occupational competence. Furthermore, the DHH participants perceived highly prestigious occupations as unsuitable for DHH adults even if communication considerations were not relevant. These findings are consistent with a study of Australian adolescents who prematurely ruled out career options and showed a lack of awareness of helpful strategies and job accommodations (Punch et al., 2006). Changing DHH students' attitudes about potential career choices will be a challenge for educators and parents.

COMMUNICATION IN THE WORKPLACE

A variety of resources are available for employers to learn how to communicate with DHH employees, and DHH individuals have access to a host of material about ways to advocate for reasonable accommodations. However, the increasing diversity of DHH individuals entering the labor force who used modern hearing aid technology or cochlear implants throughout their school years has the potential to alleviate some of the need for communication accommodations. The purpose here is to understand that, historically, communication barriers have limited career advancement among DHH individuals (Luft, 2000). Foster and MacLeod (2003) stated that effective workplace communication "can enhance opportunities for personal as well as professional success, including access to social networks, increased productivity and promotions. Poor communication may result in a stagnant career, social isolation, or even dismissal" (p. 137). DHH individuals encounter unique challenges when searching for jobs, and subsequently face higher rates of unemployment (Johnson, 1993). When employed, they encounter a variety of assimilation and socialization challenges in the workplace. Persistent communication difficulties with supervisors and coworkers are a primary reason DHH people leave jobs (Luft, 1998).

DHH workers might not understand hearing culture or communication protocol in the work environment, just as hearing coworkers often do not understand deafness or deaf culture. Again, the changing diversity of DHH workers in terms of increased higher educational levels, the use of digital hearing aids or cochlear implants throughout their school years, and developing social experiences have the potential to temper cultural differences. However, because the historical challenges remain for a significant portion of the DHH population, it is still important for all DHH graduates to understand the communication challenges and cultural differences as they face the future. Belknap et al. (1995) contended that DHH employees are disadvantaged because they lack "access to incidental information (that which is not conveyed explicitly to an individual but is overheard or inferred intuitively)" (p. 22). In addition, Foster (1992) noted DHH employees "experience difficulty joining informal interactions and conversations such as those involving the office grapevine" (p. 18). Belknap et al. (1995) further observed, "[I]t is not uncommon for people to make erroneous negative assumptions about a deaf person's intelligence based solely on his or her speech or English language skills, or in reaction to behavior such as touching and facial expressions not considered acceptable in the hearing work milieu" (p. 24). This view is reinforced by the research findings of Most (2010) that demonstrated the importance of speech intelligibility in hearing people's perceptions of DHH people's personalities and abilities. From the DHH employees' view, they report feeling isolated and devalued at work (Wells, 2008), spend break time alone (Lussier et al., 2000), and feel they are assigned tasks that do not use their potential.

When DHH people secure jobs, have a supportive supervisor, are comfortable with coworkers, and are provided reasonable accommodations, it is no surprise why they might choose to stay in one position longer. But, what about individuals who want career growth? How can DHH individuals use their communication skills to earn a promotion or find a job with more responsibility in another organization? What strategies can DHH individuals use to become more fully functioning and invaluable members of an organization?

Employers Value Communication Competence

Communication skills are essential in the workplace. Surveys of employers consistently identify communication competencies as important in hiring and promotion decisions. Morreale and Pearson (2008) found 73 references between 1955 and 2006 that suggested communication skills are fundamental to workplace success. This is also consistent with the literature on career growth and leadership that emphasizes the importance of clear communication. Broadly stated, however, communication competencies usually involve speaking, writing, and listening.

Speaking in the Workplace

In this context, the term *speaking* does not refer to spoken language but involves how one shares points of view and ideas, as well as presents one's self to others. Important workplace "speaking" skills involve building interpersonal relationships, conversing with others, delivering presentations, handling customer complaints, resolving conflict, working in teams, and getting along with others. Managerial communication competencies include interviewing employees, managing teams, providing instructions, leading meetings, motivating others, and giving feedback. DHH individuals face challenges in many of these situations.

Scherich (1996) identified six workplace situations in which hearing loss appears to limit DHH individuals' ability to participate effectively: work-related social functions, meetings, training, socializing with coworkers, receiving instructions and supervision, and performance evaluations. Interactive skills are essential in most careers, and DHH people who are perceived to have challenges when interacting with hearing coworkers, supervisors, or clients/customers may not be as competitive or marketable in their quest for professional positions. The research of Boutin and Wilson (2009) on job outcomes of DHH people who received vocational rehabilitation services showed that fewer deaf people (31%) obtained competitive professional employment compared with hard-of-hearing people (69%), presumably because there is a greater expectation for interactive communication with hearing people in professional positions. A follow-up study by Boutin (2010) using the new Standard Occupational Classification showed that hard-of-hearing people (74.1%) had the competitive advantage across all job categories compared with deaf individuals (25.9%). Kelly et al. (2015) found that workplace communication consisted of 78% to 80% talking, writing, or using sign language with speech (simultaneous communication) when DHH individuals interact and communicate with hearing coworkers.

Writing in the Workplace

Writing competencies include the ability to write clearly and concisely; find, evaluate, and organize information for a particular audience; use appropriate grammar, punctuation, and mechanics; and demonstrate accurate spelling. DHH individuals' writing ability is associated with their employment outcomes. Belknap et al. (1995) observed:

> Some graduates of postsecondary training programs achieve high levels of technical expertise although their English literacy skills

approximate 8th or 9th grade level . . . however . . . inability to understand highly specialized and constantly revised technical manuals and procedures can seriously impede career mobility and advancement. (p. 24)

Hartmann (2010) found that DHH individuals with higher quality written English skills were more likely to be employed, whereas the findings of Wells (2008) showed that poor writing skills among DHH employees limited promotion opportunities.

Listening in the Workplace

Research also links listening ability to positive career outcomes. In this context, the term *listening* is not meant audiologically, but refers to making a concerted effort to understand the perspectives of others within the work environment. Better listeners are promoted at a faster rate (Sypher et al., 1989). Listening competencies become more critical as individuals advance in their careers and are perceived by managers as important to career development (Brownell, 1994). In fact, when judging coworkers' communication competence, one study found listening competency accounted for almost one-third of the overall evaluation (Haas & Arnold, 1995).

Wolvin and Coakley's (1993) taxonomy of listening and Welch and Mickelson's (2013) Listening Competency Scale help distinguish listening from hearing and understand the importance of workplace listening competencies. The base level of Wolvin and Coakley's (1993) taxonomy includes discriminative and comprehensive listening. Discriminative listening includes processing auditory and visual cues, identifying feelings, distinguishing between truths and untruths, and interpreting facial expressions. Depending on the degree of hearing loss, auditory reception may be limited, but most DHH individuals are assumed to be particularly attuned to reading facial expressions.

Comprehensive listening includes understanding the main idea of a message: paying close attention, recalling information after the communication exchange, and asking clarifying questions. Research suggests that when miscommunication occurs, DHH individuals tend to avoid asking for clarification (Stinson & Antia, 1999). Jeanes et al. (2000) examined profoundly deaf children's ability to request clarification when miscommunication occurred and found they exhibited significantly fewer attempts to clarify any misunderstandings in their face-to-face interactions. These authors also found that children who used spoken languages were more likely than those who signed to request clarification and/or recognize misunderstandings. At the college level, Marschark et al. (2007) used a question–answer game to examine the frequency of requests for clarification when misunderstanding occurred between paired DHH college students who relied on American Sign Language, spoken language, or a mixed-mode pairing in which one used sign and the other relied on spoken language. Regardless of communication mode, results showed that DHH college students rarely requested clarification when miscommunication occurred, or were even aware that further information was needed. It is important for DHH employees to ask for immediate clarification rather than accepting uncertainty. Higher order listening includes critical and appreciative listening. Critical listening involves evaluating and assessing the content of a message. Appreciative listening includes enjoying listening, listening with an open mind, and valuing what others have to communicate.

Attending behaviors are the final level on Wolvin and Coakley's (1993) taxonomy. Verbal attending behaviors include matching the speaker's "tone of voice" and restating or summarizing what the message sender has said. This applies to sign language as well. Nonverbal attending behaviors include maintaining eye contact and an attentive posture while someone is speaking (such as learning toward the speaker). As can be seen from this taxonomy, hearing loss should not limit a DHH individual's ability to listen to and understand others' points of view.

Communication Strategies

This section describes several research-based behavioral and cognitive communication strategies that could help DHH professionals accomplish their individual career goals. Although these strategies could benefit all employees, fair or not, DHH persons may have to be more intentional and goal directed.

Message Design Logic

Message design logic is a communication framework used to analyze how message senders select messages to communicate and how message recipients interpret the meaning of messages. Message creators have many thoughts from which to choose before sending a message, and recipients can interpret expressed messages a variety of ways. O'Keefe (1988) argued that individuals have three different ways of selecting thoughts for expression and construction. These design logics are expressive, conventional, and rhetorical.

Empirical studies suggest that message design logics range in sophistication from expressive (being the least) to rhetorical (being the most). Rhetorical message producers align their goals with the message receivers' goals. In contrast, expressive message producers view language as a way to express feelings and thoughts. The expressive view leads to messages that are often overly direct—to the point of being impolite (O'Keefe, 1988). As a result, individuals using expressive design logic are perceived as less competent by others (O'Keefe &

McCornack, 1987). Luft (2000) noted: "Inappropriate communication strategies and responses often lead to serious job repercussions for deaf employees" (p. 51). DHH individuals are often perceived as being very direct—approaching communication in a way most characterized as expressive or the least sophisticated in design logic. Mindess et al. (2006) described this very direct approach to communication as "straight talk." They observed "it may be the hardest part of Deaf culture for hearing people to accept" (p. 87). American Sign Language does not tend to incorporate many politeness strategies (Mindess et al., 2006). In fact, for deaf people, being direct is valued and being indirect is often seen as inappropriate (Lane, 1992). This cultural discourse strategy is widely understood within deaf culture, but when used in the workplace within a hearing culture it could contribute to negative career outcomes.

Self-Monitoring

Self-monitoring, a behavior associated more commonly with the rhetorical and conventional design logics than the expressive design logic, is associated positively with promotions. High-self-monitoring individuals are more sensitive to role expectations than low self-monitors. High-self-monitoring individuals use social cues to guide personal behavior in contrast to low self-monitors, who are less attuned to what is appropriate in different contexts (Snyder, 1974). Sypher and Sypher (1983) found self-monitoring to be related positively to an employee's level in an organization. High self-monitors are more likely to achieve cross-company promotions and, for those who remain with their first employer, within-company promotions (Kilduff & Day, 1994).

Self-monitoring is related to executive function, and there is a fairly consistent body of literature indicating challenges among deaf individuals (Hauser et al., 2008). For example, Hintermair (2013) examined the frequency of executive function disorders in German DHH students compared with a U.S. normative sample of hearing students, and revealed highly significant differences in all domains of executive functioning for the DHH students, with a 3.5- to 5-fold increase in their rate of dysfunctions. Within the context of self-monitoring of learning, the lack of self-monitoring by DHH students has been discussed with respect to numerical cognition, language learning, and knowledge comprehension (Bull, 2008; Marschark & Wauters, 2008). Inability to develop good self-monitoring skills by DHH students most likely will impact their future careers and professional growth opportunities.

Extroversion

Extroversion is one of the Big Five personality factors associated with career success. An extrovert is someone who is outgoing and has a tendency to be assertive and energetic. In a meta-analysis, Ng et al. (2005)

found extroversion to be related positively to career satisfaction, salary, and promotion. It is important to recognize, however, that not all work environments require employees to be extroverted. Companies that value a quiet atmosphere or jobs that involve more individual work might be a better fit for introverts. In fact, Johnson (1993) contended that DHH employees perform better on individual tasks than on tasks involving social interaction. However, for those individuals who desire a management position, for which interpersonal communication is a requirement of the job, it is important to understand that individuals with extroverted personalities are perceived as more leader-like (Hogan et al., 1994).

Silence and withdrawn behavior may lead supervisors and coworkers to perceive DHH individuals mistakenly as introverts, especially within group situations. However, the following list provides examples of ways DHH employees can take what they know about extroverts and learn to use extrovert behavior when necessary:

- Build rapport with others; engage coworkers in "small talk."
- Focus on the positive; maintain an optimistic attitude (don't complain or gossip).
- Volunteer; offer to take on coordinating roles whenever the opportunity arises.
- Be enthusiastic; use eye contact, posture, and facial expressions to communicate positive energy.

Proactive Behavior and Career Outcomes

Having a proactive personality in the workplace has been linked to positive career outcomes. Crant (2000) defined proactive behavior as "taking the initiative in improving current circumstances or creating new ones; it involves challenging the status quos rather than passively adapting to present conditions" (p. 436). Individuals with proactive personalities are known for going beyond normal role expectations and job requirements to engage in proactive behaviors such as gathering information from their formal and informal workplace network, assuming responsibility for their own careers, and developing innovative ideas. These proactive behaviors are associated positively with job and career promotions (Seibert et al., 2001).

One way DHH employees can take initiative in the workplace is to educate hearing coworkers about deafness. Foster and MacLeod (2003) interviewed a relatively highly skilled group of DHH professionals, and one of the themes that emerged included strategies deaf employees use to overcome communication barriers that stressed the importance of taking the lead to create "the best possible environments for themselves" (p. 135).

Seeking information is a second proactive behavior DHH employees can use in the workplace. They should identify and cultivate relationships with formal and informal networks (Foster & MacLeod, 2003). These individuals can be supportive supervisors, trusted coworkers, interpreters, administrative assistants, or others who are willing to share information. DHH employees can take responsibility for their own careers by searching proactively for a mentor. Foster and MacLeod (2004) found that having a mentor was an important factor for DHH people who were promoted to supervisory positions in primarily hearing work environments. A trusted colleague need not always be a supervisor. A mentor can help DHH employees learn about the organizational culture, how decisions are made, and about opportunities for additional training or advancement (Myers & Danek, 1990).

Using proactive workplace strategies has never been more important. Traditionally, careers have been characterized by employee–employer relationships. However, what it means to have a career is changing, and contemporary career theory has put forth a variety of concepts that speak to the importance of thinking beyond one's current job and employer. The protean career is one that is driven by the individual and not the organization; a protean person's own personal career choices and search for self-fulfillment are the unifying or integrative elements (Hall, 1976, 2004). The word *protean* comes from the mythical Greek sea god Proteus, who could predict the future and adapt successfully to his envisioned future. Boundaryless careers are the opposite of organizational careers with a common factor of independence rather than dependence on organizational career arrangements (Arthur, 1994; Arthur & Rousseau, 1996). A boundaryless career emphasizes that individuals must take an active role in developing their career. In fact, one study found a boundaryless mind-set to be correlated with a proactive personality (Briscoe et al., 2006). The postcorporate career concept also emphasizes the importance of being self-directed. Peiperl and Baruch (1997) contended that increasingly more careers take place outside of large organizations in small firms and entrepreneurial ventures.

DIGITAL TECHNOLOGY AND ONLINE MARKETING

There is no question that digital technologies are radically changing the nature of business practice for marketing and communication that will increasingly affect the career experiences for most individuals. These changes are happening at an accelerating pace, and employees in organizations around the globe are expected, more and more, to reinvent work processes, develop new products, and create new organizations to succeed in this shifting environment. The new nature of work created by the adoption and use of information and communication technologies (ICTs) has been studied extensively. Among the many new business processes, the domain of marketing (which manages the understanding of and communication with customers) may be the most transformed by the advent of new technologies. Digital marketing and digital business invariably bring new capabilities as well as challenges for the contemporary organization and its employees, both DHH and hearing.

Digital technologies and communication are inextricably intertwined. The Digital Marketing Institute defines digital marketing as the use of digital technologies to create an integrated, targeted, and measurable communication that helps to acquire and retain customers while building deeper relationships with them (Smith, 2007). From social media to mobile technologies, digital marketing professionals are rapidly adapting to new communication patterns to address more fully the needs of their customers, as well as interact with their coworkers. As noted by Ragu-Nathan et al. (2008), "the adoption and use of ICTs . . . have altered the means of interaction among and between individuals and the organization" (p. 417). The infusion of ICTs across a wide range of work environments provides a greater emphasis on interactive communication (more text than voice) that requires clear written language skills. For DHH people, the increased use of digital technologies to communicate and interact with colleagues and customers offers a potential level playing field for direct online communication that bypasses the use of an intermediary such as a sign interpreter, relay service, or having hearing coworkers and customers/clients develop sufficient expressive and receptive sign language skills to interact effectively.

The transformative nature of information technology across the employment spectrum suggests that many DHH individuals may be challenged to compete for jobs that require increasingly sophisticated literacy skills. However, consider the example of Alicia Lane-Outlaw, chief creative officer for AllOut Marketing, Inc. Alicia is a deaf professional who built an online marketing career by combining her undergraduate knowledge in biology with her love of the visual arts and graphics, to develop expertise in multimedia communications. Digital technology dominates her work environment, and most of her professional interactions are conducted via online communication with coworkers in other locations. In a short video (Lane-Outlaw, 2012), she describes the factors that helped her adapt and succeed in this field.

The influence of information technology on organizations impacts both current and future employees, including DHH individuals who aspire to work for those organizations. They will be applying for positions in organizations in which information technology and business strategy are aligned (Broadbent & Weill, 1993; Ullah & Lai, 2013) to achieve successful organizational performance (Chan & Reich, 2007; Leonard & Seddon, 2012). In some businesses, there will be one "digital business strategy" that represents a fusion of the two strategic initiatives as advocated by Bharadwaj et al. (2013). Importantly, as products and services become more digital and available, the data and interpretation that surround them will also become a valuable asset. These substantial changes will inevitably impact and result in new responsibilities for the people of the organization and new opportunities for future employees. DHH students preparing to enter the labor force and become competitive in information fields dependent on digital technologies will have to possess the requisite literacy in language and mathematics, as well as data analysis skills.

Employees working in the era of digital business are experiencing new expectations, practices, and careers compared with their predecessors. The advent of collaboration tools, cloud hosting for software and content, video conferencing, and advanced smartphone technologies means that distributed work teams are more common than ever. For example, the software company Mozilla is a global community with multiple teams of people distributed worldwide collaborating, communicating, and interacting daily with digital tools. Early research on virtual teams (Jarvenpaa & Leidner, 1998) found challenges with interpersonal trust in a computer-mediated environment. Virtual team performance is now known to be affected by a wide range of factors such as task inputs, including culture and training; socioemotional processes of cohesion and trust; and task processes involving communication and coordination (Powell et al., 2004). Given the lack of literature on how DHH people adapt to and perform within the context of virtual collaborative teams, this would be an ideal focus for future research.

These changes point to a new set of skills and additional multiple literacies required for the next generation of workers. Although the pace and magnitude of digital transformation are daunting, young people are succeeding at embracing this new environment to achieve success. As an exemplar of the new generation of successful individuals, consider Eva Skolvi. Eva is a highly motivated, young DHH entrepreneur from Norway who describes in a video the factors that contributed to her success as a young entrepreneur (Skovli, 2012). As a teenager, she began selling a curated group of products targeted at women age 15 to 30 years old. Curated commerce helps shoppers discover products based on their personal preferences; it is basically the online version of shopping in exclusive and personal boutiques. This effort ultimately launched as the online storefront Kipekee.com (Swahili for "unique"). On the first day in business, almost no one visited the online store. However, by using online digital tools such as e-mail, blogs, social media, and traditional websites, Eva began to attract an audience. Since that time, Kipekee has experienced steady growth. Attracting customers to her website required a familiarity with a variety of different tools, but especially an understanding of how people might best be engaged through the communities that surround the online digital tools. By contributing content to a select group of blogging websites,

Eva connected with a group of individuals who ultimately praised her store and attracted more customers.

Like Eva, many individuals are pursuing careers that leverage digital tools. A quick scan of career-focused websites (e.g., Hotjobs, Indeed, or Monster) reveals an increase in the number and diversity of such jobs. Although it may go unstated in these job descriptions, current and future generations will need to manage computer-mediated communication through a large number of communication channels: web, e-mail, social media, mobile technologies (more text than voice), instant messaging, and dedicated sharing tools (such as Microsoft Sharepoint, DropBox, or GitHub). Their skills need to extend beyond multiple literacies and technical competency toward mastering the human dimension. They will learn to establish trust and a positive culture through this new set of digital tools, while tracking, measuring, and advancing project goals.

In the absence of any substantive body of literature on DHH individuals' use of digital tools in the workplace, this is a prime area for future research. Specifically, new research should focus on how DHH individuals are managing computer-mediated communication via the various available channels. Another focus should be on whether they have the technical abilities to track, measure, interpret, and advance project goals of a company. Currently, it is unknown how many DHH people work in information technology fields. A body of research literature needs to be developed on DHH people in 21st-century digital work environments.

Furthermore, marketing professionals will build awareness of offerings through search engine optimization, establish relationships with customers through social media marketing, and measure their success using available tools such as Google Analytics. Many individuals will learn software programming, and database and web design to serve their goals. Last, as digital business strategies become the norm, employees will look for opportunities in the data that have historically been locked within a company. Novel data discovery applications such as Qlikview, Splunk, and Tableau are making data available and more salient across organizations, rather than being restricted to a group of analysts or research professionals. In this new environment, an ability to capture, analyze, visualize, and interpret data is becoming a standard expectation for all information careers. Needless to say, excellent written language skills and mathematical knowledge are critically important to success in pursuing careers that involve digital tools and online marketing, as well as the ability to measure and analyze data.

DHH adults already working who cannot read or write sufficiently to communicate effectively in the workplace should consider taking adult literacy courses to function successfully in the digital work world. DHH students who are preparing for careers need to be cognizant of the multiple literacy requirements of the ever-evolving digital world and plan accordingly to develop appropriate skills if they are to be competitive in the 21st-century labor market dominated by digital technologies.

ENTREPRENEURSHIP

Entrepreneurs develop a business from the ground up—coming up with an idea and turning it into a profitable business (Brooks, 2015). Although the terms *entrepreneur* and *small-business owner* are often used interchangeably, what distinguishes them is that an entrepreneur generally focuses on innovation and big ideas, and has a willingness to take on more than an ordinary degree of risk (Spiropoulos, 2014; Spring, 2014).

DeMartino et al. (2011, manuscript submitted 2015) explored the nature of DHH entrepreneurship by comparing DHH and hearing alumni with similar academic degrees from a large university. The rate of DHH entrepreneurship was half that of the hearing comparison group, and their new ventures were smaller, with many being single-person (micro) enterprises. The most educated individuals within the DHH study sample, arguably those with the greatest potential for career advancement, were not pursuing entrepreneurial outcomes to the same degree as their hearing peers. Interestingly, there was no difference between DHH and hearing alumni expressing the desire to become entrepreneurs within the next 5 years. The findings of DeMartino et al. (2011, manuscript submitted 2015) also revealed that general self-efficacy (GSE)—the general self-confidence individuals' possess to accomplish tasks—was uniformly lower in the DHH sample compared with the hearing sample. DHH entrepreneurs' GSE, in particular, was also lower than that of hearing entrepreneurs, but there was no difference in the level of entrepreneurial self-efficacy (ESE) between DHH and hearing entrepreneurs—the self-confidence individuals' possess to accomplish entrepreneurial-oriented tasks successfully.

The ESE scale developed by McGee et al. (2009) best describes the characteristics associated with becoming an entrepreneur:

- *Opportunity recognition search*: Involves one's ability to identify the need for a new product, to brainstorm a new idea for a product or service, and to design a product or service that will satisfy what customers' need or want
- *Venture creation planning*: Involves one's ability to estimate customer demand, to determine competitive prices, to project the amount of startup funds, and to design an effective marketing/advertising campaign
- *Marshalling resources*: Involves one's ability to convince others to identify and believe in one's vision, to network to make

contacts and communicate, as well as to communicate clearly and concisely in written and verbal form
- *Venture implementation of people*: Involves one's ability to supervise employees, to recruit and hire, to delegate tasks, to deal with day-to-day problems, to inspire and encourage, and to train employees
- *Venture implementation of finances*: Involves one's ability to maintain financial records, to manage financial assets, and to understand financial documents (pp. 977–982)

Entrepreneurship is about personal empowerment. Regardless of individuals' rationales for pursuing an entrepreneurial career, they gain a unique degree of professional empowerment to manage their affairs in a way most consistent with their personal career desires and barriers they face, and they use their unique strengths. The general entrepreneurship literature identifies a lack of traditional career options and low career satisfaction as important factors promoting entrepreneurial outcomes. Given the career-growth challenges faced by DHH people, an understanding of the potential of entrepreneurship seems uniquely appropriate. However, to date, very little is known about the prevalence, drivers, and critical factors associated with DHH entrepreneurship.

Career motivation theory as applied to entrepreneurial activity has generally focused on motivators such as the need for achievement, willingness to take risks, tolerance for ambiguity, locus of control, self-efficacy, and goal setting (Shane et al., 2003). It has also been theorized that individuals are either pulled (in a positive manner) or pushed (in a negative manner) toward career choices (Gilad & Levine, 1986). The entrepreneurship literature classifies factors such as discrimination, unemployment, underemployment, and passive unemployment (layoffs or firings) as factors that push individuals toward entrepreneurship (Shane et al., 2003). Hessels et al. (2008) described this type of entrepreneurship as "necessity or refuge based." Others have noted push factors such as the inability to obtain needed working flexibility or infrastructure accommodations (Dawson & Henley, 2012) as well as job dissatisfaction (and future perceived satisfaction) driving entrepreneurial career decisions (Hisrich & Brush, 1986). The few studies conducted on DHH entrepreneurship suggest underemployment and periods of unemployment are important considerations driving DHH entrepreneurial outcomes (DeMartino et al., manuscript submitted 2015).

Pull-related factors in career motivation theory are related to self-realization and independence, among other variables and personal factors associated with starting a new venture (Cassar, 2007; Douglas & Shepherd, 2002). Dennis (1996), for example, found that "greater personal control" served as an essential aspect of self-employment, whereas Smeaton (2003) reported that "independence" and "being one's own boss" served as the primary motivating force. Carter et al. (2003) also included the important impact of self-realization that aligns internal visions with actions.

The entrepreneurship push/pull literature provides insights for future research of DHH entrepreneurship. First, push and pull factors are not mutually exclusive; one can be pulled and pushed simultaneously. For example, a high degree of ESE could "pull" DHH individuals to become entrepreneurs whereas at the same time underemployment and unemployment could "push" them in that direction. Second, low satisfaction with one's job or career does not always lead to entrepreneurial outcomes. Schjoedt and Shaver (2007) found that job security may counter and suppress considerations promoting entrepreneurship. Other potentially hindering factors for DHH people interested in entrepreneurial activities may be personal life and family considerations such as quality of life, spouse/partner co-career issues, and child/school requirements. Kelly et al. (2015) found that DHH study participants showed a significantly stronger orientation for personal life/family compared with hearing peers with similar educational levels.

In an early study of DHH people's entrepreneurial motivations, Pressmen (1999) found that most DHH entrepreneurs had started home-based, nonemployer businesses and were driven by the intrinsic motivation to be one's own boss, rather than the extrinsic motivation to make more money. Research into the nature of DHH entrepreneurship was explored qualitatively through a subsequent phenomenological study (Atkins, 2011). Atkins (2011) observed that many professional fields had been opened to the DHH community through the Americans with Disabilities Act. This legislation provided the impetus to remove employment barriers for DHH workers, including accommodations that would mitigate communication barriers. But it is unknown whether greater access and accommodation resulting from Americans with Disabilities Act promotes or impedes DHH entrepreneurial activities.

The limited research on DHH entrepreneurship suggests entrepreneurial activity in the DHH population is less than that of the general population. Furthermore, DeMartino et al. (manuscript submitted 2015) showed that most DHH entrepreneurs are pushed toward entrepreneurship as a result of negative work factors such as underemployment and unemployment. Pull factors related to self-actualization, greater independence, and a desire to advance their careers do not play a significant role.

SUMMARY OF KEY FACTORS FOR CAREER SUCCESS AMONG DHH INDIVIDUALS

Study after study has demonstrated a strong relationship between education level and salary, promotions, and career satisfaction. Earning a university or college bachelor's degree or higher has been shown consistently to provide positive employment and financial benefits for DHH people (Schley et al., 2011; Schroedel & Geyer, 2000; Walter et al., 2002; Welsh & MacLeod-Gallinger, 1992). Two critical areas associated with attending college and graduating are English language skills and mathematical knowledge/skills (Cuculick & Kelly, 2003; Garberoglio et al., 2014). However, the long-term evidence for DHH students in the United States acquiring sufficient English literacy and mathematical skills during their K–12 school years is not encouraging, as evidenced by the existing research (Qi & Mitchell, 2012; Shaver et al., 2011). This results in the majority of DHH students entering college underprepared in English, reading, mathematics, and science reasoning (Kelly, 2008). Not surprisingly, most DHH students have less confidence in their verbal, mathematical, and science skills compared with typical students entering college (Albertini et al., 2011).

Although there was a considerable increase in DHH people's earning university and college degrees at the bachelor's level or higher during the second half of the 20th century, research has long shown a lack of vertical mobility in the workplace (Welsh & Walter, 1988) that continues to this day (Kelly et al., 2015). Assuming equivalent educational levels of a bachelor's or graduate degree, if DHH individuals want to be recognized and compete for promotions to advance their careers, they will have to understand and attend to the same factors that contribute to career success for all people, hearing status notwithstanding.

Regardless of field or industry, communication skills are critical to employment success, career growth, and career advancement. Specifically, these involve four important aspects of communication: (a) "listening" to understand others' points of view, (b) interacting to share one's views or ideas and build interpersonal relationships, (c) writing clearly and concisely, and (d) reading. All four are essential workplace communication competencies. How one presents one's self to others by using these skills is critical to job success and career growth. Communicators who tailor the messages they send to their audiences and understand workplace organizational culture will be perceived as more competent. Using behaviors characteristic of high self-monitoring, extroversion, and proactivity will help DHH people accomplish their goals for career growth and advancement.

Digital technologies and communication are inextricably intertwined. Along with computer-based work environments comes computer-mediated communication requiring the use of e-mail, blogs, social media, mobile technologies (more text than voice), and websites. The advent of collaboration tools and related technologies have increased the use of distributed work teams collaborating from different locations, possibly worldwide, requiring daily interactive communication using digital tools. Furthermore, an ability to capture, analyze, visualize, and interpret data is becoming a standard expectation for all information careers. All of this points to the increased importance of clear written language skills and mathematical knowledge if one is to interact effectively and develop the ability to measure and analyze data. This is a potentially fertile area for future research given the lack of substantive literature on DHH individuals working in information careers with the related expectations for sophisticated interactive communication skills, as well as data capture, analysis, and data interpretation knowledge/skills.

For DHH people, the increased use of digital technologies to communicate and interact offers a potential level playing field for direct online communication that bypasses the use of intermediaries such as a sign interpreter or relay service. However, it also carries the expectation of having solid literacy skills, especially writing skills and reading comprehension—two skill areas that have presented consistent challenges for DHH students. DHH students preparing for careers in fields that involve digital technologies to communicate and process information need to be cognizant of the expectations and literacy requirements for such positions

Research exploring DHH entrepreneurship and its empowering potential are at the early stage of development. The small extant literature suggests DHH entrepreneurship is limited, driven by push-oriented variables, and not currently viewed as a mainstream DHH career option. Despite these findings, entrepreneurship provides a potential, if not unique, option for DHH people who continually face employment and career growth barriers related to communication, outsider status, and discrimination. Understanding the career paths, barriers, and activities of successful DHH entrepreneurs represents a new area of research with the potential of expanding career empowerment for DHH people.

Regardless of hearing status, when it comes to being successful on the job, achieving promotions, and especially advancing one's career, everyone must play by the same rules. Attaining higher educational levels and developing strong interactive communication skills (sharing one's ideas, listening to understand other points of view, communicating with clear writing, reading), as well as mathematical literacy, all contribute to being a successful employee. If one wants to obtain promotions and grow her or his career, then being proactive and extroverted with good self-monitoring skills are important behaviors to develop. And, last but not least, developing self-confidence is also critical to career growth—the general self-confidence to accomplish tasks (GSE) and the more specific self-confidence to accomplish entrepreneurial-oriented tasks successfully (ESE). The question is whether the educational enterprise (K–12 through postsecondary), parents, and DHH students themselves can meet the challenge together to develop such skills for them to be competitive and successful in the jobs of the future.

REFERENCES

ACT (2005). *What are ACT's college readiness benchmarks?* Iowa City, IA: ACT. Retrieved from http://www.act.org/path/policy/pdf/benchmarks.

Albertini, J. A., Kelly, R. R., & Matchett, M. K. (2011). Personal factors that influence deaf college students' academic success. *Journal of Deaf Studies and Deaf Education, 17*(1) 85–191.

Allen, T. E. (1994). Who are the deaf and hard-of-hearing students leaving high school and entering postsecondary education? Paper submitted to Pelavin Research Institute as part of the project "A Comprehensive Evaluation of the Postsecondary Educational Opportunities for Students Who Are Deaf or Hard of Hearing." Washington, DC: U.S. Office of Special Education and Rehabilitative Services. Retrieved from http//:research.gallaudet.edu/AnnualSurvey/whodeaf.php.

Arthur, M. B. (1994). The boundaryless career: A new perspective for organizational inquiry. *Journal of Organizational Behavior, 15,* 295–306.

Arthur, M. B., & Rousseau, D. M. (1996). *The boundaryless career: A new employment principle for a new organizational era.* New York, NY: Oxford University Press.

Atkins, W. S. (2011). Exploring the lived experiences of deaf entrepreneurs and business owners. PhD dissertation, University of St. Thomas.

Aud, S. D., Hussar, W., Kena, G., Bianco K., Frohlich L., Kemp, J., & Tahan, K. (2011). *The condition of education 2011.* Washington, DC: U.S. Department of Education, National Center for Education Statistics.

Belknap, P. J., Korwin, K. A., & Long, N. M. (1995). Job coaching: A means to reduce unemployment and underemployment in the deaf community. *JADARA, 28*(4), 21–38.

Bharadwaj, A., El Sawy, O. A., Pavlou, P. A., & Venkatraman, N. (2013). Digital business strategy: Toward a next generation of insights. *MIS Quarterly, 37*(2), 471–482.

Blatto-Vallee, G., Kelly, R. R., Gaustad, M. G., Porter, J., & Fonzi, J. (2007). Visual-spatial representation in mathematical problem solving by deaf and hearing students. *Journal of Deaf Studies and Deaf Education, 12,* 432–448.

Boutin, D. L. (2010). Occupational outcomes for vocational rehabilitation consumers with hearing impairments. *Journal of Rehabilitation, 76*(3), 40–46.

Boutin, D. L., & Wilson, K. B. (2009). Professional jobs and hearing loss; A comparison of deaf and hard of hearing consumers. *Journal of Rehabilitation, 75*(1), 36–40.

Briscoe, J. P., Hall, D. T., & DeMuth, R. L. F. (2006). Protean and boundaryless careers: An empirical exploration. *Journal of Vocational Behavior, 69,* 30–47.

Broadbent, M., & Weill, P. (1993). Improving business and information strategy alignment: Learning from the banking industry. *IBM Systems Journal, 32*(1), 162–179.

Brooks, C. (January 2015). What is entrepreneurship? *Business News.* Retrieved from www.businessnewsdaily.com/2642-entrepreneurship.html.

Brownell, J. (1994). Managerial listening and career development in the hospitality industry. *Journal of the International Listening Association, 8,* 31–49.

Bull, R. (2008). Deafness, numerical cognition, and mathematics. In M. Marschark & P. Hauser (Eds.), *Deaf cognition: Foundations and outcomes* (pp. 171–200). New York, NY: Oxford University Press.

Burkhauser, R. V., Houtenville, A. J., & Tennant, J. R. (2014). Capturing the elusive working-age population with disabilities: Reconciling conflicting social success estimates from the Current Population Survey and the American Community Survey. *Journal of Disability Policy Studies, 24*(4), 195–205.

Carter, N. M., Gartner, W. B., Shaver, K. G., & Gatewood, E. J. (2003). The career reasons of nascent entrepreneurs. *Journal of Business Venturing, 18*(1), 13–39.

Cassar, G. (2007). Money, money, money? A longitudinal investigation of entrepreneur career reasons, growth preferences and achieved growth. *Entrepreneurship and Regional Development, 19*(1), 89–107.

Chan, Y. E., & Reich, B. H. (2007). IT alignment: An annotated bibliography. *Journal of Information Technology, 22*(4), 316–396.

Crant, J. M. (2000). Proactive behavior in organizations. *Journal of Management, 26*(3), 435–462.

Cuculick, J. A., & Kelly, R. R. (2003). Relating deaf Students' reading and language scores at college entry to their degree completion rates. *American Annals of the Deaf, 148*(4), 279–286.

Dawson, C., & Henley, A. (2012). "Push" versus "pull" entrepreneurship: An ambiguous distinction? *International Journal of Entrepreneurial Behaviour & Research, 18*(6), 697–719.

DeMartino, R., Atkins, W. S., Barbato, R. J., & Perotti, V. J. (2011). Entrepreneurship in the disability community: An exploratory study on the deaf and hard of hearing community. *Frontiers of Entrepreneurship Research, 31*(4), 5 [abstract].

DeMartino, R., Perotti, V. J., Atkins, W. S., Barbato, R. J., Murthy, R., & Stromeyer, W. R. (2015). Entrepreneurial proclivities in the deaf and hard of hearing communities: A mixed method exploration. Manuscript submitted for publication.

Dennis, J. (1996). Self-employment: When nothing else is available? *Journal of Labour Research, 17*(4), 645–661.

Douglas, E. J., & Shepherd, D. A. (2002). Self-employment as a career choice: Attitudes, entrepreneurial intentions, and utility maximization. *Entrepreneurship Theory and Practice, 26*(3), 81–90.

Foster, S. (1992). *Working with deaf people: Accessibility and accommodation in the workplace.* Springfield, IL: Charles C. Thomas.

Foster, S., & MacLeod, J. (2003). Deaf people at work: Assessment of communication among deaf and hearing persons in work settings. *International Journal of Audiology, 42*(Suppl. 1), 128–139.

Foster, S., & MacLeod, J. (2004). The role of mentoring relationships in the career development of successful deaf persons. *Journal of Deaf Studies and Deaf Education, 9*(4), 432–458.

Garberoglio, C. L., Cawthon, S. W., & Bond, M. (2014). Assessing English literacy as a predictor of post-school outcomes in the lives of deaf individuals. *Journal of Deaf Studies and Deaf Education, 19*(1), 50–67.

Gaustad, M. G., & Kelly, R. R. (2004). The relationship between reading achievement and morphological word analysis in deaf and hearing students matched for reading level. *Journal of Deaf Studies and Deaf Education, 9*(3), 269–285.

Gaustad, M. G., Kelly, R. R., Payne, J. A., & Lylak, E. (2002). Deaf and hearing students' morphological knowledge applied to printed English. *American Annals of the Deaf, 147*(5), 5–21.

Geyer, P. D., & Schroedel, J. G. (1998). Early career job satisfaction for full-time workers who are deaf or hard of hearing. *Journal of Rehabilitation, 65*, 33–37.

Gilad, B., & Levine, P. (1986). A behavioral model of entrepreneurial supply. *Journal of Small Business Management, 24*(4), 45–54.

Haas, J. W., & Arnold, C. L. (1995). An examination of the role of listening in judgments of communication competence in co-workers. *The Journal of Business Communication, 32*(2), 123–139.

Hall, D. T. (1976). *Careers in organizations*. Pacific Palisades, CA: Goodyear.

Hall, D. T. (2004). The protean career: A quarter-century journey. *Journal of Vocational Behavior, 65*, 1–13.

Hartmann, E. A. (2010). Evaluating employment outcomes of adults who are deaf and hard of hearing. PhD dissertation, Teachers College, Columbia University.

Hauser, P. C., Luomski, J., & Hillman, T. (2008). Development of deaf and hard-of-hearing students' executive function. In M. Marschark & P. Hauser (Eds.), *Deaf cognition: Foundations and outcomes* (pp. 286–308). New York, NY: Oxford University Press.

Hessels, J., Van Gelderen, M., & Thurik, R. (2008). Entrepreneurial aspirations, motivations, and their drivers. *Small Business Economics, 31*(3), 323–339.

Hintermair, M. (2013). Executive functions and behavioral problems in deaf and hard-of-hearing students in general and special schools. *Journal of Deaf Studies and Deaf Education, 18*(3), 344–359.

Hisrich, R. D., & Brush, C. (1986). Characteristics of the minority entrepreneur. *Journal of Small Business Management, 24*(1), 1–8.

Hogan, R., Curphy, G. J., & Hogan, J. (1994). What we know about leadership: Effectiveness and personality. *American Psychologist, 49*, 493–504.

Jarvenpaa, S. L., & Leidner, D. E. (1998). Communication and trust in global virtual teams. *Journal of Computer-Mediated Communication, 3*(4). Retrieved from http://onlinelibrary.wiley.com/doi/10.1111/j.1083-6101.1998.tb00080.x/full. Accessed January 26, 2016.

Jeanes, R. C., Nienhuys, T. G. W. M., & Rickards, F. W. (2000). The pragmatic skills of profoundly deaf children. *Journal of Deaf Studies and Deaf Education, 5*(3), 238–247.

Johnson, V. A. (1993). Factors impacting the job retention and advancement of workers who are deaf. *The Volta Review, 95*(4), 341–354.

Karmel, C. A. (1982). 'Rubella bulge' of the 60's reaches the colleges. *The New York Times*. Retrieved from http://www.nytimes.com/1982/04/25/education/rubella-bulge-of-the-60-s-reaches-the-colleges.html. Accessed January 26, 2016.

Kelly, R. R. (2008). Deaf learners and mathematical problem solving. In M. Marschark & P. Hauser (Eds.), *Deaf cognition: Foundations and outcomes* (pp. 226–249). New York, NY: Oxford University Press.

Kelly, R. R., & Gaustad, M. (2007). Deaf college students' mathematical skills relative to morphological knowledge, reading level, and language proficiency. *Journal of Deaf Studies and Deaf Education, 12*(1), 25–37.

Kelly, R. R., Quagliata, A. B., DeMartino, R., & Perotti, V. (July 2015). Deaf workers: Educated and employed, but limited in career growth. Paper presented at the 22nd International Congress on the Education of the Deaf. Athens, Greece.

Kilduff, M., & Day, D. V. (1994). Do chameleons get ahead? The effects of self-monitoring on managerial careers. *Academy of Management Journal, 37*(4), 1047–1060.

Lane, H. (1992). *The mask of benevolence: Disabling the deaf community*. New York, NY: Knopf.

Lane-Outlaw, A. (2012). *Breaking the glass ceiling with Alicia Lane-Outlaw* [video]. Rochester, NY: National Technical Institute for the Deaf at Rochester Institute of Technology. Retrieved from http://www.rit.edu/ntid/reach/success-stories/alicia-lane-outlaw. Accessed January 26, 2016.

Leonard, J., & Seddon, P. (2012). A meta-model of alignment. *Communications of the Association for Information Systems, 31*(11), 230–259.

Lewis, G. B., & Allee, C. L. (1992). The impact of disabilities on federal career success. *Public Administrations Review, 52*(4), 389–397.

Lewis, L., Farris, E., & Greene, B. (1994). *Deaf and hard of hearing students in postsecondary education: Statistical analysis report*. NCES 94-394. Washington, DC: U.S. Department of Education, National Center for Education Statistics.

Luft, P. (2000). Communication barriers for deaf employees: Needs assessment and problem-solving strategies. *Work: A Journal of Prevention, Assessment and Rehabilitation, 14*(1), 51–59.

Luft, P. (April 1998). Difficulties of deaf/hard of hearing supported employees in comparison with other disability groups. Paper presented at the meeting of the American Educational Research Association, Policy to Practice in Special Education Session. San Diego, CA.

Lussier, R. N., Say, K., & Corman, J. (2000). Need satisfaction of deaf and hearing employees. *The Mid-Atlantic Journal of Business, 36*, 47–61.

Marschark, M., Convertino, C. M., Macias, G., Monikowski, C. M., Sapere, P., & Seewagen, R. (2007). Understanding communication among deaf students who sign and speak: A trivial pursuit? *American Annals of the Deaf, 152*(4), 415–424.

Marschark, M., Knoors, H., & Tang, G. (2014). Perspectives on bilingualism and bilingual education for deaf learners. In M. Marschark, G. Tang, & H. Knoors (Eds.), *Bilingualism and bilingual deaf education* (pp. 445–476). New York, NY: Oxford University Press.

Marschark, M., Sapere, P., Convertino, C., & Pelz, J. (2008). Learning via direct and mediated instruction by deaf students. *Journal of Deaf Studies and Deaf Education, 13*(4), 546–561.

Marschark, M., Sapere, P., Convertino, C., & Seewagen, R. (2005). Access to postsecondary education through sign language interpreting. *Journal of Deaf Studies and Deaf Education, 10*(1), 38–50.

Marschark, M., & Wauters, L. (2008). Language comprehension and learning by deaf learners. In M. Marschark & P. Hauser (Eds.), *Deaf cognition: Foundations and outcomes* (pp. 309–350). New York, NY: Oxford University Press.

McGee, J. E., Peterson, M., Mueller, S. L., & Sequeira, J. M. (2009). Entrepreneurial self-efficacy: Refining the measure. *Entrepreneurship Theory and Practice, 33*(4), 965–988.

Mindess, A., Holcomb, T. K., Langholtz, D., & Moyers, P. P. (2006). *Reading between the signs: Intercultural communication for sign language interpreters* (2nd ed.). Boston, MA: Intercultural Press.

Mitchell, R. E. (2006). How many deaf people are there in the United States? Estimates from the Survey of Income and Program Participation. *Journal of Deaf Studies and Deaf Education, 11*(1), 112–119.

Morreale, S. P., & Pearson, J. C. (2008). Why communication education is important: The centrality of the discipline in the 21st century. *Communication Education, 57,* 224–240.

Moores, D. F. (1987). Higher education. In J. V. Van Cleve (Ed.), *Gallaudet encyclopedia of deaf people and deafness* (Vol. 1, pp. 403–404). New York, NY: McGraw-Hill.

Most, T. (2010). How does speech intelligibility affect self and others' perceptions of deaf and hard-of-hearing people? In M. Marschark & P. E. Spencer (Eds.), *The Oxford handbook of deaf studies, language, and education* (Vol. 2, pp. 251–263). New York, NY: Oxford University Press.

Myers, P. C., & Danek, M. M. (1990). Deaf employment assistance network: A model for employment service delivery. *Journal of the American Deafness and Rehabilitation Association, 24*(2), 59–67.

Ng, T. W. H., Eby, L. T., Sorensen, K. L., & Feldman, D. C. (2005). Predictors of objective and subjective career success: A meta-analysis. *Personnel Psychology, 58,* 367–408.

National Technical Institute for the Deaf (2006). *Annual report: October 1, 2005–September 30, 2006.* Rochester, NY: National Technical Institute for the Deaf at the Rochester Institute of Technology. Retrieved from http://www.ntid.rit.edu/sites/default/files/annual_report2006.pdf.

National Technical Institute for the Deaf (2014). *Annual report: October 1, 2013–September 30, 2014.* Rochester, NY: National Technical Institute for the Deaf at the Rochester Institute of Technology. Retrieved from http://www.ntid.rit.edu/sites/default/files/annual_report_2014.pdf.

O'Keefe, B. J. (1988). The logic of message design: Individual differences in reasoning about communication. *Communications Monographs, 55*(1), 80–103.

O'Keefe, B. J., & McCornack, S. A. (1987). Message design logic and message goal structure effects on perceptions of message quality in regulative communication situations. *Human Communication Research, 14*(1), 68–92.

Peiperl, M. A., & Baruch, Y. (1997). Back to square zero: The post-corporate career. *Organizational Dynamics, 25*(4), 7–22.

Powell, A., Piccoli, G., & Ives, B. (2004). Virtual teams: A review of current literature and directions for future research. *ACM Sigmis Database, 35*(1), 6–36.

Pressman, S. (1999). A national study of deaf entrepreneurs and small business owners: Implications for career counseling. PhD dissertation, Virginia Polytechnic Institute and State University.

Punch, R., Creed, P. A., & Hyde, M. B. (2006). Career barriers perceived by hard-of-hearing adolescents: Implications for practice from a mixed-methods study. *Journal of Deaf Studies and Deaf Education, 11*(2), 224–237.

Qi, S., & Mitchell, R. E. (2012). Large-scale academic achievement testing of deaf and hard-of-hearing students: Past, present, and future. *Journal of Deaf Studies and Deaf Education, 17*(1), 1–18.

Ragu-Nathan, T. S., Tarafdar, M., Ragu-Nathan, B. S., & Tu, Q. (2008). The consequences of technostress for end users in organizations: Conceptual development and empirical validation. *Information Systems Research, 19*(4), 417–433.

Richardson, J., Marschark, M., Sarchet, T., & Sapere, P. (2010). Deaf and hard-of-hearing students' experiences in mainstream and separate postsecondary education. *Journal of Deaf Studies and Deaf Education, 15*(4), 358–382.

Rivera-Batiz, F. (1992). Quantitative literacy and the likelihood of employment among young adults in the United States. *The Journal of Human Resources, 27*(2), 313–328.

Rose, H., & Betts, J. R. (2001). *Math matters: The links between high school curriculum, college graduation, and earnings.* San Francisco, CA: Public Policy Institute of California.

Rosenbaum, J. E. (1984). *Career mobility in a corporate hierarchy.* Orlando, FL: Academic Press.

Scherich, D. L. (1996). Job accommodations in the workplace for persons who are deaf or hard of hearing: Current practices and recommendations. *Journal of Rehabilitation, 62*(2), 27–35.

Schjoedt, L., & Shaver, K. G. (2007). Deciding on an entrepreneurial career: A test of the pull and push hypotheses using the panel study of entrepreneurial dynamics data1. *Entrepreneurship Theory and Practice, 31*(5), 733–752.

Schley, S., Walter, G. G., Weathers, R. R., II, Hemmeter, J., Hennessey, J. C., & Burkhauser, R. V. (2011). Effect of postsecondary education on the economic status of persons who are deaf or hard of hearing. *Journal of Deaf Studies and Deaf Education, 16*(4), 524–536.

Schroedel, J. G., & Geyer, P. D. (2000). Long-term career attainments of deaf and hard of hearing college graduates: Results from a 15-year follow-up study. *American Annals of the Deaf, 145,* 303–314.

Seibert, S. E., Kraimer, M. L., & Crant, J. M. (2001). What do proactive people do? A longitudinal model linking proactive personality and career success. *Personnel Psychology, 54*(4), 845–874.

Shane, S., Locke, E. A., & Collins, C. J. (2003). Entrepreneurial motivation. *Human Resource Management Review, 13*(2), 257–279.

Shaver, D., Newman, L., Hang, T., Yu, J., & Knokey, A. (February 2011). *Facts from NLTS2: Secondary school experiences and academic performance of students with hearing impairments.* Menlo Park, CA: SRI International. Retrieved from http://www.nlts2.org/fact_sheets/nlts2_fact_sheet_2011_02.pdf. Accessed January 26, 2016.

Skovli, E. (2012). *Breaking the glass ceiling with Eva Skovli* [video]. Rochester, NY: National Technical Institute for the Deaf at Rochester Institute of Technology. Retrieved from http://www.rit.edu/ntid/reach/success-stories/eva-skovli. Accessed January 26, 2016.

Smeaton, D. (2003), Self-employed workers: Calling the shots or hesitant independents? A consideration of the trends. *Work, Employment & Society, 17*(2), 379–391.

Smith, K. (2007). What is digital marketing? Retrieved from http://digitalmarketing101.blogspot.com/2007/10/what-is-digital-marketing.html. Accessed January 26, 2016.

Snyder, M. (1974). Self-monitoring of expressive behavior. *Journal of Personality and Social Psychology, 30*(4), 526–537.

Spiropoulos, R. (May 2014). Small business owners vs entrepreneurs: Which one are you? Black Enterprise. Retrieved from www.blackenterprise.com/small-business/small-business-owners-vs-entrepreneurs-which-one-are-you/.

Spring, M. (May 2014). Are you a small-business owner or an entrepreneur? The difference is important. *Entrepreneur*. Retrieved from www.entrepreneur.com/article/233919.

Stinson, M. S., & Antia, S. D. (1999). Considerations in educating deaf and hard-of- hearing students in inclusive environments. *Journal of Deaf Studies and Deaf Education*, 4(3), 163–175.

Sypher, B. D., Bostrom, R. N., & Seibert, J. H. (1989). Listening, communication abilities, and success at work. *Journal of Business Communication*, 26, 293–303.

Sypher, B. D., & Sypher, H. E. (1983). Perceptions of communication ability self-monitoring in an organizational setting. *Personality and Social Psychology Bulletin*, 9(2), 297–304.

Toossi, M. (2002). A century of change: The U.S. labor force, 1950–2050. *Monthly Labor Review*, May, 15–28.

Toossi, M. (2012). Labor force projections to 2020: A more slowly growing workforce. *Monthly Labor Review, January*, 43–64.

Ullah, A., & Lai, R. (2013). A systematic review of business and information technology alignment. *ACM Transactions on Management Information Systems (TMIS)*, 4(1), 1–29.

U.S. Census Bureau. (2010). American Community Survey. http://www.census.gov/acs. Accessed January 26, 2016.

U.S. Census Bureau. (2011). Educational attainment in the United States: 2011– Detailed tables. Current Population Survey, 2011 annual social and economic supplement. Retrieved from www.census.gov/hhes/socdemo/education/data/cps/2011/tables.html.

U.S. Department of Labor. (2015). Standard Occupational Classification. Retrieved from http://www.bls.gov/soc/. Accessed January 26, 2016.

Walter, G. G., Clarcq, J. R., and Thompson, W. S. (2002). Effect of degree attainment on improving the economic status of individuals who are deaf. *JADARA*, 35(3), 30–46.

Weisel, A., & Cinamon, R. G. (2005). Hearing, deaf, and hard-of-hearing Israeli adolescents' evaluations of deaf men and deaf women's occupational competence. *Journal of Deaf Studies and Deaf Education*, 10(4), 376–389.

Wells, A. G. (2008). Deaf world, that's where I'm at: A phenomenological study exploring the experience of being a deaf employee in the workplace. PhD dissertation, University of Memphis.

Welch, S. A., & Mickelson, W. T. (2013). A listening competence comparison of working professionals. *International Journal of Listening*, 27(2), 85–99.

Welsh, W. A. (1993). Factors influencing career mobility of deaf adults. *The Volt Review*, 95, 329–339.

Welsh, W., & MacLeod-Gallinger, J. (1992). Effect of college on employment and earnings. In S. B. Foster & G. G. Walter (Eds.), *Deaf students in postsecondary education* (pp. 185–209). New York, NY: Routledge.

Welsh, W. A., & Walter, G. G. (1988). The effect of postsecondary education on the occupational attainments of deaf adults. *Journal of the Deafness and Rehabilitation Association*, 22(1), 14–22.

Willoughby, L. (2011). Sign language users' education and employment levels: Keeping pace with changes in the general Australian population. *Journal of Deaf Studies and Deaf Education, 16*(3), 401–413.

Winn, S. (2007). Employment outcomes for people in Australia who are congenitally deaf: Has anything changed? *American Annals of the Deaf, 152*(4), 382–390.

Wolvin, A. D., & Coakley, C. G. (1993). A listening taxonomy. In A. D. Wolvin & C. G. Coakley (Eds.), *Perspectives on listening* (pp. 15–22). Norwood, NJ: Ablex.

18

Recognizing Diversity in Deaf Education: Now What Do We Do With It?!

Marc Marschark and Greg Leigh

No one who has worked with a significant number of deaf learners will have any doubt with regard to the considerable diversity among them. Although it may not be obvious to the parents of a (single) deaf child or to adults who happen to know only a deaf person or two, the individual differences among deaf children and, of particular importance for our current purposes, the individual differences likely to affect formal and informal learning, are such that deaf education remains very challenging for both teachers and students, regardless of the age of the learner. This chapter examines the scope of factors that appear most likely to affect learning and academic outcomes among deaf learners, regardless of whether they really do (discussed later in the chapter). Given the wealth of knowledge available in this regard, even if it is not always acknowledged in educational decision making (Archbold & Mayer, 2012), this chapter is not intended to provide a comprehensive, in-depth analysis of all the relevant variables. Rather, the focus is on academically related factors for which there is empirical evidence pointing toward both (a) a better understanding of how those factors affect learning and (b) directions for accommodating those factors in the methods and materials of instruction—or not.

The suggestion that there are some factors affecting the education of deaf and hard-of-hearing (DHH) learners that might not or should not be accommodated is not meant to be facetious, but has two levels of meaning. First, even if we accept the assertion that "deaf children are not hearing children who can't hear" and that we should not teach them as such (Knoors & Marschark, 2014), the reality is that the deaf students of today are the citizens of tomorrow with all the rights, privileges, and responsibilities thereof. Whether or not they believe it (or like it), they will need to be competent, and preferably fluent, in the written (if not spoken) vernacular of their workplaces and their communities (see Chapter 11). They will need problem-solving skills that allow them to be flexible in the physical and intellectual contexts of their employment and have communication and social skills that allow them to be engaged both occupationally and socially (see Chapter 17). We can facilitate access for DHH individuals and educate hearing individuals about living and working with them—and vice versa—but that does not remove the onus on the former to fulfill the familial, employment, and civil responsibilities of members of society. There are ways that DHH learners, therefore, are going to have to accommodate the society in which they live, even if they see that as "the hearing world."

A second reason why some factors affecting academic performance and outcomes of DHH learners might not be accommodated, frankly, pertains to their complexity. There are some factors associated with educating DHH learners that simply are beyond the scope of teachers or researchers, at least in any broad sense. For example, a variety of reports have indicated that family characteristics including race, household income, maternal level of education, and individual characteristics such as gender and temperament are associated significantly with academic achievement of DHH students just as they are for hearing students, but they are beyond our control (see Marschark et al., 2015b; Mitchell & Karchmer, 2011; Stinson & Kluwin, 2011). Furthermore, an estimated 40% to 50% of DHH learners have secondary disabilities (Blackorby & Knokey, 2006), including cognitive and behavioral disabilities that are likely to affect classroom learning (Knoors & Vervloed, 2011). Variability in the individual characteristics of DHH learners thus is a much greater challenge for teachers of DHH students compared with teachers of hearing students, if for no other reason than the added complexity of their jobs in the classroom. In a study involving more than 500 DHH secondary school students in the nationally representative sample of the National Longitudinal Transition Study 2 (NLTS2), Marschark et al. (2015b) found that DHH students being diagnosed with dyslexia or a learning disability was a major (negative) predictor of academic achievement across the curriculum (reading, mathematics, social studies, and science), second only to whether they had attended regular schools only (a positive predictor) as opposed to special schools or a mix of regular and special schools. But, more about that later.

The lack of any detailed discussion on the impact of secondary disabilities on DHH learners' academic outcomes follows largely from the fact that the variability they add to other academically relevant factors does not fit into convenient "boxes" that can be labeled and distinguished or on a scale of severity or risk that can be quantified. Marschark et al. (2015b), for example, found that being diagnosed with attention deficit disorder/attention deficit hyperactivity disorder (ADD/ADHD) was not a significant predictor of DHH secondary school students' academic achievement when other factors were controlled, whereas having a secondary disability other than dyslexia/learning disability or ADD/ADHD was a significant predictor of achievement in mathematics and social studies but not reading or science. Why mathematics and social studies and not reading or science? Secondary disabilities are not all or none; how does the severity of ADD/ADHD or various neuropsychological impairments affect learning? How do they interact with variability in language fluency, parental hearing status, family socioeconomic status, and so on?

Similar complexities are the reason why this chapter also does not consider etiologies of hearing loss (see Chapter 14). How it is that an individual comes to be born deaf or have a progressive or acute hearing loss—with or without a secondary disability—certainly can affect language development, social development, cognitive development, and a variety of interactions with people and things in the environment. Whether a particular etiology is genetic or adventitious, syndromic or nonsyndromic, and affects only hearing or also other physical and/or neuropsychological functioning may well have bearing on the growth and development of a child as well as day-to-day functioning in the family and in school. Nevertheless, the variety of these factors, not to mention the myriad possible interactions among them, are such that they result in (currently) unknown variability in educationally relevant foundations, abilities, and outcomes. This is one reason why the development and education of DHH children with secondary disabilities is such a difficult area and why there is so little by way of an evidence base for parents and teachers of these children to build on (see Van Dijk et al., 2010). This is not to say that investigations into specific sequelae of hearing loss-related etiologies are unimportant or that such research could not be informative with regard to fostering the development and education of DHH children. It is only to say that, given the heterogeneity of that population, the work would be difficult, expensive, and likely of only limited generalizability.

A related factor, degree of hearing loss, is another variable that is not considered here at any length, although the reasons for that omission are rather different. Calderon (1998) suggested that the relatively high rate of co-occurrence of hearing loss and learning disabilities suggests shared etiologies. It appears to be unknown whether there is any relation between the *degree* of hearing loss and the *severity* of secondary disabilities, but at face value, Calderon's observation would suggest that such an association is likely. Nevertheless, within the literatures pertaining to education, early intervention, and psychology (both cognitive and psychosocial) involving DHH learners, it is most common to see DHH individuals grouped together without reference to hearing thresholds. We know that even minimal hearing losses can have a measurable impact on children's literacy (Goldberg & Richburg, 2004; Moeller et al., 2007), and it generally is assumed that the greater the hearing loss, the poorer the academic (and especially literacy) outcomes (e.g., Karchmer et al., 1979). In any sample of DHH learners, however, hearing thresholds typically are confounded with communication modality (Allen & Anderson, 2010; Wagner et al., 2002), with the use (and benefit) of assistive listening devices (Blackorby et al., 2002), and with school placement (Shaver et al., 2014; Stinson & Kluwin, 2011).

In the representative sample of secondary school students in NLTS2, when other factors were controlled, Marschark et al. (2015b) found that reported mild hearing loss was a significant predictor of poor performance in reading, mathematics, and social studies, but moderate or severe/profound losses were not. This finding may reflect the assumption by teachers that students with better hearing, and thus often with good speech intelligibility, are less in need of additional support compared with students with greater hearing losses (Archbold, 2015). (An interesting question for future research is whether *students* with lesser hearing losses think they are less in need of additional support [Marschark et al., 2016].) Possible support for this interpretation can be found in results from the Special Education Elementary Longitudinal Study (SEELS). Blackorby and Knokey (2006) reported that, among DHH elementary and middle school students, those with severe/profound hearing losses outperformed peers with moderate hearing losses on Woodcock-Johnson III Passage Comprehension and Mathematics subtests. However, the investigators did not report results for students with mild hearing losses and did not consider the impact on results of cochlear implant (CI) use among children with profound hearing losses. In a sample of DHH students just entering college, however, Marschark et al. (2015c) found no significant correlations between either aided or unaided hearing thresholds and college entrance scores (reading comprehension, mathematics, English, or composite scores) regardless of whether the students used CIs. Convertino et al. (2009) found hearing thresholds and CI use also unrelated to learning in college classrooms. The issue of long-term benefits of CI use is discussed later. The point here is that, although hearing thresholds, like other student and family characteristics, are likely to affect academic outcomes, variability in that measure (with regard both to intensity and frequency) has only rarely been investigated with regard to various aspects of academically relevant cognitive functioning or with regard to academic achievement when other factors are controlled. This work, too, would be difficult and expensive given the sample sizes needed; but, if early findings from SEELS and NLTS2 hold up, it might well be of considerable importance and benefit to educating learners with various levels of hearing loss.

THREE THINGS WE THINK WE KNOW ABOUT DEAF EDUCATION BUT REALLY DON'T

Having touched on several aspects of the diversity among DHH learners that we are unable to discuss in any depth at this point, we next describe three factors that also are relevant to academic outcomes among DHH learners but remain in need of further investigation. One thing that makes these three areas interesting (at least to us) is that there are popular assumptions that we already have the answers to the relevant questions, when the reality is not so clear. In raising (or reraising) questions about what we know and what we don't know in these areas, we necessarily need to leave aside ways in which each of them might be affected by the factors noted earlier: family variables such as parents' education, household income, race/ethnicity, and a priori child characteristics including secondary disabilities and hearing thresholds. In fact, all these factors may be intertwined in some subtle and not-so-subtle ways, but there are some larger issues to be addressed first.

What Is the Long-Term Impact of Early Intervention for DHH Children?

Sass-Lehrer and Young (see Chapter 2) noted that the effectiveness of various early intervention methods vary as a function of children, families, and cultures. It would be worthwhile to add to that list something akin to the "state-of-the-art" in the field as well. For example, Calderon and Greenberg (1997) reported that DHH children who had participated in early intervention programming that included sign language fared better in early language, social development, and cognitive functioning than those who had participated in oral-only programming. Twenty years later, with the remarkable success of CIs for many deaf children, it is unlikely their generalization is still valid. No doubt it is true for some children, but if the history of the "war of methods" (Lang, 2011) with regard to deaf education tells us anything, it is that any one-size-fits-all approach to language does most DHH children a disservice (see Chapter 8). Beyond broader use of sign language, technology (Segers & Verhoeven, 2015), improved methodologies with regard to speech and hearing therapies (Fagan, 2016), recognition that sign language and spoken language can be mutually supportive rather than mutually exclusive (e.g., Giezen et al., 2014; Yoshinaga-Itano & Sedey, 2000), and family-centered early intervention methods (e.g., Brown & Nott, 2006; see also Chapter 2), all have contributed to improvements in the developmental trajectories of DHH children.

Calderon and Naidu (1999) found that the age at which intervention services were first provided predicted DHH children's receptive and expressive language and speech scores and, likely not coincidentally, also was associated with greater mother–child interaction. More specifically, Yoshinaga-Itano et al. (e.g., Yoshinaga-Itano & Sedey, 2000; Yoshinaga-Itano et al., 2001) have documented consistent findings indicating that children identified and receiving intervention before six months of age show normal language development, even if "normal" in those studies frequently refers to "low-normal" functioning relative to hearing norms. What appears to be lacking in this rich area of investigation are studies of the long-term impact of early intervention services on the language, social functioning, and especially academic achievement of DHH learners. One would expect transitivity insofar as if early intervention facilitates early language development, and better language abilities are associated with greater academic achievement, then early intervention should be associated with greater academic achievement. A missing piece in that nonequation, however, is a link between early language development and better later language abilities, an issue to be discussed at some length later in this chapter. But, we are now more than several decades into the "early intervention movement." There are large numbers of DHH individuals who were involved in early-intervention programming and now have reached secondary school, postsecondary education, and the workplace. What are the long-term effects of early-intervention programming at large and perhaps even different forms of early-intervention programming?

So, why do we not know about the long-term effects of early intervention, aside from the assumption that they are undoubtedly positive? Although they were not focusing on the longer term questions being raised here, Sass-Lehrer and Young (see Chapter 2) suggested that the relative paucity of evaluation studies with regard to early-intervention programming might reflect concerns that any evaluation might be "too reductionist" in seeking the critical factors in early-intervention programming, differing opinions on "what counts as an outcome," and "whether we might have a limited view of best outcomes for deaf and hard-of-hearing children (which focus more on language/communication and less on social–emotional well-being)." They noted that because of the diversity among DHH children and their familial contexts, results of such studies may not be generalizable across contexts. More important, however, Sass-Lehrer and Young (Chapter 2) emphasized that "[w]e may find the same fundamental evidence-based principles still hold true but simply have to be applied differently. Or, better evidence arising from new research may cause us to cast off long-held truths about best practice" (p. 25). The same could be said for questions about long-term impact on language fluencies, psychosocial functioning, and academic outcomes. The data are out there, but no one seems to be asking the "long-term questions," apparently in the belief early benefits are undoubtedly durable. The important thing is to ask the questions and then decide how best to live with the answers.

What Is the Long-Term Impact of Bilingual Educational Programming for DHH Children?

Among the many points of agreement in a field that frequently appears dysfunctional, and a point alluded to earlier, is that DHH learners who primarily use sign language for interpersonal communication also will benefit from and in many ways require the ability to communicate in the language of the community in which they live. To a greater or lesser extent (a convenient hedge given the sensitivity of the issue), the written form of the vernacular may well be sufficient for the needs, or at least the desires, of some DHH adults. That is, the claim here is not that DHH individuals need to use spoken language, but they need to be competent at least in the written form of the vernacular—that signing deaf individuals need to be bilingual. The argument from the other direction, that DHH learners who primarily use spoken language for interpersonal communication will benefit from having sign language skills, may be less obvious or persuasive, but it has been made in several ways. One is in terms of the importance of sign language to deaf youth's finding their identities and having better quality of life (e.g., Holcomb, 2013; see also Chapter 12), although the findings of Kushalnagar et al., (2011) and Marschark et al. (2015a) fail to support this argument. Other arguments for deaf children who might be using a spoken language to acquire a sign language as well include the possibility that the acquisition of spoken language ultimately might be insufficient or unsatisfactory for an individual's needs (Caselli et al., 2012; Humphries et al., 2012) and that the potential benefits of sign language in addition to spoken language outweigh the risks (Mellon et al., 2015).

This is not the place to debate the personal or cultural benefits of bilingualism among deaf individuals. This is not the intention, and the point does not even appear debatable as long as no universals are invoked. The relatively brief consideration of bilingual deaf education here is only to suggest that, even when recognized as potentially beneficial, if not essential, for many deaf learners, the case for the benefits of sign language to *academic outcomes* has yet to be made. Bowe (1992), Stewart (1993), and Moores (2008) all lamented the lack of research on the impact of sign language-based instruction on student learning and academic outcomes. More recently, Spencer and Marschark (2010) and Marschark and Knoors (2015) noted that, despite the continuing lack of evidence, theoretical and philosophical arguments for bilingual programming continue to be raised. In particular (only because it is the area in which the vast majority of research has been conducted), Marschark and Knoors (2015) argued that, although being fluent in sign language will likely better support a child's acquisition of literacy skills than if the child is lacking fluency in any language, the theoretical and practical paths from sign language to print literacy remain obscure and confounded (Mayer & Akamatsu, 1999; Mayer & Leigh, 2010). As Mayer (see Chapter 10) noted, claims that proficiency in sign language can provide DHH learners with access to print literacy in the vernacular "runs counter to the available evidence from other bilingual contexts in which it is well established that L2 proficiency is necessary to effectively and readily construct meaning in text in L2" (p. 275).

On the assumption that effective bilingual education requires the learner to be immersed in a bilingual language environment, there are at least two obvious challenges facing DHH learners in that regard. One is the school environment characterized internationally by a lack of certified deaf teachers, the lack of sign language fluency among many (deaf as well as hearing) teachers of the deaf who are usually nonnative signers, and the "Catch-22" of deaf learners being among deaf peers who are not fluent signers. The other challenge, as noted by Knoors and Marschark (2014; see also Hermans et al., 2009), is that despite the abundance of evidence indicating the importance of parent–child language development and the fact that more than 95% of DHH children have hearing parents, we know very little about how to provide these parents with sufficient sign language skills to support the sign skills of their children, their language abilities at large, their knowledge of the world, and their academic achievement (see Chapter 4). But, we do know that less than full access to language early on leaves DHH children with lags in both their sign language and literacy skills that cannot be remediated later (Cormier et al., 2012; Mayberry & Lock, 2003).

The issue here is not just one of deaf learners having hearing parents. The study by Marschark et al. (2015b) mentioned earlier involving a (U.S.) nationally representative sample of DHH secondary school students found that neither sign language skills nor parental hearing status were significant predictors of academic achievement among DHH secondary school students (see also, Lange et al., 2013). Related to this, an ongoing project by Marschark and colleagues (e.g., Marschark et al., 2015c) is examining the abilities of DHH college students in sign language, spoken language, several cognitive domains, and psychosocial functioning, as well as interactions among these factors. Thus far, neither having deaf parents nor being a native signer has been associated with significantly better academic achievement as indicated by college entrance scores.

Nover et al. (2002) summarized findings from a 5-year project at a school for the deaf that used bilingual programming. Stanford Achievement Test reading comprehension scores were reported for more than 150 students, more than a third of whom had deaf parents. Only students age 8 to 12 years old scored (slightly) higher than the national norms for DHH students. Knoors and Marschark (2012), however, reported scores from another school for the deaf on the same test for students of the same age, who were born in the same years as those in the study by Nover et al. (2002). The students in that Total Communication program, few of whom had deaf parents, scored higher than those in the bilingual program of Nover et al. (2002), exceeding their scores in all but one of the five age groups.

Apparently, there are only two published studies providing explicit evidence of a positive impact of bilingual programming on DHH students' academic outcomes. Heiling (1998) described a 1980s cohort of deaf eighth-grade students in Sweden that had received signed instruction throughout their school years and were reported to be "fluent" in sign language. In fact, those students had been exposed primarily to simultaneous communication (speech and sign together) rather than Swedish Sign Language, but they demonstrated greater reading and mathematics achievement compared with an earlier cohort educated exclusively through spoken language. Heiling (1997, cited in Bagga-Gupta, 2004), however, reported that those advantages were not found in a 1990s cohort that had received instruction through Swedish Sign Language. Moreover, later research by Rydberg et al. (2009) found that although achievement levels of deaf individuals had increased since Sweden had adopted bilingual education for deaf learners, achievement among hearing individuals had increased even more, so deaf learners continued to lag behind their hearing peers (see Bagga-Gupta [2004] and Swanwick et al. [2014] for the lack of evidence in support of bilingual programming in Scandinavia). In other words, Heiling's (1998) results did not demonstrate the effectiveness of bilingual education, but reflected general improvements in the outcomes of Swedish education.

In the second published study, Lange et al. (2013) compared reading and mathematics achievement of groups of DHH students in a bilingual program with norms from a group composed primarily of hearing students who had the same starting points in achievement and grade levels. After at least 4 years in the program, 41% of the DHH students in one group were reading at or above average; 55% of those in another group were performing at or above average in mathematics. The researchers concluded that "[w]hereas some groups are lobbying for a one-size-fits-all model to deaf education, research demonstrates a variety of paths for D/HH students to develop academically," and advocated continuing research into alternative educational options for DHH learners (Lange et al., 2013, p. 543). These results augur well for the potential of bilingual programming for at least some DHH students, although it is important to note that students in the program studied by Lange et al. (2013) who had levels of achievement below the national norms were excluded from the study. It also is noteworthy that, although approximately 40% of the students in each of the groups had at least one deaf parent, there were no significant differences between their scores and scores of peers without deaf parents. Their study thus leaves us with the diversity-related questions of which DHH students will benefit from bilingual programming and for which of them will bilingual programming lead to better academic outcomes than any other education model given that parental hearing status (and thus presumably sign language skill) does not appear to be associated with greater achievement in the long term. (Lange et al. [2013] did not report the ages of the students in their study, only their grades.)

Are Deaf Students Really Visual Learners?

This is another question to which it is generally assumed we already have the answer. Of course deaf people are visual learners (e.g., Dowaliby & Lang, 1999; Hauser et al., 2008; Marschark & Hauser, 2012). How could it be otherwise? Like some of the other questions raised earlier, however, this one is more complex than it first might appear. Consider just three complicating factors. First, if it is assumed that deaf students are visual learners because of their lesser dependence on auditory information, it should follow that their likelihood of being visual learners would be correlated with their hearing thresholds (Tharpe et al., 2002). Aside from the challenge this would create in the classroom, this relation that has not yet been demonstrated empirically. Second, there have been indications of deaf individuals surpassing hearing peers on some visual–spatial skills (e.g., Corina et al., 1992; Rettenbach et al., 1999), but more often than not other factors, including use of sign language or being a (deaf or hearing) native signer, have qualified those results.

Furthermore, there have now been a number of studies demonstrating that hearing individuals perform as well or better than deaf peers across a variety of visual–spatial processing and memory tasks (e.g., Blatto-Vallee et al., 2007; Marschark et al., 2013; Marschark et al. 2015c; Van Dijk et al. 2013). López-Crespo et al. (2012) went further, arguing there is no evidence that deaf individuals have better visual memory than hearing individuals, and the findings of Marschark et al. (2015c) suggest this conclusion might apply to visual cognition more broadly. Even in domains where DHH individuals appear to demonstrate better spatial skills than hearing individuals, both language ability (but not its modality) and executive functioning appear to be mediating factors (Marschark et al., 2015c; Stiles et al., 2012; Talbot & Haude, 1993). With regard to classroom learning, however, Dowaliby and Lang (1999) found that adding neither sign language nor visual animation improved significantly DHH students' learning of a science lesson presented in text.

A third, and the most significant qualifier to the suggestion that, in some general sense, deaf students might be visual learners centers on what it means to be a visual learner in the first place. Using one's eyes to take in information does not make one a visual learner. Being a visual learner or verbal learner refers to learning styles, normally identified through the administration of standardized assessments or questionnaires. Importantly, the two styles are not mutually exclusive, and there is little support for the assumption that "visual learners" learn better with visual instruction methods or materials whereas "verbal learners" learn better with verbal instruction methods or materials (Pashler et al., 2008). Specifically with regard to DHH students, there do not appear to be any published studies that have evaluated their visual, nonverbal learning styles, let alone have considered them in the context of hearing thresholds or language fluencies. Such studies currently are underway, but identifying visual and verbal learning styles used across different academic subjects and settings would require additional steps. The one academic domain that has yielded suggestive evidence in this regard is mathematics.

Zarfaty, Nunes, and Bryant (2004) examined the ability of 3- and 4-year-old deaf children to remember the number of colored "bricks" they saw on a computer screen. A variety of studies has indicated deaf individuals' difficulties in processing and remembering sequential/temporal information relative to hearing peers, consistent with the neurophysiological and neuropsychological underpinnings of sequential/temporal processing, audition, and hearing loss (see Mayberry, 2002; Marschark et al., 2015c). Zarfaty et al. (2004) asked their preschool participants to reproduce the number of "bricks" on each trial after the blocks had been presented either together, in a spatial array, or sequentially, one at a time. The deaf children performed as well as a hearing comparison group when the objects were presented sequentially, but performed better than their hearing peers when the objects were presented in a spatial array. The researchers concluded that deaf preschoolers understood number concepts as well as their hearing age-mates, and that their learning of mathematics would benefit from the use of spatially organized materials.

Among older learners, Blatto-Vallee et al. (2007) found that DHH students in middle school through college were less likely than hearing peers to use visual–spatial information to represent conceptual aspects of mathematics problems. Their primary task involved the solving of mathematical word problems accompanied by diagrams. These researchers found that the hearing students tended to use "schematic" mental representations that preserved relational information and supported problem solving. The DHH students treated the diagrams essentially as pictures, less frequently using relations depicted in them to help with problem solution. The use of "schematic" representations was associated with better performance on a pair of visual–spatial tasks for both deaf and hearing students, tasks on which hearing students outperformed their deaf peers. However, the use of schematic representations was the single best predictor of the deaf students' performance on the mathematics task, whereas that variable did not predict the hearing students' performance. If representing mathematics-related diagrams as "pictures" is an example of being a visual learner, it is not a quality we would wish for deaf learners.

Marschark et al. (2013) replicated and extended the results of Blatto-Vallee et al. (2007). Although hearing college students equaled or surpassed the performance of DHH students on all their visual–spatial tasks, DHH students' scores were related more strongly to performance on mathematics problems involving diagrams than those of the hearing students. In short, regardless of whether DHH learners excel in various visual–spatial tasks, they appear to use their visuospatial abilities in ways somewhat different than their hearing peers. Marschark et al. (2015c) and Castellanos et al. (2016) provided evidence that the deployment of such abilities and task performance are related to executive function as well as language. Marschark et al. (2015c), for example, found that visual–spatial performance was related more to the level of DHH students' language abilities rather than language modality (signed or spoken). When it comes to education, the point is that not only is there no evidence that deaf students are visual learners, but also a full understanding of how, when, and for whom visual materials in the classroom are best used is yet to be determined. The available evidence points to the potential of using DHH students' spatial abilities to enhance their performance in mathematics. Yet, given the diversity in their hearing thresholds, language modalities and fluencies, learning styles, and cognitive abilities, any one-size-fits-all approach, again, is unlikely to be optimal for many.

THINGS WE KNOW ABOUT DEAF EDUCATION (BUT NOT ENOUGH)

The preceding section likely made some readers uncomfortable, either because skewering three long-held beliefs about educating DHH learners suggests the task is even more difficult than we thought or simply because they do not believe the results described. With regard to both, it is important to note the lack of evidence concerning an aspect of deaf education (or anything else) does not mean it is not valid. It seems highly likely that early intervention and bilingual education will have significant benefits for a variety of DHH children, and some (as yet unknown) proportion of them likely will be characterized as visual learners. However, finding the results described in the previous section uncomfortable or unbelievable does not mean they can be ignored unless equally contradictory evidence is obtained. Most educators and investigators familiar with the literature in deaf education recognize they can find at least one published study to support almost any methodology or perspective. All too frequently, such studies involve small and/or select groups either for the purposes of experimental control (such as native signers) or because of attrition (for example, individuals successful with an intervention such as CIs or auditory–verbal therapy continue in the program whereas those who are unsuccessful drop out).

The foregoing is not an unrealistic call for randomized controlled trials in deaf education or the stringent stipulations for establishing an evidence base according to the U.S. Department of Education's What Works Clearinghouse. Given the low incidence of significant hearing loss in children, parental preferences, and educational bureaucracies, this is not going to happen. Nevertheless, it is worth noting that large, government-supported studies in the United States, the Special Education Elementary Longitudinal Study (SEELS; www.seels.net) and NLTS2 (www.NLTS2.org), which were designed to be statistically representative, have yielded data indicating that DHH students have better academic outcomes than suggested by other sources, such as the Gallaudet Research Institute's Annual Survey of Deaf and Hard-of-Hearing Children and Youth (e.g., Blackorby et al., 2007; Marschark et al., 2015b). The annual survey involves a large sample, but it is weighted toward DHH learners with greater hearing losses who are more likely to use sign language and attend schools and programs for the deaf (Allen & Anderson, 2010; Holt, 1993). Yet, regardless of its generalizability, it is the most frequently cited source of information on DHH students' academic achievement in the United States (e.g., Qi & Mitchell, 2012; Traxler, 2000). Given the knowledge diversity among deaf learners, large unbiased samples, replications, and/or appropriate statistical procedures are necessary if we are to draw valid conclusions about any of the issues addressed in this chapter.

Previous sections have alluded to the need for longitudinal studies or at least large-sample investigations to determine whether factors influencing academic achievement for diverse DHH children have long-term effects. More precisely, the question is the extent to which early advantages or gains are maintained throughout the school years and into postsecondary education and lifelong learning. Perhaps because of the strictures of research funding and education legislation in some countries, and because of concerns about the welfare of young children, the largest volume of literature with regard to deaf education appears to be focused on achievement during the preschool and primary school years. Many such studies also have taken place in schools and programs designed for DHH children—a situation that seems likely to yield less than broadly generalizable results given the dispersal of DHH students associated with the move to inclusive education in many countries.

At the other end of the educational continuum are studies concerned with what might be considered academic *outcomes*: the achievements of DHH learners entering or enrolled in postsecondary programs. These studies have come from a relatively limited number of programs designed specifically for DHH students, most of them from the National Technical Institute for the Deaf, including both separate and inclusive classrooms at Rochester Institute of Technology, and the stand-alone programs of Gallaudet University. Studies conducted at such institutions may be limited insofar as they include samples more restricted in terms of prior achievement, cognitive abilities, and the possible presence of secondary disabilities relative to individuals in K–12 programs. At the same time, they provide valuable evidence with regard to long-term effects of childhood and early school factors as well as the opportunity to follow DHH graduates and investigate the impact of schooling on employment and life in the real world (see Chapter 17).

With these caveats in mind, three more issues in the literature relating to DHH learners are important areas for consideration. These are areas in which findings are consistent both in replications and in convergent evidence from related studies. What makes these topics worthy of consideration here (having been discussed in other venues) is their potential both for clarifying other findings with regard to deaf education and offering directions for academically relevant interventions. In particular, all three areas of investigation suggest we need to look carefully at what teachers are doing (and not doing) in classrooms designed for DHH students as well as those designed for hearing students, no matter how inclusive they may seek to be. Importantly, the three domains considered in this section are yielding consistent information at both the secondary and postsecondary levels, so it appears we can have some confidence in the findings, even if their source is unclear.

Long-Term Academic Benefits of Cochlear Implantation

Tsach and Most (see Chapter 13) note that various studies have indicated that, among students with comparable hearing losses, students with CIs demonstrate greater academic skills than peers who use hearing aids. Some studies have found children with CIs, on average, to be functioning at grade level (e.g., Damen et al., 2006; Geers, 2002, 2003; Spencer et al., 2004) whereas others have found them to be functioning better than peers without CIs but still delayed relative to hearing peers (Archbold et al., 2008; Spencer et al., 2003; Vermeulen et al., 2007). Most such studies, however, have included only preschool- or primary school-age students. The study by Spencer et al. (2004) is one notable exception because it included only secondary school students who had received their CIs relatively late, at least by current standards, between 2 years and 13 years of age (mean, 6.4 years). Testing conducted when they were at least 16 years of age indicated that 63% of the sample who were consistent users (≥8 hours per day) were reading at grade level, and the entire sample was reading within the normal range. This study is also atypical, however, because the students were supported by sign language interpreters throughout their school years.

More commonly, it appears that the early benefits of CIs to reading achievement (the most frequently examined academic domain among CI users) are not as long-lasting as the benefits to hearing and speech.

In a follow-up to Geers's (2002, 2003) earlier studies, Geers et al. (2008) found that individuals who had been reading, on average, at grade level when they were 8 to 9 years of age were almost 2 years behind grade level when they were 15 to 16 years of age. More important, there was greater variability at the later ages, with reading levels ranging from grade 2 to beyond grade 12 among the 15- to 16-year-olds. Archbold et al. (2008) found that 7 years after cochlear implantation, more than 50% of children who had received their CIs between 1 year and 3 years of age were reading within a year of grade level or higher, although about 40% were more than 1 year delayed. In contrast, among those who had received their CIs between 4 years and 7 years of age, 80% to 100% were at least 1 year delayed in reading. Considering the NLTS2 data, CI use was not a significant predictor of achievement for secondary school students in reading, mathematics, social studies, or science in the study by Marschark et al. (2015b). In the sample of incoming college students evaluated by Marschark et al. (2015c), students with CIs were found to have no higher college entrance scores than their deaf peers without CIs in reading comprehension, mathematics, or English. Other studies have found deaf learners with hearing aids to demonstrate better reading skills than peers with CIs for a variety of hypothesized reasons (e.g., Geers & Hayes, 2011; Harris & Terlektsi, 2010; Nittrouer et al., 2012).

Archbold (2015) suggested that "it is still uncertain whether the early encouraging results continue as deaf learners move into adolescence, with the more demanding and subtle skills required to achieve age-appropriate reading levels (e.g., inferencing)" (p. 36). As CI users move from primary to secondary school and beyond, the length of time using their implant increases, a variable that usually is seen as a positive predictor of academic and other outcomes from cochlear implantation, but there seems to be some kind of asymptote in academic gains. Among the "demanding and subtle" requirements for secondary and postsecondary academic functioning are the content and structure of educational materials, which are more complex and abstract than those intended for primary school. Vocabulary, also, becomes more abstract and low frequency as children progress through school (Wauters et al., 2006).

With regard to vocabulary and language more generally, DHH learners' challenges are often attributed to less incidental learning because they are unable to overhear the language of others in their environments. The expectation that CIs would ameliorate the situation has not yet been demonstrated. Stelmachowicz et al. (2004) and Connor et al. (2000) reported accelerated growth in young children's vocabularies after cochlear implantation, especially if they received them early. The possibility that greater, early exposure to spoken language, and incidental learning in particular, might allow vocabulary repertoires of children with CIs to catch up to their hearing peers is a different question. Convertino et al. (2014) investigated the vocabulary and world knowledge of deaf college students with and without CIs. With regard to vocabulary, Peabody Picture Vocabulary Test-4 scores indicated not only that students with CIs had not caught up to their hearing peers by college age, but also their vocabularies were no larger than those of deaf peers without CIs. There also were no significant differences in Peabody Picture Vocabulary Test-4 scores between students who had received their CIs earlier (before 3.5 years of age) or later.

Convertino et al. (2014) observed patterns of scores similar to those obtained in the vocabulary task in other tasks that examined world knowledge that typically is obtained incidentally: chronological ordering of historical events, classifications of famous names by profession, or identifying the magnitudes of real-world objects (such as the weight of a chicken egg or the height of a basketball hoop). The same pattern observed in estimates of number and magnitude among objects directly in front of them (for example, the number of candies in a jar or the circumference of a clock on the wall) also indicated the importance of incidental learning of skills (estimation) rather than facts. Importantly, the deaf (with and without CIs) and hearing groups did not differ in their ability to locate U.S. states on a map—an ability learned explicitly by school children in the United States. Taken together, the results demonstrate there is no impediment to deaf learners' with or without CIs acquiring world knowledge comparable with their hearing peers. When such knowledge depends on incidental learning, however, it cannot be left to chance.

In addition to DHH learners' having difficulty in overhearing or "overseeing" the conversation of others (see Chapter 4), much of our word and world knowledge is acquired through reading, and we know that DHH learners generally read less than their hearing age-mates. The cumulative and interactive effects of having less knowledge, making reading more difficult and thus less likely, also contributes to the lags observed in reading achievement of DHH learners, even if they use CIs. Nittrouer and Caldwell-Tarr (2016) therefore emphasized the importance of going beyond "early" intervention and continuing to provide additional academically related interventions for CI users throughout the school years (e.g., Nunes et al., 2014). This issue and the associated issues of ensuring systems are in place to provide such service, and the training and deployment of appropriate teachers within such systems are, we would argue, particularly important considerations.

Long-Term Academic Benefits of Early Sign Language

If research concerning the long-term benefits of cochlear implantation is just beginning, this situation is understandable. CIs have not been around that long. In the United States, they have been available to children as young as 18 months only since 1998 and 12 months since 2002, so the youngest recipients are just now reaching secondary school. The reasons why investigators have not explored the long-term impact of early sign language are far less clear. A number of studies have indicated that deaf children with deaf parents and, to a lesser extent, deaf children whose hearing parents created a sign language-rich environment for their deaf children demonstrate early reading skills on par with grade-level expectations, or at least better than that typically seen among young DHH learners (Chamberlain et al., 2000). Those studies, however, have focused exclusively on readers of primary school age.

Several findings suggest the benefits of early access to sign language provided by deaf parents may be as limited in their long-term effects as the benefits of early access to spoken language provided by CIs. An early study by Jensema and Trybus (1978), for example, indicated that deaf children of deaf parents demonstrated higher achievement than those with hearing parents. The small differences in achievement scores between 14- and 18-year-old DHH children with zero, one, or two deaf parents, however, were not significant. In fact, the investigators found that parent–child sign language was associated negatively with vocabulary, reading comprehension, and mathematics achievement scores, whereas parent–child spoken language was associated positively with those scores. This may reflect the relatively poor reading abilities of deaf adults during the 1970s (Qi & Mitchell, 2012), making them less than ideal reading models for their deaf children.

More recently, as noted earlier, neither parental hearing status nor sign language use was associated with secondary school achievement in the nationally representative sample of DHH students in the NLTS2 database (Marschark et al., 2015b). Convertino et al. (2009) similarly found parental hearing status unrelated to DHH students' learning in mainstream college classrooms (n = 794). Marschark et al. (2015c) found that the native signers in their study of first-year college students scored significantly higher than deaf peers who were nonnative signers on expressive and receptive measures of American Sign Language skill, but there were no differences between the native and nonnative signers on English, reading, or mathematics college entrance scores.

It thus appears that, even when DHH learners have early access to language either through audition (CIs) or sign language (deaf parents), the early benefits that accrue to reading and other aspects of the curriculum are not necessarily maintained into the secondary school years. The locus of this consistent finding might lie in the nature of materials intended for older learners, lesser vocabulary and world knowledge, or a more general lack of fluency in either the vernacular or sign language. For both CI users and deaf children of deaf parents, however, their access to language both directly and indirectly (in other words, incidentally) is going to be less than that available to normally hearing peers to a greater or lesser extent. That "greater or lesser extent" will be related to hearing thresholds, language fluencies, prior knowledge, and the other sources of diversity described earlier. What is surprising in this situation is that the long-term impact of early access to sign language (from deaf parents) has not been explored. Unlike the situation with CIs, sign language-oriented schools for the deaf and bilingual education have been around long enough that the issue should have been addressed earlier. Is it a sensitive issue? Yes. But advocates of sign language as the language of instruction (including bilingual education) have the same responsibility as advocates of CIs: demonstrating the long-term benefits to DHH learners.

Academic Benefits of Appropriately Trained Teachers

One implication of DHH students having less knowledge of the world than their hearing classmates has emerged from a number of studies concerning their learning through text, sign language, and spoken language. In examining factors contributing to learning both through direct instruction (teachers signing for themselves) and mediated instruction (via sign language interpreting or real-time text), Marschark et al. (e.g., Borgna et al., 2011; Marschark et al., 2008) found that college-age DHH students consistently come in to the classroom with less content knowledge than their hearing peers. Although this finding might explain in part why it is that DHH students appear to learn less in the classroom than their hearing classmates, several of these studies found that, when taught by skilled teachers of the deaf, DHH students learned just as much as their hearing peers given their own starting points. That is, controlling for prior knowledge either statistically or through the use of gain scores indicated that DHH and hearing students receiving the same instruction acquired comparable amounts of new information regardless of whether the teacher was signing (or signing and speaking) or using an interpreter, and regardless of whether the teacher was deaf or hearing. In conducting these studies, however, the investigators regularly noticed that it was not only classroom content that created challenges for DHH students; students also were less familiar with common words (such as *summarize, confirm,* or *drowsy*) and knowledge of the world that would support learning. It remains unclear precisely what the teachers familiar with teaching deaf students were doing that the (award-winning) mainstream teachers were not (see Chapter 8 for some possibilities).

Thirty years ago, Kluwin and Moores (1985) suggested that at least 50% of the variability in deaf students' achievement in mathematics might be the result of instructional factors. Among other things, experienced teachers of deaf learners are more likely to understand what their DHH students know and how they learn, and are more accustomed to teaching in very diverse classrooms. Regrettably, few studies have been undertaken to determine the characteristics of those most effective teachers other than asking teachers and students what they think those characteristics are (e.g., Lang et al., 1993; but see Chapter 8). Given findings in various studies indicating that DHH students had relatively poor awareness of how much they understood and were learning in the classroom (Borgna et al., 2011; Marschark et al., 2008), student assessments of what contributed to their learning (or not) should be treated with some caution. Interestingly, the fact that such results have been found consistently to be independent of whether DHH students relied primarily on sign language or spoken language suggests the primary factor in these findings cannot be attributed to language modality or the use of sign language interpreters. Rather, it emphasizes that the variety of factors affecting DHH students' learning described earlier, including lesser world knowledge obtained incidentally, is cumulative over time.

Another teacher-related factor affecting DHH students' learning over time relates to social–emotional functioning. Although it is rarely considered in studies conducted in North America, a variety of European studies has demonstrated the importance of student–teacher relations and classroom management in DHH students' academic achievement (e.g., Wolters et al., 2011; for reviews see Chapter 8, this volume, and Knoors and Marschark [2014], Chapter 7). DHH learners have been found to be less satisfied with their teachers' classroom management (such as time on task and classroom control [Hermans et al., 2014]), but the warmth and strength of student–teacher bonds may turn out to be more important for DHH learners than their hearing peers. The fact that teachers of the deaf are more comfortable with DHH learners than the typical mainstream teacher, thus likely contributing to greater student–teacher closeness, may be one factor that contributes to DHH students' greater gains when taught by the former. We know the issue is not simply one of direct (signed or spoken) versus mediated (interpreted or real-time text) instruction (Marschark et al., 2008). But, direct communication between teachers and DHH students likely would engender greater social–emotional bonds between them. More internationally based work clearly needs to be done in this area.

Changing Times and School Placement

Studies conducted during the 1980s and 1990s indicated that DHH students enrolled in inclusive programs with hearing peers frequently did not feel very included (e.g., Cappelli et al., 1995; Stinson & Antia, 1999; Stinson & Liu, 1999). For the most part, this situation was attributed to communication issues (e.g., Punch & Hyde, 2005). With the influx of DHH students into mainstream settings and more of them using CIs and spoken language, one might expect the situation to be changing, but if it is, change is coming slowly. Some studies have found deaf youth to report better communication with friends and family after cochlear implantation (Christiansen & Leigh, 2002; Wheeler et al., 2007). Spoken language outcomes, both expressive and receptive, are extremely variable after implantation, however (Caselli et al., 2012; Niparko et al., 2010), and true social inclusion appears limited to those CI users who gain better speech and hearing benefits (Bat-Chava & Deignan, 2001; Jambor & Elliott, 2005; Most & Aviner, 2009). As in other aspects of deaf education, however, the situation is far more complex.

In the Netherlands, Wauters and Knoors (2008) found no differences in peer acceptance, social status, or the number of mutual friendships among DHH and hearing primary school students. Wolters et al. (2011), in contrast, found that DHH students in their final year of primary education were less well accepted and less popular than their hearing peers. In absolute terms, Wolters et al. (2011) found that DHH students in mainstream settings were less popular with their peers than DHH students in special schools, and they scored lower than hearing peers regardless of whether they were in mainstream or special schools. This situation may reflect the greater burden on students who are "different" as they enter the teen years, a time when subtleties of spoken language—jokes, nonliteral language, sarcasm, and whispering—become more important (see Punch & Hyde, 2005). This situation notwithstanding—and in contrast to the implication from studies indicating that DHH students may benefit more from skilled teachers of the deaf than equally skilled mainstream teachers—by secondary school age, most DHH students report preferring to be enrolled in regular schools rather than schools for the deaf, and to use spoken language rather than sign language (O'Neill et al., 2014; Van Gent et al., 2012; cf. Chapter 12). (Interestingly, it does not appear this question has been asked of DHH learners in the United States other than in studies conducted at the National Technical Institute for the Deaf.)

In their review of the literature, Stinson and Kluwin (2011) noted that school placement for DHH students accounts for as little as 1% to 5% of the variance in achievement scores. This figure is consistent with the 7% obtained by Marschark et al. (2015b), but they found that attendance in mainstream schools only was the single best predictor of secondary school students' achievement across the curriculum when other factors were controlled. Although DHH students' social preferences in secondary school clearly have sociocultural and hormonal roots, it also appears that by secondary school, DHH students in mainstream schools and those who use spoken language demonstrate greater classroom participation (e.g., Stinson & Whitmire, 1991) and better social–emotional functioning (Punch & Hyde, 2005; Van Gent et al., 2012) than peers in special schools. But it's complicated. Punch and Hyde (2005), for example, found that deaf students attending mainstream secondary schools reported having few close friends at school, largely because of communication barriers, but there were no differences in their reported loneliness or social acceptance relative to hearing age-mates. Wolters et al. (2011) found that after the transition from primary to secondary school, DHH students in mainstream classrooms demonstrated lesser communication skills than hearing classmates but better psychosocial adjustment relative to DHH peers in schools for the deaf. When other factors were controlled, Schick et al. (2013) found that reported quality of life among deaf 11- to 18-year-olds was unrelated to school placement, communication modality, degree of hearing loss, or CI use.

What are we to make of these apparently contradictory findings? Reviews by Stinson and Kluwin (2011), Knoors and Marschark (2014, Chapter 11), and Hintermair (2011) indicated that the influence of school placement on social–emotional functioning is far more complex than has been considered here, and may differ for DHH learners in primary school versus secondary school (and/or in some countries). No doubt, early family and school environments, temperament, communication skills, hearing thresholds, the presence of secondary disabilities, self-esteem, cultural expectations, and a variety of other factors play into the ability of DHH students to fit in to and cope with the social milieu of school, and interactions among such factors will change with age and experience. For all stakeholders in deaf education, the point is that we not only have to give greater attention to diversity among DHH learners with regard to the link between social–emotional functioning in academic achievement in school (see Chapter 8), but also we may need to give greater attention to the preferences of the learners themselves. When 75% of DHH 18- to 27-year-olds in the United Kingdom indicate they prefer to use spoken language only (O'Neill et al., 2014) and DHH Australian teens prefer poor communication to using assistive listening devices (Punch & Hyde, 2005), it tells us a lot about the lives of many DHH youth as well as the society in which they live. Other DHH youth, in contrast, may be reported to be exploring their Deaf identities and their potential roles as Deaf adults in society, but little attention has been paid to how individuals balance such opposing forces (Marschark et al., 2015a). Only by understanding the diverse factors that feed into the social–emotional functioning of DHH learners at different ages can we appreciate and accommodate the ways in which it influences their academic functioning at various points.

DIVERSITY: WHAT DO WE DO ABOUT IT?

The foregoing was intended to summarize the need for consideration diversity on several dimensions relating to deaf education, regardless of how "comfortable" that sometimes might be. There are various of factors contributing to diversity, only some of which have been investigated empirically and not all of which will turn out to be tractable to teachers or researchers. The point is that we have to ask the right questions (assuming we can determine what they are) and then live with—and make appropriate use of—the answers. Anecdotes and research involving carefully selected samples may contribute to our understanding of the strengths and needs of DHH learners, but we need to look beyond hearing thresholds, language modalities, and literacy skills (see Chapter 8). The findings summarized in this chapter suggest that our obsession with single factors such as language modality, CI use, or school setting may be blinding us to the "tricky mix" of methods and materials necessary to educate DHH students optimally (Nelson et al., 1993).

All stakeholders in deaf education have the same goal—helping DHH learners to reach their full academic potential—even if we may have different methods and priorities. We all would like to be able to identify *the* factor that would allow us to guarantee that goal. Unfortunately, it's complicated.

REFERENCES

Allen, T. E., & Anderson, M. L. (2010). Deaf students and their classroom communication: an evaluation of higher order categorical interactions among school and background characteristics. *Journal of Deaf Studies and Deaf Education, 15*, 334–347.

Archbold, S. (2015). Being a deaf student: Changes in characteristics and needs. In H. Knoors, & M. Marschark (Eds.), *Educating deaf learners: Creating a global evidence base* (pp. 23–46). New York, NY: Oxford University Press.

Archbold, S. M., Harris, M., O'Donoghue, G. M., Nikolopoulos, T. P., White, A., & Richmond, H. L. (2008). Reading abilities after cochlear implantation: The effect of age at implantation on outcomes at five on seven years after implantation. *International Journal of Pediatric Otorhinolaryngology, 72*, 1471–1478.

Archbold S., & Mayer, C. (2012). Deaf education: the impact of cochlear implantation. *Deafness and Education International, 14*, 1–14.

Bagga-Gupta, S. (2004). *Literacies and deaf education: A theoretical analysis of the international and Swedish literature.* Stockholm: The Swedish National Agency for School Improvement.

Bat-Chava Y., & Deignan, E. (2001). Peer relationships of children with cochlear implants. *Journal of Deaf Studies and Deaf Education, 6*, 186–199.

Blackorby, J., & Knokey, A.-M. (2006). *A national profile of students with hearing impairments in elementary and middle school: A special topic report from the Special Education Elementary Longitudinal Study.* Menlo Park, CA: SRI International.

Blackorby, J., Wagner, M., Cadwallader, T., Cameto, R., Levine, P., & Marder, C. (with Giacalone, P.). (2002). *Engagement, academics, social adjustment, and independence: The achievements of elementary and middle school students with disabilities.* Menlo Park, CA: SRI International.

Blatto-Vallee, G., Kelly, R., Gaustad, M., Porter, J., & Fonzi, J. (2007). Visual–spatial representation in mathematical problem solving by deaf and hearing students. *Journal of Deaf Studies and Deaf Education, 12*, 432–448.

Borgna, G., Convertino, C., Marschark, M., Morrison, C., & Rizzolo, K. (2011). Enhancing deaf students' learning from sign language and text: Metacognition, modality, and the effectiveness of content scaffolding. *Journal of Deaf Studies and Deaf Education, 16*, 79–100.

Bowe, F. G. (1992). Radicalism vs reason: Directions in the educational use of ASL. In M. Walworth, D. Moores, & T. J. O'Rourke (Eds.), *A free hand: Enfranchising the education of deaf children* (pp. 182–197). Silver Spring, MD: T. J. Publishers.

Brown, P. M., & Nott, P. (2006). Family-centered practice in early intervention for oral language development: Philosophy, methods, and results. In P. E. Spencer & M. Marschark (Eds.), *Advances in the spoken language development of deaf and hard-of-hearing children* (pp. 136–165). New York, NY: Oxford University Press.

Calderon, R. (1998). Learning disability, neuropsychology, and deaf youth: Theory, research, and practice. *Journal of Deaf Studies and Deaf Education, 3*, 1–3.

Calderon, R., & Greenberg, M. (1997). The effectiveness of early intervention for deaf children and children with hearing loss. In M. J. Guralnik (Ed.), *The effectiveness of early intervention* (pp. 455–482). Baltimore, MD: Paul H. Brookes.

Calderon, R., & Naidu, S. (1999). Further support of the benefits of early identification and intervention with children with hearing loss. *The Volta Review, 100*, 53–84.

Cappelli, M., Daniels, T., Durieux-Smith, A., McGrath, P. J., & Neuss, D. (1995). Social development of children with hearing impairments who are integrated into general education classrooms. *The Volta Review, 97*, 197–208.

Caselli, M. C., Rinaldi, P., Varuzza, C., Giuliani, A., & Burdo, S. (2012). Cochlear implant in the second year of life: Lexical and grammatical outcomes. *Journal of Speech, Language, and Hearing Research, 55*, 382–394.

Castellanos, I., Pisoni, D. B., Kronenberger, W. G., & Beer, J. (2016). neurocognitive function in deaf children with cochlear implants: early development and long-term outcomes. In M. Marschark & P. E. Spencer (Eds.), *The Oxford handbook of deaf studies in language* (pp. 264–275). New York, NY: Oxford University Press.

Chamberlain, C., Morford, J., & Mayberry, R. (Eds.) 2000. *Language acquisition by eye*. Mahwah, NJ: Lawrence Erlbaum Associates.

Christiansen, J., & Leigh, I. (2002). *Cochlear implants in children: Ethics and choices*. Washington, DC: Gallaudet University Press.

Connor, C. M., Hieber, S., Arts, H. A., & Zwolan, T. A. (2000). The education of children with cochlear implants: Total or oral communication? *Journal of Speech, Language, and Hearing Research, 43*, 1185–1204

Convertino, C. M., Borgna, G., Marschark, M., & Durkin, A. (2014). Word and world knowledge among deaf students with and without cochlear implants. *Journal of Deaf Studies and Deaf Education, 19*, 471–483.

Convertino, C. M., Marschark, M., Sapere, P., Sarchet, T., & Zupan, M. (2009). Predicting academic success among deaf college students. *Journal of Deaf Studies and Deaf Education, 14*, 324–343.

Corina, D. P., Kritchevsky, M., & Bellugi, U. (1992). Linguistic permeability of unilateral neglect: Evidence from American Sign Language. In *Proceedings of the Cognitive Science Conference* (pp. 384–389). Hillside, NY: Lawrence Erlbaum Associates.

Cormier, K., Schembri, A., Vinson, D., & Orfanidou, E. (2012). First language acquisition differs from second language acquisition in prelingually deaf signers: Evidence from sensitivity to grammaticality judgement in British Sign Language. *Cognition, 124,* 50–65.

Damen, G. W., van den Oever-Goltstein, M. H., Langereis, M. C., Chute, P. M., & Mylanus, E. A. (2006). Classroom performance of children with cochlear implants in mainstream education. *The Annals of Otology, Rhinology, and Laryngology, 115*(7), 542–552.

Donne, V., & Zigmond, N. (2008). Engagement during reading instruction for students who are deaf or hard of hearing in public schools. *American Annals of the Deaf, 153*(3), 294–303.

Dowaliby, F., & Lang, H. (1999). Adjunct aids in instructional prose: A multimedia study with deaf college students. *Journal of Deaf Studies and Deaf Education, 4,* 270–282.

Fagan, M. K. (2016). Spoken vocabulary development in deaf children with and without cochlear implants. In M. Marschark & P. E. Spencer (Eds.), *The Oxford handbook of deaf studies in language* (pp. 132–145). New York, NY: Oxford University Press.

Geers, A. (2002). Factors affecting the development of speech, language, and literacy in children with early cochlear implantation. *Language, Speech, and Hearing Services in the School, 33,* 172–183.

Geers, A. E. (2003). Predictors of reading skill development in children with early cochlear implantation. *Ear & Hearing, 24,* 59S–68S.

Geers, A., & Hayes, H. (2011). Reading, writing, and phonological processing skills of adolescents with 10 or more years of cochlear implant experience. *Ear & Hearing, 32,* 49S–59S.

Geers, A., Tobey, E., Moog, J., & Brenner, C. (2008). Long-term outcomes of cochlear implantation in the preschool years: From elementary grades to high school. *International Journal of Audiology, 47*(Suppl. 2), S21–S30.

Giezen, M., Baker, A., & Escudero, P. (2014). Relationships between spoken word and sign processing in deaf children with cochlear implants. *Journal of Deaf Studies and Deaf, 19,* 107–125.

Goldberg, L. R., & Richburg, C. M. (2004). Minimal hearing impairment: Major myths with more than minimal implications. *Communication Disorders Quarterly, 25,* 152–160.

Harris, M., & Terletski, E. (2011). Reading and spelling abilities of deaf adolescents with cochlear implants and hearing aids. *Journal of Deaf Studies and Deaf Education, 16,* 24–34.

Hauser, P. C., Lukomski, J., & Hillman, T. (2008). Development of deaf and hard-of-hearing students' executive function. In M. Marschark & P. C. Hauser (Eds.), *Deaf cognition: Foundations and outcomes* (pp. 286–308). New York, NY: Oxford University Press.

Heiling, K. (1998). Bilingual vs. oral education. In A. Weisel (Ed.), *Issues unresolved: New perspectives on language and deaf education* (pp. 141–147). Washington, DC: Gallaudet University Press.

Hermans, D., Knoors, H., & Verhoeven, L. (2009). Assessment of sign language development: The case of deaf children in The Netherlands. *Journal of Deaf Studies and Deaf Education, 15,* 107–119.

Hermans, D., Wauters, L., de Klerk, A., & Knoors, H. (2014). Quality of instruction in bilingual schools for deaf children. In M. Marschark, G. Tang, & H. Knoors (Eds.), *Bilingualism and bilingual deaf education* (pp. 272–291). New York, NY: Oxford University Press.

Hintermair, M. (2011). Health-related quality of life and classroom participation of deaf and hard-of-hearing students in general schools. *Journal of Deaf Studies and Deaf Education, 16,* 254–271.

Holcomb, T. K. (2013). *An introduction to American deaf culture*. New York, NY: Oxford University Press.

Holt, J. (1993). Stanford Achievement Test—8th edition: Reading comprehension subgroup results. *American Annals of the Deaf, 138,* 172–175.

Humphries, T., Kushalnagar, P., Mathur, G., Napoli, D. J., Padden, C., Rathmann, C., & Smith, C. R. (2012). Language acquisition for deaf children: Reducing the harms of zero tolerance to the use of alternative approaches. *Harm Reduction Journal, 9,* 16.

Jambor, E., & Elliott, M. (2005). Self-esteem and coping strategies among deaf students. *Journal of Deaf Studies and Deaf Education, 10,* 63–81.

Jensema, C. J. & Trybus, R. J. (1978). *Communicating patterns and educational achievements of hearing impaired students*. Washington, DC: Gallaudet College Office of Demographic Studies.

Karchmer, M. A., Milone, M. N., & Wolk, S. (1979). Educational significance of hearing loss at three levels of severity. *American Annals of the Deaf, 124,* 97–109.

Kluwin, T., & Moores, D. (1985). The effect of integration on the achievement of hearing-impaired adolescents. *Exceptional Children, 52,* 153–160.

Knoors, H., & Marschark, M. (2012). Language planning for the 21st century: Revisiting bilingual language policy for deaf children. *Journal of Deaf Studies and Deaf Education, 17,* 291–305.

Knoors, H., & Marschark, M. (2014). *Teaching deaf learners: Psychological and developmental foundations*. New York, NY: Oxford University Press.

Knoors, H., & Vervloed, M. P. J. (2011). Educational programming for deaf children with multiple disabilities. In M. Marschark, & P. E. Spencer (Eds.), *The Oxford handbook of deaf studies, language and education* (pp. 82–96). New York, NY: Oxford University Press.

Kushalnagar, P., Topolski, T. D., Schick, B., Edwards, T. C., Skalicky, A. M., & Patrick, D. L. (2011). Mode of communication, perceived level of understanding, and perceived quality of life in youth who are deaf or hard of hearing. *Journal of Deaf Studies and Deaf Education, 16,* 512–523.

Lang, H. (2011). Perspectives on the history of deaf education. In M. Marschark, & P. Spencer, (Eds.), The Oxford handbook of deaf studies, language, and education (2nd ed., Vol. 1, pp. 7–17). New York, NY: Oxford University Press.

Lang, H. G., McKee, B. G., & Conner, K. N. (1993). Characteristics of effective teachers: A descriptive study of perceptions of faculty and deaf college students. *American Annals of the Deaf, 138,* 252–259.

Lange, C. M., Lane-Outlaw, S., Lange, W. E., & Sherwood, D. L. (2013). American Sign Language/English bilingual model: A longitudinal study of academic growth. *Journal of Deaf Studies and Deaf Education, 18,* 532–544.

López-Crespo, G. A., Daza, M. T., & Méndez-López, M.(2012). Visual working memory in deaf children with diverse communication modes: Improvement by differential outcomes. *Research in Developmental Disabilities, 33,* 362–368.

Marschark, M., & Hauser, P. C. (2012). *How deaf children learn*. New York, NY: Oxford University Press.

Marschark, M., & Knoors, H. (2015). Educating deaf learners in the 21st century: What we know and what we need to know. In H. Knoors & M. Marschark (Eds.), *Educating deaf learners: Creating a global evidence base* (pp. 617–647). New York, NY: Oxford University Press.

Marschark, M., Machmer, E., & Convertino, C. (2016). Understanding language in the real world. In M. Marschark & P. E. Spencer (Eds.), *The Oxford handbook of deaf studies in language* (pp. 431–451). New York, NY: Oxford University Press.

Marschark, M., Machmer, E. J., Spencer, L. J., Borgna, G. L. J., A. Durkin, A., & Convertino, C. (2015a). Psychosocial functioning, language, and academic achievement among deaf and hard-of-hearing students. Unpublished manuscript.

Marschark, M., Morrison, C., Lukomski, J., Borgna, G., & Convertino, C. (2013). Are deaf students visual learners? *Learning and Individual Differences, 25,* 156–162.

Marschark, M., Sapere, P., Convertino, C. M., & Pelz, J. (2008). Learning via direct and mediated instruction by deaf students. *Journal of Deaf Studies and Deaf Education, 13,* 446–461.

Marschark, M., Shaver, D. M., Nagle, K., & Newman, L. (2015b). Predicting the academic achievement of deaf and hard-of-hearing students from individual, household, communication, and educational factors. *Exceptional Children, 8,* 350–369.

Marschark, M., Spencer, L., Durkin, A., Borgna, G., Convertino, C., Machmer, E., Kronenberger, W. G., & Trani, A. (2015c). Understanding language, hearing status, and visual-spatial skills. *Journal of Deaf Studies and Deaf Education, 20,* 310–330.

Mayberry, R. I. (2002). Cognitive development in deaf children: The interface of language and perception in neuropsychology. In S. J. Segalowitz, & I. Rapin (Eds.), *Handbook of neuropsychology* (2nd ed., Vol. 8, part II, pp. 71–107). Philadelphia, PA: Elsevier.

Mayberry, R. I., & Lock, E. (2003). Age constraints on first versus second language acquisition: Evidence for linguistic plasticity and epigenesis. *Brain and Language, 87,* 369–383.

Mayer, C., & Akamatsu, C. T. (1999). Bilingual–bicultural models of literacy education for deaf students: Considering the claims. *Journal of Deaf Studies and Deaf Education, 4,* 1–8.

Mayer, C., & Leigh, G. (2010). The changing context for sign bilingual education programs: Issues in language and the development of literacy. *International Journal of Bilingual Education and Bilingualism, 13,* 175–186.

Mellon, N. K., Niparko, J. K., Rathmann, C., Mathur, G., Humphries, T., Napoli, D. J., et al. (2015). Should all deaf children learn sign language? *Pediatrics, 136*(1), 170–176.

Mitchell, R., & Karchmer, M. (2011). Demographic and achievement characteristics of deaf and hard-of-hearing students. In M. Marschark & P. Spencer (Eds.), *The Oxford handbook of deaf studies, language, and education* (2nd ed., Vol. 1, pp. 18–31). New York, NY: Oxford University Press.

Moeller, M. P., Tomblin, J. B., Yoshinaga-Itano, C., Connor, C. M., & Jerger, S. (2007). Current state of knowledge: Language and literacy of children with hearing impairment. *Ear & Hearing, 28*(6), 740–753.

Moores, D. (2008). Research on Bi–Bi instruction. *American Annals of the Deaf, 153,* 3–4.

Most, T., & Aviner, C. (2009). Auditory, visual, and auditory-visual perception of emotions by individuals with cochlear implants, hearing aids, and normal hearing. *Journal of Deaf Studies and Deaf Education, 14,* 449–464.

Nelson, K. E., Loncke, F., & Camarata, S. (1993). Implications of research on deaf and hearing children's language learning. In M. Marschark and D. Clark (Eds.), *Psychological perspectives on deafness* (pp. 123–152). Hillsdale, NJ: Lawrence Erlbaum Associates.

Niparko, J. K., Tobey, E. A., Thal, D. J., Eisenberg, L. S., Wang, N. Y., Quittner, A. L., & Fink, N. E. (2010). Spoken language development in children following cochlear implantation. *Journal of the American Medical Association, 303*(15), 1498–1506.

Nittrouer, S., Caldwell, A., Lowenstein, J. H., Tarr, E., & Holloman, C. (2012). Emergent literacy in kindergartners with cochlear implants. *Ear & Hearing, 33,* 683–697.

Nittrouer, S., & Caldwell-Tarr, A. (2016). Language and literacy skills in children with cochlear implants: Past and present findings. In N. Young, & K. Kirk (Eds.), *Cochlear implants in children: Learning and the brain.* New York, NY: Springer.

Nover, S., Andrews, J., Baker, S., Everhart, V., & Bradford, M. (2002). *ASL/English bilingual instruction for deaf students: Evaluation and impact study.* Final report 1997–2002. Retrieved from http://www.gallaudet.edu/Documents/year5.pdf. Accessed January 26, 2016.

Nunes, T., Barros, R., Evans, D., & Burman, D. (2014). Improving deaf children's working memory through training. *International Journal of Speech & Language Pathology and Audiology, 2,* 51–66

O'Neill, R., Arendt, J., & Marschark, M. (2014). *Achievement and opportunities for deaf students in the United Kingdom: From research to practice.* Retrieved from http://www.nuffieldfoundation.org/sites/default/files/files/EDU%2037468%20-%20Nuffield%20Report%20MASTER%20v3.pdf. Accessed January 26, 2016.

Pashler, H., McDaniel, M., Rohrer, D., & Bjork, R. (2008). Learning styles: Concepts and evidence. *Psychological Science in the Public Interest, 9,* 106–119.

Punch, R., & Hyde, M. (2005). The social participation and career decision-making of hard of hearing adolescents in regular classes. *Deafness and Education International, 7,* 122–138.

Qi, S., & Mitchell, R. E. (2012). Large-scale academic achievement testing of deaf and hard-of-hearing students: Past, present, and future. *Journal of Deaf Studies and Deaf Education, 17,* 1–18.

Rettenbach, R., Diller, G., & Sireteneau, R. (1999). Do deaf people see better? Texture segmentation and visual search compensate in adult but not in juvenile subjects. *Journal of Cognitive Neuroscience, 11,* 560–583.

Rydberg, E., Gellerstedt, L. C., & Danermark, B. (2009). Toward an equal level of educational attainment between deaf and hearing people in Sweden? *Journal of Deaf Studies and Deaf Education, 14,* 312–323.

Schick, B., Skalicky, A., Edwards, T., Kushalnagar, P., Topolski, T., & Patrick, D. (2013). School placement and perceived quality of life in youth who are deaf or hard of hearing. *Journal of Deaf Studies and Deaf Education, 18,* 47–61

Segers, E., & Verhoeven, L. (2015). Benefits of technology-enhanced learning for deaf and hard-of-hearing students. In H. Knoors, & M. Marschark (Eds.),

Educating deaf learners: Creating a global evidence base (pp. 23–46). New York, NY: Oxford University Press.

Shaver, D., Marschark, M., Newman, L., & Marder, C. (2014). Who is where? Characteristics of deaf and hard-of-hearing students in regular and special schools. *Journal of Deaf Studies and Deaf Education, 19,* 203–219.

Spencer, L., Barker, B., & Tomblin, J. B. (2003). Exploring the language and literacy outcomes of pediatric cochlear implant users. *Ear & Hearing, 24,* 236–247.

Spencer, L. J., Gantz, B. J., & Knutson, J. F. (2004). Outcomes and achievement of students who grew up with access to cochlear implants. *Laryngoscope, 114,* 1576–1581.

Spencer, P. E., & Marschark, M. (2010). *Evidence-based practice in educating deaf and hard-of-hearing students.* New York, NY: Oxford University Press

Stelmachowicz, P. G., Pittman, A. L., Hoover, B. M., & Lewis, D. E. (2004). Novel-word learning in children with normal hearing and hearing loss. *Ear and Hearing, 25,* 47–56.

Stewart, D. (1993). Bi-Bi to MCE? *American Annals of the Deaf, 138,* 331–337.

Stiles, D. J., McGregor, K. K., & Bentler, R. A. (2012). Vocabulary and working memory in children fit with hearing aids. *Journal of Speech, Language, and Hearing Research, 55,* 154–167.

Stinson, M., & Antia, S. (1999). Considerations in educating deaf and hard-of-hearing students in inclusive settings. *Journal of Deaf Studies and Deaf Education, 4,* 163–175.

Stinson, M., & Kluwin, T. (2011). Educational consequences of alternative school placements. In M. Marschark, & P. Spencer (Eds.), *The Oxford handbook of deaf studies, language, and education* (2nd ed., Vol. 1, pp. 47–62). New York, NY: Oxford University Press.

Stinson, M., & Liu, Y. (1999). Participation of deaf and hard-of-hearing students in classes with hearing students. *Journal of Deaf Studies and Deaf Education, 4,* 191–202.

Stinson, M., & Whitmire, K. (1991). Self-perceptions of social relationships among hearing-impaired adolescents in England. *Journal of the British Association of Teachers of the Deaf, 15,* 104–114.

Swanwick, R., Hendar, O., Dammeyer, J., Kristoffersen, A.-E., Salter, J., & Simonsen, E. (2014). Shifting contexts and practices in sign bilingual education in northern Europe: Implications for professional development and training. In M. Marschark, G. Tang, & H. Knoors (Eds.), *Bilingualism and bilingual deaf education* (pp. 292–310). New York, NY: Oxford University Press.

Talbot, K. F., & Haude, R. H. (1993). The relationship between sign language skill and spatial visualizations ability: Mental rotation of three-dimensional objects. *Perceptual and Motor Skills, 77,* 1387–1391.

Tharpe, A., Ashmead, D., & Rothpletz, A. (2002). Visual attention in children with normal hearing, children with hearing aids, and children with cochlear implants. *Journal of Speech, Hearing and Language Research, 45,* 403–413.

Traxler, C. (2000). The Stanford Achievement Test, 9th edition: National norming and performance standards for deaf and hard-of-hearing students. *Journal of Deaf Studies and Deaf Education, 5,* 337–348.

Van Dijk, R., Klappers, A. M. L., & Postma, A. (2013). Haptic spatial configuration learning in deaf and hearing individuals. *PLoS One, 8,* e61336.

Van Dijk, R., Nelson, C., Postma, A., & van Dijk, J. (2010). Assessment and intervention of deaf children with multiple disabilities. In M. Marschark & P. Spencer (Eds.), *Oxford handbook of deaf studies, language, and education* (Vol. 2, pp. 172–191). New York, NY: Oxford University Press.

Van Gent, T., Goedhart, A. W., Knoors, H., Westenberg, P. M., & Treffers, P. D. (2012). Self concept and ego development in deaf adolescents: A comparative study. *Journal of Deaf Studies and Deaf Education, 17,* 333–351.

Vermeulen, A. M., van Bon, W., Schreuder, R., Knoors, H., & Snik, A. (2007). Reading comprehension of deaf children with cochlear implants. *Journal of Deaf Studies and Deaf Education, 12*(3), 283–302.

Wagner, M., Marder, C., Blackorby, J.,& Cardoso, D. (2002). *The children we serve: The demographic characteristics of elementary and middle school students and their households.* Menlo Park, CA: SRI International.

Wauters, L. N., & Knoors, H. (2008). Social integration of deaf children in inclusive settings. *Journal of Deaf Studies and Deaf Education, 13,* 21–36.

Wauters, L. N., Van Bon, W. H. J., Tellings, A. E. J. M., & Van Leeuwe, J. (2006). In search of factors in deaf and hearing children's reading comprehension. *American Annals of the Deaf, 151,* 371–380.

Wheeler, A., Archbold, S., Gregory, S., & Skipp, A. (2007). Cochlear implants: The young people's perspective. *Journal of Deaf Studies and Deaf Education, 12,* 303–316.

Wolters, N., Knoors, H. E. T., Cillessen, A. H. N., & Verhoeven, L. (2011). Predicting acceptance and popularity in early adolescence as a function of hearing status, gender, and educational setting. *Research in Developmental Disabilities, 32,* 2553–2565.

Yoshinaga-Itano, C., Coulter, D., & Thompson, V. (2001). Developmental outcomes of children born in Colorado hospitals with universal newborn hearing screening programs. *Seminars in Neonatology, 6,* 521–529.

Yoshinaga-Itano, C., & Sedey, A. (2000). Speech development of deaf and hard-of-hearing children in early childhood: Interrelationships with language and hearing. *Volta Review, 100,* 181–212.

Zarfaty, Y., Nunes, T., & Bryant, P. (2004). The performance of young deaf children in spatial and temporal number tasks. *Journal of Deaf Studies and Deaf Education, 9,* 315–326.

Index

Note: Page numbers followed by "f" and "t" denote figures, tables respectively.

ABC stories, 96–97
academic inclusion, 359–60, *see also* inclusion/inclusive education
access-participation theory, 336–37
adaptation vs. translation (of assessment tools), 210
adult basic education (ABE), 420–21, 433t, 435, 436
adult-mediated communication, 83–86
affective disorder, 393–95
age of child
   and impact of parental personality and stress on child adjustment, 125–26
   at time of intervention, 9
Agreeableness (A), 123, 124
allies (hearing-deaf/hard-of-hearing alliances)
   defined, 338
   importance of, 337–43
American Sign Language (ASL), 419, *see also* sign language
   ASL stories, 96–97
   communication-rich schooling and, 94–95
   interactive educational media in, 97–99
   proficiency in, 306
     reading proficiency and, 173, 306
   strategic and interactive writing instruction (SIWI) and, 94–95, 102
American Sign Language Assessment Instrument (ASLAI), 179–84
American Sign Language Phonological Awareness Test (ASL PAT), 195–99
American Sign Language Production Test (ASL PT), 192–93
American Sign Language Receptive Skills Test (ASL RST), 186–87
American Sign Language Vocabulary Test (ASL VT), 204–6
Analogies task, 182
Archbold, S., 276
Articulation, *see* oral methods/oral communication
ASCB (Social Conversational Skills Rating Scale), 250–51
assistive technologies, use of, 31–34
attachment, 385–87
attention deficit hyperactivity disorder (ADHD), 392–93, 508–9
auditory ability and inclusion, 356
auditory rehabilitation and inclusion, 356–57
Australia, 7
   inclusion of DHH students in higher education in, 444–47
Australian Sign Language, 444
autism spectrum disorder (ASD), 389–92

Belgium, *see* Flanders
Belknap, P. J., 483–85
best-practice documents, 21, 22, 26, *see also* Best Practices international consensus statement
best practices
   for DHH children struggling to learn syntax, 310
   in early-intervention services, 21–22, 25, 26, 32
   best-practice recommendations, 21–22, 26, 32, 36
   documents on, 22–23
   evidence-based practice, 23–25

best practices (*Cont.*)
  goals for implementation of, 41–42
  principles of, 26–38
  recommendations for research and further action, 38–40
  for typically hearing ELLs struggling to learn syntax, 308
Best Practices in Family-Centered Early Intervention, 23
  foundational principles of, 43
Best Practices international consensus statement, 23–24, 27, 30, 34
Big Five-Factor Model of personality, 123–25
bilingual educational programming for DHH children, 159, 171, 223, 227, 231, 233–34, 406, 524
  long-term impact of, 512–16
bilingualism, bimodal, 12–16, 99, 275, *see also* linguistic diversity
  assessment tools and, 171, 173, 199
Blamey, P., 111
blended classroom, 427–28
bonding social capital, 326
  strategies for building, 343–45
Bosso, E., 425
Bowe, F., 513
bridging social capital, 326–27
  strategies for building, 346–50
Britain, 137
British Sign Language Nonsense Sign Repetition Test (BSL NSRT), 193–95
British Sign Language Production Test (BSL PT), 190–92
British Sign Language Receptive Skills Test (BSL RST), 184–86
  steps in adapting it to German Sign Language, 188, 189t
British Sign Language Vocabulary Test (BSL VT), 199–204
Bronfenbrenner, Urie, 55–57

Calderón, Margarita, 233
Calderon, Rosemary, 113–14, 119–21, 511
Caldwell-Tarr, A., 522
captioning, 442–43, 457–63
career motivation theory, 494–95

career success among DHH individuals, *see also* workplace
  entrepreneurship, 493–95, 497
  key factors for, 480–82, 495–97
Chandler, M. J., 121
CHARGE syndrome/CHARGE association, 37–38, 390
chromogenic color print, *see* C-Print
Classifier Category Sorting task, 182
classroom, acoustical conditions in, 358
classroom interaction (with DHH students), *see also* interaction(s)
  classroom management, instructional, and emotional support, 229–33
  importance of, 223–25
  and learning, 225–29
classroom participation of mainstream DHH students, 361–65, 367–74, *see also* mainstream DHH students
  classroom variables and, 372–73
  and communication and academic and social performance, 373–74
  compared with participation of hearing students, 365–67
Classroom Participation Questionnaire (CPQ), 232, 367–68, 373
closed captioning, *see* captioning
closed-class words, *see* function words
Coakley, C. G., 485–86
cochlear implants (CIs)/cochlear implantation, 111–13, 387, 510, *see also specific topics*
  and child adjustment, 126
  and development of pragmatic skills, 249–52
  early, and global outcomes, 11
  long-term benefits of, 520–22
  and mental health problems, 404–7
  need for new competencies for speech-language therapists working in an age of, 148–52
  and pragmatic skills, 252–58
  prevalence, 7
  sign language and, 150–52, 234, 387, 407
cognitive ability, 8–9
cognitive appraisal, 119
College Reading Readiness Program, 418, 425–29, 431–37
  review of the reading data, 431–33, 433f

college-ready student skills, 423–25
colleges, *see* higher education
communication
    pedagogy driven by authentic, 100–104
    in workplace, 482–89
communication competence valued by employers, 483–86
communication-rich schooling, impact of, 91–96
communication strategies and the workplace, 486–89
communication technologies, *see* information and communication technologies
communities of practice, 334
community of learners, 334
competencies for teachers of the deaf (ToDs) and other qualified professionals, 135–36, 161–67
    are necessary but not guaranteed, 157–59
    categories of, 139, 142–46
    core, 142–46
    development of a survey of, 139–40
    need for, 140–41
    need for family-centered, 153–57
    need for pan-European, 137–40
    ranking of, 141–48
composing model (model of the composing process), 272–74, 273f
comprehension test, 183
computer-based interventions, 301, *see also* information and communication technologies
conscientiousness, parental, 123, 124
constant inquiry, stance of, 39
contact theory/contact hypothesis, 328
content space vs. rhetorical space (writing process), 273f, 273–74, 282, 284–85
content words, *see* lexical words
Convention on the Rights of People with Disability, 157–58, 441, 462
conversational balance and maintenance, 260, 261t, 262, 266
conversational turn type, 260, 262, 263t, 264, 266

conversation analysis (CA), 254–55, 258
conversations, 250–51, *see also* Instructional Conversation; pragmatic skills
    maintaining mutual engagement during, 252–58
coping
    defined, 124
    in parents of deaf children, 118–21
    personality and, 123–24
coping behaviors, emotion- vs. problem-focused, 119–20
C-Print, 457–63
cultural background, 9
cytomegalovirus (CMV), congenital, 383, 384

deaf and hard-of-hearing (DHH) adults as resource for families, 29–30
deaf and hard-of-hearing (DHH) children, *see also specific topics*
    addressing the needs of "all deaf children," 4, 6–8
    contrasted with other "disabled" populations, 7
    early identification of, 7–11
    factors associated with better outcomes for, 10–12
Deaf Culture Art/De'VIA Art, 347
deaf identity theorists, 332
Deaf parents, DHH children of, 15
    sign language acquisition and development in, 110–11, 326
Deaf role models, 97–99
Deaf Student Support Program (DSSP), 444, 445
depression, 394, 395
Deunk, M., 238
developing systems, 49
De'VIA Art/Deaf Culture Art, 347
dialogic pedagogy, 87–90
dialogic reading, 301–2
differentiated approach to instruction, 12–16
    language use and, 235–40
    timing of differentiation (reactive vs. proactive), 238–40
digital technology, 489–93

disabilities, *see also* Convention on the Rights of People with Disability
   additional/secondary
      presence of, viii, 8
      severity of, 509
"disabled" populations, DHH population contrasted with other, 7
disruptive behavior disorder, 392–93
diversity, viii–ix, 4
   accounting for, 8–9
   vs. difference, 274–76
   in the population of learners, 276–78
   reading intervention and, 418–19
   recognizing diversity in the modern era, 6–12
   what to do about, 527–28
Dorminy, J. L., 329–32
Dutch, sign-supported, 234–35, 237
Dutch DHH students, 230, 306–7, *see also* Flanders

Early Childhood Technical Assistance Center/Early Childhood Outcomes Center, 39
Early Hearing Detection and Intervention (EHDI) programs, 23
early intervention, 56, *see also* best practices; transition to school
   early and timely access to, 26–27
   long-term impact of, 511–12
early-intervention programs, evaluation of, 39–40
early-intervention specialists, core competencies of, 34
Easterbrooks, Susan R., 298–99, 313–14
ecological learning theory, 222–23
ecological systems perspective/ ecological framework, *see* transition to school
education, *see also specific topics*
   deaf, viii
      things we know about it (but not enough), 518–27
      things we think we know about it but don't, 510–18
   nature of, vii
   views and perspectives on, vii
educational attainment, factors that influence, 480–82

educational placement decisions, 54–55, *see also* school placement
effectiveness, defined, 38
efficacy, defined, 38
emotional support, 27–31
emotion- vs. problem-focused coping behaviors, 119–20
employment, *see also* career success among DHH individuals; workplace
   factors that influence, 480–82
engineering, *see* STEM
engines of development, 56
English language learners (ELLs), 302
entrepreneurial self-efficacy (ESE), 493–94, 497
entrepreneurship, 493–95
equal status, 328
Europe
   see also *specific countries*, 137–41
   competencies of teachers of the deaf (ToDs) in, 137–41
evidence-based practice, *see* best-practices
evidence-informed practice, 25, *see also* best-practices
evoked production, modeling with, 308
expectations for students, high, 425
extraversion, 487–88
   parental, 123–25

families, supporting
   and deaf student success, 126–28
familly-centered competencies (FCCs)
   evaluating, 154–56
   of professionals working as home-based service providers, 153–56
   parents' experience of, 156–57
familly-centered practices, *see also* Best Practices in Family-Centered Early Intervention
   relational and participatory components of, 155
Family-Centered Practices Checklist, 154, 155
   Flemish version of, 155–56, 156t
family members, *see also* individual family service plans
   wanting them to learn and use sign language, 340

Family Stress Scale (FSS), 117
family support, 27–31
family-to-family support networks, 30
feedback, modeling with, 308
finances, venture implementation of, 494
five factor model, *see* Big Five-Factor Model of personality
Fixsen, Dean L., 425
Flanders, Belgium, 136, 138, 141, 142, 145t, 146, 147, 154, 154–55, 158–59
Folkman, S., 118–19
fourth environments, 331
freewriting, 335–36
frequency modulation (FM) systems and equipment, 227, 228, 236, 357, 358
function words, 310–11
    successful interventions for any student struggling to learn, 311–12
    universals in, 311

Gallaudet, Edward Miner, 4, 6
general self-efficacy (GSE), 493, 497
German Sign Language, 306–7
German Sign Language Receptive Skills Test (DGS RST), 188–90
German Switzerland, 207
Gill, C. J., 338
Glickman, N., 332
Global Coalition of Parents of Children who are Deaf or Hard of Hearing (GPOD), 29, 40
global factor scores, 10–11
grammar, 191, 391, 396
Greece
    inclusion of DHH students in higher education in, 447–51
    speech-language therapists in, 149
    practices of, 151
Greek Sign Language (GSL), 448–50
Greenberg, M., 113–14, 119, 511

Halliday, M. A. K., 286, 286t
hard-of-hearing students, 466, *see also* deaf and hard-of-hearing (DHH) children
Hattie, John, 224
hearing abilities, providing equitable services to children with all levels of, 36–38

hearing aids, 10, 32–33
    deaf learners with cochlear implants vs., 112, 150, 157, 251, 357, 360, 369, 405, 406, 520, 521
    and learning, 112, 157, 251, 357, 360, 369, 520, 521
    and mental health problems, 405, 406
    psychopharmacological treatment and, 403
hearing allies, *see* allies
hearing loss
    degree of, 509
    effect of, 110–11
hearing screening, 26–27
    need for new competencies for speech-language therapists working in an age of newborn, 148–52
Hermans, D., 231
higher education, *see also* inclusion/inclusive education; postsecondary enrollment; training
    reading intervention and community and technical college placements, 419–21
    staff development in, 466–67
    transition from secondary education to, 464–65
home-based service providers (HBSPs), need for family-centered competencies for professionals working as, 153–57
Home Intervention Hearing and Language Opportunities Parent Education Services (HI HOPES), 33–34
home intervention to support transition to school, 58–62
home life and home support, 55–56
home-school relationship and transition to school, 63–66
Hopper, Mindy, 333–37, 348
hybrid teaching model (blended classroom), 427–28
Hyde, Merv B., 444–47

identity development, identity theories, and social capital, 331–33
incidental learning opportunities, lack of access to, 333–37

inclusion/inclusive education, 347, 441,
    see also mainstream DHH students
    of DHH students in higher
        education, 441–43
    a case in Australia, 444–47
    a case in Greece, 447–51
    a case in New Zealand, 451–56
    a case in the United States, 456–62
    as cost vs. investment, 464–65
    factors that contribute to, 356
        educational setting, 358–59
        student factors, 356–58
    and the future, 462–67
    measures of successful, 359–61
    from segregation to, 355–56
individual family service plans (IFSP), 62, 63, 67, 154
informal learning, see incidental learning opportunities
information and communication technologies (ICTs), 31–33, 489–90
Instructional Conversation (IC), 87–90
instructional methods in deaf education, constant search for new, viii
instructional scaffolding, see scaffolding
intelligence, 399–400
interaction(s), see also classroom interaction; peer interactions; strategic and interactive writing instruction; Teaching through Interaction model
    and learning, 223
interactive educational media to broaden language input, 96–100
International Classification of Functioning, Disability and Health (ICF), 153
International Congress on Education of the Deaf (ICED), vii–ix, see also Milan Congress resolutions
    history of, 1–2
    22nd, 1
    Vancouver statement: responding to Milan, 2–3
Internet, see information and communication technologies
Interpreters, see sign language interpreter(s)
Intervention, see also specific topics
    type and quality of, 9

Jamieson, Janet R., 72
Jervell and Lange-Nielsen syndrome, 395
Johnson, V. A., 488
Joint Committee on Infant Hearing (JCIH) 2013 document (position statement), 22–24, 26, 27, 30, 34, 38, 40

Kelly, Ronald R., 481
Knoors, Harry, 233, 513–14
knowledge (and understanding)
    of speech-language therapists (SLTs), 150–51
    of ToDs, 139
Konstantrareas, M. M., 114–15
Korthagen, F. A., 231–32

Lampropoulou, Venetta, 114–15
Lane-Outlaw, Alicia, 490
language development
    exposure to sign language and, 99, 511
    sociocultural perspective on, 83
language impairment, see specific language impairment
language input, use of interactive educational media to broaden, 96–100
language intervention(s)
    how we got off track in designing evidence-based, 298–99
    in the school years, 297–98
language learning, natural
    vs. direct teaching of language, 100–101
language skills and inclusion, 357
language socialization, peer-supported, 81–83
language subsystems, 247
language use (in classroom), 240–41, see also classroom interaction
    accommodating the needs of diverse DHH learners, 233–35
    classroom interaction and, 223–29
    and differentiated instruction, 235–40
    functions of language in the classroom, 220–21
    and learning, 219–20
language zone, 91–94
Lave, J., 333–34
Lazarus, R. S., 118–19

learning disabilities and inclusion, 358
learning styles, visual vs. verbal, 516–18
lexical words, 311
　successful interventions for any
　　student struggling to learn, 311–12
Lexile Framework for reading, 428, 430
Lexile reading levels, 428, 429, 429t, 432, 432f, 433t, 434–37
linguistic background, 9
linguistic diversity, 222–23
linguistic skills, *see* pragmatic skills
listening in the workplace, 485–86
listening technologies, *see* assistive technologies
Longitudinal Outcomes of Children with Hearing Impairment (LOCHI) study, 9–12
long QT syndrome, 395
Lytle, Linda Risser, 346–49

MacKenzie, M. J., 121–22, 126–27
mainstream DHH students, *see also* classroom participation; inclusion/inclusive education
　vs. hearing students
　　communication, social functioning, and academic performance, 368–72
　　how they feel during class, 367–68, 372–73
Maiorana-Basas, M., 298–99, 313–14
Mann, W., 209–10
marketing, digital technology and online, 489–93
Marschark, Marc, 24, 233, 508, 513–14
marshalling resources, 493–94
maternal level of education, 9
maternal sensitivity, 111
mathematics, *see* STEM
Mather, S. A., 227–28
Matthews, T. J., 227–28
McCrae, R. R., 123–24
McDonough, S. C., 121–22, 126–27
McGee, J. E., 493–94
Melick, A. M., 332
mental class maps (MCMs), 239
mental health examination
　diagnostic process, 396–97
　physical examination in relationship to, 400
　psychiatric assessment, 397–99
　psychological assessment and testing, 399–400
mental health problems
　of children with cochlear implants, 404–7
　developmental aspects of, 385–88
　differential diagnostic aspects of
　　clinical picture, 388–90
　　specific disorders and raise specific complexities, 390–96
　epidemiology of deafness and, 381–82
　etiology and pathogenesis related to
　　environmental influences, 384–85
　　genetic factors, 382–83
　　neurobiological factors, 383–84
　interventions for
　　psychopharmacological treatment, 402–4
　　psychotherapy and other psychological interventions, 402
　　specialized services vs. generic, 400–402
message design logic, 486–87
metacognition skills, 422–23
metalinguistic interventions, 308, 309
metasyntactic therapy, 308
Milan Congress resolutions
　deconstructing the, 3–6
　responding to the, 2–3
Millen, Kaitlyn, 344
modeling with evoked production and feedback, 308
Moores, D., 513
morphemes, 299
morphological development, evidence-based practices in, 299–304
morphology
　nature of, 299–300
　successful interventions for DHH children struggling to learn, 302–4
　successful interventions in typically hearing children struggling to learn, 300–302
　explicit instruction, 302
　universals in, 300
mutual engagement, 333–34

narrative content and structure, 191
National Black Deaf Advocates, 344
National Technical Institute for the Deaf at Rochester Institute of Technology (NTID/ RIT), 443, 456–57, 477, 519–20
NEO Five-Factor Inventory-3, 124–25, *see also* Big Five-Factor Model of personality
Netherlands, 231, 232, 237, 388–89, 526, *see also* Dutch
neuroticism, parental, 123–25
"New Era: Deaf Participation and Collaboration, A," 2
Nittrouer, S., 522
Nonsense Sign Repetition Test (NSRT), 193–95
nonverbal intelligence, 111

Oliva, Gina A., 346–49
"one-size-fits-all" approach, viii–ix, 12–13, 126, 225, 241, 467, 515, 518
open-class words, *see* lexical words
openness to experience, parental, 123
opportunity recognition search, 493
oppressors–oppressed distinction, 339, *see also* allies
oral methods/oral communication, 4, *see also* spoken language
  vs. sign language, 2

Paatsch, Louise, 253–54
parent advisors, 34
Parental Distress, 118
parental level of education, 9
parental personality and stress, 122–24
  and child adjustment, 124–26
Parental Stress Index (PSI), 117, 118
parenting stress, 113–14
  factors linked to, 114–16
parenting stress levels with deaf vs. hearing children, 116–18
parents of deaf children, *see also* Deaf parents
  coping in, 118–21
  parental personality, stress and child adjustment, 124–26
  use of sign language, 304
parent-to-parent support, 29

pedagogical model to address diversity, 288–90, *see also* process writing model
Pedagogy of the Oppressed (Freire), 339
peer group entry task, 112–13
peer interactions, 248, 252, 257–60, 262, *see also* pragmatic skills
peer note-taking, 445
peer-supported language socialization, 81–83
peer tutors, 449–51
peripheral participation, 333–34
personal attributes (of ToDs), 139
personality, *see also* communication strategies and the workplace; parental personality and stress and coping, 123–24
  definition and nature of, 122–23
Peter's Picture video series, 97–99, 102
phonology, signed language, 193, 196, 197, *see also* American Sign Language Phonological Awareness Test
Pianta, R. C., 55–56
Pipp-Siegel, S., 114–15
Plotkin, Rachael M., 124–26
policy context of school, 56
policy influences on home, early intervention, and school contexts, 66–68
postsecondary collaboration, 421
postsecondary enrollment, *see also* higher education
  placement testing as barrier to, 420–21
postsecondary obstacle, reading as, 419–20
Power, Desmond "Des" J., 225–27, 444–47
practice wisdom, 25
practitioners, *see also* speech-language therapists
  qualified, 34–36, *see also* competencies for teachers of the deaf (ToDs) and other qualified professionals
pragmatic skills
  development of, 247–49, 266–67
  from childhood to adolescence, 258–66
  in toddlers with cochlear implants, 249–52

of school-age children with cochlear
    implants vs. their hearing
    peers, 252–58
preschool, 56
proactive behavior and career
    outcomes, 488–89
problem- vs. emotion-focused coping
    behaviors, 119–20
process writing model, 280–83, *see also*
    pedagogical model to address
    diversity
  elements and implementation of
    a, 282–88
professional skills, 139, *see also*
    competencies for teachers of the
    deaf (ToDs), and other qualified
    professionals
professional training, *see* training
proximal processes, 56
psychopharmacological treatment
  of children, general and ontogenic
    factors in, 402
  deafness-related factors, 402–4
  effects and side effects of, 402–4
  psychoeducation during, 404
psychotic disorders, 395–96
Putnam, Robert, 326–27

Quittner, A. L., 118

Radical Middle, 297
  reading in the, 313–14
Ramsey, C. L., 330
reading, dialogic, 301–2
Reading for Life (Fennessy & Dorling), 430
reading growth, measuring, 428–29
reading intervention, 437–38, *see also*
    College Reading Readiness
    Program
  methodology: constructing the
    learning and delivery, 426–31
  authentic academic reading
    material, 429–30
  blended classroom/hybrid
    teaching, 427–28
  building vocabulary and
    background knowledge, 430–31
  instructional minutes, 426–27
  measuring reading growth, 428–29

the need for, 417–21
program design principles, 421–25
student case studies, 433–36
systemic change and, 425–26
reading material, authentic
    academic, 429–30
reading skills/proficiency, *see also* Lexile
    reading levels
  academic, 422–23
  and ASL proficiency, 173, 306
  lack of, as postsecondary
    obstacle, 419–20
reading text difficulty based on grade
    level, 428, 429t
reasoning skills test, 182
receptive skills tests, 184–90
Reich, C. F., 227–28
relationships of child, 56–57, 111, *see also*
    teacher-student relationships
relegated periphery, 337
rhetorical space vs. content space (writing
    process), 273f, 273–74, 282, 284–85
Rimm-Kaufman, S. E., 55–56
Rogoff, B., 334
role models, 97–99

Sameroff, A., 121
Sarant, J. Z., 111
Sass-Lehrer, M., 34
scaffolding, 84, 334–35
school placement, *see also* educational
    placement decisions
  changing times and, 525–27
  community and technical
    college, 419–21
  placement testing as barrier to
    postsecondary enrollment, 420–21
school-related variables and the
    transition to school, 56, *see also*
    transition to school
science, technology, engineering, and
    mathematics (STEM), 457–61
self-efficacy, 493–94, 497
self-monitoring, 487
semantics vs. syntax, 312–13
sentence repetition test (SRT), 207–9
sign bilingualism, *see* bilingualism
signed first language (L1) and second
    language (L2), 275

signed language acquisition data, 172–74, *see also* sign language acquisition and development
signed language phonology, 196, 197
  research into the development of, 193
signed language skills, accurate measurement of, 211–12, *see also* sign language assessment tools in Europe and North America
sign language, 82, 207, 227, 419, 485, 515, *see also* American Sign Language; bilingualism; *specific topics*
  grammar and syntax in, 391, 396
  Instructional Conversation (IC) and, 88, 90
  linguistic diversity and, 222
  mental health problems and, 391, 396
  morphology of, 300, 302
  parental use of, 304
  used to support the development of spoken language, 14–15
  wanting hearing family members and friends to learn and use, 340
  and the workplace, 475, 484–87, 490
sign language acquisition and development, 83, 86, 111, 227, *see also* signed language acquisition data; sign language assessment tools in Europe and North America; sign language instruction
  cochlear implants (CIs) and, 150–52, 234, 387, 407
  in deaf children with deaf parents, 110–11, 326
  importance of, 387
  long-term benefits of early, 99, 234, 511, 522–24
  measures of, 211–12
  research in, 211
  sequential acquisition of spoken language and sign language, 15–16
  speech-language therapists' (SLTs) attitudes toward, 150–52
  visual technologies and, 33
sign language assessment tools in Europe and North America, *see also* sign language acquisition and development

educational and research contexts, 171–72
  challenges related to, 172–74
  example of a responsive sign language test interface, 210, 211f
  new technologies, 210–12
  normative samples, 174
  test adaptation, 209–10
  test descriptions, 174, 175–77t, 178–209
  test formats, 173
sign language instruction, 234–37, 347, 348, *see also* sign language acquisition and development
sign language interpreter(s), 443, 463, 478
  as allies, 341, 349
  competencies and training as a, 146, 148, 158, 450, 463
  importance of, 341, 342, 407, 443
sign language interpreting, 442–43
  models of, 341–42
Sign Language of the Netherlands, 234–35, 237
sign language proficiency of parents, 387
sign-supported Dutch, 234–35, 237
sign-supported English, 234, 419
simultaneous communication, 14–15
situated learning, 333–34
Skolvi, Eva, 491–92
social capital, 326
  forms of, 326–27, 343–50
  and human development, 326–31
  impoverished, in general-education settings, 327–31
  research directions regarding, 350–51
  theories related to identity and, 331–33
Social Conversational Skills Rating Scale (ASCB), 250–51
social-emotional development, 387–88
social functioning of mainstream DHH students vs. hearing students, 368–72, *see also* mental health problems
social inclusion, 360–61
socialization, language, *see* language socialization
social performance, classroom participation and, 373–74
social skills and pragmatic skills, 248
socioeconomic status, 9
South Africa, 33–34
  hearing screening in, 26–27

speaking in the workplace, 484
specific language impairment (SLI), 239–40, 300, 301, 308
speech intelligibility and inclusion, 357–58
speech-language therapists (SLTs), 136, 141, 142, 144, 146, 147, 156–59
  experience of, 150
  knowledge and professional views of, 150–51
  questionnaire for, 149–50
  training of, 150
    need for active involvement in interdisciplinary teams and advanced, 151–52
speech-to-text (speech recognition), 457
Spencer, P. E., 24
spoken language, *see also* oral methods/oral communication
  and sign language, sequential acquisition of, 15–16
  use of sign language to support the development of, 14–15
STEM (science, technology, engineering, and mathematics), 457–61
Stewart, D., 513
stories, 86, 430, 431
  writing, 265, 345, 360
story-based interventions, 300–302
storybooks, 302, 312
storytelling, 96–99, 190–93
strategic and interactive writing instruction (SIWI), 91–95, 102
  sign language and, 92, 94–95, 102
student-teacher relationships, *see* teacher-student relationships
summer camps, 344–45
support services in higher education, DHH student use of, 465–66
supralexical unitization, 314
Swiss German Sign Language Sentence Repetition Test (DSGS SRT), 207–9
syntax
  the form of English syntax, 305–6
  nature of, 304–5
  vs. semantics, 312–13
  in sign language, 391, 396
  successful interventions for DHH children struggling to learn, 308–10
  successful interventions in typically hearing children struggling to learn, 307–8
  universals in, 306–7
syntax test, 182–83

teachers and inclusion, 359, *see also* inclusion/inclusive education
teachers of the deaf (ToDs), 139, *see also* competencies for teachers of the deaf (ToDs) and other qualified professionals
  qualifications and experience of, 144–46
  skills of, 142
  training of, 142
    academic benefits of appropriately trained ToDs, 524–25
    formal and postgraduate, 159–60
teacher-student relationships, 230–32, 525
Teaching through Interaction model, 223–25, 229
teaching writing, 271–72
  diversity and, 274–78
    addressing diversity in practice, 280–88
    diversity of outcomes, 278–80
    a pedagogical model to address, 288–90
  theoretical underpinnings of, 272–76
technology, *see also* information and communication technologies; STEM
  digital, 489–93
  use of, 463–64
tele-intervention, 33
think-alouds, 284
training, *see also* sign language interpreter(s)
  of speech-language therapists (SLTs), 150
    need for advanced, 151–52
  of teachers of the deaf (ToDs), 142, 524–25
    formal and postgraduate, 159–60
transactional model of development, 121–22
transition to school, 49–50, 72
  barriers to, 59, 60, 62–68
  for children with special needs, 52–53

transition to school (*Cont.*)
   for DHH children, 53–55
      home and early intervention to support, 58–62
      relational aspects of stakeholder contexts, 57–68
      facilitators of, 59, 60, 62–67
      pretransition period, 58–59, 61–64, 66–67
   for typically developing children, 51–52
   understanding it from an ecological systems perspective, 55–57
   what we know about, 50–55
   working together toward a smooth transition using an ecological framework, 68, 69–71t
translation vs. adaptation (of assessment tools), 210
Trueba, H. T., 84

underachievement of DHH learners, viii
United Nations (UN) Convention on the Rights of People with Disability, 157–58, 441, 462
universal newborn hearing screening (UNHS), 7–9, 11
universities, *see* higher education

Vancouver Congress, statement at, 2–3
VECTOR transition program, 417–19, 421, 422, 424, 426, 432, 434–36
venture creation planning, 493
venture implementation of people and finances, 494
verbal vs. visual learners, deaf students as, 516–18
videos, *see* interactive educational media to broaden language input
Vietnam Intergenerational Deaf Education Outreach Project, 30–31
visual (vs. verbal) learners, deaf students as, 516–18
visual supports, 309
vocabulary, building, 430–31
vocabulary tests, 180, 182, 182f, 199–206
Vocational Education, Community Training, and Occupational Relations (VECTOR) transition program, 417–19

Web-based American Sign Language Vocabulary Test (ASL VT), 204–6
Welsh, W. A., 482
Wenger, E., 333–34
Wolvin, A. D., 485–86
Wood, David, 225–26
Wood, Heather, 225–27
Workplace, *see also* career success among DHH individuals
   communication in, 482–89
   digital technology and online marketing, 489–93
   education, employment, and job/career satisfaction of DHH people in U.S., 476–80
   sign language and the, 475, 484–87, 490
writing, *see also* teaching writing
   in the workplace, 484–85
writing process, a model of the, 272–74, 273f